MW00905138

Essentials of

Gerontological Nursing

Adaptation to the Aging Process

Essentials of Gerontological Nursing

Adaptation to the Aging Process

Angela Simon Staab, RN, MN, CS
Gerontological Nurse Practitioner
Annie Penn Hospital
Reidsville, North Carolina

Adjunct Assistant Professor
University of North Carolina at Chapel Hill
University of North Carolina at Greensboro

Linda Compton Hodges, RN, EdD
Dean and Professor
College of Nursing
University of Arkansas for Medical Sciences
Little Rock, Arkansas

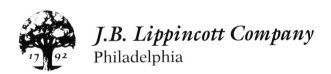
J.B. Lippincott Company
Philadelphia

Sponsoring Editor: *Jennifer E. Brogan*
Coordinating Editorial Assistant: *Danielle J. DiPalma*
Project Editor: *Barbara Ryalls*
Indexer: *Katherine Pitcoff*
Design Coordinator: *Melissa Olson*
Cover Designer: *Larry Pezzato*
Production Manager: *Helen Ewan*
Production Coordinator: *Nannette Winski*
Compositor: *Pine Tree Composition, Inc.*
Printer/Binder: *R. R. Donnelly & Sons Company/Crawfordsville*
Cover Printer: *Lehigh Press*

Library of Congress Cataloging-in-Publication Data

Essentials of gerontological nursing : adaptation to the aging process
 / [edited by] Angela Simon Staab, Linda Compton Hodges. — 1st ed.
    p. cm.
    Includes bibliographical references and index.
    ISBN 0–397–54973–3
    1. Geriatric nursing.   I. Staab, Angela Simon.   II. Hodges, Linda
Compton.
    [DNLM: 1. Geriatric Nursing—methods. 2. Nursing Process. WY
152 E78 1994]
RC954.E87 1996
610.73′65—dc20
DNLM/DLC
for Library of Congress   93–783
                                                                   CIP

The material contained in this volume was submitted as previously unpublished material, except in the instances in which credit has been given to the source from which some of the illustrative material was derived.

Any procedure or practice described in this book should be applied by the health-care practitioner under appropriate supervision in accordance with professional standards of care used with regard to the unique circumstances that apply in each practice situation. Care has been taken to confirm the accuracy of information presented and to describe generally accepted practices. However, the authors, editors, and publisher cannot accept any responsibility for errors or omissions or for any consequences from application of the information in this book and make no warranty, express or implied, with respect to the contents of the book.

The authors and publisher have exerted every effort to ensure that drug selection and dosage set forth in this text are in accordance with current recommendations and practice at the time of publication. However, in view of ongoing research, changes in government regulations, and the constant flow of information relating to drug therapy and drug reactions, the reader is urged to check the package insert for each drug for any change in indications and dosage and for added warnings and precautions. This is particularly important when the recommended agent is a new or infrequently employed drug.

Materials appearing in this book prepared by individuals as part of their official duties as U.S. Government employees are not covered by the above-mentioned copyright.

9 8 7 6 5 4 3 2 1

This book is dedicated to our parents, Angela and Frank Simon and Jimmy and Mary Compton, who were inspiring examples of how to adapt to the aging process with dignity, grace, and wisdom. The book is also dedicated to our many friends, colleagues, and patients who are members of the chronologically gifted community. In touching our lives they have helped us to gain insight into life's priorities.

Acknowledgments

We would like to thank our family, friends, colleagues, patients, and students, who have supported us during the writing of this text. A special thank-you goes to the men and women who make up a nationally known group of contributing authors whose expertise and positive approach to the project made its creation a pleasurable experience. We are particularly appreciative of the editorial guidance and professional support given to us by Jennifer Brogan of J. B. Lippincott. We would also like to thank our Developmental Editors Carol Wonsiewicz and Maryann Foley for their candid critique and suggestions for manuscript improvement. We would like to acknowledge Barbara Renn and Wentzi Haskin for their professional assistance in coordinating this project.

Contributors

Doris Ballard-Ferguson, *PhD, RNC*
Associate Professor
University of Arkansas for Medical
Sciences
Little Rock, AR
Chapter 4—Promoting Physical
Functioning in the Older Adult

Cornelia Beck, *PhD, RN, FANN*
Associate Director
Center for Outcomes Research and
Effectiveness
Associate Dean for Research and Evalu-
ation/Professor
College of Nursing
Associate Professor
Department of Psychiatry
University of Arkasas for Medical
Sciences
Little Rock, AR
Foreword

Norman D. Brown, *EdD, RN*
Associate Professor
College of Nursing
University of Arkansas for Medical
Sciences
Little Rock, AR
Chapter 31—Future Trends in the Care of
the Older Adult

Mary Carolyn Cooper, *PhD, MSN, RN*
Clinical Assistant Professor
School of Nursing
University of North Carolina
Chapel Hill, NC

Chapter 26—Problems Associated With
Issues of Death and Dying

Nancy Fleming Courts, *PhD, RN, NCC*
Assistant Professor of Nursing
University of North Carolina at
Greensboro
Greensboro, NC
Chapter 14—Problems With Circulation

Mary Jean Etten, *BSN, MA, MSN, EdD*
Instructor
St. Petersburg Junior College
St. Petersburg, FL
Chapter 13—Problems With Skin, Hair,
and Nails

Barbara Haight, *DrPH, RNC, FAAN*
Professor of Nursing
Medical University of South Carolina
Charleston, SC
Chapter 27—Problems With Changing
Roles in the Family

Millicent H. Hair, *RN, BSN, MSN*
Service and Rehabilitation Coordinator
Rockingham County Unit
American Cancer Society
Volunteer Hospice Rockingham County
Education/Growth Chairperson
North Carolina Baptist Nursing
Fellowship
Eden, NC
Chapter 25—Problems Associated With
Abnormal Cell Growth

C. Hope Hartz, RNP, CS, MSN
Instructor/Nurse Practitioner
College of Nursing
Department of Family and Community
    Medicine
University of Arkansas for Medical
    Sciences
Little Rock, AR
Nurse Practitioner
Former Director
ARGENTA Health Care Services
North Little Rock, AR
*Chapter 17—Problems With Endocrine
    Function*

Dana Hull Hickman, MSN, FNP-C
Family Nurse Practitioner
Shelby, NC
Chapter 18—Problems With Continence

Carolyn Hoskins, RN, MSN
Department of Nursing Faculty
Rockingham Community College
Wentworth, NC
Chapter 19—Problems With Elimination

Joan M. Iannone, MSN, RN, C
Associate Director, Nursing Education
Greensboro Area Health Education
    Center
Greensboro, NC
Appendix

Mary Louise Icenhour, RN, PhD
Assistant Professor
School of Nursing
Duke University
Durham NC
*Chapter 30—Problems With Community
    Resources*

Faye Ivey, BSN, MSN, JD
Attorney at Law
Greensboro, North Carolina
Lecturer
School of Nursing
University of North Carolina at
    Greensboro
Greensboro, NC

*Chapter 26–Problems Associated With Is-
    sues of Death and Dying*

Carolyn M. Jenkins, RNC, RD, DrPH
Assistant Professor
College of Nursing, Medical University
    of South Carolina
Charleston, SC
Chapter 11—Problems With Nutrition

Donald D. Kautz, PhD, RN, CS
Instructor
North Central Technical College
Wausau, WI
Chapter 23—Problems With Sexuality

Suzanne Vollrath Keogh, MS, RN, CS
Quality Coordinator
Lila Doyle Nursing Care Facility
Seneca, SC
*Chapter 28—Problems with Abuse and
    Neglect*

Kelly H. Leech, BSN
Captain, Army Nurse Core
Walter Reed Medical Center
Washington, DC
*Chapter 27—Problems With Changing
    Roles in the Family*

Priscilla Mackenzie Kline, EdD, RN
Associate Professor
College of Nursing
Clemson University
Clemson, SC
Chapter 22—Problems With Cognition

Ruth Miller, BA, MPA, RN, FNP-CS
Family Nurse Practitioner
Division of Hematology-Oncology
East Carolina University, School of
    Medicine
Greenville, NC
*Chapter 24—Problems With Substance
    Abuse*

Joyce A. Moser, BSN, MSN, RN
Staff Nurse
North Carolina Baptist Hospital
Outpatient Surgery

Winston-Salem, NC
*Chapter 9—Problems With Speaking and
Swallowing*

Elizabeth Murrow, *PhD, MSN*
Professor
Clemson University
Clemson, SC
*Chapter 2—Demographics in Aging:
Implications for Nursing*

Mariana Newton, *PhD*
Associate Professor, Division of
Communication Disorders
University of North Carolina at
Greensboro
Greensboro, North Carolina
*Chapter 3—Promoting Communication
in Older Adults*

Doris Nolan, *RN, BSN, MS, MPH, EdD*
Gerontologist
Milton, MA
*Chapter 15—Problems With Respiratory
Function*

Melodie Olson, *PhD, RN*
Associate Professor
College of Nursing
Medical University of South Carolina
Charleston, SC
*Chapter 20—Promoting Healthy
Psychosocial Functioning in the Older
Adult*

Linda M. Patterson, *MA-CCC*
Independent Speech Pathologist
High Point Regional Hospital
High Point, North Carolina
Home Care of Central Carolina
Greenboro, North Carolina
*Chapter 9—Problems With Speaking and
Swallowing*

Mary Ann Placey, *MSN, FNP-C*
Tannenbaum Medical Associates PA
Greensboro, NC
*Chapter 10—Problems With Drug
Administration*

Carla Gene Rapp, *MNSc, RN, CRRN*
Doctoral Student
University of Iowa College of Nursing
Iowa City, Iowa
*Chapter 29—Problems With Living
Arrangements*

Sue V. Saxon, *PhD*
Professor of Gerontology
University of South Florida
Tampa, FL
*Chapter 6—Problems With Other Senses,
Temperature Regulation, and Pain
Perception*

Kathryn Polski Schindler, *BSN, RN, MS*
Clinical Nurse Specialist
Public Health Department
Anderson, SC
*Chapter 2—Demographics in Aging:
Implications for Nursing*

Elizabeth Jean Shook, *MNSc, RNP*
Gerontological Clinical Nurse Specialist
Clinical Instructor
College of Nursing
University of Arkansas for Medical
Sciences
Little Rock, AR
Chapter 7—Problems With Sight

C. Sue Snyder, *RN, PhD*
Associate Professor
Indiana University of Pennsylvania
Indiana, PA
*Chapter 16—Problems With Tissue
Oxygenation*

Jeanne Merkle Sorrell, *RNC, PhD*
Associate Professor
College of Nursing and Health Science
George Mason University
Fairfax, VA
*Chapter 12—Problems With Sleep, Rest,
and Consciousness*

Deborah Warford Stokely, *RN-CS, MSN, FNP*
Family Nurse Practitioner
Thomasville Family Practice
Thomsville, NC
Chapter 5—Problems With Mobility

Elizabeth Jean Shook, MNSc, RNP
Gerontological Clinical Nurse Specialist
Clinical Instructor
College of Nursing
University of Arkansas for Medical
  Sciences
Little Rock, AR
Chapter 7—Problems With Sight

C. Sue Snyder, RN, PhD
Associate Professor
Indiana University of Pennsylvania
Indiana, PA
*Chapter 16—Problems With Tissue
  Oxygenation*

Jeanne Merkle Sorrell, RNC, PhD
Associate Professor
College of Nursing and Health Science
George Mason University
Fairfax, VA
*Chapter 12—Problems With Sleep, Rest,
  and Consciousness*

Deborah Warford Stokely, RN-CS, MSN, FNP
Family Nurse Practitioner
Thomasville Family Practice
Thomasville, NC
Chapter 5—Problems With Mobility

Reviewers

Barbara Metcalf, RN, BScN, MHSC
Gerontological Clinical Nurse Specialist
Mt. Royal College
Calgary, Alberta, Canada

Maryann Anderson, MS, RNC, CNA
Assistant Professor of Nursing
Weber State University
Ogden, VT

Mary Ellen Simmon, RNC, MS
Professor of Nursing
Oakton Community College
Des Plaines, IL

Whitney A. Nash, RN, BSN
Director of Nurses
Community Skilled Care Center
Medical Center of Southern Indiana
Charlestown, IN

Eileen M. Kaslatas, RN, MSN
Professor
Macomb Community College
Clinton Township, MN

Nancy K. O'Quinn, MSN, MEd
Assistant Professor
Albany State College
Albany, GA

Carolyn Castelloe, RNC, BSN, MAEd
First Level Coordinator/Instructor
Roanoke Chowan Community College
Ahoski, NC

Dolly Meilinger, RN, MSN
Assistant Professor of Nursing—
   Associate Degree Program
Gardner-Webb University
Boiling Springs, NC

Verle Waters, MA, RN
Dean Emerita
Ohlone College
Fremont, CA

Foreword

The care of the older adult poses a unique challenge to nurses in a multitude of settings, from the technological complexity of the intensive care unit to the psychosocial and environmental complexity of the patient's home. It involves nurses who not only have a variety of educational degrees but also have a diversity of educational experiences in gerontological nursing within the same educational degree. The editors of this textbook have effectively addressed this kaleidoscopic challenge of providing essential information needed to provide quality nursing care.

Essentials of Gerontological Nursing: Adaptation to the Aging Process distinguishes itself by addressing four movements significant to nursing's contemporary agenda. One—the editors' approach mirrors an important effort within the profession to organize nursing knowledge around problems for which the effectiveness of nursing interventions is demonstrated in measurable outcomes rather than organizing knowledge around a medical model. Two—this textbook reflects a holistic approach to the older adult by carefully addressing physiologic functioning along with recognizing the importance of psychosocial functioning and environmental influences, such as living arrangements and comunity resources. Three—a positive philosophy of aging, rather than a decrement model, permeates the text, as reflected in the emphasis on survivorship and changing roles. Four—the text reflects a model of shared control in which older adults assume more responsibility for their health behaviors by the inclusion of important information for instructing patients in self-care.

This book achieves its goal of providing essential knowledge of gerontological nursing within a contemporary framework. It is especially timely in view of the escalating need for nurses who have the special knowledge and clinical expertise to care for an exponential increase in older adults within our society.

Cornelia Beck, PhD, RN

Preface

Older adults challenge nurses to provide the ultimate in nursing care. They are survivors who have endured environmental, emotional, and social stressors, and physical wear and tear. Therefore, the complexity of their needs far exceeds those of other age-related populations. Older adults are the major consumers of health care services. As this group increases, they will make greater financial demands on an already taxed health care system. The nurse is challenged to find new ways to address their multiple needs in an era where quality care, access, and cost demand health care reform.

Essentials of Gerontological Nursing: Adaptation to the Aging Process offers the nurse insights for meeting the challenges of this growing population. It is designed as a basic text for undergraduate students and the practicing nurse. The book focuses on a nursing model based on functional areas of care. The primary framework is a problems approach that incorporates adaptation to the aging process. This approach was selected because nurses and students apply the nursing process to resolving the problems and concerns of their patients through nursing care strategies. We have named the text "essentials" because it contains essential nursing information needed to provide quality care in all clinical settings and in the home. Most of the book emphasizes clinical application of knowledge and clinical skills. The text is designed to be incorporated into any nursing course that deals with the care of the older adult in a variety of settings or to be used as a basic text for a course in gerontological nursing. It serves as a ready reference for the nurse practicing in settings where older adults receive care.

The text is divided into five components. Part I introduces the reader to the role of nursing in the care of the older adult emphasizing demographics of the population and standards of care. Part II focuses on problems associated with physiologic functioning. These chapters are designed to emphasize biologic aspects of care. Emphasis is placed on the physiologic changes associated with aging, the adaptation to these changes, common health care problems confronted by the older adult. Part III focuses on psychosocial functioning. These chapters address the ability of the older adult to adapt and cope with problems associated with the last decades of life and the resolution of the last developmental stage. Part IV centers on problems associated with role change, living arrangements, and utilization of community resources. The final chapter in this section bridges the current state of nursing care delivery for the older adult with trends for the future. The appendix provides the reader specific laboratory based on norms for the older adult.

The majority of chapters are based on a common framework. This framework includes a discussion of the physiologic and psychological changes related to a specific area of functioning. A heavy emphasis is placed on assessment since this serves as the foundation for appropriate planning and nursing interventions. A list of current NANDA nursing diagnoses related to altered functioning in defined areas serves as the foundation for a discussion of the problems associated with the specific adaptation to the aging process. Common "nursing problems" are addressed and interventions and expected outcomes are identified.

The major features of the book emphasize current and concise guidelines for approaching gerontological nursing practice. They provide a comprehensive and new approach to gerontological nursing with emphasis on communication, health promotion, survivorship, and changing roles. The chapters contain objectives, assessment tools, bulleted lists of critical information, and patient teaching boxes that provide concise points to emphasize when instructing patients in self-care. Each chapter contains Clinical Pearls that are little-known tips the authors present as "pearls of wisdom" from their patient care experience. Most chapters end with in-depth Nursing Care Plans that address major problems confronted in the care of older adults. References and a Bibliography that represent the author's selection of a combination of classic and current literature on clinical practice issues conclude each chapter.

The goal of this book is to provide the student and practicing nurse with a current, easily read text that emphasizes the problems associated with adaptation to the aging process. Contributing authors include teachers and practicing clinicians known nationally for their contributions to the field of gerontological nursing. It is our hope that this text will serve to educate current and future generations of nurses to provide care that will enhance the lives of our growing, older population.

Contents

P A R T   **3**

Problems With Psychosocial Functioning

P A R T   **4**

Problems in the Home and Community

Aging Population

The Older Adult

Objectives

1. Examine definitions of aging.
2. Describe the scope of gerontological nursing practice.
3. Discuss the biologic theories of aging.
4. Discuss the psychological theories of aging.
5. Explain the role of nursing in the care of the older adult.

INTRODUCTION

AGING IS A COMPLEX AND DYNAMIC PROCESS with intricately interrelated and inseparable physiologic, psychological, and sociologic components. It is a normal process that implies continued growth, development, and adaptation until death. The older adult has a multitude of needs and problems that require gentleness and caring from the nurse to promote health, well-being, recovery from illness or disability, and successful development toward senescence. Persons age in different ways and at different rates. Because aging changes occur at an uneven rate in different parts of the body, these changes can only be used as guidelines for nursing care and the problems presented by the aging process.

With aging comes a gradual and progressive slowing of behavior and functioning. Because the older adult faced with stress and change has a narrower margin for reserve capacity, this decrease is generally not evident during the body's resting state. Not all functional changes in older adults are due to aging—some are due to disease. Aging presents a gradual, increased vulnerability to disease. The nurse should be concerned with keeping the older adult at his or her optimal functional level. The goal is wellness, regardless of the level of physical, cognitive, or emotional impairment.

Much of the fear about growing older is due to society's perception of aging and a fear that disability is inevitable. There are many fears about safety and security, love and belonging, and threats to self-concept. Older adults, however, have proven their ability to adapt and survive. They have greater life experiences, courage, wisdom, and endurance and an independent spirit that aids them in adapting to the process of aging. Older adults seldom regard themselves as being old—they just say that others are getting younger!

Nurses must identify and resolve personal feelings about aging, especially about their own aging process. They must develop a philosophy that is contrary to the negative views held by society toward aging. This philosophy must reinforce a growth-oriented view of aging rather than reinforcing the current trend of viewing aging as the last half of life—a downward, degenerating process that leads to incompetence, negative self-worth, and low self-esteem, with death as the ultimate outcome. This is necessary if they are to assist the older adult in meaningful ways to adapt to the normal aging process and the problems it can present.

GERONTOLOGY

Gerontology is a branch of science that deals with the problems of adaptation and diseases of aging people and old age. Geriatrics focuses on the diseases and disabilities associated with older people rather than their health. Gerontological nursing is concerned with assessing nursing needs of older people, planning and implementing nursing care to meet those needs, and evaluating the effectiveness of such care to achieve and maintain a level of wellness consistent with the limitations imposed by the aging process (American Nurses' Association, 1987).

AGING

Aging is an objective and subjective universal process. Objectively, aging begins at birth, but it is most associated with the elderly or older adulthood. Chronologically and legally, 65 years of age and older is considered old. Subjective age can be related to personal feelings, identity age, cognitive age, social age, serotype age, comparative age, and perceived or self-perceived age (Miller, 1990).

The 1965 amendment of the Social Security Act identified senior citizens, or "Silver or Golden Agers," as persons 65 years of age or older. Medicare established age 65 as the minimum age criterion for eligibility for retirement and health care benefits in the United States. Some gerontologists further divide aging into chronologic categories of "young-old" (65–74 years), "middle-old" (75–84 years), and "old-old" (85 years or older). Because this categorization may cause health professionals to differentiate the way they treat persons by age alone, most gerontologists prefer to classify people according to functional age.

Definitions of functional age should be related to health, physical independence, and social and psychological functioning. Functional age emphasizes that abilities and changes occur at different rates; all older adults of the same chronologic age do not function at the same level. Besides being individual, functional age tends to be associated less with negative attitudes about aging. Functional abilities are associated with well-being. The functional age pro-

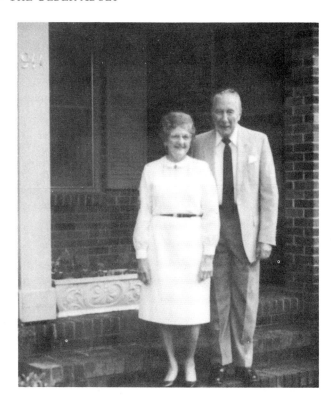

vides a better basis of care for the nurse, because nurses address the responses of older adults to actual or potential health problems. Asking people's chronologic age does not give as much information as asking how they feel, the condition of their health, or what activities they can accomplish in a day. An assessment of functional age answers all of these questions.

Clinical Pearl

Assessment: Functional age is very individual.

AGEISM

Ageism, as a gerontological concept, is defined as the process of systematic stereotyping and discrimination against people because they are old. Old age is viewed by different cultures in various ways. Some cultures view it as a thing to look forward to, because with age comes wisdom, whereas other cultures dread it, viewing it as a time of less respect. Ethnic and racial affiliations help to determine not only individual attitudes, but also the considerable strengths many minority members exhibit in adapting to old age. The problem arises when becoming older is viewed in prejudicial terms of uselessness or functional incapability. Nurses must assess their personal attitudes toward aging if they are to have a positive influence on others.

THE NURSE'S ROLE

Aging, like pregnancy, is not a disease. It is a normal evolutionary state. Therefore, disability and dysfunction are not normal or inevitable occurrences of aging. The role of the nurse must be as an autonomous health care professional who coordinates complex care of older adults and their families and who assumes a leadership role on the multidisciplinary health care team. Gerontological nursing is among the most specialized areas of nursing practice. Many of the problems of the aged are associated with daily functioning and are therefore more responsive to nursing models of care than to medical management. These gerontological nursing models are based on the following principles.

- Patients have the right to self-determination and independent decision making.
- Patients are holistic in nature, and their health and well-being are affected by the interaction of physiologic, pathologic, psychological, social, financial, and environmental factors.
- Nursing has a role in assisting patients to optimize health, to improve the quality of life, to achieve comfort, and to facilitate personal growth (Phillips, 1990).

Older adults are more vulnerable than younger adults to many problems. Physiologic changes make it difficult to maintain and regain homeostasis when presented with physiologic stressors. Often, there are psychological deficits and a sociologically imposed preoccupation with memory deficits. The information-processing requirement of a lifetime of memories may alter perceptions of cognitive function and memory. Life circumstances may alter the view the older adult has of self and can increase the possibility of depression. With time, the social network is altered, with decreasing numbers of persons available for interaction as friends and family members die. Therefore, loneliness may occur as relationships with significant others change. Economically, decreases in assets imposed by retirement, coupled with the cost of health care, introduce the possibility of impoverishment. Frail older adults are those who often have social, economic, physical, or mental limitations and who are ill or incapacitated most of the time and require assistance from others to perform ordinary tasks of daily living. Because of these circumstances, they consume the most health care time, space, and dollars.

Designing nursing interventions for the older adult can be complex, because they are complicated by the many dimensions of aging. Diversity among older adults is also intensified by the large age span involved as well as differential genetic endowments, cohort experiences, health habits, and functional deficits.

The nurse needs creativity and resourcefulness to implement a plan of care, especially if the patient is experiencing sensory deficits. Older patients' benign short-term forgetfulness can be a major problem, for example, when teaching them about their medications. Intelligence is not affected by aging, but older adults are more capable of using their experience in solving problems and learning new content than are younger people. The nurse must capitalize on the existing sensory capabilities and facilitate growth of the older adult through adaptation.

Clinical Pearl

Implementation: The nurse can teach the older adult "new tricks" or new information, but this must be accomplished slowly and with attention to sensory deficits.

Gerontological nursing requires sophisticated assessment and intervention skills, coordination and care management skills, and an intimate relationship between the nurse and the older adult. The nurse has the potential for more contact with the older adult than any other health care professional. Nurses have the assessment, counseling, support, education, and coordination skills needed to care for the older adult in a variety of settings. Nurses can best help older adults reach their greatest potential rather than face slow or rapid deterioration. The nurse provides assessment, guidance, teaching, and support; cares for older adults in the home and the community; directs them to other types of care when needed; and cares for them as they undergo sophisticated treatments, if needed.

In all settings, the establishment of goals or plans is important to the care of older adults. The nurse must respond to the direction specified by the medical plan of care while creating a comprehensive nursing perspective that incorporates goals related to health promotion, rehabilitation, and the maintenance of optimal functional ability or support of decline. Nurses must be geared to the responses of persons to actual or potential health problems. Older people respond differently to disease, the manifestation of disease states, and the functional consequences of illness (Miller, 1990). Older adults require special management by nurses who are trained to understand their unique needs. Caregiver education and program development will continue to be a large portion of the role of the gerontological nurse.

To make discriminate judgments about changes that occur in patient care, the nurse must know the various theories of aging and understand the needs and life space of the aging person. The nurse needs to be aware of the effect of age-related problems and chronic disease. It is essential that the nurse understand the losses that occur with normal aging, such as the loss of loved ones and the sense of loss associated with retirement. The nurse is also challenged to find cost-effective ways to provide quality long-term care for the chronically ill and aging population in this era of limited resources. The use of medical technology and special issues, including the needs and rights of the terminally ill and those with chronic disease and severe medical complications, can have legal implications and present moral dilemmas. Nurses must be prepared to participate in the debate of consumer and provider choices. Emphasis must be placed on helping older adults understand their choices.

THEORIES OF AGING

Aging may be defined as the sum of all the changes that occur in humans with the passage of time that lead to functional impairment and death. An alternate definition might be a decreasing ability to survive stress. Stress is regarded as any factor or process that tends to shift the internal environment away from its normal equilibrium, with the end point of homeostatic impairment in an internal environment incompatible with life. Aging includes those changes that occur in any cell or organ system as a function of time, independent of any external or pathologic influences, such as disease. Disease is a pathologic or abnormal state found in any cell, organ, or organ system in a unit of time or extending over many units of time. Unfortunately, many consider aging to be a pathologic state or disease process. Aging is neither a disease process nor the result of a summation of multiple disease states. Aging and death, like birth and maturation, are a part of the normal life cycle.

Aging is viewed from biologic, psychological, and social theories. Biologic theories attempt to explain the physiologic processes and structural alterations in living organisms that determine mental developmental changes, longevity, and death. Aging can be defined as biologic age, psychological age, and social age. Therefore, it is a highly complex phenomenon that requires viewing the aging person as a whole in relationship to his or her environment. This perspective lends understanding to the multiple aspects of the care required by the older adult. Psychological theories try to describe and explain aging behavior among and between persons. Biologic and environmental factors are believed to influence the process of behavioral change. Theory development related to sociologic aspects of aging has focused largely on ways that older adults adapt during later life and on their status as a group compared with other age groups in this society. Some theories compare the elderly across societies.

The theories underscore the importance of planning care in diversified and individualized ways, with consideration for the person's functional and physical limitations, preferences, lifestyle, and personality. They accentuate the influences of culture, family, education, community, roles, and patterns of responses and disease states.

Gerontological nurses need to understand the difference between age-related changes and risk factors that affect the function of older adults. They need to understand the influence that biologic, psychological, and social aging has on the improvement of the older adult's ability to function and on life expectancy.

BIOLOGIC THEORIES OF AGING

Biologic theories attempt to explain the physiologic processes that occur independent of external or pathologic influences, that occur gradually, and that are automatic and universal. Each of the current biologic theories of aging contains a body of data that provides some evidence that makes it universally acceptable and lends support to the underlying hypothesis. Most of the theories are not mutually exclusive. Indeed, all or some may operate simultaneously.

Programmed Aging Theory (Cellular Aging). Programmed aging theories state that manifestations of senescent changes are the result of genetic programs containing "aging genes" responsible for the senile changes preceding the demise and death of the organism. Therefore, contained within the cellular genetic code is the information that probably programs normal cellular aging. Similar cells in specific species and organisms may age at different rates, just as different cells within the same organism may age at different rates (Hayflick, 1965).

Cross-Link Theory. Cross-link theory, a genetic theory, suggests that a strong chemical bonding between organic molecules in the body causes increased stiffness, chemical instability, and insolubility of connective tissue and DNA (Rockstein & Sussman, 1979). Evidence to support this theory is based on the rate of DNA repair as it relates to the life span of the species. In cultured human cells, the rate of DNA repair decreases as the cells age.

Theories of Random Deterioration. A major theory of random deterioration, also a genetic theory, is free radical reactions (Harman, 1981). This theory proposes that an increase in unstable free radicals (unstable molecules possessing an extra electrical charge, or free electron) causes deterioration in biologic systems. When free radicals attack molecules, they damage cell membranes. Aging occurs because of accumulated cell damage that interferes with function.

Immunologic Theory (Autoimmunity Theory). With age, the ability of the immunologic system to quantitatively and qualitatively produce antibodies diminishes. As normal immune responses decline, autoimmune manifestations increase greatly with age. The immune system becomes less able to discriminate between self and nonself, resulting in an increase in autoimmune diseases. Advocates of the immunologic theory of aging argue that most of the diseases of old age or late life arise with greater frequency in aging and are characterized by some degree of immune dysfunction. This may explain the adult onset of such conditions as cancer, maturity-onset diabetes, rheumatic heart disease, senile dementia, arthritis, and several vascular diseases.

Stress and Viral Theories. There are numerous stress- and viral-based theories. The wear-and-tear theory conceptualizes that body structures stop functioning as a result of their wearing out or being overused (Hayflick, 1988). Organs have a fixed amount of energy available and they wear out. When cells wear out, the body will not function well. Repeated injury or insult to the tissues and overuse is thought to enhance the process of aging.

Similarly, the stress adaptation theory supposes that the effects of residual damage resulting from stress accumulate, and the body no longer is able to resist the stress and dies (Selye, 1976). Stress reactions produce changes in the structure and chemicals of the body that can cause irreversible damage to the organism. The theory incorporates internal and external stressors of life, including physical, psychological, social, and environmental.

Viral theories are similar to those promoting viral diseases. These theories assume that a slow virus or ordinary virus is present in the body and may play a part in the aging process. They assume that the virus is present in the body at birth and grows as aging occurs.

Neuroendocrine Theory. Followers of the neuroendocrine theory argue that decrements in a system so essential to survival and homeostasis as neurons and hormones must play a profound role in the regulation of the aging process. No part of the body acts in isolation from neurologic and endocrine systems. These more recent and less developed theories link aging to a centralized control in the brain, specifically the hypothalamus and the pituitary, and to the immune system.

PSYCHOLOGICAL AND SOCIAL THEORIES OF AGING

Some researchers indicate that genetic endowment and physiologic factors are not the primary determinants of longevity. They argue that age of parents at death shows little correlation with longevity of offspring. They propose that lifestyle, personality, and environmental factors are more important.

Activity Theory. Activity theory is a commonsense or lay theory that encourages a positive role adjustment to aging and is reflected in legislation, newspapers, and science programs. Persons who achieve optimal age, according to this theory, are those who stay active and manage to resist the shrinkage of their world (Havighurst & Allrecht, 1953). As roles change, the person finds substitute activities for these roles. The major difficulty with the activity theory is that it does not deal adequately with personality differences.

Disengagement Theory. Disengagement theory states that, under normal conditions of health and economic independence, aging involves a natural, systematic, inevitable withdrawal, or "disengagement," of the aging person from others in the social system. Forces shrink the older adult's world. This withdrawal, when complete, leads to a new equilibrium characterized by increased distance and a less role-connected style of interaction. The withdrawal is mutually satisfying for both parties. For the older adult, it brings releases from social pressures; for society, it allows younger persons who are more energetic to assume functional roles to provide an orderly transition of power (Cumming & Henry, 1961).

This theory does not address the influence of personality type, nor does it explain the many older adults who remain extremely active and creative until death or the dissatisfaction of those who are forced to withdraw from social involvements. It does, however, explain the relatively high morale of older adults, even under great duress, and their apparent acceptance of a more contemplative life.

Continuity Theory. Continuity theory states that a person develops habits, commitments, preferences, and a number of other dispositions that become a part of his or her personality in the process of becoming an adult (Havighurst, Neugarten, & Tobin, 1963). With aging, there is a predisposition toward maintaining continuity in these dispositions. Therefore, aging is dependent on the aging person's life, personality type, the ability to adjust to stress, and on his or her social milieu remaining stable over the life span. Parts of continuity theory suggest that people, as they age, gravitate toward increased inner orientation and increased separation from the environment. People become more individual as they age. As such, the person's lifestyle and personality will be reflected in old age as it is in younger years.

Interactionist Theory. Interactionist theory proposes that age-related changes result from interaction between the biologic and psychological personal characteristics of the person, societal circumstances, and the older adult's history of social interaction patterns (Lemon, Bingston, & Peterson, 1972). The roles the person fulfills over a lifetime are called "careers" by the interactionist theorist. Career development and progression can be disrupted by accident or unexpected illness, but, in general, people tend to try to balance their careers. Interactionists believe that although persons change roles or career involvement in later years as they choose, the significance of the middle years' "career set" remains.

Minority Group Theory. Minority group theory suggests that older adults are a minority group. The theory is based on the premise that by showing visible characteristics of biologic aging, the older adult becomes susceptible to discrimination similar to that which affects racial or sexual minority groups (Rose, 1962).

Human Needs Theory. Human needs theory emphasizes the concept of motivation and human needs. The most famous of these is Maslow's theory of basic human needs arranged in a hierarchy of physiologic needs, safety and security, love and belonging, self-esteem, and self-actualization. Persons move between the levels, but are always striving toward the higher needs. The older adult should therefore be a fully mature person who has autonomy, creativity, independence, and a positive relationship with family and society (Maslow, 1954).

SUMMARY OF THEORIES

The biologic and psychological theories have important implications for nursing practice, because they underscore the importance of planning care in diversified and individualized ways, with consideration for the person's functional and physical limitations, preferences, lifestyle, and personality. They accentuate the influence of culture, family, education, community, roles and patterns of responses, and disease states. The nurse can use these theories as a basis to plan intervention in the care of older adults.

DEVELOPMENTAL TASKS OF AGING

Erickson's theory of development is based on freudian dynamics. According to Erickson, each stage of life has a psychosexual crisis that must be overcome in order to lay the foundation for a new stage (Erickson, 1963). His theory does not clearly explain why the organism moves from one state to the next. It assumes that certain inner biologic and outer sociologic conditions are required for progression to the next task. These concepts are somewhat cultural and class bound. There seems to be, however, some tasks that are accomplished by successfully aging persons that need to be viewed by the nurse in planning care of the older adult. These may increase the problems associated with aging or may facilitate the adaptation of the older adult to the aging process. Some of these tasks include:

- Adjusting to full or semi-retirement
- Accepting help from others graciously and comfortably as dependency increases
- Learning new affectionate roles with one's children, who are now mature adults
- Establishing ongoing, satisfying affectionate roles with grandchildren and other members of the extended family

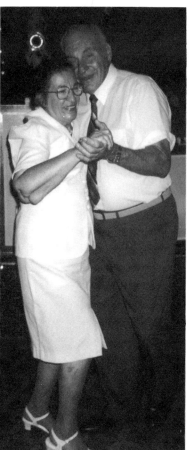

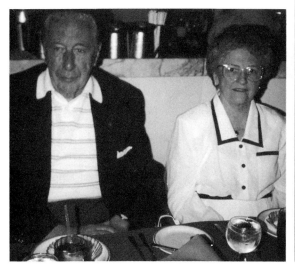

- Being a good companion to an aging spouse
- Facing the loss of one's spouse
- Finding and preserving mutually satisfying friendships outside the family circle
- Choosing and maintaining ongoing social activities and functions appropriate to health, energy, and interests
- Maintaining a sense of moral integrity in the face of disappointments and disillusionments in life's hopes and dreams
- Making a good adjustment to failing powers as aging diminishes strength and abilities
- Adapting interests and activities to reserves of vitality and energy of the aging body
- Mastering new awareness and methods of dealing with physical surroundings as a person with occasional or permanent disabilities
- Keeping mentally alert and effective
- Preparing for eventual and inevitable cessation of life by adopting a philosophy of life that allows one to live and die in peace

STANDARDS OF PRACTICE

The practice of gerontological nursing involves a commitment to provide health care to meet the needs of the older population. Current gerontological nursing practice is a dynamic, evolving process governed by a set of regulatory standards that serve as a model for professional practice. The standards apply to all gerontological settings and are meant to be a resource for assessment tools, plans of care, and outcome determination. They are useful in the process of peer review, evaluation, and improvement of care. The standards as published by the American Nurses' Association include rationale, structure, process, and outcome criteria. The following standards and scope of gerontological nursing practice are meant to assist nurses in providing care of the highest quality to older adults. Rationales provide further definition of the standards. Display 1-1 shows the Standards of Gerontological Nursing Practice as put forth by the American Nurses Association (1987).

Display 1-1
STANDARDS OF GERONTOLOGICAL NURSING PRACTICE

Standard I. Organization of Gerontological Nursing Services

All gerontological nursing services are planned, organized, and directed by a nurse executive. The nurse executive has baccalaureate or master's preparation and has experience in gerontological nursing and administration of long-term care services or acute care services for older clients.

Standard II. Theory

The nurse participates in the generation and testing of theory as a basis for clinical decisions. The nurse uses theoretical concepts to guide the effective practice of gerontological nursing.

Standard III. Data Collection

The health status of the older person is regularly assessed in a comprehensive, accurate, and systematic manner. The information obtained during the health assessment is accessible to and shared with appropriate members of the interdisciplinary health care team, including the older person and the family.

Standard IV. Nursing Diagnosis

The nurse uses health assessment data to determine nursing diagnoses.

Standard V. Planning and Continuity of Care

The nurse develops the plan of care in conjunction with the older person and appropriate others. Mutual goals, priorities, nursing approaches, and measures in the care plan address the therapeutic, preventive, restorative, and rehabilitative needs of the older person. The care plan helps the older person attain and maintain the highest level of health, well-being, and quality of life achievable, as well as a peaceful death. The plan of care facilitates continuity of care over time as the client moves to various care settings, and is revised as necessary.

(continued)

Display 1-1
STANDARDS OF GERONTOLOGICAL NURSING PRACTICE *(Continued)*

Standard VI. Intervention

The nurse, guided by the plan of care, intervenes to provide care to restore the older person's functional capabilities and to prevent complications and excessive disability. Nursing interventions are derived from nursing diagnoses and are based on gerontological nursing theory.

Standard VII. Evaluation

The nurse continually evaluates the client's and family's responses to interventions in order to determine progress toward goal attainment and to revise the data base, nursing diagnoses, and plan of care.

Standard VIII. Interdisciplinary Collaboration

The nurse collaborates with other members of the health care team in the various settings in which care is given to the older person. The team meets regularly to evaluate the effectiveness of the care plan for the client and family and to adjust the plan of care to accommodate changing needs.

Standard IX. Research

The nurse participates in research and uses and disseminates research findings.

Standard X. Ethics

The nurse uses the code for nurses established by the American Nurses Association as a guide for ethical decision making in practice.

Standard XI. Professional Development

The nurse assumes responsibility for professional development and contributes to the professional growth of interdisciplinary team members. The nurse participates in peer review and other means of evaluation to ensure the quality of nursing practice.

Reprinted with permission from *Standards and Scope of Gerontological Nursing Practice* © 1987, American Nurses Association, Washington, DC.

FRAMEWORK FOR PRACTICE

Gerontological nursing provides special management of older adults by nurses who understand their special needs and devise skilled geriatric care and rehabilitation plans. These plans must include resolution of any pathologic processes plus restoration to the level of function attained before any illness. In all cases, the needs and wishes of family caregivers must be included in the care planning process. The nurse must be aware of referral services and resources available to meet individual and family needs based on an appropriate total patient assessment.

Functional assessment of the older adult acts as an appropriate framework for gerontological nursing practice. It focuses on a person's abilities and disabilities regardless of chronologic age or medical diagnosis. Each individual problem in the older adult must be assessed functionally. Assessment for function will uncover the hidden problems often not mentioned because of embarrassment, negativity, modesty, ignorance, or lack of perception as a problem. For example, the older adult with hypothyroidism or congestive heart failure, instead of manifesting symptoms of shortness of breath and easy fatigability, may cease to go shopping or climb stairs or take part in fewer social outings.

Functional assessments can influence conventional medical management decisions. For example, it may not be necessary to treat elevated blood pressure if the effect of therapy will be to the patient's detriment. If the patient gets woozy every time he or she stands quickly to do housework, treatment may not be advantageous. Collaborative information sharing with other members of the health care team ensures the highest functional outcomes.

Assessment tools are varied and generally include a complete history and physical examination, a basic self-care activities inventory, and more complex instrumental activities of daily living inventory. Other instruments include the Lawton (Lawton, 1972); Older Adult Resources and Services (OARS) (Duke, 1978); Fillenbaum (Fillenbaum, 1985); the Katz Index (Katz, 1963), developed to measure and record the ability of the older adult to function independently; and the Barthol Index (Mahoney, 1965), designed for use in rehabilitation settings. Other areas included in the functional assessment are cognitive function, affective function (determines whether depression is present), nutritional status, financial status, caregiver evaluation (including a caregiver stress level assessment), social function, and rehabilitative potential. Total assessment should include the need for supportive services, preventive measures, and evaluation for placement in a long-term-care setting.

Functional assessment of the older adult should incorporate physical, psychological, and socioeconomic factors interacting to influence a comprehensive evaluation of the person's health status. A wide range of history, physical, and mental status examination forms are available for use with older adults. The nature of the assessment process, including the history and physical exam, is dictated by the purpose, setting, and timing of the assessment. Specific questions for history and physical exam techniques are suggested in the context of this text. Diagnostic, physical, and laboratory findings are incorporated to determine overall health, well-being, and need for health and social services. The nurse will need to use the information as deemed appropriate.

The nurse must be aware of special considerations for history taking of the older adult to avoid inaccurate or confusing data. The assessment should be conducted in an area that is private, comfortable, well-lit, and has a minimum of background noise to compensate for sensory losses of aging. Lighting should not be glaring, and the older adult should be provided a study chair with arms. The nurse should be close enough to be seen and heard while respecting the patient's need for personal space. Ample time should be permitted for slower responses, but attention should be paid to limiting the interview time to reduce fatigue. If the patient has a memory impairment, anxiety state, or psychological disturbance, arrange for a family member to be present to fill in missing or inaccurate information. Be aware of the patient's underreporting of symptoms by assuming that they are a normal part of aging. An important part of the history taking in a functional assessment is determining how the older adult spends the day. Asking the patient to relay the day's activities will provide information about lifestyle and life problems and more particularly about life satisfaction, chief concerns, and desire for change.

No one instrument has been shown to be better than others, and there are pitfalls in the use of standardized assessment instruments. Their accuracy depends on patient and caregiver honesty. Observation of the patient may increase the validity of the tool. The functional assessment team should use instruments that fit the purpose and setting for which they are intended. The minimal amount of information contained in a total assessment should include assessments of the home living arrangements, finances, sociocultural patterns, medications, nutrition, and a supporter person inventory along with mental status and physical examination. It is important that there be a link between the assessment process and the provision of patient care planning and services.

REFERENCES

American Nurses Association. (1987). *Standards and scope of gerontological nursing practice.* Kansas City, MO: American Nurses Association.

Cumming, E., & Henry, W. (1961). *Growing old: The process of disengagement theory.* New York: Basic Books

Duke University Center for the Study of Aging and Human Development. (1978). *Multidimensional functional assessment: The OARS methodology.* Durham, NC: Duke University Press.

Erickson, E. H. (1963). *Childhood and society* (2nd ed.). New York: W. W. Norton.

Folstein, M. F., Anthony, J. C., & Parhad, I., (1985). The meaning of cognitive impairment in the elderly. *Journal of the American Geriatrics Society, 33*(4), 228–235.

Harman, D. (1981). The aging process. *Procedures of the National Academy of Science, USA, 78*(11), 7124.

Havighurst, R. J., & Allrecht, R. (1953). *Older people.* New York: Longmans, Green.

Havighurst, R. J., Neugarten, B. L., & Tobin, S. S. (1963). Disengagement, personality and life satisfaction in the later years. In P. Hansen (Ed.), *Age with a future* (pp. 419–425). Copenhagen: Munksgood.

Hayflick, L. (1988). Why do we live so long? *Geriatrics, 43*(10), 77–87.

Hayflick, L. (1965). The limited in vitro lifetime of human diploid cell strains. *Experimental Cell Research, 37,* 614–636.

Katz, S., Ford, A., Moskowit R., Jackson, B., & Jaffe, M. (1963). Studies of illness in the aged: The index of ADL, a standard measure of biological and psychosocial function. *Journal of the American Medical Association, 185,* 914–919.

Lawton, M. P. (1971). The functional assessment of elderly people. *Journal of the American Geriatrics Society. 19*(6), 465–481.

Lemon, B. W., Bingston, V. L., & Peterson, J. (1972). An exploration of the activity theory of aging: Activity types and life satisfaction among in-movers to a retirement community. *Journal of Gerontology, 127,* 511–523.

Maslow, A. H. (1954). *Motivation and personality.* New York: Harper and Row.

Miller, C. A. (1990). *Nursing care of older adults.* Glenview, IL: Scott, Foresman/Little Brown Higher Education.

Phillips, L. R. (1990). The elderly, the nurse, and the challenge. In D. M. Corr & C. A. Corr (Eds.), *Nursing care in an aging society.* New York: Springer.

Rockstein, M., & Sussman, M. (1979). *Biology of aging.* Belmont, CA: Wadsworth.

Rose, A. M. (1962). The subculture of aging: A topic for sociological research. *Gerontologist, 12,* 123–127.

Selye, H. (1976). *The stress of life.* New York: McGraw Hill.

BIBLIOGRAPHY

Erickson, E. H. (1982). *The life cycle computed: A review.* New York: W. W. Norton.

2

Demographics in Aging: Implications for Nursing

Objectives

1. Identify demographic trends that influence the health and well-being of older adults.
2. Describe the relationships among health, income, and education in older persons.
3. Explain the role of the nurse in providing care to older adults whose health and well-being may be negatively affected by changing demographic patterns.
4. Develop a plan of nursing care that includes demographic factors that may affect the health care of older adults.

INTRODUCTION

GROWING OLD IS AN EXPERIENCE OF RECENT years. In the past, people didn't age—they died (Gibbs, 1988). The American Association of Retired Persons (AARP) reported that about 2.1 million Americans celebrated their 65th birthday in 1992, resulting in approximately 6,000 birthdays each day (Fowles, 1993). During this same year, about 1.6 million persons aged 65 years or older died, an increase of more than 521,000 persons (1,420 daily).

There are approximately 31 million older adults in the United States (U.S. Bureau of the Census, 1991), constituting about 12.7% of the population (Fowles, 1993). Not only is the older age group increasing in number and as a percentage of the population, but they are also getting older as a group. In 1992, the 65- to 74-year-old group, or the "young-old," as they are referred to by gerontologists, included 18.5 million and was eight times larger than the same age group in 1900 (Fowles, 1993). The 75- to 84-year-old "middle-old" group was 10.6 million larger, or 14 times greater, than the same age group in

Staab, AS and Hodges, LC: ESSENTIALS OF GERONTOLOGICAL NURSING,
© 1996 J. B. Lippincott Company

1900 (Fowles, 1993). The greatest increase was among the "old-old," those persons 85 years of age and older. The old-old age group, which includes approximately 3 million persons (Fowles, 1993), increased 26 times more than did this same age group at the turn of the century. The increase in the older population is a major result of improved disease prevention and health care in this century (U.S. Senate Special Committee on Aging, 1984).

This aging of the aged has implications for health care and nursing. There are more older adults who will need health care, and they will be among the very old. The old-old age group will have more complex, chronic health care needs than the young-old, who are expected to remain well if they pursue a healthy lifestyle. Nurses will need to provide a continuum of care for older adults that includes preventive, restorative, and maintenance services.

Aging of the population is a worldwide concern. Most developed countries have a high percentage of aging persons. The aging population is expected to continue to grow. In the United States, the older population is expected to represent approximately 20% of the population by the year 2030 (Fowles, 1993).

Statistics on aging populations suggest that all older people are alike and have the same needs. However, older adults are an extremely heterogenous group, with variations in age, culture, and socioeconomic conditions. Older adults are much more diverse than younger persons who have had fewer life experiences. Health care policy based exclusively on chronologic age may fail to accommodate the diversity that exists among older adults.

Aging can be defined both in chronologic terms and as a process. As a process, aging begins at conception and results in a sequence of events (maturation) that occur in all persons throughout their life span but at different rates. Aging may vary among persons based on a variety of biopsychosocial factors, such as environmental conditions, nutrition, and genetics. In contrast, chronologic aging, the number of years passed since birth, has been the basis for legislation using age 65 years as the onset of old age. Chronologic age continues to guide public policy decisions affecting the older adult. However, the age limit differs in Title VII of the Older Americans Act, the nutrition program, which set 60 years as the eligibility age, and the Department of Housing and Urban Development, which considers age 62 as the lower limit (Rempusheski, 1991).

▷ *Clinical Pearl*

Assessment: Health care decisions for older adults should be based on factors other than chronologic age because of the diversity that exists among this age group. Similarly, in nursing, care should not be based on chronologic age as the only criterion. A complete assessment is necessary before care is implemented to accommodate the different rates at which people age.

LIFE EXPECTANCY

The length of time that a person is expected to live represents life expectancy. Life expectancy is based on mortality rates. A person born in 1900 could expect to live an average of 48 years, whereas a person born in 1987 could expect to live 74.7 years (U.S. Senate Special Committee on Aging, 1984). Differences in life expectancy exist among races and between men and women. In the United States in 1985, the life expectancy for males was less than for females. In 1987, a white person could expect to live 6 years longer than a black person, until they reached the age of 65, when the differences between the races are small and the actual death rates for persons older than age 75 are higher for whites than for blacks (U.S. Senate Special Committee on Aging, 1984). Life expectancy after age 65 years varies internationally as well.

GENDER AND MARITAL STATUS

As the population grows older, women increasingly outnumber men. The cause of this disparity between mortality rates of men and women is unknown, but it is thought to be related to biologic (hormonal) and sociologic reasons. Because of the differences in life span for men and women, the nurse working with older adults should be knowledgeable in women's health issues and understand the social implications that could result from women living longer than men.

A social difference between men and women that has been reported concerns marital status. In 1992, 76% of older men were married, but only 41% of older women had a living spouse (Fowles, 1993). There were five times as many widows as widowers. Older black men and Hispanic men are more likely to be widowers than are white men (Atchley, 1994). The divorce rate represented only 5% of older persons in 1992, but the number of divorces in this age group is increasing rapidly, especially among women (Fowles, 1993). This difference in marital status has important economic, social, and health-related implications. Atchley (1994) suggested that most older men have a spouse to rely on, but many older women had to find other sources of social support.

ETHNICITY

In 1992, approximately 86% of persons older than 65 years of age in the United States were white, 8% were black, and 6% were other races (Fowles, 1993). According to Atchley (1994), the proportion of white elderly is declining, black elderly is increasing, and other groups are remaining the same. In the future, a large number of Asian refugees will join the 65+ age group and present unique challenges to the health care system because of their language and cultural backgrounds. According to Cavanaugh (1993), one of the problems in understanding ethnic variations in aging is the lack of research. Nurses should be aware of the special needs of each culture and make adjustments in their nursing care to accommodate this diversity, such as:

- Giving special attention to personal hygiene practices to accommodate a variety of approaches
- Providing interpreters
- Serving traditional foods, if possible
- Creating ways to acknowledge the customs and celebrations of persons of diverse cultures.

LIVING ENVIRONMENTS

Most older adults (94%) live independently in the community, whereas about 6% live in institutions (Atchley, 1994). However, as age increases, about 20% of older adults will need to spend some time in a nursing home. Most older adults (80%) living in the community own their homes (Carp, 1991). Other older adults live in rented homes and substandard housing, including single-room hotels. Some live on the streets because of a lack of available housing, mental condition or choice.

There is less migration among the elderly (5%) than in younger (17%) age groups (Carp, 1991). The majority stay and age in one place. Those who do move do not go far, with only 20% moving to another state. Florida and California are the top two destination states, with Arizona a distant third (Carp, 1991). The migration patterns of the young tend to be to urban areas, leaving the rural elderly isolated, lacking many amenities and health care services.

Older adults usually relocate to be nearer to other family members. Contrary to public opinion, family members do not abandon older members, even when they are institutionalized. Close contact is usually maintained over the years between generations. Four of every five older persons have living children (Fowles, 1993). Most (66%) older adults have one child living within 30 minutes of them (Fowles, 1993). Most older adults prefer to live independently as long as possible and usually do not live with their children until they are forced to because of failing health.

▷ *Clinical Pearl*

Assessment: Relocation by older persons to be near their adult children may result in strained relationships and less support than anticipated.

Many older adults live alone. Older adults who live alone represent 33% of the population 65 years of age and older, and their numbers are expected to increase (Kasper, 1988). In 30 years, the number of elderly people living alone will have increased from 8.5 to 13.3 million, and 85% of them will be women (Kasper, 1988). There is controversy about the desirability and satisfaction of older adults who live alone. Some have suggested that living alone causes alienation and decreases the quality of life (Kasper, 1988), but others indicated that living alone is less stressful than living with a spouse and does not negatively affect mental health (Aldersberg & Thorne, 1990; Preston & Dellasega, 1990). Most older adults prefer to live in the community and remain in their homes, thus most nursing care may be provided in the home, and family caregivers may or may not be available.

Cost of care is a major factor in the delivery of health care. Home health care is more cost-effective, both in human and financial terms, than institutionalization. Maintaining independence and a healthy lifestyle depends greatly on the availability of adequate funds.

FINANCIAL ASPECTS

Probably in no other area is there so much difference among older adults than in income. The elderly are more sharply stratified into rich and poor than are younger age groups. Income tends to concentrate among a very few who are extremely wealthy, in contrast to younger age groups, where money is more evenly divided. For family units 65 years of age and older, one-fifth of the older persons had over half (53%) of the total income for all the aged (Catchen, 1989).

The median income of older persons in 1992 was $14,548 for men and $8,189 for women (Fowles, 1993). Older adults receive their income primarily from Social Security and other federal entitlement programs, private pensions, earnings, and assets. Poor older persons depend on Social Security or other federal retirement programs for most of their income (Catchen, 1989). The death of one person in a married couple will usually result in a dramatic reduction in income because of the loss of Social Security checks. Unfortunately, living costs for the remaining spouse are not significantly less. This is especially the case if the husband dies first, because his check is usually the larger of the two (Catchen, 1989). In 1992, about 4 million older persons (13%) lived in poverty in the United States (Fowles, 1993). The highest poverty rates are in nine Southern states, where more than 17% of the population over 65 years of age are living in poverty. Poverty is more commonly a problem for women and minority groups.

Medicare, initiated in 1965, is a national health insurance program for most persons older than age 65 years. Medicare is administered by the Social Security Administration and pays for selected costs in hospital and medical bills. The deductibles and excluded services in Medicare have increased dramatically over the last few years, reducing services and increasing the out-of-pocket expenditures of the older adult for health care services. Consequently, many older adults are forced to spend down to Medicaid eligibility levels to obtain the care they need. Because most older adults have experienced material deprivation or economic problems during the Great Depression, they may refuse to obtain needed health care services if they do not have or believe they do not have sufficient funds to pay for them.

Medicaid, a national health care plan for the poor, is administered by the Department of Health, Education, and Welfare. Medicaid covers more services than Medicare but is available only to those who are very poor. It is unfortunate that to become eligible for health care benefits, the person or couple must first become destitute.

Nurses need to know where health care dollars are spent and who pays for them. In 1987, of the $162 billion spent on health care, older adults accounted for 36% of the total personal health care expenditures and represented 12% of the total U.S. population (Fowles, 1993). Government programs paid approximately 63% of the health care expenditures of older persons in 1987, compared with only 26% for younger persons (Fowles, 1993). Home health care continues to receive very little financial support from government sources. Older adults paid approximately $1,500 (out-of-pocket), or one-fourth the cost of health care (Fowles, 1993). Many older adults use Medigap insurance to pay for some health care costs that are not covered by Medicare. Medigap or Supplemental Insurance coverage is available from a variety of vendors, including the AARP.

Retirement and employment of older adults influences their financial status. Most older persons prefer to retire from paid employment when they are eligible. However, some choose to continue working, and others need to work for financial reasons. In 1992, approximately 12% of all older adults in the United States were working or actively seeking employment (Fowles, 1993). Unfortunately, those who choose to work and those who must work for economic reasons are often forced to take low-paying and strenuous jobs, such as working in fast food and retail establishments.

Statistics indicate that older persons are loyal employees and dependable workers (Atchley, 1994). Many older persons work part-time. For most older adults, the decision to work part-time is determined by the amount a person is permitted to earn before Social Security benefits are taxed.

There is an emphasis at the governmental level to retain and retrain older workers. In addition, federal legislation has changed the retirement age from 65 years to 68 years beginning in the year 2000. This policy will increase the number of people in the workforce, which is declining internationally. With increased numbers among the aged who are unable or who do not desire to work, it is projected that as the baby boomers reach retirement age, the ratio of working-age persons will decrease. This has implications for health care providers and policy planners. Health care resources that are already limited will become more scarce, and there will be fewer professionals to meet the increased demands. Bahr (1994) suggested that such issues as allocation of scarce resources, availability of jobs, and payment for needed health care services will become more pressing and demand answers from health care personnel, policymakers, and individuals.

Older adults fill important roles in society. They often perform volunteer work, filling the void left in service agencies as younger women, who traditionally held these positions, seek paid employment. The Older Americans Act has provided increased volunteer activities for older adults through several programs, including the Retired Senior Volunteer Program, which places volunteers in schools and community organizations; the Service Corps of Retired Executives, which helps small businesses; and the Senior Companion Program, in which older adults help other disabled older persons. Older persons also serve as caregivers for grandchildren both on a part-time and permanent basis.

Political action is another area that the older adult is affecting. Atchley (1994) suggested that because tenure is so important in politics, the older members can have considerable power as well as considerable strength in special interest groups. The AARP has 28 million members (Gibbs, 1988). The Gray Panthers has 80,000 members. These organizations have considerable influence and pressure Congress on issues important to older persons. Pressure from older persons was effective in 1990 in reversing a federal surtax that required only the aged to pay for catastrophic health insurance that would have been used by a small percentage of this age group. This is a form of ageism in which a person would have been taxed based only on age. Little attention was given to the fact that older adults pay taxes for all levels of formal education but use very few of these resources. Older adults are more likely to vote than younger adults. It is anticipated that the political clout of older Americans will increase.

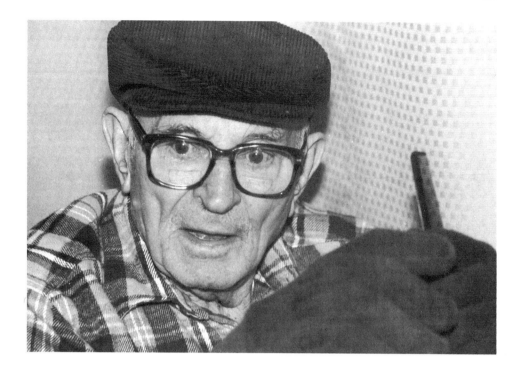

RELIGIOUS ACTIVITIES

Spirituality is an important part of the lives of many aging persons. Older persons not only volunteer frequently but also attend more religious activities than younger persons. According to Atchley (1994), religious participation declines in later life, but not in-home religious activity. This suggests that attendance at religious services may be difficult or impossible for some older persons, but that lifelong spiritual interest and devotion continues. Involvement in religious activities may vary by race and culture. Older blacks display a high degree of involvement in religious activities, and church attendance may indicate the amount of support available in times of need (Burnside, 1988).

EDUCATIONAL LEVEL

Educational level and income are related to health status. Persons with higher educational levels can expect to live healthier lives. According to Fowles (1993), the educational level of the older population is increasing. Between the years 1970 and 1993, the percentage of older persons who had completed high school increased from 28% to 60%, to include approximately 63% of whites, 33% of blacks, and 26% of Hispanics. In 1992, about 12% had 4 or more years of college. By the year 2009, nearly 20% of the older population will be college graduates, compared with about 10% in 1979 (Atchley, 1994). This increased education will affect the social, economic, and political climate in the United States. Many older persons with no or very limited formal education are self-educated and highly motivated to learn. Consequently, it would be a mistake to draw inferences about what the older person has learned or is capable of learning based on years of schooling. Educational opportunity and intellectual ability may be very different in this age group. Older adults who experienced the Great Depression in the 1930s may have had to stop going to school to work.

HEALTH STATUS

Three national goals established for older adults by the U.S. Department of Health and Human Services will influence nursing care by the year 2000: increased life expectancy, reduced disability caused by chronic conditions, and increased healthy years of life to at least 65 years (Abdellah, 1991).

The first goal, to increase life expectancy from birth to at least 78 years of age, is closely related to the third goal to increase the healthy years of life. These goals suggest that quantity of years and quality of life are important for older persons.

The second goal, to reduce disability caused by chronic conditions, implies that health care providers will need to help older adults make lifestyle adjustments to prevent disability from chronic conditions. Most older persons have one or more chronic conditions, but the majority (69%) assessed their health as better than fair (Fowles, 1993). This statistic suggests that despite chronic conditions, most older persons have learned to live with long-term challenges.

Chronic illness has been described as the major health care problem in this country (Baines & Oglesby, 1991). The most frequently occurring chronic conditions in older patients in 1991 were arthritis (48%), hypertension (37%), hearing impairments (32%), heart disease (30%), cataracts (17%), orthopedic impairments (18%), sinusitis (14%), diabetes (10%), and tinnitus and varicose veins (8% each) (Fowles, 1993). According to Fowles (1993), approximately 6 million older adults needed assistance from another person in managing self-care activities of daily living. Home management or instrumental activities include preparing meals, shopping, managing money, using the telephone, and doing housework. Assistance with these activities is needed by 7.6 million older persons (Fowles, 1993). Most older adults who require aid in home management reported receiving assistance. In contrast, less than half who had difficulty with personal care had help (Fowles, 1993).

The increasing incidence of acquired immunodeficiency syndrome (AIDS) in the older adult will require more formal (professional) and informal (family) health care assistance for those afflicted. According to the Centers for Disease Control HIV/AIDS Surveillance Report, in 1990 there were 1,718 reported cases of AIDS in persons aged 65 years and older in the United States (Baines & Oglesby, 1991). Most older adults with AIDS are men (1,326), and the primary route of transmission of the human immunodeficiency virus is transfusion.

An estimated 15% to 25% of all elderly persons have serious symptoms of mental disorders. The number of persons with mental disorders living in nursing homes continues to rise, and approximately 27% of patients in state mental institutions are 65 years of age and older (U.S. Senate Special Committee on Aging, 1984). Alzheimer's disease is the leading cause of cognitive impairment in the older adult population (U.S. Senate Special Committee on Aging,

1984). Approximately 6% of older adults have Alzheimer's disease, and the percentage who have this affliction is expected to double by the year 2040.

Not only do older adults experience more chronic illnesses than younger age groups, but they are also hospitalized more frequently for acute care. Older people accounted for 35% of all hospital admissions in 1991 (Fowles, 1993). The average length of stay was 8.6 days for older persons, compared with 5.2 days for younger persons (Fowles, 1993). Older adults also visited a physician more frequently than did younger people. Although older persons stay in the hospital for longer periods than younger age groups, they are now being discharged sooner and with more complex problems. (Baines & Oglesby, 1991). The reason for this is the use of diagnosis-related groups (DRG), in which hospitals are paid a fixed amount for the treatment of medical conditions. For most patients, the length of time spent in the hospital does not determine how much the government will pay; consequently, hospitals are encouraged to discharge patients as quickly as possible. This has resulted in patients going home to family caregivers with more complicated health care needs and many needing increased services from home health care nurses. It has also raised the acuity level in nursing homes, which often are unprepared to cope with older patients who are seriously ill. In addition, some states report an acute shortage of nursing home beds, especially for persons who must depend on Medicaid for payment of long-term-care services.

Because of illness, approximately 8% of all older adults are home bound. Most health care (80%) in the United States is provided by family members, even in the presence of professional health care services (Baines & Oglesby, 1991). Demographic changes that may influence the availability of caregivers include more women in the workforce who provide the majority (72%) of the caregiving, increased mobility, decreased family size, and increased divorce rate. About half of all care provided to an older person is given by another older adult who may also be in ill health. Relief for families, such as adult day and respite care, is the focus of legislation at the state and national levels (Stone, 1987).

Health care providers, particularly nurses, whose role it is to assist persons who are physically and mentally challenged in a variety of settings, will be among those affected by the changing patterns of family composition. Nurses will need to educate informal family caregivers and assist those persons who do not have family caregivers.

REFERENCES

Abdellah, F. (1991). Public policy impacting on nursing care of older adults. In E. Baines (Ed.). *Perspectives on gerontological nursing* (pp. 155–169). Newbury Park, CA: Sage.

Adlersberg, M., & Thorne, S. (1990). Emerging from the chrysalis. *Journal of Gerontological Nursing, 16*, 4–8.

Atchley, R. (1994). *Social forces and aging.* Belmont, CA: Wadsworth.

Bahr, R. T. (1994). Ethical issues. In M. Hogstel (Ed.), *Nursing care of the older adult.* Albany, NY: Delmar.

Baines, E., & Oglesby, F. (1991). Conceptualization of chronicity in aging. In E. Baines (Ed.), *Perspectives on gerontological nursing* (pp. 251–274). Newbury Park, CA: Sage.

Burnside, I. (1988). *Nursing and the ages: A self-care approach.* New York: McGraw-Hill.

Carp, F. (1991). Living environments of older adults. In E. Baines (Ed.), *Perspectives on gerontological nursing* (pp. 185–197). Newbury Park, CA: Sage.

Catchen, H. (1989). Generational equity: Issues of gender and race. *Women & Health, 14*, 21–38.

Cavanaugh, J. (1993). *Adult development and aging.* Pacific Grove, CA: Brooks/Cole Publishing Co.

Fowles, D. (Ed.). (1993). *A profile of older Americans.* Washington, DC: American Association of Retired Persons.

Gibbs, N. (1988, February 22). Grays on the go. *Time, 131,* 66–75.

Kasper, J. (1988). *Aging alone.* Report of the Commonwealth Fund Commission on Elderly People Living Alone, Baltimore.

Preston, D., & Dellasega, C. (1990). Elderly women and stress, does marriage make a difference? *Journal of Gerontological Nursing, 16,* 26–32.

Rempusheski, V. (1991). Historical and futuristic perspectives on aging and the gerontological nurse. In E. Baines (Ed.), *Perspectives on gerontological nursing* (pp. 3–28). Newbury Park, CA: Sage.

Stone, R. (Ed.). (1987). *Exploding the myths: Caregiving in America.* A study by the subcommittee on Human Services of the Select Committee on Aging, U. S. House of Representatives (Report No. 99-611). Washington, DC: U.S. Government Printing Office.

U.S. Bureau of the Census. (1991). *Statistical Abstract of the United States.* Washington, DC: U.S. Government Printing Office.

U.S. Senate Special Committee on Aging. (1984). *Aging America: Trends and projections* (No. 101-E). Washington, DC: U.S. Government Printing Office.

BIBLIOGRAPHY

Taeuber, C. (1992). *Sixty-five plus in America.* U.S. Bureau of the Census. Washington, DC: U.S. Government Printing Office.

Promoting Communication in Older Adults

Objectives

1. Describe the dynamic nature of communication development throughout life.
2. Explain the changing communication needs and capabilities of older adults.
3. Describe several facilitative communication techniques.
4. Describe ways to improve the environment for and methods of communication.

INTRODUCTION

COMMUNICATION IN OLDER ADULTS WAS previously believed to remain essentially unchanged throughout one's life, barring severe hearing impairment or changes related to illness, such as stroke, dementia, or cancer. Now, however, observations reveal that communication development and change continues throughout the life span. Effective communication is essential to one's independence, compliance, socialization, and feelings of satisfaction and well-being. When communication fails, the needs of the older person remain unmet and the stress on others increases.

Communication breakdown threatens satisfying interpersonal relationships with family, friends, and professional caregivers. Broken relationships lead to social isolation and, eventually, further communication breakdown. Communication changes occur in essentially healthy older adults. Such changes are even more pronounced in those older adults who experience generalized slowing of motor functions and thought processes. Memory loss and depression experienced by some older adults also appear to be related to communication

Staab, AS and Hodges, LC: ESSENTIALS OF GERONTOLOGICAL NURSING,
© 1996 J. B. Lippincott Company

function. The longer people live, the more likely it will be that communication will change along with the biologic, psychological, and social changes that are a part of normal aging. Effective communication with the older adult, whether patient, spouse, family member, or colleague, is essential to successful gerontological nursing.

An increasing number of older adults are living longer than ever. Many enjoy essentially good health and active daily lives. The communicative competencies of these older adults are usually remarkably well preserved. Nevertheless, some changes in communication do occur. These changes are to communication like wrinkles, gray hair, and a slow gait are to the body; they are relatively minor changes in form and function.

NORMAL PHYSIOLOGIC CHANGES

In some very old adults, the cumulative effect of these relatively minor changes is sufficient to require adjustment by family and friends of their communication exchanges. Communication problems that might be experienced by the older adult include the following:

- Word retrieval difficulties. These problems are reflected in the inability to recall the name of someone one knows well, calling one's children by the wrong name, and not being able to think of specific familiar information.
- Decrease in fluency (generation) and flexibility (elements). *Fluency* is the ability to think of and name a large number of different elements within a class, for example, naming animals in a zoo or words beginning with F. *Flexibility* concerns the variability of the elements, for example, different ways to solve a problem or unique uses for an object. These characteristics are of the same nature, although not as severe, as those seen in patients with dementia.
- Overall slowing of rate. Generalized slowing is the most, and perhaps the only, common change seen in older adults. It is manifested by a slower rate of speaking, slower response times to the utterances of others, and slower retrieval of words and thoughts.
- Changes in voice quality. These changes reflect the physiologic and psychological status of the older patient. The fundamental frequency, or pitch, of the voices of older women becomes lower with increasing age; frequency stays the same or gets slightly higher in older men. Moreover, perturbation (disturbance of steadiness of pitch and volume) increases with age, resulting in tremor in the voices of older adults.
- Imprecise articulation. Imprecise articulation results from difficulty or errors in planning the production of speech sounds, slowness or poor coordination of the movement of the speech articulators (lips, tongue, lower jaw, soft palate, pharynx), or both planning and production problems. Speech sounds may sound jumbled or mumbled to the listener, making the speaker difficult to understand.
- Decrease in communication efficiency. A combination of the above changes results in decreased communication efficiency between speaker and listener. That is, the rate at which messages can be sent and received accurately is markedly reduced and uneven, making communication laborious.

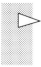

Clinical Pearl

Assessment: Telling a person something doesn't automatically mean that he or she received and understood the message as the speaker intended it.

ABNORMAL CHANGES

Gradual disturbances in communication, memory, judgment, and orientation may occur in some very old adults, even without specific dementing illness. The communication of older adults with cognitive changes is quite different from that of those who have had a stroke or other focal lesions of the central nervous system. In those older adults who have conditions associated with dementia, the changes are more apparent, although the patients are often minimally aware of their difficulties.

Communication problems associated with cognitive changes are usually worse late in the day, when the patient is tired and/or when the communication exchanges are frequent and complex. The most common communicative characteristics associated with cognitive change include those associated with comprehension, memory, and expression (Au & Bowles, 1991; Ripich, 1991). Some communication problems associated with cognitive changes are as follows:

- Poor recognition and comprehension. Declining ability to recognize familiar words and understand the meaning of spoken words is a distinguishing feature of communication in older adults who have early mild dementia.
- Semantic-episodic memory problems. These result in "empty speech." With this characteristic, older adults speak words clearly and construct utterances grammatically. The content, or meaning, however, of what they say is vague and limited.
- Decrease in fluency (generation) and flexibility (elements). These characteristics are of the same nature, although usually more severe, as those described above. Reductions in fluency and flexibility result in reduced verbal output, contrary to descriptions of talkativeness in older adults without cognitive impairment.
- Overuse of pronouns without clear referents. A patient might say, for example, "Someone came to see me today" instead of "Mr. Jones came to see me today." The use of pronouns without clear referents makes it difficult for the listener to understand about whom or what the older adult is talking. The lack of referent appears to be related to difficulty in recalling or retrieving the specific name of a person, place, or thing.
- Frequent repetition, triggered by visual presence of long-term recall. The decline in semantic-episodic memory for recent events causes the older adult to rely heavily on images or sounds within the immediate environment to prompt topics of conversation, comments, or questions. If the environment remains constant, older adults may begin to repeat utterances because they are unable to remember the content of recent remarks or episodes.
- Verbal disguise. Many patients engage in cover-up communicative behaviors to hide their difficulties. For example, they may overuse or misuse

stereotypic conversational remarks ("I haven't seen you in a long time" when they saw the person just a short time before). Sometimes patients use denial ("I don't feel well" or "I'm not hungry; I just ate") to avoid social situations with which they think they can't cope.

PSYCHOSOCIAL ISSUES

Certain communication problems often accompany depression. Loss, loneliness, generalized slowing of function, health problems, medication side effects, and changes in many other facets of living may contribute to feelings of depression and despair. Many causes of depression are reversible; others can be modified with medical treatment. Hence, obtaining a complete medical evaluation is essential for the depressed older person.

Depression in older adults often occurs with dementia, making differential diagnosis sometimes difficult. Unlike dementia, the onset of symptoms of depression is usually rapid and definitive. Some communicative problems that occur with depression are similar to those that occur with dementia, but others can help distinguish the two. Some communication problems associated with depression are as follows:

- Communicative withdrawal. Depressed patients make very little effort to participate. Whereas patients with dementia in early stages make every effort to prove communication and social adequacy, the depressed patient rejects social contact and refuses to try.
- Decrease in the quantity and complexity of communication. The most obvious manifestation of communicative and social withdrawal, aside from physical absence, is the paucity of communicative attempt and participation. Clinically, the depressed patient's performance is highly variable on tasks of comparable difficulty, whereas the patient with dementia's performance is predictable and consistent.
- Reliance on body language and other nonverbal signals. In the absence of verbal communication, some depressed patients rely heavily on nonverbal communication (body language and facial expressions) to convey feelings or needs.

NURSING ASSESSMENT

Although analysis of the patient's behavior is important, observation of interactions between the nurse and the patient is equally important. Communication breakdowns involve both partners, who must serve as senders of and responders to messages.

When verbal communication of older persons is inefficient or impaired, nonverbal behaviors such as yelling, pushing, or refusing to move often function as communication devices. These behaviors may be annoying to the nurse or caregiver, creating negative feelings toward the patient and increasing the stressfulness of caregiving. Examples of these patient behaviors and some of the intended messages are listed in Table 3-1. Family and caregivers should be instructed about such nonverbal behaviors and their possible meanings.

Awareness of the communicative messages underlying nonverbal behaviors helps caregivers to respond insightfully. However, unrecognized or misunderstood nonverbal behaviors are a major source of stress for gerontological

Table 3-1	NONVERBAL BEHAVIORS AND POSSIBLE MEANINGS	
	Behavior	Function/Message
	Ringing bell, yelling	I want immediate attention.
	Whining	I don't like my situation.
	Hitting, slapping, pushing, turning away, pretending to be asleep, refusing to move	I don't want to be dependent. I'm in control. I want to do things my way by myself in my own time.
	Collecting things that don't belong to him or her	I'm loved, I'm important. I can control myself and others.
	Moving things to new locations	I'm in control; my world makes sense to me.
	Taking things from other people	I'm connected to others; I can meet my own needs. I control others.
	Untying restraints on others	I'm in control of others.

nurses and other caregivers. Signs of stress are physical, such as unsteady gait, nausea, and headaches, and mental or emotional, such as unclear thinking, frustration, and absentmindedness.

NURSING DIAGNOSES

The nurse must be aware of changes in communication with the older adult. Changes must be made in the environment through use of facilitative strategies, activities, and communicative behavior. Some nursing diagnoses related to promoting communication in the older adult might include:

- Impaired Verbal Communication related to altered physical or mental processes
- Impaired Verbal Communication related to depression
- Noncompliance related to impaired comprehension of communication
- Impaired Social Interaction related to communication problems
- Social Isolation related to loss of communication competencies
- Self-Esteem Disturbance related to communication impairment
- Ineffective Individual Coping related to communication problems
- Diversional Activity Deficit related to impaired communication abilities and resulting social interaction problems
- Ineffective Family Coping: Compromised related to communication problems.

NURSING INTERVENTIONS

Communication involves at least two people who act in partnership to achieve balance of power by adjusting to each other, alternatively taking and relinquishing control. The strategy for balancing communicative partnership involves analysis of communication breakdown and adjustment of each partner to maximize the contribution of the other.

Although the communication of older adults may be inefficient and even disruptive and aberrant, the needs of nurses and other caregivers in the relationship should not be denied. The nurse and/or caregiver needs to feel cooperation, appreciation, approval, safety from personal injury, and the opportunity to improve the condition of those for whom he or she cares. Ineffective communication leads to conflict and stress for the patient, nurse, and caregiver. Minimizing conflict can be accomplished through facilitative communicative strategies. Careful attention should be given in the nursing plan to achieving effective and productive communication.

Consultation with a speech-language pathologist provides the gerontological nurse with a valuable resource in the analysis of communicative partnerships and development of strategies for balancing the communicative relationship. Individual speech-language therapy may be helpful, but perhaps even more important is the coaching function the speech-language pathologist can provide to nurses and other caregivers, including family members. Communication partnerships must be balanced sensitively and smoothly to avoid conflict triggered by fear, anger, guilt, and feelings of powerlessness, as depicted in the nursing care plan for an older adult experiencing communication problems.

COMMUNICATION STRATEGIES

When one partner is an older person whose communication patterns are changing, the gerontological nurse needs to facilitate communication by using strategies that encourage expressions of love, needs, and control and responding with expressions of comfort, security, love, and understanding. The nurse should accept expressions of anger, fear, distrust, and confusion as situation-directed rather than person-directed. When nurses give people choices, they are giving them power within their abilities. By communicating structure or routines, the nurse or caregiver is fostering feelings of security and trust in the patient.

There are many strategies for building trust and understanding between the nurse and older adult that will enhance the relationship. The following are several communication circumstances and examples of facilitative and nonfacilitative responses.

- Label the feelings the patient expresses. Labeling feelings encourages the expression of feelings by acknowledging and naming them. The patient may correct the responder with the name of another feeling if the label chosen wasn't exactly right.
  Example: The older person says to the nurse, "I'm not going to take that medicine. I've been taking it for 3 weeks and the pain isn't any better."
  Facilitative response: "It's discouraging when you take medicine and then you don't feel better." This names the feeling: discouragement.
  Nonfacilitative response: "Oh, yes, you have to take this medicine. The doctor ordered it." This response ignores the feeling and emphasizes the patient's lack of control.

- Acknowledge nonverbal messages as communication attempts.
  Example: The nurse walks into a patient's room to find the patient tearing and tugging at his clothing.
  Facilitative response: "You feel uncomfortable. You want me to pay attention to you. These clothes are bothering you."
  Nonfacilitative response: "I want you to stop that. You're going to ruin

your clothes if you keep tearing them." These statements may be true, but they don't acknowledge the behavior as a communicative attempt.

- Avoid "why" questions. Why questions suggest fault with the patient's judgment and cause defensive feelings and reactions.
  Example: The nurse encounters Mr. Jones, who is walking around public areas not wearing any clothes.
  Facilitative response: Redirect him physically, accompanied by "I'll help you get your clothes on so that you can be here with your friends. The bathroom is this way."
  Nonfacilitative response: "Mr. Jones, why are you in here without any clothes on?" Mr. Jones probably can't answer your question and he perceives your disapproval or alarm.

- Confirm or validate what a patient says first to clarify your understanding and then ask the patient to say more.
  Example: Mrs. Smith speaks in a soft voice and it is difficult to understand her. Only a few words are discernible—"daughter," "party," "this week."
  Facilitative responses: "Let me see if I understood what you said. You are telling me about your daughter and a party this week. Is that right?" "Tell me about the party."
  Nonfacilitative responses: "That's nice." This response is so general that it does not communicate that the message was really understood. "I like parties." This response changes the topic. "Your daughter is going to have a birthday party this week?" This response is expanded before understanding of the patient's message is confirmed.

- Take responsibility for breakdown in communication and attempts to correct it.
  Example: Mrs. Smith responded to your request with a response that sounded like several words, but only one word—"party"—was understandable.
  Facilitative responses: "I'm sorry. I didn't quite understand." "I'm having a hard time hearing you today. I'm going to listen more carefully." "It's difficult for me to understand you. Give me another chance."
  Nonfacilitative responses: "You're not talking very well today." "I can't understand you when you mumble." "Maybe you can tell me later."

- Tell the older adult what is needed in order to be understood, for example, to speak louder, face the partner, speak more slowly, or demonstrate by pointing or gesturing.
  Example: Mrs. Smith smiles, acknowledging the nurse's efforts and willingness to correct the breakdown.
  Facilitative responses: Move closer to the patient and take her hand. This communicates nonverbally that the nurse is trying to make a communication connection—a partnership. Then, "Tell me again. This time try to talk louder so I can hear you better." "Look at me when you talk; I can understand you better." "Say it slowly for me." "Tell me another way."
  Nonfacilitative responses: "What was that?" "Uh-huh." "Oh." "Party?"

- Relieve tension with humor directed toward self.

Example: The older person resists the nurse's help in getting out of bed in the morning, indicating that she doesn't want to get up.

Facilitative response: "Oh, some days it just seems like too much trouble to get up, doesn't it?" This statement acknowledges the message and the feeling. Then, "Some days my get-up-and-go feels like it already got up and went."

Nonfacilitative response: "C'mon you've got to get up. It's nearly 8 o'clock." "You have to get up to eat your breakfast." These statements ignore feelings and impose the nurse's choices and control on the patient.

PATIENT AND FAMILY EDUCATION

Family members, visitors and other communicative partners can also facilitate communication in meaningful, functional ways. The nurse may suggest facilitative communication activities, such as those included in the teaching box, to others who are communicative partners of older adults.

Patient Teaching Box
FACILITATIVE COMMUNICATION ACTIVITIES

Instruct patients and communicative partners in the following facilitative activities:

Partnership Balance	Facilitative Communication Activities
Caregiver is sender; older adult is receiver	Read aloud to the older adult. Short articles from the newspaper or magazines such as *Reader's Digest* will hold interest. Report the news in your own words.
Caregiver is receiver; older adult is sender	Encourage the older adult to reminisce; ask him or her to expand on events and ideas. Listen to life stories of older adults. Make a tape recording of their stories for their grandchildren or for children at a school. Write letters dictated by the older adult.
Joint routines	Eat a meal together. Talk about topics of mutual interest. Look at pictures together (albums of family or travel, slides, videos) and tell each other about them. Sing familiar songs together. Paint, draw, or color together; talk about resulting pictures. Visit while completing craft or handwork projects together. Plan an imaginary or real trip that the older adult would like to take. Discuss the itinerary, what to take, etc. Care for plants, animals, and others. Construct a care package as a gift. Plan a dinner party. Discuss the decorations, food, guest list, activities. Walk in a nearby park. Discuss the plant and animal life. Plant a flower bed or box. Discuss plans, materials, and tools needed, plant care. Go on errands together.

COMMUNICATION ENVIRONMENT

The communication of the older adult will be facilitated further by improving the environment for communication and the manner with which the nurse or other communicative partner speaks. This too helps balance the communication and relieve stress of both patient and partner.

- Enhance the communication environment. Reducing background noise from such sources as radio, television, other talkers, and dishes clattering reduces audible distraction and competition.
- Position yourself at eye level with your older partner, face to face. Reading facial expressions and lips facilitates hearing and comprehension.
- Lower the pitch of your voice. A lower pitch takes less effort and makes listening easier.
- Slow your rate of speech. A slower rate is relaxing and affords more time for the older adult to process and understand spoken messages.
- Reduce the complexity of your language. Complex, long sentences are more difficult to process. Be careful, however, not to "talk down" to the patient. Even if the behavior of the patient is childlike, convey respect and dignify conversation by speaking to older adults as adults.
- Actively listen. Undivided attention to the older adult's messages will reduce frequency of breakdowns and the need for repairs.

COMMUNICATION SYSTEMS

Some older adults may experience increasingly impaired communication related to progressive neurologic disease. Such patients in the absence of or with minimal cognitive impairment may benefit from augmented communication systems. These systems may include manual or gestural communication, letter or picture displays that the patient uses by pointing to symbols, and speech output devices activated by keyboards or switches of various kinds. The nurse should arrange for evaluation by a speech-language pathologist to determine the need for and appropriateness of augmented communication systems, make and facilitate implementation of recommendations, and provide training in the use of such systems.

 Clinical Pearl

Intervention: Effective communication is satisfying communication; it takes time, planning, and practice.

Communication with older adults can be a satisfying and rewarding experience. Changes require adaptation of the communication environment and the employment of facilitative strategies, activities, and communication behaviors by the gerontological nurse to balance communication partnerships. The nurse's role as a teacher of other communicative partners will extend and expand the opportunities for older adults for successful communication throughout their lives.

Nursing Care Plan

FOR AN OLDER ADULT WITH IMPAIRED VERBAL COMMUNICATION

Nursing Diagnosis: Impaired Verbal Communication: Impaired comprehension, use of language, and production of speech related to altered physical and/or mental processes.

Definition: Reduction in functional communication competence possibly resulting in social isolation, loss of independence, noncompliance, and inability to cope.

Assessment Findings:
1. Difficulty in comprehending speech communication due to mental confusion, memory loss, and slow mental processing
2. Difficulty in producing clear speech due to motor slowing, poor motor control of articulators, missing teeth
3. Difficulty in speaking loudly enough to be heard and understood by others due to general weakness, poor respiratory support
4. Confusion of thought and language
5. Reduction in communication attempts and participation
6. Excessive reliance on nonverbal communication

Nursing Interventions with Selected Rationales:
1. Identify behaviors that may signal communicative difficulty.
   Rationale: Behavior identification aids in assessment and patient teaching.
2. Acquire consultation with a speech-language pathologist to determine the need for individual evaluation and treatment.
   Rationale: A speech-language pathologist may assist with identifying appropriate strategies to improve communication and provide ongoing evaluation of the patient's progress.
3. Identify nonfacilitative responses of nurses and other communicative partners.
   Rationale: Nonfacilitative responses block communication and impair an already impaired state.
4. Initiate communication facilitation strategies by nurses and other caregivers.
   Rationale: Communication facilitation strategies build trust and enhance the relationship between the older adult and the nurse or caregiver.
5. Teach families about communication facilitation strategies and activities.
   Rationale: Family education allows for continuation of interventions to improve the patient's status.
6. Evaluate effectiveness through objective and subjective measures.
   Rationale: Evaluation allows for a determination of the patient's progress and readjustment of and institution of new strategies for improvement.

Desired Patient Outcomes/Discharge Criteria:
1. Patient will be able to communicate more effectively and efficiently.
2. Patient and family will experience improved quality of life.

REFERENCES

Au, R., & Bowles, N. (1991). Memory influences on language in normal aging. In D. Ripich (Ed.), *Handbook of geriatric communication disorders.* Austin, TX: PRO-ED.

Ripich, D. (1991). Language and communication in dementia. In E. Ripich (Ed.), *Handbook of geriatric communication disorders.* Austin, TX: PRO-ED.

BIBLIOGRAPHY

Hoffman, S. B., & Platt, C. A. (1990). *Comforting the confused: Strategies for managing dementia.* Owings Mills, MD: National Health Publishing.

Nussbaum, J. F., Thompson, T., & Robinson, J. D. (1989). *Communication and aging.* New York: Harper and Row.

Problems in Physiologic Functioning

4

Promoting Physical Functioning in the Older Adult

Objectives

1. Discuss the role of physical functioning in the promotion of health of the older adult.
2. Describe musculoskeletal changes that may exert major influences in the physical functioning of the older adult.
3. Describe several functional parameters used to accurately assess the older adult's physical functioning.
4. Compare and contrast the nursing interventions used in promoting exercise and physical functioning in community-based and institutionalized older adults.
5. Discuss the concept of "safe exercise."
6. Discuss the role of rest, relaxation, and sleep in promoting well-being in the older adult.
7. Describe several nursing interventions/strategies used to promote rest, relaxation, and sleep in institutionalized and community-based older adults.

INTRODUCTION

PHYSICAL FUNCTIONING IN THE OLDER ADULT requires the ability to integrate fine and gross motor skills needed to perform self-care activities and activities of daily living, such as toileting, feeding, dressing, grooming, bathing, and ambulation. Ability to perform these skills is crucial to maintaining physical independence and self-determination and promoting overall health status and general well-being. As with all adults, especially the older adult, physical functioning is maintained by constant use. Lack of physical functioning can cause a number of movement problems, including pain, stiffness, weakness, and deformity, which not only limit movement and functional abilities, but also may cause falls. Consequently, the lack of physical functioning is the leading cause of institutionalization of the older adult. Accurate assessment of the older adult's musculoskeletal function is essential in preventing deconditioning and helping the older adult develop the capacity for independent motor activity.

NORMAL PHYSIOLOGIC CHANGES

In the process of normal aging, muscles, bones, and articulating surfaces undergo changes resulting in decreased muscle mass, strength, coordination, and alterations in cartilage. Reduced tissue elasticity, caused by increased muscle collagen, results in joint and muscle stiffness. Muscle strength and movement are decreased, especially in the arm and leg muscles. Oxygen and nutrient perfusion to the muscles is reduced, resulting in decreased spread of muscle contraction, leading to slower movements.

Bone mass and mineral absorption, such as calcium absorption, are reduced. Bone mass decreases progressively, characterized by gradual resorption of the internal surface of long and flat bones and a slower accretion of new bone on the outside surface. Consequently, the long bones are externally enlarged but internally hollowed out. The vertebral end plates are thinned, and the skull becomes slightly enlarged. There is a loss of trabeculae, resulting in weaker bone. Increased flexion occurs at the wrist, hips, and knees, and joint movements are limited because of the deterioration of the cartilage surface of the joints. As the cartilage is eroded, the bone makes direct contact with bone, resulting in arthritis with pain, a crackling sound (crepitation) on movement, and/or a lack of movement. A loss of water from the cartilage results in narrowing of intervertebral discs and contributes to loss of height. Slight flexion of the head, neck, hips, and knees affects gait and results in slower, shortened, wider steps.

The result of these overall changes is an older person whose posture and appearance looks more curved and bent, who perhaps appears shorter, and whose gait is slower with shortened and widened steps. The individual also experiences reduced overall mobility, flexibility, and stability in movements. These changes not only limit movement and functional abilities in some, but also can contribute to falls, which can lead to other more serious injuries, such as broken bones or head injuries.

Over time, stress, a common human experience, can seriously damage a person's overall well-being. As in other age groups, the older adult experiences and adjusts to stress in a variety of ways. Several of the ways older adults reduce stress and fatigue is by resting and relaxing. Rest and relaxation have been shown to increase feelings of energy, vitality, and self-control (Pender, 1987). In the older adult, disturbances in rest and relaxation may cause damage in biochemical processes within the brain and can lead to progressive disorientation of the mind and of behavioral activities of the central nervous system, causing multiple psychological and physical problems (Byyny & Speroff, 1991; Chenitz, 1991; Ebersole & Hess, 1990; Eliopoulos, 1992).

ABNORMAL PHYSIOLOGIC CHANGES

Various abnormal changes result in a number of physical disorders that can affect the older adult's physical functioning. Problems related to the musculoskeletal system affect the older adult's mobility. Cardiac and pulmonary disorders can affect the older adult's endurance level, thereby affecting his or her ability to perform activities of daily living. A problem affecting any body system ultimately can affect the older adult's ability to function.

PSYCHOSOCIAL CHANGES

The inability to physically function has a serious effect on psychological functioning and well-being. Inability to perform basic self-care activities and activities of daily living leads to loss of independence and feelings of low self-esteem and hopelessness in older adults. Low morale and depression have been found to be prevalent in those with declining physical functioning. However, most older adults who exercise report that they feel better. Exercise improves body functioning and one's body image, which in turn affects morale. Exercise is advocated as one method of preventing and/or reducing stress. Exercise enhances movement and improves self-confidence, self-concept, and overall well-being (Knortz, 1991; Larson & Bruce, 1987).

NURSING ASSESSMENT

For the older adult, assessment of physical functioning must include both quality and quantity of movement. The quality component addresses the older person's actual ability to ambulate, the characteristics of gait, the ability to rise from a chair and toilet, and the ability to climb stairs. The quantity component of the assessment considers the length of time the person is able to ambulate without discomfort or fatigue.

HISTORY AND PHYSICAL EXAMINATION

Using appropriate questions during the nursing history and through physical examination techniques, the nurse should assess the function of all limbs for pain, contractures, spasms, arthritis, weakness, and paralysis. Additionally, the nurse should assess the hand dominance and the degree of joint motion, flexion, and extension of fingers, wrists, and elbows (Eliopoulos, 1992). A baseline assessment on physical functioning should also include the following:

- How much time is spent standing, sitting, and walking
- How far the older adult walks
- Whether assistive devices are used

There are several reliable and valid measurement scales for assessing overall physical function in the older adult, including the Barthel Index (Appendix 4-1, Mahoney & Barthel 1965) and the PULSES Profile (Appendix 4-2, Moskowitz, 1985.) The Barthel Index identifies degrees of physical independence in self care abilities such as feeding and dressing, and mobility abilities such as distance walking, climbing stairs, or propelling a wheelchair. The Barthel Index uses direct observation to evaluate the older person's level of functioning. Items are individually weighted and the maximum score of 100 indicates independence and a score of 40 or less indicates dependence.

The PULSES profile evaluates functioning in six categories: physical condition, upper extremities, lower extremities, sensory function, excretory functions, and social and mental status. Each category is scored on a scale of 1 (no gross abnormalities) to 4 (severe abnormalities or variations)—the higher the score, the more impaired the physical functioning. The PULSES profile and Barthel index are both used to augment the nursing process and complement clinical judgment.

To prevent the sequela of rest and relaxation deprivation, the nurse should assess for any correlating stressors, such as physical discomfort (pain), situational stress (personal/family), and environmental changes (shift changes), as well as correlating medical problems/diagnoses, including metabolic disorders, neuromuscular disorders, depression, and cardiovascular disease.

For the older adult in an institutional setting, the natural sleep-wake pattern may not coincide with the institution's schedule. Assessment of rest and relaxation patterns should include usual rest and relaxation patterns, relaxation and meditation patterns, distribution of rest patterns throughout the day, use of sleep aids, and frequency and length of naps (Pender, 1987).

RISK FACTORS

During assessment, the nurse must be aware of certain risk factors that may affect the older adult's ability to function. Older adults adjust to alterations in musculoskeletal functioning by taking a longer time to complete a task. With some persons, muscular weakness along with arthritic changes and joint stiffness may make learning to use canes, crutches, and walkers a little more difficult. The older adult is more easily awakened, takes longer to fall asleep, awakens often during the night, and spends more time lying in bed awake. Consequently, an older adult deprived of rest and relaxation may become depressed, sensitive to pain, irritable, apathetic, disoriented, and confused.

DIAGNOSTIC TESTS

As with any problem, appropriate diagnostic tests including blood tests, scans, and X-rays should be performed to rule out any pathologic problems, such as metabolic disorders, neuromuscular disorders, cardiovascular disease, and depression. These should be corrected if at all possible.

NURSING DIAGNOSES

Potential nursing diagnoses for a patient with alterations in physical functioning may include the following:

- Activity Intolerance related to muscle weakness
- Diversional Activity Deficit related to isolation
- Health Seeking Behaviors related to impaired mobility
- Impaired Physical Mobility related to degenerative changes

NURSING INTERVENTIONS

Optimal physical functioning is a survival need in the older adult. Physical functioning increases a general sense of well-being, aids recovery from some illnesses, and prolongs psychological and physical independence in the older adult. The ability to function physically allows for control over activities of daily living and enhances self-care ability. Therefore, nursing interventions are focused on promoting and maintaining optimal physical functioning in older adults.

EXERCISE

One modifiable aspect of increasing physical endurance, strength, and optimal functioning is exercise (Marsiglio & Holm, 1988; O'Brien & Vertinsky, 1990; Topp, 1991). Exercise is the key to consumption of body fat, reduction of blood pressure, reduction of blood sugar, and enhancement of musculoskeletal strength. Exercise can help control weight, blood pressure, and blood sugar in conditions of obesity, hypertension, and diabetes, respectively, and can improve flexibility and range of motion in those who have arthritis. It increases blood flow and keeps tissues healthy. For minimal loss of muscular strength, it is imperative that all older adults exercise, even those who are wheelchair bound and bedridden.

Positive benefits of exercise can be achieved from mild exercise. Engaging in light to moderate physical activity for at least 30 minutes a day will benefit physical functioning in the older adult, especially in those who have never exercised regularly. For example, low-impact aerobics has been found to be successful in improving the physical conditioning of sedentary older women.

Some older adults may avoid exercise, perhaps because they are unaware of its potential benefits. They may also harbor misconceptions about exercise, for example, that it will increase appetite, that it is no longer necessary or safe, and that once retired they should rest. Exercise for the older adult should be planned with an outcome to improve the older adult's functional status. Tailoring exercise to an individual's level of ability and preferences can help motivate the older person to become more active. In addition to walking, classes in water walking, dancing, martial arts, weight training, bowling, or dance clubs may also appeal to a variety of preferences for safe exercises within the older adult population (see Patient Teaching Box 4-1).

For those adults who cannot walk, wheelchair exercises should be implemented. Classes for wheelchair exercises should be separated from other exercise classes. This allows for older adults to be grouped by ability and lessens embarrassment by their limitations and feelings of being out of place. Wheelchair exercises accompanied by music, to which the older adult can relate, such as big band or ethnic music, adds to the fun and satisfaction important to health-promoting exercise programs.

Clinical Pearl

Intervention: Whenever possible, it is helpful to relate exercises to the functions that older adults need to perform, such as lifting, bending, shopping, and bathing.

Patient Teaching Box 4-1
SAFE EXERCISE

When instructing older patients how to exercise safely, include the following points:

- Consult with the health care provider (physician or nurse practitioner) before undertaking any physical program.
- Engage in an exercise program of low to moderate activity from 20 to 30 minutes at least three times a week.
- Sweating and breathing a little harder than normal are not unusual or necessarily harmful reactions to exercise.
- Building up to your goals gradually and warming up and cooling down will minimize any adverse reactions.
- Be alert to the signs and symptoms of exertion in yourself and others with whom you walk or exercise: dizziness; extreme shortness of breath or labored breathing; sore, painful muscles; irregular or fluttering heartbeat; nausea; chest pains; feeling very hot; low abdominal pain; extremely heavy perspiration; blue lips or fingers; and lack of coordination.
- If you have any of these symptoms, slow down.
- If symptoms persist, stop walking and rest.
- If you feel dizzy or nauseous, lower your head or lie down.
- If the symptoms do not go away, get immediate medical attention.

PATIENT EDUCATION

Range of motion and in-bed exercises (quadriceps sets, gluteal sets, and straight leg raising) should be taught. Some important considerations in joint range-of-motion exercises are as follows:

- Extremities are supported and held at the joints.
- All movements are done slowly and smoothly and without discomfort to the older adult.
- A joint should not be moved beyond its free range of motion; movement should be stopped if there is pain.
- When holding an extremity, avoid grasping the muscle unless absolutely necessary, as with some older adults with arthritis.

Nurses also play a major role in teaching older adults about safe exercise. Regardless of the type of exercise, the older adult needs to be cautioned about tailoring the exercise to his or her ability level.

Walking, an example of a safe form of exercise, is usually the preferred form of exercise for the older adult. Walking provides for simple stretching, range of motion, and deep breathing without aerobics. For the physically independent older adult, walking provides for maximal health benefits (see Patient Teaching Box 4-2).

For the physically impaired, in addition to range of motion and in-bed exercises, teaching should include transfer activities such as moving the patient from bed to chair or stretcher, teaching walking (gait training) and use of adaptive devices such as a cane or walker. Transfer training, gait training and use of adaptive devices should be referred to the physical and occupational therapist, respectively. For the physically impaired older adult living at home, rather than being sedentary, assisting with household chores not only enhances good functioning of their body systems but also promotes a sense of

Patient Teaching Box 4-2
GUIDELINES FOR WALKING

To get the most benefit from walking, the following guidelines should be included:
• Walk naturally.
• Let arms hang loosely at sides.
• Wear good, comfortable shoes that fit well and give feet good support. Break in walking shoes and experiment with the most comfortable weight of socks to avoid any problems with feet.
• Hands, knees, and ankles should be relaxed.
• Heels should strike the surface first.
• Use heel-to-toe rolling motion.
• Breathe naturally.
• Find a friend to walk with for at least 30 minutes daily.
• Map out a route that's interesting and fits goals for distance or time.

self worth by providing them an opportunity to be productive. Therefore, teaching wellness to the caregivers of the physically impaired older adult should stress the importance of physical activity for them.

REST, RELAXATION, AND STRESS REDUCTION

Although older persons tend to sleep fewer hours at night than when they were younger, they continue to need rest. Nurses must plan for periods of decreased activity for rejuvenation. For example, daily activities need to be planned to accommodate an afternoon nap. Promoting relaxation and rest periods during the day should be a common nursing intervention for the older adult. Patient Teaching Box 4-3 demonstrates the sequence for progressive relaxation. Nursing interventions that can assist the hospitalized older adult to achieve rest and relaxation include comfort measures, such as back rubs, oral hygiene, soft music, and relaxation tapes, and environmental measures, such as decreased noise (voices, alarms), closed doors, pulled curtains, and lowered lights or night-lights. Some general measures for community-based older adults include increasing daytime activities and exercise and teaching techniques to enhance rest and relaxation. Relaxation techniques most helpful in the older adult in-

Patient Teaching Box 4-3
PROGRESSIVE RELAXATION

Older adults need to establish a specific time for relaxing and to proceed in the following sequence:
• Loosen tight clothes.
• Remove glasses and shoes, if applicable.
• Assume comfortable position in a chair.
• Breathe slowly and deeply.
• Tighten muscle groups one at a time; tighten feet for 5 seconds and relax muscles. Repeat for calves, and move up the body to the top of the head, concentrating on one muscle group at a time.

clude guided imagery, self-induced relaxation, meditation, prayer, and reading the Bible. In guided imagery, the older adult uses imagination to visualize a place where he or she feels relaxed. It is important for the nurse to emphasize that the primary focus should be on feelings and sensations rather than on details. Self-induced relaxation uses breathing and muscle relaxation to provide a feeling of peacefulness or serenity. Meditation, prayer, and reading the Bible are other ways in which older adults can manage stress and achieve relaxation.

REFERENCES

Byyny, R. L., & Speroff, L. (1991). *A clinical guide for the care of older women.* Baltimore: Williams & Wilkins.

Chenitz, C. W. (Ed.). (1991). *Clinical gerontological nursing: A guide to advanced practice.* Philadelphia: W.B. Saunders.

Ebersole, P., & Hess, P. (1990). *Toward healthy aging: Human needs and nursing response* (3rd ed.). St. Louis: Mosby.

Eliopoulos, C. (1992). *Gerontological nursing* (2nd ed.). Philadelphia: Lippincott.

Knortz, K. (Ed.). (1991). *Topics in Geriatric Rehabilitation, 6*(4), 1–70.

Larson, E. B., & Bruce, R. A. (1987). Health benefits of exercise in an aging society, *Archives of Internal Medicine, 147,* 353–356.

Mahoney, F. I. & Barthel, D. W. (1965). Functional evaluation: The Barthel Index. *Maryland State Medical Journal,* 14–65.

Marsiglio, A., & Holm, K. (1988). Physical conditioning in the aging adult. *Nurse Practitioner, 13*(9), 33–41.

Moskowitz, E. (1985). PULSES profile in retrospect. *Archives of Physical Rehabilitation, 66,* 648.

O'Brien, S. J., & Vertinsky, P. A. (1990). Elderly women, exercise and healthy aging. *Journal of Women and Aging, 2*(3), 41–65.

Pender, N. J. (1987). *Health promotion in nursing practice* (2nd ed.). Norwalk, CT: Appleton & Lange.

Topp, R. (1991). Development of an exercise program for older adults: Pre-exercise testing, exercise prescription and program maintenance. *Nursing Practitioner, 16*(10), 16–28.

BIBLIOGRAPHY

Clark, M. J. (1992). *Nursing in the community.* Norwalk, CT: Appleton-Century-Crofts.

Heckheimer, E. F. (1989). *Health promotion of the elderly in the community.* Philadelphia: W. B. Saunders.

Thomas, G. S., & Rutledge, J. H. (1986). Fitness and exercise for the elderly. In K. Dychtwald (Ed.), *Wellness and health promotion for the elderly* (pp. 165–178).

Weiler, P. G. (1986). Education and training in wellness for health care providers. In K. Dychtwald (Ed.), *Wellness and health promotion for the elderly* (pp. 71–86).

APPENDIX 4-1
The Barthel Index

The Barthel Index uses direct observation to evaluate an older person's level of functioning. Specific criteria are scored numerically. A total score of 100 indicates that the older adult is completely independent.

Note: A score of zero is given when the patient cannot meet the defined criterion.

1. Feeding
   - 10 Independent. The patient can feed himself a meal from a tray or table when someone puts the food within his reach. He must put on an assistive device if this is needed, cut up the food, use salt and pepper, spread butter, etc. He must accomplish this in a reasonable time.
   - 5 Some help is necessary (when cutting up food, etc., as listed above).
2. Moving from wheelchair to bed and return
   - 15 Independent in all phases of this activity. Patient can safely approach the bed in his

wheelchair, lock brakes, lift footrests, move safely to bed, lie down, come to a sitting position on the side of the bed, change the position of the wheelchair, if necessary, to transfer back into it safely, and return to the wheelchair.

- 10 Either some minimal help is needed in some step of this activity or the patient needs to be reminded or supervised for safety of one or more parts of this activity.
- 5 Patient can come to a sitting position without the help of a second person but needs to be lifted out of bed, or if he transfers with a great deal of help.

3. Doing personal toilet
   - 5 Patient can wash hands and face, comb hair, clean teeth, and shave. He may use any kind of razor but must put in blade or plug in razor without help as well as get it from drawer or cabinet. Female patients must put on own make-up, if used, but need not braid or style hair.

4. Getting on and off toilet
   - 10 Patient is able to get on and off toilet, fasten and unfasten clothes, prevent soiling of clothes, and use toilet paper without help. He may use a wall bar or other stable object of support if needed. If it is necessary to use a bed pan instead of a toilet, he must be able to place it on a chair, empty it, and clean it.
   - 5 Patient needs help because of imblance or in handling clothes or in using toilet paper.

5. Bathing self
   - 5 Patient may use a bathtub, a shower, or take a complete sponge bath. He must be able to do all the steps involved in whichever method is employed without another person being present.

6. Walking on a level surface.
   - 15 Patient can walk at least 50 yards without help or supervision. He may wear braces or prostheses and use crutches, canes, or a walkerette but not a rolling walker. He must be able to lock and unlock braces if used, assume the standing position and sit down, get the necessary mechanical aides into position for use, and dispose of them when he sits. (Putting on and taking off braces is scored under dressing.)
   - 10 Patient needs help or supervision in any of the above but can walk at least 50 yards with a little help.

6a. Propelling a wheelchair
   - 5 If a patient cannot ambulate but can propel a wheelchair independently. He must be able to go around corners, turn around, maneuver the chair to a table, bed, toilet, etc. He must be able to push a chair at least 50 yards. Do not score this item if the patient gets score for walking.

7. Ascending and descending stairs
   - 10 Patient is able to go up and down a flight of stairs safely without help or supervision. He may and should use handrails, canes, or crutches when needed. He must be able to carry canes or crutches as he ascends or descends stairs.
   - 5 Patient needs help with or supervision of any one of the above items.

8. Dressing and undressing
   - 10 Patient is able to put on and remove and fasten all clothing, and tie shoe laces (unless it is necessary to use adaptations for this). The activity includes putting on and removing and fastening corset or braces when these are prescribed. Such special clothing as suspenders, loafer shoes, dresses that open down the front may be used when necessary.
   - 5 Patient needs help in putting on and removing or fastening any clothing. He must do at least half the work himself. He must accomplish this in a reasonable time.

Women need not be scored on use of a brassiere or girdle unless these are prescribed garments.

9. Continence of bowels
   - 10 Patient is able to control his bowels and have no accidents. He can use a suppository or take an enema when necessary (as for spinal cord injury patients who have had bowel training).
   - 5 Patient needs help in using a suppository or taking an enema or has occasional accidents.

10. Controlling bladder
   - 10 Patient is able to control his bladder day and night. Spinal cord injury patients who wear an external device and leg bag must put them on independently, clean and empty bag, and stay dry day and night.
   - 5 Patient has occasional accidents or cannot wait for the bed pan or get to the toilet in time or needs help with an external device.

Reproduced from Mahoney FI, Barthel DW. Functional evaluation: the Barthel Index. Maryland State Med J 1965:14–65. With permission.

APPENDIX 4-2
PULSES Evaluation Guide

Six categories of functioning are evaluated. Each category is scored on a scale of 1 (no gross abnormalities) to 4 (severe abnormalities or variations). The higher the score, the more impaired the physical functioning.

	P	U	L	S	E	S
	Physical Condition cardiovascular pulmonary and other visceral disorders	Upper Extremities shoulder girdles, cervical and upper dorsal spine	Lower Extremities pelvis, lower dorsal and lumbosacral spine	Sensory Function vision hearing speech	Excretory Functions bowel and bladder	Social and Mental Status emotional and psychiatric disorders
Normal	1 Health maintenance	1 Complete function	1 Complete function	1 Complete function	1 Continent	1 Compatible with age
Mild	2 Occasional medical supervision	2 No assistance required	2 Fully ambulatory despite some loss of function	2 No appreciable functional impairment	2 Occasional stress incontinence or nocturia	2 No supervision required
Moderately Severe	3 Frequent medical supervision	3 Some assistance necessary	3 Limited ambulation	3 Appreciable bilateral loss or complete unilateral loss of vision or hearing. Incomplete aphasia	3 Periodic incontinence or retention	3 Some supervision necessary
Severe	4 Total care Bed or chair confined	4 Nursing care	4 Confined to wheelchair or bed	4 Total blindness Total deafness Global aphasia or aphonia	4 Total incontinence or retention (including catheter and colostomy)	4 Complete care in psychiatric facility

*Adapted from Moskowitz E. PULSES Profile in retrospect. Arch Phys Rehabil 1985;66:648.

5

Problems With Mobility

Objectives

1. Describe the physiologic changes of aging associated with mobility problems.
2. Identify steps in the nursing assessment of an older adult with a mobility problem.
3. Discuss the roles and responsibilities of the physical therapist/occupational therapist in conjunction with the nurse in the care of the older adult.
4. Identify nursing diagnoses related to problems with mobility in the older adult.
5. Design nursing interventions for the older adult with a mobility problem.
6. Design a nursing care plan for the older adult with a mobility problem.

INTRODUCTION

MOBILITY PROBLEMS IN THE OLDER adult can have serious and far-reaching physical and psychological effects. The ability to move about and care for one's self can mean the difference between independence and dependence and remaining at home or being institutionalized. Mobility not only affects the musculoskeletal system but also nutrition, elimination, circulation, and skin integrity. Mobility problems can cause older adults to lose confidence in their abilities and to feel "old." Restoring mobility and encouraging older adults to use their existing abilities are vital. An assessment of the older adult's functional abilities, a knowledge of the aging process, and an individualized plan of care are essential to attaining these goals. The nurse can provide teaching, support and referrals for the patient and family. Proper intervention can increase independence and activity and decrease social isolation.

NORMAL PHYSIOLOGIC CHANGES

Due to normal physiologic changes and alterations in health, the older adult is at high risk for mobility problems. Through careful observation, planning, and intervention, the older adult can maintain mobility and can lead an independent life.

Staab, AS and Hodges, LC: ESSENTIALS OF GERONTOLOGICAL NURSING,
© 1996 J. B. Lippincott Company

As a person ages, the number of muscle fibers generally decreases and become smaller (atrophy) and weaker. Muscle strength, tone, and endurance decrease. Ligaments and tendons stiffen with age, decreasing joint flexibility and range of motion, especially in the knees, hips, and spine. The synovium in joints loses elasticity, resulting in more wear and tear on articular surfaces. Decreased activity levels and disuse tend to exacerbate these changes. There is also a decrease in the density of bones (osteoporosis), which weakens them.

Motor neurons decrease, causing a slower reaction time and diminished coordination and balance. All of these changes can result in decreased endurance and make the older adult more vulnerable to injury. For example, the force of stepping off a sidewalk curb may be enough to cause a hip fracture.

 ▷ *Clinical Pearl*

Intervention: Encourage the older adult to use ramps in public buildings and at street corners rather than risk the stress of stepping and stair-climbing–like motions.

Thinning intervertebral disks and shortening vertebrae of the spine result in a loss of height, which decreases by approximately 1.2 cm for every 20 years of life. The thoracic and cervical curves of the spine become more pronounced, leading to a stooped posture with head and neck thrust forward and hips and knees slightly flexed. As a result of these anatomic changes, the stance of the older adult becomes wider, movement is cautious and deliberate, and the height of each step is decreased. These changes may cause difficulty with walking and maintaining balance.

ABNORMAL PHYSIOLOGIC CHANGES

Aging persons experience declines in mobility that are only partially due to the aging process. Changes in joint structure, muscle weakness and stiffness, and mental status as well as other physical changes may result in such problems as osteoarthritis, gait disturbances, and falls.

OSTEOARTHRITIS

The presence of worn and inflamed joints in the older adult, as in osteoarthritis and degenerative joint disease, is common. It is estimated that at least 90% of the population older than age 60 have some degree of osteoarthritis (Bates, 1991). The cartilage cushion in the joints becomes frayed and begins to wear away, allowing the ends of the bones to touch. Osteoarthritis usually occurs in weight-bearing points, and the overweight older person compounds the stress placed on these already compromised joints. This can result in the pain and stiffness associated with osteoarthritis. These symptoms cause the older adult to move these joints less often, resulting in further muscle weakness and stiffness. Joints most affected are the hips, knees, spine, and distal fingers. Surgical replacement of the hip and knees is a common procedure used when the older adult has severe restriction of joint movement or severe pain. Total joint replacement or arthroplasty is the surgery of choice because of the high success rate in restoring mobility and joint comfort with minimal healing time. Discharge planning should begin at or before admission in older adults to coordinate multiple services associated with rehabilitation and home care.

GAIT DISTURBANCE

Gait disturbance is a major cause of mobility problems among the older adult population and may be one of the primary reasons for an older adult's being institutionalized. The cause of a gait disturbance is multifactorial and may include musculoskeletal disorders, nervous system disorders, anxiety, medications, visual impairment, and normal physical changes. Figure 5-1 depicts some gait disturbances. Gait disturbance, a major cause of falls among older adults, may result in injury, disability, decreased mobility, and decreased confidence in abilities.

FALLS

Falls may be multifactorial in origin. Common causes are physical problems, environmental factors, and medications (see Display 5-1). The hospitalized older adult is at great risk of falling. The average age of a patient at risk to fall in the hospital is 65 years (Tieaskie, 1989). These patients usually have a cardiovascular problem and are awake and oriented when they fall.

PSYCHOSOCIAL ISSUES

Mobility is considered a prerequisite to independence. The inability to move about in the environment requires the presence of others to meet basic needs, such as daily hygiene and toileting. As functional dependency increases, the immobile older adult often experiences loss of self-esteem, a change in self-concept, hopelessness, powerlessness, and depression. The inability to handle self-care tasks attributed to immobility often requires a family member or caregiver to assume new responsibilities involving intimate personal care. This may generate feelings of conflict and role reversal for the caregiver. The nurse should provide support to the caregiver as he or she works through feelings resulting from demands of the immobile person. Special efforts may be needed to include the immobile older adult in social situations.

NURSING ASSESSMENT

Detection of mobility problems requires astute observation and assessment skills by the nurse. Many problems with mobility are attributed to old age and are not reported by patients or family unless specifically asked. Some patients will try to hide mobility problems for fear of being labeled "unsafe" and possibly institutionalized. The key to mobility problems is the ability to function.

HISTORY AND INTERVIEW

The nurse needs to obtain reliable and valid information concerning a patient's functional abilities. Use the following questions as a guide when assessing the older adult's functional abilities.

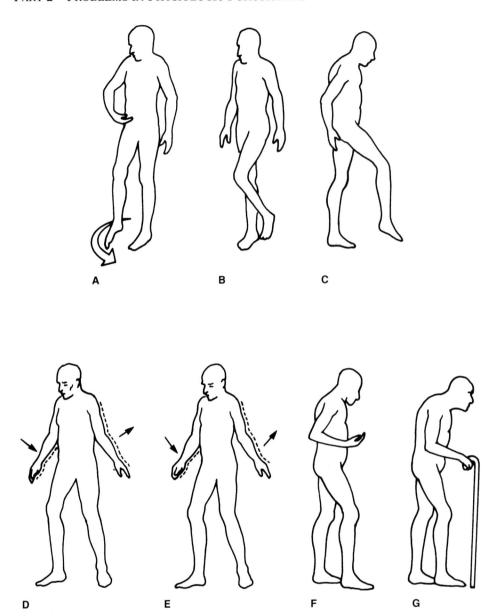

Figure 5-1. (A) Spastic hemiparesis: Unilateral foot drop and foot dragging; leg circumducted; arm immobile and close to side of body with joints flexed. **(B)** Scissors: Slow, short steps; gait stiff, legs cross while stepping. **(C)** Steppage (foot slapping): Wide-based with feet dragging or lifted high; knees flexed, feet down to floor with slapping motion; no staggering or weaving. **(D)** Sensory ataxia: Unsteady, wide-based; feet thrown forward and outward on heels and then toes with a double tapping sound, watches ground while walking, cannot stand steadily with eyes closed. **(E)** Cerebellar ataxia: Staggering, unsteady, wide-based, cannot stand steadily with eyes open or closed. **(F)** Parkinsonian: Trunk forward, hips and knees slightly flexed, short shuffling steps; without arm swinging while stepping. **(G)** Gait of old age: Diminished speed, balance, and grace; short, uncertain steps; possible knee and hip flexion.

Display 5-1
CAUSES OF FALLS IN THE OLDER ADULT

Physical Problems

Epilepsy
Syncope
Transient ischemic attack/
    cerebrovascular accident (stroke)
Postural hypotension   usually loss of consciousness
Hypoglycemia
Cardiac arrhythmias
Hypocalcemia
Hyperventilation

Vertigo (acute labyrinthitis or Meniere's disease)
Parkinson's disease
Arthritis (osteo or rheumatoid)
Dementia (acute or Alzheimer's)
Amputation
Decreased sensation in feet and legs
Decreased circulation in feet and legs
Impaired vision
Impaired hearing
Incontinence
Foot problems (corns, bunions, deformities)
Gait disturbances
Advanced age
Delayed reaction time

Environmental Factors

Trailing wires or extension cords
Loose rugs
Lack of stair railings
Slick or wet floor
Uneven flooring
Inadequate lighting
Cluttered environment
Lack of bath rails
Slippery tub/shower floors

In the past month, have you had any difficulties with the following:

- Turning in bed?
- Getting out of bed?
- Standing up?
- Sitting down?
- Getting on or off the toilet?
- Getting in or out of the tub/shower?
- Getting around the house?
- Preparing your meals?
- Cleaning your house?
- Dressing yourself?

- Doing your laundry?
- Getting up or down steps?
- Driving or using public transportation?
- Doing errands (grocery store, drugstore)?
- Attending any social functions (church, club)?

Any positive answers need to be explored as to frequency of occurrence, what or how much difficulty was involved, possible causes of the difficulty, and possible solutions. This information provides an excellent baseline for recognizing future changes.

Clinical Pearl

Assessment: Do not assume that mobility problems and/or muscle or joint pain are an inevitable sign of old age. Pursue these complaints for a possible underlying disease process.

RISK FACTORS

Nursing assessment should include evaluating the person for the presence of risk factors for falls. The risk of falls is increased with certain categories of drugs, including hypnotics, antipsychotics, tricyclic antidepressants, and some anticonvulsant agents. Vestibulotoxic drugs, such as salicylates, can cause tinnitus and imbalance. A useful assessment tool for evaluating fall potential and a checklist to help prevent falls in the hospitalized older adult are provided in Displays 5-2 and 5-3.

PHYSICAL EXAMINATION

After assessing the patient's functional abilities, the nurse needs to evaluate general areas of the musculoskeletal system. This requires inspection and palpation of the joints and surrounding tissues. The nurse should note any of the following:

- Swelling in or around a joint
- Tenderness in or around a joint
- Redness of the skin overlying a joint
- Increased heat in or around a joint
- Crepitation (a feeling or sound of crunching when the joint is moved)
- Symmetry of changes—compare each side of the body

After assessing the joints and surrounding tissues, the nurse needs to assess the patient's range of motion. It is important to compare one side of the body with the other. A general assessment of range of motion can be done visually, but the most accurate method of assessing progress and detecting early, slight changes in range of motion is the use of the goniometer. This is a measuring tool that is used more by the physical therapist but is useful for the nurse as well. The arms of the goniometer are placed parallel with the axis of each bone that makes up the joint. Display 5-4 provides the normal range-of-motion

Display 5-2

EVALUATING FALL POTENTIAL IN OLDER ADULTS

Diagnosis:
Primary:
Secondary: **Age:**

I. Patient history of falls
___ Fall prior to admission
___ Fall during previous admission
___ Fall during this admission

II. Physical status
___ Dizziness
___ Weakness
___ Vision impaired
___ Paresis (partial or complete paralysis)
___ Altered gait and/or need for ambulatory device
___ Joint difficulties
___ Seizure disorder
___ Syncope/transient ischemic attacks

III. Mental status
___ Confusion (illogical thinking)
___ Impaired memory or judgment
___ Disoriented to persons, places, things, or times
___ Lack of familiarity with immediate surroundings
___ Inability to understand/follow directions (may be due to a communication problem)

IV. Medications
___ Antiemetics
___ Drugs that have a diuretic effect
___ Drugs that increase GI mobility (laxatives, cathartic, enemas)
___ Psychotropic drugs (tranquilizers, antidepressants)
___ Narcotic analgesics
___ Hypnotic or sedative
___ Hypotension inducing: anti-Parkinson drugs; antihypertensive drugs; cardiac drugs, including Inderal

Display 5-3

CHECKLIST FOR PREVENTING FALLS

Patient's Name: **Diagnosis:** **Age:**

	Yes	No	Comments
1. Are restraints needed? If yes, what type?	___	___	_____
2. Are side rails up?	___	___	_____
3. Is the bed in a low position?	___	___	_____
4. Are bed wheels locked?	___	___	_____
5. Is call light within patient's reach?	___	___	_____
6. Does the patient understand how to use the call light?			
7. Is the night-light on?	___	___	_____
8. Are water, tissues, urinal, and phone within reach?			
9. Is appropriate footwear available?	___	___	_____
10. Have analgesics, hypnotics, or sedatives been given?	___	___	_____
11. Is telemetry secured?	___	___	_____

Display 5-4

NORMAL RANGE OF MOTION FOR EACH OF THE MAJOR JOINTS

Neck

    Flexion: 45 degrees
    Extension: 55 degrees
    Lateral flexion: 40 degrees
    Rotation: 70 degrees

Shoulder

    Flexion: 180 degrees
    Extension: 50 degrees
    Abduction: 180 degrees
    Adduction: 50 degrees
    External rotation: 90 degrees
    Internal rotation: 90 degrees

Elbow

    Flexion: 160 degrees
    Extension: 0 degrees

Wrist

    Flexion: 90 degrees
    Extension: 70 degrees
    Ulnar deviation: 55 degrees
    Radial deviation: 20 degrees
    Pronation: 90 degrees
    Supination: 90 degrees

Hip

    Flexion: 120 degrees
    Extension: 15 degrees
    Abduction: 45 degrees
    Adduction: 45 degrees
    External rotation: 40 degrees
    Internal rotation: 40 degrees

Knee

    Flexion: 130 degrees
    Extension: 0 degrees

Ankle

    Plantar flexion: 45 degrees
    Dorsiflexion: 20 degrees
    Inversion: 30 degrees
    Eversion: 20 degrees

Torso

    Flexion: 75 to 90 degrees
    Extension: 30 degrees
    Lateral flexion: 35 degrees
    Rotation: 30 degrees

degrees found in joints. Range of motion will vary with individuals and normally decreases slightly with aging.

Next, the nurse should assess the patient's muscle strength by providing resistance to a muscle group or muscle while the patient pushes against it. When exercising the patient, the nurse should continually assess the patient's muscle function to advance the patient to the next level of exercise. A grading system using a scale of 0 (no muscle strength) to 5 (able to oppose maximum resistance) should be documented, including appropriate active and passive exercise needed for each grade.

The nurse also should observe the patient performing some simple maneuvers, such as:

- Sitting: Look for the patient's ability to maintain an upright posture. Note any leaning to one side or the other.
- Getting to a sitting position and rising from a sitting position
- Standing: Evaluate posture and any signs of instability.
- Rising from a supine position
- Walking, to determine gait.

A simple test for instability is to have the patient stand unsupported with feet close together. Observe for swaying of the body. Gently nudge the sternum to cause the patient to move the upper body or sway. If unable to regain posture or withstand the displacement, the patient is considered to be unstable. Be prepared to hold the body steady for the unstable patient.

DIAGNOSTIC TESTS

Diagnostic tests are an important part of assessment for people of all ages. Various tests, such as blood studies, scans, computed tomography, and magnetic resonance imaging, can help identify any pathologic problems responsible for immobility. However, the significance of diagnostic results in the older adult must be tempered by age-related changes in these values. Such tests as sedimentation rate, antinuclear antibodies, and rheumatoid factor are normally elevated in later years and may not be significant for diagnosing a specific disease when looking at mobility problems.

NURSING DIAGNOSES

Based on the nursing assessment and physical findings, common nursing diagnoses associated with problems with mobility can be identified. Some of these include the following:

- Activity Intolerance related to weakness, stiffness, and pain
- Body Image Disturbance related to a mobility problem
- High Risk for Disuse Syndrome related to a mobility problem
- Diversional Activity Deficit related to immobility, pain, and weakness secondary to a mobility problem
- Altered Health Maintenance related to a mobility problem
- Impaired Home Maintenance Management related to a mobility problem
- High Risk for Injury related to a mobility problem
- Chronic Pain related to a mobility problem
- Impaired Physical Mobility related to pain, weakness, and deformities
- Altered Role Performance related to a mobility problem
- Self-Care Deficit (specify activity of daily living) related to a mobility problem
- High Risk for Impaired Skin Integrity related to immobility
- Social Isolation related to restricted mobility.

NURSING INTERVENTIONS

With the many causal factors for mobility problems, the nurse can call on numerous interventions to help the patient. Self-care is the mainstay for treatment for preventing disability and dysfunction. Once the patient's deficits have been identified and his or her strengths assessed, an individualized plan of care can be implemented.

ASSISTIVE DEVICES

It is most important to keep the older adult as independent as possible. This may be accomplished with the use of assistive devices. However, some patients may require the assistance of another person to help them to move. When this occurs, it is important that the patient be moved safely. One excellent way to assist the patient with moving is with a gait belt, a 2-inch wide canvas belt. A gait belt allows the assistant to move the patient easily and safely, without grasping the fragile skin and body parts of the older adult, thereby decreasing the likelihood of injury to the patient and the assistant. The gait belt is excellent to use while walking with an unstable patient, because it provides a ready place to grasp if assistance is needed.

Adaptive equipment and assistive devices are available for making dressing, bathing, and preparing meals easier. The patient and the family should be encouraged to discuss these possible needs with health care providers and nurses so that appropriate referrals and equipment can be obtained. Figure 5-2 shows some adaptive equipment that can be used.

Clinical Pearl

Intervention: A wheeled cart is an inexpensive and helpful device. The patient can use it to move objects, such as dishes and food, from one place to another while having something stable and supportive to grasp.

ENVIRONMENTAL MODIFICATION AND SAFETY

Maintaining the patient's safety and preventing falls in the home is of the utmost importance. The nurse needs to evaluate the patient's environment for factors that may contribute to falls. Making the environment safe and less likely to contribute to a fall includes the following:

- Removing scatter rugs and securing loose carpeting
- Removing extension cords and tacking down long trailing cords along walls to prevent tripping
- Providing secure railings on all steps
- Providing adequate lighting, especially in halls and stairways
- Uncluttering the environment and storing unnecessary items
- Arranging furniture for walking ease
- Placing nonslip decals or mats in tub or shower bottoms
- Providing handrails on tubs, showers, and commodes.

It may be necessary to observe the patient actually moving about in his or her environment to look for any potential problems. If the patient must use an assistive device, such as a cane, walker, or wheelchair, the environment may require further modifications. Ramps may need to be installed or living arrangements may need to be changed to accommodate these ramps. It is imperative that the patient and his or her family have proper instruction in the use and care of assistive devices and can actually use them safely and properly.

PATIENT EDUCATION

The nurse needs to make sure that mobility problems do not hamper the ability to meet basic needs, such as nutrition, hygiene, and toileting. Many factors must be considered when trying to meet these basic needs.

The nurse needs to assess the patient's current dietary practices and identify necessary changes. If the patient is unable to provide his or her own meals,

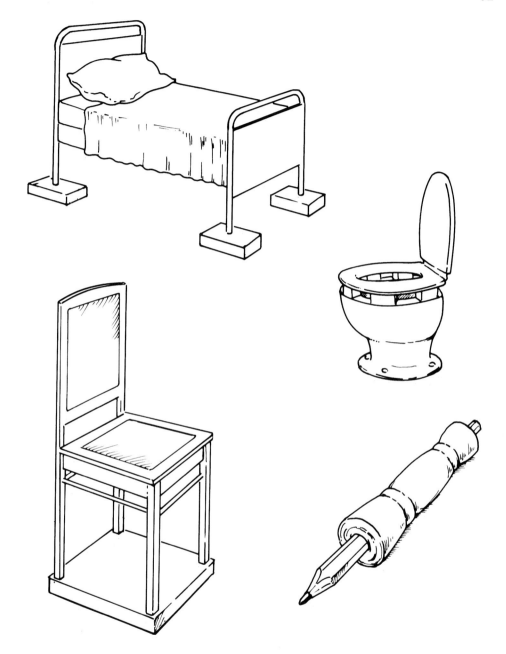

Figure 5-2. Types of adaptive equipment.

arrangements need to be made for home delivery. Family or friends may be able to supply the needed help. If this is not possible, the nurse may need to contact community resources, such as Meals On Wheels. Foods need to be rich in calcium, vitamins, and protein to promote maintenance of healthy bones and muscles. Special dietary considerations and modifications may need to be instituted if the patient has other health problems as well. For example, if the patient has osteoarthritis and is overweight, dietary measures should focus on helping the older adult lose weight to minimize the stress placed on the joints.

The nurse needs to complete a comprehensive assessment of the home and living arrangements. Some interventions may require the older adult and/or the family to learn a new method of accomplishing a task. Many of these interventions center on protecting the patient and the joints. The Patient Teaching Box lists interventions to use in accomplishing a task.

Adherence to these guidelines may require modifications to the home, including adding rails in halls, in tubs, or around toilets. The patient may need to rearrange cabinets and the work space so that food, utensils, tools, and personal care items are within easy reach.

The nurse can teach the patient and family how to use heat and/or cold treatments. These can provide temporary pain relief. Some patients find heat, such as warm showers or baths, an electric heating pad, or an electric blanket works best for them, whereas others prefer cold, such as ice packs or cold compresses. The patient may need to experiment to find out what works best. The nurse should emphasize the cautious use of these treatments for short periods of time to avoid any burns or skin damage.

Another important aspect of patient education involves footwear and foot care. The patient and family need guidance in choosing safe footwear. Footwear needs to be the appropriate size and style, such as low wedges and sneakers. Slippers or thongs that do not have closed heels are generally not safe. In addition, the older adult may have other health problems; the presence of diabetes mellitus or peripheral vascular disease makes foot care extremely important.

Rest, which is a treatment for joint problems in the younger person, may be hazardous for the older adult. If the older adult is bedridden for a week or two, he or she may lose the ability to walk. Therefore, with the older adult, priority should be placed on keeping him or her physically active to avoid a loss of independence (Dunkin, 1992). Numerous programs and instructional materials

Patient Teaching Box
INTERVENTIONS FOR ACCOMPLISHING A TASK

Use the following guidelines to help you perform any task:
- Use the strongest and largest joints possible.
- Distribute the load over several joints.
- Use good body mechanics.
- Organize your work.
- Sit whenever you can.
- Reduce or eliminate all unnecessary bending, reaching, and stretching.
- Avoid prolonged periods of maintaining the same joint position.

are available for planning an exercise program. The Arthritis Foundation is an excellent resource for information and suggestions.

PROFESSIONAL SERVICE COLLABORATION

Occupational therapists are trained to assist patients and their families to meet their needs within their limitations. The nurse can request a referral from the physician for the occupational therapist to evaluate the patient and his or her environment and support system to determine what plan of care is needed for the patient to remain as independent as possible. This plan may include teaching the patient and/or family, supplying equipment for the home, and fitting the patient for adaptive devices and/or joint-protecting splints.

When older adults do not move, they quickly lose their ability to do so. Because they are not always amenable to moving or being moved, the nurse may need to be creative in carrying out a planned activity regimen (Tyson, 1989). Muscle strengthening and stretching exercises have been found to be effective in the older adult to help decrease the loss of muscle function that comes with age. The physical therapist can work in conjunction with the nurse to evaluate the patient and devise an exercise plan for his or her individual needs. The physical therapist can work with the patient and family both in the home and in institutional settings. Like the occupational therapist, the physical therapist along with the nurse can provide assistance with environmental modifications and adaptive devices. The physical therapist and nurse are skilled in assisting the patient and family with the use of such devices as canes, walkers, crutches, and wheelchairs and in teaching about exercise and techniques for moving.

Nursing Care Plan

FOR PATIENTS WITH MOBILITY PROBLEMS

Nursing Diagnosis: Impaired Physical Mobility related to weakness, stiffness, and pain secondary to musculoskeletal disorder.

Definition: A state in which the individual experiences or is at risk of experiencing limited physical movement.

Assessment Findings:
1. Inability to move purposefully in the environment
2. Inability to move due to imposed restrictions (eg, bed rest, traction, casts, medical protocols)
3. Range of motion limitations
4. Limited muscle strength or control
5. Impaired coordination
6. Nonfunctioning or missing limb

Nursing Interventions with Selected Rationales:
Degenerative Joint Disease
1. Assess the functional use of each joint and the patient's ability to perform activities of daily living.

(continued)

Nursing Care Plan

FOR PATIENTS WITH MOBILITY PROBLEMS *(Continued)*

Rationale: Assessment of functional ability provides a baseline for evaluating patient's progress.
2. Assess the level of pain and stiffness present.
Rationale: Assessment of pain and stiffness helps determine degree of limitation and patient discomfort.
3. Teach patient and family to exercise each joint through its normal range of motion.
Rationale: ROM (range-of-motion) exercises help maintain functional use.
4. Teach patient and family to position joints in good alignment during rest periods to maintain functional position.
Rationale: Proper alignment prevents deformity and further injury.
5. Teach patient and family the use of massage and hot/cold treatments for pain and stiffness.
Rationale: Treatments help alleviate pain and stiffness, promoting ease in use of the joint.
6. Suggest appropriate environmental adaptations if needed.
Rationale: Environmental adaptations promote safety and prevent injury.
7. Make referrals to physical/occupational therapists as needed.
Rationale: Referrals to physical therapist and occupational therapist provide additional personnel to develop appropriate treatment regimes to enhance functioning.
8. Make referrals to appropriate agencies as needed for support services (Meals On Wheels, home health, etc.).
Rationale: Outside referrals provide continued support and follow-up.

Desired Patient Outcomes/Discharge Criteria:
1. Patient maintains functional use of joints.
2. Patient performs activities of daily living within limitations.
3. Patient will be as independent as possible within imposed restrictions (physical or medical) and not develop complications.
4. Environmental changes are made to increase independence and reduce risk of falls.
5. The patient will participate in meaningful social activities.
6. Patient and family comply with therapeutic regimen.

REFERENCES
Bates, B. (1995). *A guide to physical examination and history taking* (6th ed.). Philadelphia: J. B. Lippincott.
Dunkin, M. A. (1992). Arthritis in the later years. *Arthritis Today, 1,* 26–29.
Tieaskie, L. (1989). Preventing falls. *Journal of Practical Nursing, 4,* 32–35.
Tyson, B. (1989). For want of a nail. *Geriatric Nursing, 10,* 84–85.

BIBLIOGRAPHY
Andersen, G. P. (1989). A fresh look at assessing the elderly. *RN, 6,* 28–39.
Carnevalli, D. L., & Patrick, M. (1993). *Nursing management for the elderly* (3rd ed.). Philadelphia: J. B. Lippincott.
Conn, V. S. (1990). Joint self-care by older adults. *Rehabilitation Nursing, 4,* 182–186.

Herschen, S. J. (1989). Getting a handle on patient mobility. *Geriatric Nursing, 10,* 146–147.

Matteson, M. A., & McConnell, E. S. (1988). *Gerontological Nursing.* Philadelphia: W. B. Saunders.

Pellino, T. A. (1994). How to manage hip fractures. *AJN, 94*(4):46–50.

Pless, B. S., et al. (1993). Physical health measurement of older adult: new instrumentation. *Journal of the American Academy of Nurse Practitioners, 5*(3), 114–118.

Smith, M. (1993). Two legs to stand on. *AJN, 93*(12), 42–44.

Staab, A. S., & Lyles, M. F. (1990). *Manual of geriatric nursing.* Illinois: Scott, Foresman, Little, Brown.

Problems With Other Senses, Temperature Regulation, and Pain Perception

Objectives

1. Describe the physical and psychosocial implications of age-related changes in other senses and temperature regulation.
2. Identify steps in the nursing assessment of a patient with a problem with other senses and temperature regulation.
3. List nursing diagnoses associated with problems with other senses and temperature regulation.
4. Design nursing interventions for the patient with a problem with other senses and temperature regulation.
5. Describe the psychosocial implications of chronic pain.
6. Identify steps in the nursing assessment of a patient with chronic pain.
7. List nursing diagnoses associated with pain.
8. Design nursing interventions for a patient with chronic pain.

INTRODUCTION

PROBLEMS WITH SENSATION CAN HAVE a pervasive effect on a person's life. The senses of smell, taste, and touch (tactile) are extremely important to the perception and enjoyment of the world around us. The effect of these problems is not usually fully understood or appreciated by others. Not only are physical restrictions or limitations difficult for the person but the numerous physiologic and social implications are extremely disruptive to one's life and lifestyle. Older adults with altered sensation need to learn strategies with which to cope and adapt. Families need to be taught about the dynamics of loss and sensation to better understand and support affected older adults.

Smell and taste are considered to be sensory systems of minor importance compared to vision and hearing. Age-related changes and dysfunction in these sensations are usually less obvious than those of vision and hearing. These senses are essential for adequate coping and adapting to an ever-changing environment and add immeasurably to an appreciation and enjoyment of the world in which we live. Smell and taste are involved in the pleasures of eating and therefore are crucial to proper nutrition. These senses help protect us against injury. They alert us to danger by helping us detect such hazards as smoke from fires, escaping gas, and spoiled food. The sense of touch is extremely important as a protective mechanism, in that it signals our bodies to respond to specific tactile stimulation, including temperature regulation and pain. It is also psychosocially significant as an adjunctive form of communication.

Key sensations that older adults often have problems with include temperature regulation and pain. Because their temperature-regulating mechanisms become less sensitive and less discriminatory to both internal and external stimuli, they experience more problems with environmental factors, such as heat and cooling regulation, and control of body hemostasis. Diminished tactile sensation associated with chronic illness, such as neuropathies, decreases the normal warning pain signals associated with injury. This requires increased awareness of safety factors.

NORMAL PHYSIOLOGIC CHANGES AFFECTING OTHER SENSES

Although the research is inconsistent, the preponderance of available evidence indicates a decline in smell sensitivity with age (Russell, Cummings, Profitt, Wysocki, Gilbert, & Cotman, 1993). Whether such a decline is strictly attributable to aging or whether changes are due to factors associated with aging, such as the cumulative effect of various viruses or repeated exposure to environmental pollutants over the years, is not clear. It seems that older adults have more difficulty detecting odors at low concentrations and identifying or recognizing odors. In general, odor identification declines significantly after the seventh decade, smokers are less able to identify odors than nonsmokers, and older women are better able to identify odors than older men.

Although research on the effects of aging on the sense of taste is inconsistent, most studies agree that the number of taste buds decreases starting in middle age (age 40 to 60), but taste is probably not appreciably affected until after age 60, and then with wide individual differences. In general, the sense of taste appears to be most affected by age, as is the sense of smell. Because research results are so variable, each older adult should be evaluated individually.

The skin contains a variety of receptors that respond to pressure and initiate the sensation of touch. Although there is a lack of research of tactile changes with age, the preponderance of evidence indicates a decrease in tactile sensitivity and in number of tactile receptors as a function of age (Stevens, 1992).

ABNORMAL PHYSIOLOGIC CHANGES

Several other factors are likely to impair the sense of smell in older adults. Upper respiratory viral infection is the most common cause of permanent decreased smell perception in those 50 years of age or older. Whether this is due to age-related lack of resistance to the cumulative effect of repeated viral infections is not known. Nasal sinus disease is another common reason for decreased olfactory perception in older adults. Head trauma resulting in shearing of olfactory axons is a common cause of loss and smell. The anatomic changes associated with Alzheimer's disease are associated with significant impairments in smell, especially in odor detection and odor identification. Odor recognition memory is often impaired as well (Serby, Larson, & Kalkstein, 1991). Parkinson's disease and Huntington's disease, which are more common in older adults, produce dysfunction in smell, particularly in odor recognition memory tasks.

How much of a change in taste sensitivity is due to the aging process and how much is due to other factors is unknown. Factors prevalent in older age that affect taste are periodontal disease, gingivitis, loss of teeth, dentures, drugs, excessive smoking, and changes in the sense of smell. Changes in taste sensitivity affect food choices and nutrition. Nutritional deficiencies and/or exacerbation of disease states may occur if taste is significantly impaired. Taste impairment may also affect digestion, because taste stimulants affect salivary and pancreatic flow, gastric contractions, and intestinal motility.

Some changes in touch sensitivity are related to neuropathies caused by injury, circulatory impairment, and disease.

PSYCHOSOCIAL ISSUES

Older adults who cannot discriminate various danger signals in the environment, such as smoke from fire, escaping gas, or spoiled food, are at risk for serious and life-threatening accidents. Such increased vulnerability may result in anxiety and fear, especially in older adults who live alone. An equally serious problem is that many older adults are not aware that their sensory systems have changed, so they are not sufficiently attuned to these potential dangers. Because sensory changes with aging occur gradually and because smell is not considered to be an especially important sense, many persons are not aware of the gradual changes in smell acuity. Furthermore, older adults who have decreased smell sensitivity may not be aware of body odor or of odors in the home that other people would find offensive. Social relationships and interactions may be altered if others believe the older adult is simply careless about personal cleanliness or does not care.

The most profound psychological effect of change in the sense of taste relates to nutrition. It is difficult for many older adults to be motivated to eat appropriate diets if foods are unappealing. It is easier to eat only one type of food to become satiated (eg, a can of soup) rather than choose or prepare a variety of foods. Food choice is dictated largely by the variety of taste sensations involved. If food all tastes essentially the same, why bother with variety? Overseasoning of foods is another possible compensation for lack of taste but can have serious health consequences for those with medical problems requiring dietary restrictions.

Because age-related changes in touch sensation often result in clumsiness, the older adult may drop, spill, or break items. This clumsiness may affect the person's feelings of competency and sense of self-esteem. Impaired sensitivity to touch may result in gait and mobility changes, making accidents more likely. Pain sensitivity is closely associated with touch. An injury could result in altered sensation, which could be dangerous; for example, the older adult may be unable to detect hot water.

Because touch is usually viewed as another of the minor senses, its effect on quality of life is not always appreciated. With age, the need for touch may increase. As other sensory systems become less responsive, older adults may need to augment their environmental and personal/social interactions with touch. However, for many older adults, opportunities for touch interactions, such as with children or a spouse, are reduced as one grows older. Touch can be used effectively with patients to establish rapport and to convey caring and concern. All patients may not respond to touching in the same way. Nurses should be aware of large individual differences in patients' responses to touch based on each patient's family history, individual life experiences, culture, and personal preferences as well as the nurse's personal feelings regarding touching and closeness.

Clinical Pearl

Intervention: The nurse can use touch as an effective adjunct to communication and to increase the older adult's sense of comfort, care, affiliation, and safety.

NURSING ASSESSMENT

An assessment of the other senses should be included as part of the nursing history and physical examination of all older adults. Assessment of these senses should include examination of the nose and oral cavity.

HISTORY AND INTERVIEW

The history and interview should address areas of the head, nose, and mouth. Additional areas involving the sense of touch should also be addressed. Use the following areas as a guide to formulate specific questions:

- History of head trauma, skull surgery, or jaw or facial fractures
- Sinus infection, tenderness, or facial swelling
- Nasal discharge
- Use of over-the-counter drugs, prescription medications, or recreational substances
- History of mouth lesions, ulcers, or cold sores
- Smoking history
- Dental care habits
- Neurologic problems
- Nutritional habits.

Throughout the history and interview, pay particular attention for specific indicators that may point to a deficit in smell or taste. Smell deficit indicators include:

- Frequent complaints that food doesn't "taste right" or that most foods taste bland. These complaints may stem from an impaired sense of smell as well as taste.

- Adding flavor enhancers excessively to foods (eg, salt, sugar)
- Ignoring or being unaware of strong odors of the body or in the environment
- Excessive use of perfume

Taste deficit indicators include:

- Frequent complaints about the taste of foods
- Adding flavor enhancers excessively
- Reduced interest in and motivation to eat.

PHYSICAL EXAMINATION

Visually inspect the nose. Note any asymmetry that might interfere with breathing or smell. Look for any swelling, trauma, or congenital anomalies. Examine the color and texture of the nose surface. Palpate the nose for raised bumps, hard nodes, or frontal bone depressions. Inspect the nares for flaring or discharge. Palpate the frontal and maxillary sinuses to reveal tenderness indicative of sinusitis. Avoid pressure on the eyes.

Determine patency of the nasal cavities by asking the patient to close the mouth, exert pressure on one naris with the finger, and breathe through the opposite naris. Evaluate each naris. Examine nasal cavities using a nasal speculum otoscope or manually using the thumb of the left hand to push the nose upward while shining a light into the nasal cavity.

Inspect the lower and upper portions of the nose, repositioning the patient's head several times during the examination to inspect all areas. Tip the patient's head back to inspect the inferior and middle turbinates. Inspect the septum for deviations, exudate, and perforation. Examine all areas for polyps, swelling, exudate, and change in color. The nasal mucosa is usually redder than the oral mucosa. Excessive redness indicates infection. Redness plus edema of the turbinates indicates localized infection, whereas pale turbinates reflect allergy. Secretions should be noted. Normal secretion in nasal cavities is mucoid. Watery secretions suggest upper respiratory infection or allergic rhinitis.

Assess smell and sensitivity using various aromatic substances, asking the patient to identify the odor. Test each side separately. Test substances should be volatile, nonirritating, and unambiguous, such as cloves, coffee, vanilla, chocolate, lemon, and lime. Keep test substances in tightly closed test tubes until presentation. Record the number of substances used, the number of correct responses, and any differences in sensitivity from one nostril to the other.

Examine the tongue for any swelling, change in color, coating, or ulceration. Inspect the teeth for caries, missing teeth, and malocclusions. If dentures are present, observe the fit and the condition of the dentures. Inspect gums for signs of gingivitis, inflammation, hemorrhage, or irritation from ill-fitting dentures. Inspect for more serious periodontal disease (pyorrhea) that loosens teeth in their sockets.

Assess taste sensations by applying sweet, sour (vinegar, lemon juice), salty, and bitter (quinine) solutions to the appropriate region of the tongue. Give the patient a sip of water between each tasting to avoid mixing tastes. Test twice with each substance, and test both sides of the tongue as well as the front and back.

Test light touch by lightly touching the patient with a small piece of gauze or a wisp of cotton. Ask the patient to close his or her eyes and to indicate when a touch is felt. An organized but unpatterned testing of both arms, the trunk, and both legs is useful. Compare sensations on both sides as well as distal and proximal parts of the body.

Test double simultaneous stimulation or tactile localization by having the patient close his or her eyes while asking him or her to identify where the touch occurred. Simultaneously touch two places, for example, the right cheek and the left arm, and see if the patient correctly identifies both touch stimuli.

Test two-point discrimination to determine if the patient can differentiate one stimulus from two. Assess the corresponding area on the other side of the body. Different body areas have different sensitivities.

Test stereognosis, or the ability to identify an object placed in the hand, by having the patient close the eyes and having the patient identify some object, such as a key, paperclip, pencil, or coin placed in his or her palm. Test both hands and compare findings.

DIAGNOSTIC TESTS

Various diagnostic tests, such as X-rays of the skull, sinuses, and oral cavity and scans, may be performed to rule out other pathologic conditions. Complete neurologic tests may be necessary to rule out a neurologic cause of the sensory problem.

NURSING DIAGNOSES

Many patients as well as family and caregivers are unaware of subtle changes in the senses and of the implications these changes have for quality of life. The following are potential nursing diagnoses for a patient with a deficit in smell, taste, or touch:

- Altered Nutrition: Less Than Body Requirements, related to a decreased sense of smell and taste
- High Risk for Poisoning related to diminished sense of smell and taste
- Self-Esteem Disturbance related to deficits in smell and taste
- Impaired Social Interaction related to smell and taste deficits
- Dressing or Grooming Self-Care Deficit related to smell and tactile deficits
- Sensory or Perceptual Alterations (smell and taste), related to the aging process
- High Risk for Injury related to deficit in sense of touch
- Self-Esteem Disturbance related to diminished sense of touch
- Sensory or Perceptual Alterations (touch), related to the aging process.

NURSING INTERVENTIONS

Problems with other senses affect not only the patient's health status by altering nutrition but also affect safety and interpersonal relationships. Communication with older adults must be specific to detect awareness of sensory deficits.

DIETARY MEASURES

Smell and taste are closely related to the enjoyment of food, and changes in either or both sensory systems affect food choices and motivation to eat a balanced diet involving a variety of foods. Food choices are in part determined by the smell of various foods. Personal safety is compromised if the older adult is unable to smell spoiled food. Referral to a dietitian is useful for information about attractive and appetizing food preparation. Referral to an otolaryngologist is advisable to assess specific medical conditions causing a deficit in the sense of smell or taste.

THERAPEUTIC TOUCH

The nurse should always remember that touching patients functionally and therapeutically should be individualized for each patient. The following are areas the nurse should consider in determining how and when to touch older adults:

- The need to be touched varies among patients.
- Always consider the patient's lifestyle and culture in determining touching behavior and preferences. Some ethnic groups and some families do not use touch in their interpersonal relationships. Nurses can take cues about touching from family and friends and how they relate to the patient.
- Touching can be very therapeutic for patients who have depression, low self-esteem, and reduced sense of competency.
- Patients who are disoriented, disheveled, or foul-smelling may need to be touched more than others to decrease isolation.

PATIENT AND FAMILY TEACHING

Health promotion and early discovery of changes in the senses of smell, taste, and touch are important before they interfere with proper nutrition and personal/social relationships. The changes associated with taste, smell, and touch may be subtle and go unnoticed by family or caregivers. Understanding the significance of changes will enhance compliance by patient and family. To enhance smell and taste, the patient and family can be taught to be more alert to indicators of deficits in the senses (see Patient Teaching Box: Strategies for Coping with a Deficit in Smell and Taste). To promote safety and improve social relationships, the patient and family can also be taught to install smoke detectors in the home in strategic locations, use visual gas detection indicators for gas stoves, have a family member or neighbor periodically check for spoiled food and offensive odors in the living environment, and establish a daily personal hygiene routine, including the use of deodorant.

Health promotion is important to help older adults maximize their safety by compensating for deficits in touch. They can be taught to move more slowly and carefully and to be more aware of changes in the sense of touch. Some strategies may include arranging the side rails, oxygen equipment, walkers, traction devices, and other potential barriers so the patient is easily accessible. The nurse should bend down when touching someone in a wheelchair, thus making the contact more personal and supportive. Nurses should help provide patients and their families with instructions for tactile stimulation using familiar objects, such as favorite a hairbrush or a pet, to stimulate the sense of touch and thus help keep the patient in contact with reality.

Patient and family education involves sensitizing them to the dangers of touch impairment. For example, the danger of falling increases if touch sensations from the soles of the feet are not accurate, and the danger of burning oneself increases if containers with hot liquids are not grasped firmly enough. Slower movement and conscious awareness of potential dangers assist in acci-

Patient Teaching Box
STRATEGIES FOR COPING WITH A DEFICIT IN SMELL
AND TASTE

• Use visually attractive food arrangements at meals to compensate for lack of smell
  and taste sensitivity.
• Encourage smells of cooking to permeate the area to stimulate the older adult and
  enhance motivation to eat.
• Encourage heavy smokers to stop smoking, because this may increase their deficit.
• Maintain a clean oral cavity and brush teeth at least once a day.
• Serve food warm to enhance remaining taste sensation.
• Offer food items separately rather than mashed together to preserve individual
  taste sensations.
• Suggest the use of herbs and spices in cooking rather than excessive salt and sugar.

dent prevention. The patient and family need to be taught the psychosocial significance of touch as an important mode of communication. As other sensory systems decline in efficiency, touch may be an even more valuable adjunct to communicating with older adults. Referral to a neurologist or orthopedist is helpful to assess specific central nervous system or musculoskeletal problems causing or contributing to a deficit in the sense of touch.

NORMAL PHYSIOLOGIC CHANGES RELATED TO TEMPERATURE REGULATION

Disorders of temperature regulation most likely occur in older adults because of impaired homeostatic mechanisms associated with the aging process. Older adults are less able to adjust adequately to extremes of temperature, especially adults older than age 75. They also seem less able to discriminate temperature differences accurately. Hypothalamic regulation of homeostatic mechanisms becomes less efficient with age.

ABNORMAL PHYSIOLOGIC CHANGES

Body temperature is controlled primarily by the blood flow through the vascular network of the body. The automatic nervous system, specifically the hypothalamus, controls dilation and constriction of blood vessels, which produce heat loss or heat conservation. The body obtains heat directly from the outside environment and indirectly from the process of metabolism and muscle contraction. Receptors in the skin respond to heat and cold. The body can be visualized as a core protected by several outer layers that mediate to control either heat loss or heat gain (Reuler, 1990).

DECREASED BODY TEMPERATURE

A core body temperature lower than 95°F (35°C) is defined as hypothermia. As body temperature begins to drop, there are various consequences for body organ functions (Reuler, 1990). These include the following:

- Decrease in basal metabolic rate
- Initial rise in blood pressure, but then a gradual fall; hypotension is significant below 77°F (25°C)
- Various hemodynamic effects, such as atrial fibrillation and conduction disturbances, at temperatures below 82.4°F (28°C)
- At still lower body temperatures, respiratory center depression, decreased level of consciousness, and a less efficient cough reflex leading to aspiration difficulties and respiratory insufficiency, with bronchopneumonia and aspiration pneumonia as possible later complications
- Acid–base disturbances with profound hypothermia, with acidosis from respiratory failure and tissue hypoxia
- Hypovolemia
- Central nervous system effects caused by severe hypothermia, including depressed mentation and hyporeflexia, weak pulse, and unmeasurable blood pressure.

INCREASED BODY TEMPERATURE

Heat stroke is defined as a failure to maintain normal body temperature when in a warm environment. This is caused by increases in heat, decreases in heat loss, or both. High humidity and high environmental temperatures are primary reasons for heat illness.

NURSING ASSESSMENT

Nursing assessment of thermoregulation is aimed at identifying the person's baseline body temperature, risk factors for altered thermoregulation, and early manifestations of hypothermia or hyperthermia. It involves gathering information about the patient and his or her environment and measuring body temperature.

HISTORY AND INTERVIEW

When obtaining the patient's history, questions should address the following areas:

- Response to hot and cold weather
- House temperatures
- Forms of protection, such as blankets and heat sources, used during winter months
- Any medical treatment for exposure to heat or cold
- Environmental conditions and living situation
- Activity level
- History of illnesses.

RISK FACTORS

Anyone 75 years of age or older should be considered at risk for altered thermoregulation. Other risk factors include dehydration, extremes in environmental temperatures, systemic diseases, inactivity or immobility, medications, alcohol use, and electrolyte imbalances.

In addition to exposure to cold, there are many other factors predisposing older adults to hypothermia (Abrass, 1990; Richardson, Tyra, & McCray, 1992). Disorders involving decreased heat production include hypothyroidism (especially myxedema), hypoglycemia, starvation, and malnutrition. Immobility and sedentary lifestyle caused by stroke, arthritis, parkinsonism, and other debilitating diseases add to decreased heat production. Body heat production can be significantly affected by disorders of the hypothalamus or central nervous system, such as trauma, hypoxia, tumor, or cerebrovascular disease. Drugs that commonly impair temperature regulation include ethanol, barbiturates, phenothiazines, benzodiazepines, anesthetics, and narcotics. Some medications directly affect heat-regulating mechanisms of the body; other medications impair awareness of environmental conditions. Older adults are also more prone to hypothermia as a postoperative complication because of thermoregulatory difficulties associated with aging. In addition, economic restrictions or confused and disoriented states contribute to inadequate heating in the home, thus predisposing many older adults to hypothermia.

As with hypothermia, older adults are more susceptible to hyperthermia due to age-related physiologic chances and having various diseases. Skin and fat tissue insulate the body, so those with greater fat tissue have more difficulty losing body heat in hot weather. The body is exposed to heat directly from the environment, indirectly from body metabolism and muscle contraction, and from response to infection and certain drugs. Older adults can have diminished sweating, a significantly higher core temperature at which sweating is initiated, delayed vasodilation with heating, and impaired sensitivity to change in temperature.

Many medications predispose older adults to hyperthermia. Some impair the body's ability to dissipate heat, especially by blocking sweating (Miller, 1991). These include antihistamines, anticholinergics, and phenothiazines. Some medications impair the body's cardiovascular response to excess heat, especially those interfering with peripheral vasodilation. Examples are the diuretics and beta blockers. Some medications increase body temperature, for example, and others increase metabolic rate, such as thyroid hormones.

PHYSICAL EXAMINATION

A complete review of body systems should be performed to evaluate the patient's status. A baseline body temperature should be obtained. Throughout the physical exam, the nurse should be alert to possible signs and symptoms of increased or decreased body temperature.

For older adults at risk, those showing progressive fatigue, weakness, confusion, apathy, slurred speech, ataxia, and involuntary movements should be evaluated for possible decreases in body temperature and hypothermia. Many times hypothermia is not diagnosed until serious complications develop. In the early stages, older adults may not shiver or feel cold. Low-reading thermometers are necessary to accurately assess low body temperatures. Remember that body temperature drops somewhat with age, and extremely cold temperatures are not necessary to produce hypothermia.

Early symptoms of increased body temperature or heat illness include weakness, dizziness, headache, breathlessness, confusion, anorexia, and feeling hot. Without treatment, heat illness progresses to heatstroke. Heatstroke occurs when the core temperature suddenly increases to 105°F (40.6°C) or higher (Abrass, 1990). Manifestations of heatstroke are mental confusion, delirium, coma, and anhidrosis (hot, dry skin). Complications of heatstroke include cardiac arrhythmias, tachycardia, seizures, liver failure, hypokalemia, hypovolemia, and shock.

DIAGNOSTIC TESTS

Various diagnostic tests, including serum laboratory analysis, X-rays, and scans, may be performed to rule out other possible causes and conditions associated with problems with temperature regulation.

NURSING DIAGNOSES

Based on history and physical findings, potential nursing diagnoses associated with patients having temperature regulation deficits can include:

- Ineffective Thermoregulation related to lowered or elevated body temperature
- Knowledge Deficit related to hypothermia or hyperthermia
- High Risk for Injury related to deficits in temperature regulation.

NURSING INTERVENTIONS

It is important to be aware of the very real dangers associated with problems of temperature regulation in older adults. Various factors, ranging from physical status and medications to living environments, make many older adults more vulnerable to problems associated with temperature regulation.

INCREASING BODY TEMPERATURE

For those with mild hypothermia (core temperatures higher than 92°F [33.3°C]), management consists of external rewarming and providing adequate heating in the living environment. Passive rewarming with insulating material and placing the patient in a warm environment is generally adequate for those with mild hypothermia. Active rewarming techniques using electric blankets, warm mattresses, hot water bottles, or a warm water bath work more quickly. These techniques must be used with caution because they have been associated with increased morbidity and mortality, in that cold blood may be suddenly diverted to the core, further decreasing core temperatures and possibly resulting in hypovolemic shock. In more severe hypothermia, core rewarming may be necessary. Methods used include intragastric or colonic irrigation, inhalation rewarming, extracorporeal blood rewarming, and peritoneal dialysis (Reuler, 1990).

HEALTH PROMOTION

Additional nursing interventions used for decreased body temperature include the following:

- Promote education about hypothermia among older adults and among professionals who provide services and programs for them.

- For those prone to hypothermia, have them take their temperature daily during cold weather.
- Instruct patients to eat nutritious meals and avoid alcohol.
- Encourage social interactions so that others can be aware of potentially dangerous situations during cold weather. A family member or neighbor can check on the patient daily to be sure that he or she has not fallen or become immobilized in the home.
- Encourage the patient to keep room temperature in the dwelling are at 68°F (20°C) or higher.
- Make sure the home is winterized and that blankets, quilts, or other coverings are readily available.

DECREASING BODY TEMPERATURE

Intensive nursing care is necessary in problems related to increased body temperature, because all body systems are affected. Rapid body cooling, fluid and electrolyte replacement, and careful monitoring of all body systems are necessary to prevent renal, liver, and brain damage.

HEALTH PROMOTION

Additional nursing interventions to manage increased body temperature include:

- Discouraging excessive physical activity during periods of high temperature
- Instructing the patient to wear light-colored, airy clothing to facilitate sweating
- Encouraging a diet high in carbohydrates and low in protein
- Adding fluids
- Instructing the patient to use air conditioning and fans whenever possible
- Making sure the dwelling area is ventilated adequately
- Having a telephone reassurance program, neighbor, or family member check on the patient daily during periods of high temperature
- Referring patients to community shelters to protect those especially vulnerable during prolonged heat waves.

PATIENT AND FAMILY TEACHING

Education of older adults and their families, especially those with little education and/or living in inadequate housing, is essential. Patient and family education should focus on making people more aware of the health risks in temperature regulation disorders. Older adults at risk should be specifically educated about their susceptibility to hypothermia and hyperthermia and about symptoms indicative of temperature regulation problems. At-risk older adults also need to be monitored daily during periods of extremely high or low temperatures.

Specific referrals to community programs, such as telephone reassurance, can be useful as one way to monitor vulnerable older adults daily. Referral to shelters may be necessary for some older adults who live in inadequate housing and have no other refuge from temperature extremes. Appropriate community resources may be available from the local office on aging. Prevention is the best approach, and this depends largely on education of the public, young and old.

NORMAL PHYSIOLOGIC CHANGES AFFECTING PAIN PERCEPTION

Education of health professionals about current thinking in the area of pain and pain management is a necessity, because many significant advances have been made in the past 10 to 15 years. Acute pain—mild to severe pain usually of brief duration that subsides as treatment and healing occur—can often be directly related to a disease or trauma. Chronic pain—prolonged, mild to severe pain occurring beyond a 6-month period—is not as amenable to the traditional treatments of pain.

Pain, a complex phenomenon, is highly individualized, with both objective and subjective aspects, thus it is very difficult for others to understand. It occurs in the context of various psychosocial, economic, and cultural factors that can influence the meaning, experience, and expression of pain in a given individual. "Pain is whatever the experiencing person says it is, existing whenever he says it does" (McCaffery & Beebe, 1989).

Research on the effects of aging on pain remains controversial. Some evidence indicates the perception of pain decreases with age and other evidence suggests the perception of pain increases with age. However, because pain is a complex and highly individualized experience and because aging adults are at the greatest risk of chronic disease, it is not unreasonable to expect that many older adults do indeed suffer pain.

PSYCHOSOCIAL ISSUES

Pain, especially chronic pain, can be devastating to quality of life. Depression is common in those with chronic pain, because most chronic pain conditions are unpredictable and create a pervasive sense of loss of control or helplessness. Guarding behaviors, in an effort to protect against further pain, restrict the individual's movements and activities, including social interactions and roles. Other behaviors often seen as part of a chronic pain picture include preoccupation with the pain, anxiety, loss of interest in previous activities, excessive use of analgesic medications, sleep disturbances, irritability, and disturbed interpersonal relationships. Chronic pain can have a profound and long-lasting effect on an individual's life.

NURSING ASSESSMENT

Assessment of pain is a difficult task, because pain is a personal experience known only by the individual who is in pain. Pain assessment is ongoing, not a one-time event.

HISTORY AND INTERVIEW

Assessment of older adults requires more time and a slower pace than assessment of younger individuals. For a thorough assessment, both nonverbal and verbal methods should be used. Many older adults have been taught not to complain about pain, so nurses must ask appropriate questions to elicit necessary information and must be alert to nonverbal cues providing pain information. Some older adults underreport pain because they believe it is part of aging and must be endured. For older adults, particularly those with sensory or cognitive impairments, it is necessary to first get their undivided attention in a setting free of other distractions and noise. Be sure the patient can see and hear you. Speak slowly and distinctly.

Acute and chronic pain require varied assessment techniques to determine the type of pain. Nonverbal methods of assessing acute pain include observation of the following:

- Protective or guarding behaviors in which the patient protects and guards the body area in which the pain is occurring
- Thought processes and attention distortion in that the patient may appear confused or disoriented and attention is directed only to self
- Behaviors such as crying, moaning, rubbing, restlessness, irritability, and agitation
- Facial expression indicating a pinched look, tightly clenched jaw muscles and teeth, and eyes without luster
- Increased muscle tension and complaints of nausea.

Nonverbal methods of assessing chronic pain include observation of the following:

- Protective and guarding behaviors in the patient's posture and movements
- Evidence of extreme fatigue, irritability, restlessness, anxiety, and depression
- Facial expressions resembling those of acute pain
- Changes in patient's usual activities and/or distorted interpersonal relationships.

The assessment of pain includes both verbal and written techniques. In general, assessment of pain should include type of pain, location, description, intensity, other symptoms that may accompany the pain, and mood of effective tone of the pain sufferer. Figure 6-1 provides an example of an initial pain assessment form, which helps the nurse identify pain characteristics. Other types of assessment techniques available include:

- Pain scales (verbal description scales consisting of numbers with words representing different levels of pain)
- Visual analogue scales (a 10-point scale ranging from "no pain" [0] to "most severe pain" [10])
- Pain questionnaires
- Pain charts (a drawing of the body on which the patient can mark and identify the location of pain)
- Pain diary (diary keeping may be difficult for some older adults).

PHYSICAL EXAMINATION

A complete review of body systems is essential to determine the location of the pain. Inspection, auscultation, palpation, and percussion are crucial. Throughout the physical exam, the nurse should continue to assess the patient's verbal and nonverbal responses (Fig. 6-2).

INITIAL PAIN ASSESSMENT TOOL   Date _____

Patient's Name _____ Age _____ Room _____

Diagnosis _____ Physician _____

Nurse _____

I. LOCATION: Patient or nurse mark drawing.

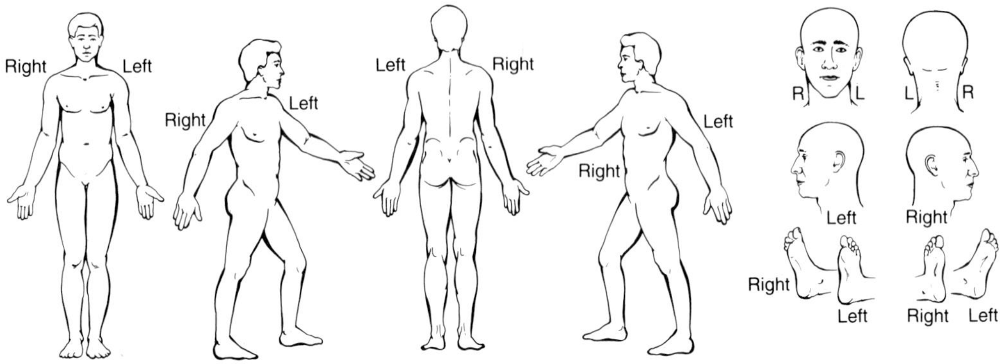

Right   Left   Right   Left   Left   Right   Left

Right   Left   Right   R L   L R

Left   Right

Right   Left   Right   Left

II. INTENSITY: Patient rates the pain. Scale used _____

     Present: _____

     Worst pain gets: _____

     Best pain gets: _____

     Acceptable level of pain: _____

III. QUALITY: (Use patient's own words, e.g. prick, ache, burn, throb, pull, sharp) _____

     _____

IV. ONSET, DURATION VARIATIONS, RHYTHMS: _____

     _____

V. MANNER OF EXPRESSING PAIN: _____

     _____

VI. WHAT RELIEVES THE PAIN? _____

     _____

VII. WHAT CAUSES OR INCREASES THE PAIN? _____

     _____

VIII. EFFECTS OF PAIN: (Note decreased function, decreased quality of life.)

     Accompanying symptoms (e.g. nausea) _____

     Sleep _____

     Appetite _____

     Physical activity _____

     Relationship with others (e.g. irritability) _____

     Emotions (e.g. anger, suicidal, crying) _____

     Concentration _____

     Other _____

IX. OTHER COMMENTS: _____

     _____

X. PLAN: _____

     _____

Figure 6-1. Initial pain assessment tool. Reprinted with permission from McCaffery, M. & Beebe, A. (1989). Pain: Clinical manual for nursing practice. St. Louis: Mosby.

FLOW SHEET–PAIN

Patient _____ Date _____

*Pain rating scale used _____

Purpose: To evaluate the safety and effectiveness of the analgesic(s).

Analgesic(s) prescribed: _____

Time	Pain rating	Analgesic	R	P	BP	Level of arousal	Other†	Plan & comments

Pain rating: A number of different scales may be used. Indicate which scale is used and use the same one each time. For example, 0-10 (0 = no pain, 10 = worst pain).

†*Possibilities for other columns:* bowel function, activities, nausea and vomiting, other pain relief measures. Identify the side effects of greatest concern to patient, family, physician, nurses.

FLOW SHEET—PAIN

Patient *Mrs. W. (Age: 92 years)* _____ Date *5/11*

Behavior indicating pain: *Behaviors indicating pain: continuous grunting, eyes tightly closed, legs pulled in toward abdomen, picks at bed covers.*

Purpose: To evaluate the safety and effectiveness of the analgesic(s).

Analgesic(s) prescribed: *Trilisate liquid 1 teaspoon (500 mg) bid; MS Contin 30 mg PO q24h*

Time	Possible behaviors	Analgesic	R	P	BP	Level of arousal	Possible comfort behaviors	Plan & comments

Figure 6-2. Pain assessment form. Reprinted with permission from McCaffery, M. & Beebe, A. (1989). Pain: Clinical manual for nursing practice. St. Louis: Mosby.

NURSING DIAGNOSES

Factors derived from a completed history and physical examination plus consideration of the interactions of psychosocial variables will help to generate nursing diagnoses. The following is a list of selected nursing diagnoses based on an older adult with pain:

- Activity Intolerance related to acute/chronic pain
- Impaired Physical Mobility related to acute/chronic pain
- Sleep Pattern Disturbance related to acute/chronic pain
- Altered Role Performance related to acute/chronic pain
- Impaired Adjustment related to acute/chronic pain
- Fatigue related to chronic pain
- Hopelessness related to chronic pain
- Impaired Social Interaction related to chronic pain
- Anxiety, related to chronic pain
- High Risk for Disuse Syndrome related to chronic pain
- Altered Family Processes related to chronic pain
- Powerlessness related to chronic pain
- Self-Esteem Disturbance, related to chronic pain
- Altered Nutrition, Less Than Body Requirements related to chronic pain.

NURSING INTERVENTIONS

The goal of nursing care for the patient in pain is to help the patient control the pain. Nurses must be knowledgeable about pharmacologic and nonpharmacologic interventions.

MEDICATION THERAPY

The most widely used method of pain management is analgesic drug therapy. Three groups of drugs used are the nonopioid analgesics, the opiate analgesics, and the adjuvant drugs.

 Clinical Pearl

Intervention: To avoid the use of opiate analgesics, which can cause respiratory and central nervous system depression, use a combination of acetaminophen and a nonsteroidal anti-inflammatory drug. These drugs augment or potentiate each other and give pain relief equal to the opioid analgesics.

The first-line agents to be used for management of mild to moderate pain are the nonopioid analgesics, especially for inflammatory conditions. These include acetaminophen (Tylenol) and the nonsteroidal anti-inflammatory drugs, such as aspirin, ibuprofen (Motrin, Advil), fenoprofen (Nalfon), and naproxen

(Naprosyn). Nonsteroidal anti-inflammatory drugs are tolerated quite well by older adults, but side effects, such as decreased platelet aggregation, prolonged bleeding time, and gastric irritation are documented.

The opioid analgesics are used for moderate or severe pain and include morphine, hydromorphone (Dilaudid), codeine (Tylenol 3, Empirin 3), and propoxyphene (Darvon, Darvocet). Narcotic drugs can become habit forming. Older adults are more sensitive to the analgesic effects of these drugs and may need much less narcotic medication than younger individuals. Side effects of narcotics include sedation, nausea, constipation, cough suppression, and most serious of all, respiratory depression. Narcotics should be constantly monitored for side effects and used only when another drug is not available.

Adjuvant drugs, a third group of drugs used to treat pain, do not have analgesic properties themselves, but have been found useful in treating some forms of chronic pain. Mild sedatives and tranquilizers can reduce anxiety and tension, and anticonvulsants can be helpful in chronic pain management.

NONPHARMACOLOGIC PAIN MANAGEMENT

Nonpharmacologic interventions are often used for older adults in the treatment of chronic pain and can be helpful in some forms of acute pain as well. Chronic pain management requires a multimodal approach, which may involve medication plus a variety of nonpharmacologic techniques. Techniques helpful in chronic pain management are imagery, distraction, self-hypnosis, physical therapy (including heat, cold, massage), relaxation, biofeedback, transcutaneous electrical nerve stimulation (TENS), exercise and cognitive strategies, or training in cognitive skills to help manage pain. Effective pain management requires a multidisciplinary and multimodal approach in which patients are taught a variety of techniques to help them gain control over and effectively manage their pain.

The nurse should reinforce the relaxation techniques with the patient until they are used effectively. Benefits of muscle relaxation for chronic pain control should be discussed with the older adult. It is important to accept the patient's statements of pain and try to understand the multiple factors involved in creating and maintaining pain situations. These factors involve not only physical parameters and limitations but also a vast array of psychosocial variables interacting in pain situations, especially in chronic pain.

PATIENT AND FAMILY TEACHING

Patient and family education will usually aid in compliance, because generally the patient and family do not understand the pain situation fully and are seeking assistance in understanding it and managing it. Patients need to understand that chronic pain is not usually cured but must be managed. Neither the patient nor the family should have unrealistic goals about being cured. This hampers the development of a positive attitude toward management. Patients must be taught specific techniques to alleviate and manage pain. Families need to be supportive of these efforts. In addition to medication, nonpharmacologic interventions such as distraction, imagery, self-hypnosis, relaxation,

Patient Teaching Box
STRATEGIES FOR PROMOTING RELAXATION
TO RELIEVE PAIN

Instruct the patient in the following strategies for promoting relaxation to relieve pain:

- Ensure that the patient is in a quiet, distraction-free environment to focus concentration and avoid feeling self-conscious.
- Position the patient comfortably, such as reclining or lying down with muscles fully supported, to facilitate relaxation.
- Have the patient start relaxing with eyes closed and taking a few deep breaths. Associate these with cue words, such as "sinking down," "letting go," or "sinking deeper and deeper" into a state of relaxation.
- Guide the patient through progressive relaxation exercises for each muscle group. A professionally prepared tape is useful for instructions. Have the patient tense each muscle group for 4 or 5 seconds and then relax them. Start with the feet and progress to head and scalp.
- Have the patient focus on how relaxed muscles feel so he or she can recognize feelings of relaxation and produce them when desired.
- At the end of the relaxation session, have the patient open eyes slowly and move slowly.
- Use caution with older adults who have musculoskeletal difficulties and do not encourage them to tense muscles too tightly.
- Be sure older adults with hearing impairments can hear and understand verbal instructions.

and cognitive therapy are useful for many pain situations. Patients need to be taught a variety of management techniques and encouraged to choose those that are most effective for them in managing their pain. The Patient Teaching Box provides strategies for promoting relaxation to relieve pain.

COMMUNITY RESOURCES

Specific referrals to pain specialists or to a reputable pain clinic are helpful if the pain is chronic and has not been controlled or managed well. These facilities have a greater array of techniques available and specific programs than those available to individuals who work with pain patients. Community support is available from organizations or support groups focusing on specific pain situations. Examples are the Arthritis Foundation or fibromyalgia support groups. Addresses and telephone numbers can be found in the telephone book, from pain clinics, or from neurologists or rheumatologists who work extensively with pain patients.

Nursing Care Plan

FOR PATIENTS WITH DEFICITS

Nursing Diagnosis: Altered Nutrition, Less than Body Requirements related to a decreased sense of smell and taste.

Definition: The state in which an individual experiences or is at risk for experiencing persistent weight loss due to reduced intake when food is available in nutritious amounts.

Assessment Findings:
1. Anorexia, weight loss
2. Offensive odors in home
3. Reduced interest and motivation to eat

Nursing Interventions With Selected Rationale:
1. Install smoke detectors in the home in strategic locations.
   Rationale: Smoke detectors sound a warning alarm to promote safety.
2. Use visual gas detection indications for gas stoves.
   Rationale: Visual detectors use another sense to give warning to decrease chance for asphyxiation.
3. Use visually attractive food arrangments at meals.
   Rationale: Visualization can be used to compensate for lack of smell and taste sensitivity to make food more palatable and to encourage increased intake.
4. Encourage smells of cooking to permeate the area.
   Rationale: Sense of smell can assist stimulation of the older adult and enhances motivation to eat.
5. Have a family member or neighbor periodically check for spoiled food and offensive odors in the living environment.
   Rationale: Checks for odors and spoiled food can decrease accidental poisoning.
6. Establish a daily oral, dental, and hygiene routine, including frequent brushing of teeth and the use of deodorants.
   Rationale: Good routine hygiene promotes a positive self image.
7. Encourage heavy smokers to stop smoking.
   Rationale: Smoking increases sensation losses.
8. Refer to a dietitian for nutritional assessment and information about attractive and appetizing food preparation.
   Rationale: The empathy and reinforcement of dietary information may increase compliance.
9. Suggest substituting herbal powders and spices on the meal table and in cooking.
   Rationale: Excessive use of salt and sugar may be avoided by substituting the spices and powders.
10. Refer to an otolaryngologist.
    Rationale: The otolaryngologist will assess specific medical conditions causing a deficit in the senses of smell and taste.
11. Evaluate medications.
    Rationale: Some medications interfere with the senses of taste or smell.
12. Provide psychosocial support and reassurance.
    Rationale: Knowledge that these are deficits and should not become totally inactive sensations may provide psychological support.

(continued)

Nursing Care Plan

FOR PATIENTS WITH DEFICITS *(Continued)*

Desired Patient Outcomes/Discharge Criteria:

1. Patient and family understand and can verbalize smell and taste deficits and implications on their lifestyles.
2. Patient is skilled in and uses nutritional management techniques that work most effectively.
3. Patient's ideal weight is maintained with no further weight loss.
4. Patient verbalizes improved interpersonal and social relationships.

REFERENCES

Abrass, I. B. (1990). Disorders of temperature regulation. In W. R. Hazard & R. Andes (Eds.), *Principles of geriatric medicine and gerontology* (2nd ed., pp. 1084—1088). New York: McGraw-Hill.

McCaffery, M., & Beebe, A. (1989). *Pain: Clinical manual for nursing practice* (7). St. Louis: Mosby.

Miller, C. A. (1991). Driving the temperature up-and-down. *Geriatric Nursing, 12,* 44–48.

Reuler, J. B. (1990). Hypothermia. In C. K. Cassel, D. E. Riesenberg, L. B. Sorensenk, & J. R. Walsh (Eds.), *Geriatric medicine* (2nd ed., pp. 579–584). New York: Springer-Verlag.

Richardson, D., Tyra, J., & McCray, A. (1992). Attenuation of the cutaneous vasoconstrictor response to cold in elderly men. *Journal of Gerontology, 47,* M211–M214.

Russell, M., Cummings, B., Profitt, B., Wysocki, C., Gilbert, A., & Cotman, C. (1993). Life span changes in the verbal categorization of odors. *Journal of Gerontology,* 49–53.

Serby, M., Larson, P., & Kalkstein, D. (1991). The nature and course of olfactory deficits in Alzheimer's disease. *American Journal of Psychiatry, 148,* 357–359.

Stevens, J. C. & Cain, W. S. (1993). Changes in taste and flavors in aging. *Critical Reviews in Food Science & Nutrition, 33,* 27–37.

BIBLIOGRAPHY

Brady, B. A., & Nesbitt, S. N. (1991). Using the right touch. *Nursing '91,* 46–47.

Brockopp, D., Warden, S., Colclough, G., and Brockopp, G. (1993). Nursing knowledge: Acute postoperative pain management in the elderly. *Journal of Gerontological Nursing, 19.*

DeGraff, C., Polet, T. & VanStaveren, W. (1994). Sensory perceptions and pleasantness of food flavors for older subjects. *Journal of Gerontology, 49*(3), 93–99.

Doty, R. L. (1990). Olfaction. In F. Boller & J. Grafman (Eds.), *Handbook of neuropsychology* (pp. 213–228). New York: Elsevier.

Ebersole, P., & Hess, P. (1990). *Toward healthy aging: human needs and nursing responses* (3rd ed.). St. Louis: Mosby.

Malsasanos, L., Barkauskas, V., & Stoltenberg-Allen, K. (1990). *Health assessment* (4th ed.). St. Louis: Mosby.

Murphy, C. (1993). Nutrition and chemosensory perception in the elderly subjects. *Critical Reviews in Food Science & Nutrition, 33,* 3–15.

Schiffman, S. (1983). Taste and smell in disease. *New England Journal of Medicine, 308,* 1275–1279.

Ship, J. A., & Weiffenbach, J. M. (1993). Age, gender, medical treatment, and medication effects on smell identification. *Journal of Gerontology, 47,* P35–P40.

Swartz, M. H. (1989). *Textbook of physical diagnosis.* Philadelphia: W. B. Saunders.

Vortherms, R. C. (1991). Clinically improving communication through touch. *Journal of Gerontological Nursing, 17,* 6–10.

Problems With Sight

Objectives

1. Identify physiologic changes that occur in the vision of an older adult.
2. Discuss common psychological changes that occur in older adults as their vision declines.
3. List appropriate patient teaching measures for nurses to include in the nursing care of visually impaired patients.
4. Demonstrate appropriate assessment techniques in evaluating an older adult's vision.
5. Demonstrate nursing care for a visually impaired patient.

INTRODUCTION

MOST OLDER ADULTS RETAIN EYESIGHT that is sufficient for activities of daily living; however, by age 70, poor vision is the rule rather than the exception. Visual changes begin precipitously around age 40 and continue to increase gradually throughout the life span. Some of these changes in vision represent natural annoyances, whereas others represent significant disease. Because the changes occur gradually, they often go unnoticed until the older adult exhibits marked changes in behavior or ability to manage daily life.

The effect of declining vision in older adults is evident in many ways. For example, declining vision makes reading labels under glaring light difficult. This may lead to an inability to buy food and cook, which may further result in poor eating habits. Alterations in depth perception may make discerning the blue steps from the blue floor almost impossible. In addition, falls occur more often with declining vision and lip reading for the hearing impaired can no longer be used to compensate for sensory changes. As these limitations occur, the sight-impaired older adult experiences loss of independence, which often results in feelings of frustration, boredom, anger, and isolation from others. As a result of visual limitations and loss, he or she may need help with activities such as driving, reading, hobbies, and work. The ability to perform these activities with assistance will bring pleasure and reinforce feelings of personal worth and ability.

Staab, AS and Hodges, LC: ESSENTIALS OF GERONTOLOGICAL NURSING,
© 1996 J. B. Lippincott Company

For those with good eyesight, it is difficult to realize the limitations imposed on an older adult's life by poor vision. Visual and hearing losses, readily apparent with age, are often taken for granted by health care professionals. As a result, many problems are missed. The nurse is in an excellent position for determining if vision problems exist while assessing the older adult's ability to perform activities of daily living. In addition, the nurse can support and assist the patient and family in making referrals for medical evaluation, locating needed resources such as low-vision aides, and counseling on how to live with vision problems. The nurse can teach specific interventions to enhance the patient's ability to remain independent and productive at home and in the community.

Clinical Pearl

Assessment: The ability to see is closely linked with the way people manage their daily lives. Loss of vision, whether limited loss or total blindness, affects an older adult's ability to function and to maintain independence.

NORMAL PHYSIOLOGIC CHANGES

Many normal physiologic changes in the eyes are associated with aging. These include diminished peripheral vision, diminished upward gaze, and decreased tear production resulting in dry eyes. Arcus senilis (a ring around the limbus of the eye), yellowing of the sclera, and a sunken appearance of the eye (due to loss of periorbital fat), is also commonly found. The four major changes affecting lifestyle are poor accommodation, altered color perception, sensitivity to light and glare, and decreased visual acuity.

POOR ACCOMMODATION

Accommodation, the ability to focus on objects at various distances, decreases from age 5 onward, and by age 40 to 50, most people recognize the need to hold objects farther away to properly focus. You may have heard an older adult say, "My arms must be growing shorter, I can't hold the paper far enough away to read it." This change in ability to accommodate is caused by the increased density and rigidity of the lens resulting from lost elasticity. The term *presbyopia* (presby meaning "old" and opys meaning "eye") is often used to describe this change in the aging eye. Presbyopia means that the near point increases or that the closest distance from the eye at which an object can be seen clearly increases. This vision problem often results in an inability to see small details, such as a buttonhole, directions on medication bottles, or telephone numbers.

ALTERED COLOR PERCEPTION

The lens of the eye yellows for unknown reasons with age and causes an inability to discriminate shortwave-length colors at the blue end of the spectrum, such as blue, violet, and green. Pastel or pale colors and dark brown, black, and dark blue may also be difficult to distinguish, because they tend to be seen as blending together. Colors most easily differentiated by older adults are yellows, oranges, and reds. Some difficulty with color perception is linked to the yellowing of the lens and impaired transmission of light through the retina with advancing age (Ebersole & Hess, 1994).

SENSITIVITY TO LIGHT AND GLARE

The ability of the aging eye to adapt to changes in light levels (too much or too little illumination) decreases. These changes occur primarily because there is a decrease in the size and elasticity of the pupil of the eye resulting from diminished elasticity of the iris. Thus, the pupil of the older adult's eye is normally small and somewhat fixed.

The small pupil size does not allow sufficient light into the eye, so more light is needed to see adequately. Older adults may need to increase the wattage of light bulbs or to carry a flashlight at night to visualize steps and keyholes. This problem is often called "night blindness." When an older adult goes from dark to light and back to dark, it takes the pupil much longer to adjust to the change than that of a younger person. This occurs because as the pupil size becomes smaller, the amount of light that reaches the retina is affected, thus limiting the efficiency of pupillary constriction and dilation.

In contrast to these lower illumination problems, increased light can produce glare. It has been suggested that increased opacity in the lens of the normal eye is the primary cause of the increasing sensitivity to glare (Burnside, 1988). Glare is a harsh, uncomfortable, brilliant light, such as sunlight. Based on this definition, it is easy to imagine the anguish and frustration such glare can promote in older adults experiencing this normal aging change in their eyes. Shiny surfaces, such as well-polished floors, can often produce a blinding glare and visual distortion to older adults. Thus, when increasing light levels, the light should be evenly distributed to minimize the glare.

DECREASED VISUAL ACUITY

Visual acuity, or the sharpness of one's vision, begins to diminish around age 40. After this time there is a sharp decline. The decline in visual acuity is probably the result of changes in the crystalline lens and vitreous humor (Corso, 1987). These changes occur because the lens gradually loses the ability to change shape. Other changes contributing to decreased visual acuity include a flattening of the cornea, which results in astigmatism and blurring of vision. Reduced ocular muscle strength resulting in diminished ability to maintain an upward gaze and sustained convergence is also common.

By age 65, most older adults have a visual acuity of 20/70 (what can be seen at 20 ft, a person with perfect vision can see from 70 ft) or less. These age-related changes in the eye have been likened to the close-up camera shot of a single flower that has a blurred background effect. Aging vision results in an image with a muted, dim backdrop behind the focal point. Older adults report that the inability to see well affects their lifestyle and prevents them from doing things they want to do.

ABNORMAL PHYSIOLOGIC CHANGES

Cataracts, glaucoma, and macular degeneration are common visual diseases caused by aging. Although these diseases are prevalent in the older adult, they can also occur in younger people and can even be present at birth. Good health habits play an important role in preventing such diseases because they can influence all aspects of the older adult's life.

CATARACTS

One of the most common vision diseases caused by aging changes in the lens of the eye is cataracts. The lens hardens and becomes compact. Opacity, or clouding of the eye's lens, blocks or changes the passage of light needed for vision. The origin is not known, however, cataracts often develop as a person ages. The tendency to form cataracts may run in families. Cataracts may also occur after an eye injury, from disease, or appear after prolonged use of certain medications, such as cortisone. As the cataract forms, the older adult may experience blurred vision without pain, possibly double vision, seeing spots or "ghost images," increased sensitivity to glare, and frequent changes of glasses that don't seem to help. Surgery is indicated to restore vision when the patient's lifestyle is affected.

GLAUCOMA

Another disease commonly affecting visual acuity in the older adult is glaucoma. This disease is manifested by increased pressure in the eye that can lead to damage to the optic nerve and to loss of vision. If untreated, it leads to progressive and irreversible loss of, peripheral vision and then central vision. This type of glaucoma, called "chronic open-angle glaucoma," is the most common type of glaucoma affecting older adults. Hereditary factors and diabetes increase the risk for glaucoma. Blacks, people taking cortisone medication, and aging individuals are at risk for glaucoma. It can also occur secondary to infections, injury, swollen cataracts, and tumors. As the pressure in the eye increases, the older adult may experience:

- Frequent changes of glasses that don't seem to help
- Loss of peripheral or side vision
- Inability to adjust eyes to darkened rooms
- Blurred or foggy vision, especially on awakening.

To relieve the pressure, a combination of oral drugs and eye drops may be prescribed and must be taken throughout life. If these are not successful, laser surgery may be necessary.

MACULAR DEGENERATION

A third common eye disease affecting visual acuity is macular degeneration. This is a condition in which the macula (a tiny portion of the retina that controls central vision) begins to degenerate. This deterioration of the macula may be caused by arteriosclerosis, a hereditary factor, trauma, or other less understood factors and results in a painless, slowly progressing loss of central vision. Peripheral vision is not lost, thus total blindness does not occur.

As the macula degenerates, the older adult may experience straight lines ap-

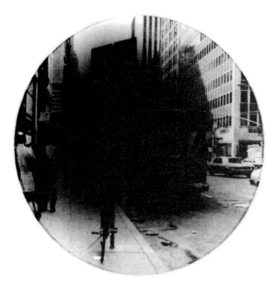

Figure 7-1. Macular degneration is a prevalent eye disease. The area of decreased central vision, called a central scotoma, is shown. The peripheral, or traveling, vision remains unaffected. (Courtesy of the Lighthouse, Low Vision Service, New York Association for the Blind.)

pearing wavy, such as a telephone pole or a distant landscape, type on a page becoming blurry, and dark or empty spaces appearing in the center of the field of vision (Fig. 7-1). Patients have difficulty with reading, sewing, driving, and recognizing faces but usually can manage independently with little difficulty when in a familiar setting. They usually do need assistance when away from familiar areas. In a very few cases, laser therapy can halt this disease. In most cases, however, no effective medicine or medical intervention is available. Low-vision aids, such as a magnifying glass, can be used to enhance remaining sight.

PSYCHOSOCIAL ISSUES

A visual impairment causes serious physical, social, and economic results that require a major adjustment to life (Allen, 1990). As persons age, they are forced to learn new styles of coping with activities and demands of daily living. Concomitant illness, memory changes, and/or other sensory losses can make these adaptations even more difficult. Thus, the older adult must cope with emotional reactions as well as physical alterations.

The major psychosocial effect of poor vision in older adults is isolation. As routine tasks become more difficult and exhausting, as usual sources of entertainment become impossible, and as the risk and fear of falling soar, older adults may feel less competent and valued. Many choose not to ask for help either from fear of becoming a burden and/or of being taken advantage of or because of ingrained personality traits. This is tragic when there is such a great need, physically and emotionally, for interaction with others.

Older adults who are isolated from adequate stimuli or interaction with others by failing sensory organs or reduced environmental stimuli can exhibit numerous psychological reactions (Ebersole & Hess, 1994). These reactions are important to note because they are often attributed to confusion or to being old. Psychological reactions resulting from declining vision may include:

- Amplification of dependent roles
- Increased need for socialization and physical stimulation due to the isolated individual's perceptual deprivation
- Diminished ability to perceive size and shape, altered motor coordination (thus enhancing falls), and diminished tactile accuracy
- Emotional reactions, such as boredom, restlessness, irritability, anxiety, and panic
- Loss of attentiveness and diminished reality testing and level of consciousness
- Decreased ability to learn and to think resulting from monotony brought on by isolation from others and from activities
- Marked behavior changes, such as inability to solve problems, hallucinations and delusions, poor task performance, increased aggression, inability to sleep or too much sleep, emotional lability, and confusion
- Isolation or sensory deprivation resulting from illness.

Most older adults tend to compensate for declining vision by using other sensory systems, making environmental modifications, and using social support systems. They have a wealth of experiences that make them less vulnerable to sensory deprivation.

NURSING ASSESSMENT

Declining vision affects a person's ability to function independently and puts him or her at risk for becoming isolated. To determine whether vision problems are occurring, the nurse must perform a functional assessment that includes the patient's ability to perform activities of daily living and an assessment of how well he or she is coping with the vision loss. In addition, because vision declines gradually with aging and symptoms may be subtle and may go undetected, a gross complete history and physical examination is performed to determine if referral to an ophthalmologist is needed.

HISTORY AND INTERVIEW

The history may be very important in assessing the extent of the visual problem, because many of the problems encountered occur gradually. The older adult may have unconsciously made some long-term adjustments. Questions that are useful in determining whether failing vision is causing functional problems include the following:

- Has there been any change in your vision?
- Do you wear glasses? Are they as helpful now as they were when you got them?
- Do you live alone? If yes, are there people nearby who assist you if needed?
- How well are you able to navigate in your place of residence?
- Is food selection at the grocery store and preparation at home a problem?
- Do you have problems meeting your personal needs, such as washing, shaving, and cleaning your teeth or dentures?
- Is it difficult to see medication labels or colors? Do you have other problems with taking medications?
- Is transportation a problem? Do you drive? If yes, are you having any problems with this? If no, how do you get where you need to/want to go?

- Do you have problems seeing at night? In ordinarily lit areas?
- Can you see the telephone dial and phone book?

The nurse will also illicit information about problems with sensory deprivation, such as boredom and loneliness. Suggested questions include the following:

- What do you do in a usual day?
- What do you do for pleasure (reading, watching TV, performing crafts, gardening, sewing)?
- Do you get out much? Does your eyesight interfere with getting out?
- Are you participating in desired recreational activities, or is visual loss restricting this?
- What other problems, if any, are you having because your vision is poor (social, concerns, fears)?

RISK FACTORS

Various factors have been suggested as contributing to vision problems. Ultraviolet rays have been associated with damage to the photoreceptor cells of the retina. Warmer environmental temperatures have been linked to the earlier age of onset of presbyopia. Numerous factors, such as lower socioeconomic status, infections, chronic disease, and certain medications, have been associated with the development of cataracts.

PHYSICAL EXAMINATION

The physical examination should include objective observations to confirm the subjective data illicited. Things to notice include the following:

- Does the patient feel the flooring cautiously with the foot before taking a step when floor coloring or texture changes?
- Is the patient's clothing soiled or spotted?
- Does the patient use hands rather than eyes to orient himself or herself (such as touching the back and seat of the chair to determine where to sit)?
- Does clothing match?
- Does the patient wear dark glasses or a hat to decrease glare?
- Does the patient look at you or just past your ear when talking as if seeing with peripheral rather than central vision? (Carnevali, 1993; Sullivan, 1983).

Physical examination of the external eye should be done by inspecting both eyes and surrounding structures for symmetry and deviations from normal. Although there may be some differences, they should be more similar than dissimilar. Eyes may appear sunken—this is considered a normal finding.

Notice if there is any swelling of the eyelids, whether they are soft and pliable, and the direction of the growth. Entropion (lid turned inward) and ectropion (lid turned outward) are significant because of the resulting dryness and irritation to the cornea and sclera. Notice any excessive tearing or inflammation around the lacrimal or tear ducts. Gently pull the eyelids back and notice whether there are lesions in the conjunctiva. Normal findings for the lids would be no lid lag, no inflammation and wrinkling in the skin of the eyelids, and soft bulges of fatty tissues seen especially in the lower lids and the inner third of the upper ones.

The color of the sclera as well as any growths should be inspected. The sclera should be white with no growths. The conjunctiva should be pink and noninflamed but may appear dry due to age-related change of diminished tear production.

The iris should be assessed for color, breaks or nicks (such as in previous cataract surgery), and whether arcus senilis is present (Fig. 7-2). The iris should be round and intact in the aging eye.

> ## Clinical Pearl
>
> *Assessment: Arcus senilis is an opaque, graying ring surrounding the cornea, caused by a deposit of fat. It is usually benign and of no consequence in older adults. It is easily assessed with the pupillary reaction.*

Note whether pupils are equal, round, and react to light and accommodation. Also, check for consensual pupil response. Pupil size may be somewhat diminished in the aged eye, causing impaired accommodation. It may be difficult to detect pupillary response because of a slowed and diminished pupillary reaction to light. Be aware that the older adult's eyes may be sensitive to light due to disease processes. The sequence for evaluating pupillary reaction to accommodation in the older adult should be done quickly and with care to avoid long periods of direct light into the eyes. Physical examination should also include use of a standard Snellen's vision chart to determine visual acuity. If the patient is unable to read letters, arrows can be used. Alternatively, the nurse can hold up fingers before the patient: identification of the number of fingers being shown will be recorded as finger perception. If the patient cannot iden-

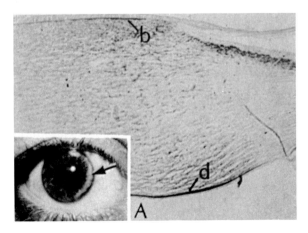

Figure 7-2. Patient with arcus senilis.

tify fingers, pass the penlight across your body. The ability to identify that a light was used is recorded as light perception. For general screening for presbyopia, ask the patient to read a newspaper held at a distance of about 12 inches from his or her face.

Visual fields should be checked to assess the scope of peripheral gaze. This test will help determine whether the patient can see peripherally or has central (tunnel) vision. Although the visual field can be precisely assessed by an ophthalmologist, the nurse can grossly evaluate any general problems with peripheral vision (Smeltzer & Bare, 1992).

Assessment of the visual fields is essential, because some loss of peripheral vision is a normal aging change. If greater than a 20-degree lateral loss of peripheral vision is present, the finding is considered abnormal. When assessing visual fields, one eye should be compared with the other. The older adult with greatly decreased visual fields should be referred to an ophthalmologist.

Extraocular movements should be evaluated to look for weakness or imbalance of the six extraocular muscles. Older adults may have difficulty focusing on near objects, so it may be necessary to make the measured distance greater for them than for young people. If nystagmus is present, it may indicate a neurologic problem, and further evaluation by an ophthalmologist is warranted.

An ophthalmoscopic examination is a very valuable part of the assessment of the fundus of the eye (that portion of the eye posterior to the lens) and should be included in evaluating the older adult's vision.

DIAGNOSTIC TESTS

The nurse must be familiar with the more common diagnostic studies and tools used in a vision assessment. Initial screening usually incorporates evaluation for intraocular pressure using tonometry, myopia, and presbyopia using a Snellen's chart and macular degeneration using an Amsler's pocket grid. These studies can be administered by the nurse and then referrals made to appropriate specialists.

Intraocular pressure, seen with glaucoma, can be measured by tonometry. The tonometer uses a puff of air to measure intraocular pressure and requires practice on the part of the operator and the older adult's cooperation during the test. The force of the air puff should be demonstrated on the patient's finger to avoid startling him or her. The normal range of intraocular pressure is 12 to 21 mm ttg.

Myopia and presbyopia are tested using a standardized Snellen's chart. The Amsler's pocket grid is used to test for macular degeneration. It is a hand-held portable device that is easy to use and has instructions printed on the card. Patients with visual acuity scores of greater than 20/50 or positive results on a test for macular degeneration are referred to the ophthalmologist.

 Clinical Pearl

Assessment: Advise anyone who cannot read newsprint from 1 ft away with glasses on to see an opthalmologist.

NURSING DIAGNOSES

Visual impairments often hinder an older adult's ability to take necessary actions to maintain self-care. The nurse must judge the patient's ability to perform activities independently and then must assist the patient and significant others as they coordinate and provide care. Some selected nursing diagnoses for a patient with a vision problem may include the following:

- Sensory or Perceptual Alterations related to vision impairment resulting from the aging process
- Social Isolation related to vision deficit and inability to drive
- Self-Care Deficits related to vision impairment
- Impaired Mobility related to vision deficit
- Altered Thought Processes related to sensory-perceptual deficits
- Knowledge Deficit related to lack of education about vision problems, resources available, visual aids, medical treatment, therapeutic interventions, how to adapt emotionally
- Altered Health Maintenance related to vision impairment
- Altered Nutrition: Less Than Body Requirements related to inability to obtain and prepare food
- Anxiety related to uncertainty of vision deficit
- High Risk for Injury related to visual losses.

NURSING INTERVENTIONS

The nurse's interventions should involve health promotion as well as disease prevention and detection activities. Nurses have a role in encouraging older adults to seek vision care. As long as the older adult thinks nothing can be done for vision problems, he or she will do nothing.

COMMUNICATION

Communication tips must be known and practiced by the older adult with vision problems and by the nurse caring for him or her. See the Patient Teaching Box for tips that nurses can teach patients about positive communication skills.

When communicating with the visually impaired older adult, the nurse should follow the guidelines listed below. These guidelines may need to be altered depending on the amount of visual loss the older adult is experiencing.

- Always identify yourself and those with you. Don't expect the older adult to remember your voice. Also state when you are leaving to make the person aware of your departure.
- Give directions before an intervention, for example, "Just two more steps and you can sit down on your bed." The nurse should speak before handing the blind person an object.
- Approach the patient from the front rather than from the rear.
- Ask if the patient wants or needs assistance. Do not assume that he or she always does.
- Help the patient locate or touch both arms of the chair when sitting. In addition, teach the patient to use his or her hands to locate the edges of tables, shelves, and chairs.

Patient Teaching Box
COMMUNICATION TIPS

1. When you walk into a room, ask a friend or nearby person to tell you who is in the room.
2. Use the talking books from your local library to keep in touch with what is going on in the world.
3. Use tape casettes to keep in touch with family and friends if writing is difficult or impossible.
4. Join a self-help group with other visually impaired older adults to share your concerns and successes in coping with your vision problems.
5. Ask a neighbor or friend to read your mail to you.
6. Use writing guides to help with such tasks as writing checks and addressing envelopes. Obtaining these may prolong independence in these areas.
7. Listen to the radio for the broadcasting of news from local newspapers and national magazines. There are special radio stations established especially to serve visually impaired listeners. These stations can be heard only through special receivers issued free to the visually impaired population by participating radio stations. To locate the station in your area, contact the Association of Radio Reading Services at 1010 Vermont Street, NW, Suite 1100, Washington, D.C. 20005; (202) 347-0992.

Adapted from AARP brochure "Aging & Vision: Making the Most of Impaired Vision" (1987).

- When walking with a visually impaired person, allow the person to place his or her arm or hand on your arm. This allows him or her to sense the direction you are going and generally to feel more secure than if you hold the arm to guide him or her.
- Teach the patient to imagine the plate of food as a clock and locate the foods in this manner. The nurse should describe what food is at each "time," such as meat at 6, cake at 12.
- Describe surroundings if they are unfamiliar. Because most visually impaired older adults were sighted at one time, describe the beauty of the surroundings when possible, so they can enjoy memories of the beauty being described (Ebersole & Hess, 1994). When the patient has changed settings, the nurse must remember to orient the patient to the layout of the room, remove clutter, simplify the setting if possible, and not to change the location of objects without the patient knowing about it.
- Encourage the patient to be assertive in letting others know what kind of help is useful and what is not (Carnevali, 1993). Remember that there are many degrees of visual impairment; allow as much independence as possible.
- Speak normally, but not from a distance. Do not raise or lower your voice. Do not alter your vocabulary; words such as "see" and "blind" are parts of normal speech.

Although enhancing communication skills will improve the health care provided for visually impaired older adults, many older adults who could be helped by glasses or other medical interventions often do not seek vision care. There are a number of prevalent theories why older adults do not seek health care for poor vision. First, insurance may not cover routine eye examinations, and the cost may be prohibitive. Second, many older adults assume that poor eyesight is normal and therefore nothing can be done to help. Third, many fear losing their independence by admitting vision problems. Last, most changes in the aging eye occur gradually, making it hard for individuals to determine when the problem is severe enough to seek medical attention.

ADAPTATION AND PATIENT TEACHING

Planning interventions includes applying knowledge of normal aging changes, the patient's unique visual problems and other problems, and the patient's level of independence and motivation. The following techniques are potential interventions for helping the older adult adapt to visual impairment:

- Use good contrast between the background and lettering of printed materials. Paper should have a dull finish, and large lettering should be used.
- Make the environment visible by enlarging certain items. Obtain large-print books or talking books for patients who enjoy reading. Information about such books is available from state and local libraries. Enlarged plastic number inserts for the telephone, large-print rulers, and measuring tapes and cups improve the visibility of items important to daily living. Games such as Scrabble, crossword puzzles, dominos, and cards are available in large, high-contrast print.
- Use contrasting colors, for example, between doorways and walls, dishes and tablecloth, and the risers and flat surfaces of steps.
- Use dots of glue or other raised material to distinguish medicine bottles or the dials on the washing machine to help find appropriate settings.
- Leave a night-light on at night and provide adequate lighting at all times. Lighting, particularly at night, should be at a similar level in all rooms. A night-light in the bedroom and bathroom might be appropriate.
- Use handrails when there is an abrupt change in lighting. Older adults should be taught to wait until they have adapted to the light before continuing to walk.
- Recommend avoiding driving at night. Be aware of poor lighting and the fact that the older person may be unable to see obstacles, read signs, or recognize familiar people when the lighting is poor.
- Avoid glare from windows and shiny surfaces, such as floors and table-tops. Provide sunglasses or a big brimmed hat when going outdoors if this seems to help.
- Avoid interpreting inability to identify colors as a sign of confusion. Likewise, do not use color coding as a mechanism for differentiating medicines or room assignments or other important information.
- Move closer to things to improve the ability to see them. Assure visually impaired older adults that it is acceptable to get closer to the object they are interested in, such as the TV or sewing.
- Provide touch often to reassure visually impaired older adults, particularly those patients confined to a wheelchair or bed. This stimulation prevents a sense of isolation and despair.

Additional nursing interventions for adapting to visual impairment include care of eyeglasses and the use of canes.

Canes serve a dual purpose for the visually impaired older adult. Canes can detect changes in surfaces and objects in the older adult's path and serve to add stability to walking. Poor compliance in using a cane is often noted, because the older adult does not want others to know that he or she needs the cane for assistance.

In teaching the older adult and the family to care for eyeglasses, emphasis should be placed on handling the glasses by the frames only, cleaning with mild soap and water or a cleaning solution, and drying with a soft cloth or tissue without fibers or other particles. The eyeglasses should be kept in a case when not worn and repaired when lens are scratched or frames bent.

Patient Teaching Box
TIPS FOR VISUAL HEALTH

- Get an eye exam every year. This helps you find out if your vision is changing and allows for prompt treatment of problems.
- See your doctor promptly if you have sudden or unexplained vision changes.
- Budget for an eye exam, even if you can't get insurance reimbursement. It's the best investment there is in good vision. Find out what free services, such as glaucoma testing, are offered in your community by contacting your state National Society for the Prevention of Blindness affiliate.
- Know the difference in kinds of eye care professionals:
  Ophthalmologists—Doctors of medicine, licensed to practice both medicine and surgery. They can prescribe glasses and contact lenses and they specialize in all aspects of eye and vision care.
  Optometrists—Doctors of optometry who are licensed specialists in select areas of eye and vision care. They may screen for vision problems and prescribe glasses. They do not prescribe medicines or perform surgery.
  Opticians—Skilled, certified professionals who make, fit, adjust, and sell glasses, contact lenses, and other optical devices prescribed by an ophthalmologist or optometrist.
- Read brochures available from your eye doctor, your local hospital, clinics, or public libraries.
- Talk to your eye doctor about your eyes and your vision. Question anything about which you feel uncertain.
- Find out if you are in a high-risk group. Certain eye conditions and diseases become more common as people get older.
- Follow prescribed eye medicine schedules. Skipping a dose or not following directions can be dangerous and lead to worsening of eye conditions.
- Make the best use of the vision you have. Devices designed for the blind or low-visioned patient are available and can enhance your ability to read, travel, and care for yourself.
- Protect your eyes against injuries. This includes reading instructions and suggested precautions for all equipment, sprays, and other supplies; knowing emergency procedures in case of an eye injury; and wearing safety glasses or goggles when appropriate.
- Avoid any driving situation that is uncomfortable for you, such as driving at night, on wet roads, during rush hour, or on long trips. Poor vision, increased sensitivity to glare, reduced night vision, diminished ability to accommodate to light changes, and other age-related changes, such as diminished coordination and slower reaction time, can combine to make accidents more likely to happen (National Society for the Prevention of Blindness, 500 East Remington Road, Schaumburg, IL 60173, (312) 843–2020).

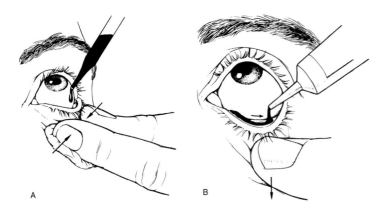

Figure 7-3. When administering eye drops, have the patient look upward while placing the eye drops into the lower conjunctival sac. When administering an eye ointment, have the patient look upward, evert the lower lid, and apply the ointment along the outer portion of the lower lid.

The National Society for the Prevention of Blindness, in a series of leaflets entitled "Life Sight," has produced a list of health promotion, prevention, and detection tips that are pertinent to older adults and should be a part of patient teaching. The Patient Teaching Box entitled Tips for Visual Health includes tips for proper prevention and detection that can help ensure good vision for a lifetime.

Administration of Eye Medications

The appropriate technique and specific patient instructions for administering eye drops and eye ointment are illustrated in Figure 7-3. The nurse should instruct the older adult and a caregiver in the proper technique.

Nursing Care Plan

FOR PATIENTS WITH VISION IMPAIRMENT

Nursing Diagnosis: Sensory or Perceptual Alterations: Visual related to uncompensated visual loss.

Definition: A state in which the invidual experiences, or is at risk of experiencing, a change in the amount, pattern, or interpretation of visual stimuli.

Assessment Findings:
1. Inability to read newsprint or identify objects or persons
2. Withdrawal, agitation, isolation
3. Refusal or inability to perform usual self-care activities
4. Inability to think clearly or express ideas clearly; confusion
5. Increase in ritualistic behaviors to enhance a sense of security
6. Fearfulness and paranoid tendencies; may blame others for their inabilities or difficulties
7. Increased dependency behaviors
8. Diminished ability to follow directions
9. Impaired memory

(continued)

Nursing Care Plan

FOR PATIENTS WITH VISION IMPAIRMENT *(Continued)*

Nursing Interventions with Selected Rationales:

1. Assess the vision loss for undetected disease, severity of visual loss, and its effect on the older adult's ability to maneuver and function in the environment and to communicate with others.
   Rationale: Assessment provides a baseline from which further changes can be detected.
2. Make referrals to appropriate clinicians for more detailed examination if problems are discovered.
   Rationale: Referrals for services provide continued support and follow-up.
3. Compensate for visual losses by adding color and contrast to the environment, such as using reds/yellows/oranges, which are more easily seen than blues/greens, or putting contrasting color strips next to stairs or changes in height or texture of the floor; avoiding glare-producing lights, floors, and large glass windows; providing multiple lights; providing night-lights to prevent dramatic changes in the amount of light available from room to room.
   Rationale: Attempts to compensate for deficiencies may help prevent injury.
4. Encourage the patient to maximize existing strengths, such as the ability to hear and touch.
   Rationale: Maximizing existing strengths promotes a positive self-image.
5. Keep pathways free of clutter, do not rearrange furniture or personal items, and avoid falls.
   Rationale: Avoiding clutter and rearranging items maintains independence.
6. Provide access to visual aides, such as talking books, large-print books, calendars and games, handrails, hand-held or table-stand magnifying glasses, and medication boxes for the visually disabled.
   Rationale: Visual aids help the patient adjust to deficit and enhance self-esteem.
7. Educate the patient and family regarding optimal care of assistive devices, including maintenance, proper fit, and cleaning. Remind patients that they should have their eyes checked annually to detect vision changes and to ensure that glasses are providing optimum assistance.
   Rationale: Patient and family education promotes compliance.
8. Provide support for the older adult patient as he or she struggles to adapt to vision losses, allowing time to ventilate and grieve over this devastating loss. Keeping a functional perspective, if possible, focusing on the patient's remaining capabilities rather than on disabilities.
   Rationale: Verbalization of feelings allows the patient to adapt to deficits.

Desired Patient Outcomes/Discharge Criteria:

1. Patient acquires glasses or other corrective aides to assist with visual deficit.
2. Patient is able to function at an optimal level of independence in the home (or in a permanent living arrangement).
3. Patient and family understand the care and maintenance of visual assistive devices.
4. Patient interacts with others socially and attends social functions in the community rather than isolating self.
5. Patient and family members voice an understanding that vision loss is a threat to security and self-esteem.
6. Patient and family demonstrate use of therapeutic approaches (including alterations in the patient's home environment that would promote independence).

REFERENCES

Allen, M. (1990). Adjusting to visual impairment. *Journal of Opthalmic Nursing and Technology,* 9(2), 47–51.

Burnside, I. (1988). *Nursing and the aged* (3rd ed.). St. Louis: McGraw-Hill.

Carnevali, D. L. (1993). *Nursing management for the elderly* (3rd ed.).

Corso, J. F. (1987). Sensory-perceptual processes and aging. *Annual Review of Gerontology and Geriatrics,* 7, 29–50.

Ebersole, P., & Hess, P. (1994). *Toward health aging* (4th ed.). St. Louis: Mosby.

Smeltzer, S. & Bare, B. (1992). In *Textbook of medical surgical nursing* (7th ed.) by Brunner & Suddarth. Philadelphia: J. B. Lippincott.

Sullivan, N. (1983). Vision in the elderly. *Journal of Gerontological Nursing,* 9(4), 228–235.

BIBLIOGRAPHY

American Association of Retired Persons (AARP). (1987). Aging and vision: Making the most of impaired vision. Pamphlet #LL3652 (9-87).

Assessing the meaning of life among older adult clients. (1992). *Journal of Gerontological Nursing,* 18(9), 19–29.

Bates, B. (1995). *A guide to physical examination* (6th ed.). Philadelphia: Lippincott.

Burggraf, V., & Stanley, M. (1989). *Nursing the elderly: A care plan approach.* Philadelphia: Lippincott.

Carotenuto, R., & Bullock, J. (1980). *Physical assessment of the gerontologic client.* Philadelphia: Davis.

Center for Health Statistics. (1988). Pacific Northwest Extension Publication #PNW 196. Oregon State University.

Colenbrander, A., et al. (1992). Low vision requirements for driving. *Journal of Opthalmic Nursing in Technology,* 11(3), 111–115.

Edmonds, S. E. (1990). Resources for the visually impaired. *Journal of Ophthalmic Nursing and Technology,* 16(1), 14–15.

Kirchner, C. (1988). *Data on blindness and visual impairment in the U.S.* New York: American Foundation for the Blind.

National Society to Prevent Blindness and Affiliates. *Healthy Habits that Promote Good Vision.* (500 East Remington Road, Schaumburg, IL 60173.)

Tavicius, D. D., & Bayne, M. V. (1991). Medical-surgical nursing: A nursing process approach. Philadelphia: W. B. Saunders.

Waterman, H. (1992). Visually impaired patient's perceptions of their needs in hospital. *Nurse Practitioner,* 5(3), 6–9.

Problems With Hearing

Objectives

1. List the physiologic changes of aging associated with hearing.
2. Describe the psychosocial changes of aging related to hearing loss.
3. Identify steps in the nursing assessment of a patient with hearing loss.
4. List nursing diagnoses associated with hearing loss.
5. Design nursing interventions for the patient with hearing loss.
6. Develop a nursing care plan for a patient with hearing impairment.

INTRODUCTION

DEAFNESS IS ONE OF THE CRUELEST FORMS of sensory deprivation. Unlike blindness, it often provokes ridicule rather than sympathy. The deaf person may appear stupid because he or she is unable to hear what is said and is often unable to control his or her own voice. The person slowly isolates himself or herself, may become depressed, and often may be greeted by unsympathetic attitudes. Listening and talking can be comforting, enlightening, and reassuring.

Hearing impairment in the older adult should be viewed not only as a loss of the ability to hear but also as a deficit that can influence perception, behavior, and personality. The changes generally become more pronounced as the person grows older, affecting activities of daily living and lifestyle. Correcting hearing problems that result from the normal aging process may present financial, social, and emotional concerns. If not corrected, hearing problems may lead to family crises, injury, physical handicaps from falls, and increased risk for trauma from pedestrian or motor vehicles due to inability to sense danger with common warning signs. Social isolation and cognitive decline may also result.

Professional nursing expertise can alter the outcome of these problems; the nurse can assist the older adult to develop coping skills needed to modify the environment. The nurse should actively assist the older adult with hearing loss detection and intervention to enhance the capability for hearing, to decrease loneliness and isolation, and to decrease potential for trauma.

Staab, AS and Hodges, LC: ESSENTIALS OF GERONTOLOGICAL NURSING,
© 1996 J. B. Lippincott Company

NORMAL PHYSIOLOGIC CHANGES

Hearing loss is one of the most prevalent conditions affecting health. With each decade, hearing loss may increase. The ability to perceive speech may be further hampered by background sounds or noises or by distorted speech, such as with unfamiliar accents and speech impediments.

▷ *Clinical Pearl*

Assessment: A common misconception is equating deafness with mental retardation. Intelligence is normally distributed in the deaf population as it is in the hearing population.

In the older adult, the tympanic membrane becomes thinner, paler, and more fibrotic, reducing transmission of sounds. Impaction of dry, hardened earwax, or cerumen, which contains more keratin as one ages, interferes with the movement of the eardrum and transmission of sound. When sound waves transmitted from outside the ear through the canal and tympanic membrane are impeded, the term "conductive hearing loss of aging" is used.

Damage to the eighth cranial nerve and associated sensory and neural structures of the inner ear are classified as sensorineural hearing loss. It is also referred to as perceptive hearing loss. If both a conductive and sensorineural loss occur, it is termed a "mixed loss."

Presbycusis, hearing loss from the effects of aging, is a common occurrence with aging beginning early in life and progressing into the older years, often affecting more men than women. It is the gradual, progressive, symmetrical loss of the ability to hear high-pitched frequencies that over time involves the loss of middle and lower-pitched frequencies. This gradual bilateral loss is due to degenerative changes in the auditory nerve neurons (eighth cranial nerve) the ossicles, and the cochlea. Degenerative changes of aging, such as neuronal loss, changes in vascular supply, and biochemical and bioelectrical changes, may impair function of the middle ear, eighth cranial nerve, cochlea, and auditory nerve pathways. Gradual atrophy and degeneration of hair cells (cilia) and decreased blood supply to the cochlea probably leads to diminished discrimination ability. This change is particularly noted in the ability to hear consonants. Consonants such as *s, z, t, f,* and *g,* composed largely of high-frequency tones, may become indiscriminate. Diminished speech discrimination may be present even with very minimal hearing sensitivity loss; therefore, conversational speech may be significantly affected. The lower frequency sounds of vowels such as *a, e, i, o,* and *u* generally remain relatively intact and are the last sounds to diminish. These changes in audibility of consonants and vowels result in impaired clarity of speech as opposed to loss of volume (loudness). Therefore, one does not have to shout to be heard by the person with presbycusis but instead needs to alter word sounds or phrases to increase hearing perception.

Clinical Pearl

Intervention: When an older adult does not hear all that you've said, simply restate the phrase more slowly, giving him or her an opportunity to hear a different selection of vowels. Stand directly in front of the person to assist lipreading. Don't shout at the person; this can be interpreted as demeaning.

ABNORMAL CHANGES

Otosclerosis is a hereditary disease that begins in youth or early adulthood but is usually not detected until middle to late adulthood. Otosclerosis refers to a form of progressive bilateral hearing loss caused by the formation of new abnormal spongy bone in the labyrinth eventually immobilizing the stapes. Because the stapes is unable to vibrate and carry the stimulus of the vibrating malleus and incus, sound transmission to the inner ear is prevented.

Tinnitus, or a ringing or buzzing in the ear, is considered a mixed loss even though it may be present without significant loss of hearing. Tinnitus can also be associated with otosclerosis, tumors, and drug toxicity, especially aspirin and streptomycin.

Meniere's disease refers to an inner ear problem resulting from a dysfunction of the labyrinth. The cause of Meniere's disease is unknown. Usually, only one ear is involved.

PSYCHOSOCIAL ISSUES

Impaired ability to communicate may lead to social isolation and a loss of independence. Because hearing gradually decreases in acuity and function, the older adult may not realize the loss until it is significant and has become obvious to caregivers and family members. Older adults often hide their failure to hear or appear unaware of the severity of their hearing loss until they have reached a late stage of social isolation. It may take time before family and friends realize that the older person has canceled all social engagements and remains at home alone most of the time. By this time, there may be communication problems requiring intervention.

Communication problems place the older adult at greater risk for loss of independence, thereby reducing the motivation to adapt to the impairment and to experience new learning. Dependent behaviors increase and rituals take on very significant meaning, providing security and relief of fear. Other symptoms of severe loss include lethargy, withdrawal, anxiety, confusion, noncommunication, and refusal to perform usual personal care behaviors (Christian, Dluhy, & O'Neill, 1989).

The older person who lives in a world of sound distortion may exhibit increased fearfulness and paranoid tendencies resulting from increased anxiety and tension (Christian, Dluhy, & O'Neill, 1989). This paranoia may be exhibited by a fear of leaving the home due to risk of personal trauma, because the person can't hear sirens or car horns. Interaction with family and friends is often affected as the individual narrows his or her environment to one that feels safe. This attempt to cope may lead to a significant change in affect or orientation. Occasionally, hearing loss is confused with dementia. Some people with hearing problems will respond to all questions with a bland expression or a polite smile, because decreased hearing can promote confusion and impairment of language comprehension. Commonly, the elderly are tested for cognitive function. They may demonstrate diminished function not because of mental disability, but because of their inability to comprehend the explanations of the tester.

Clinical Pearl

Assessment: Many cognitive tests in dementia evaluation depend on the patient's ability to hear and see.

NURSING ASSESSMENT

Assessment of any hearing loss can be accomplished on gross examination by the nurse. For medical problems, the nurse should be a patient advocate and make a referral for more sophisticated testing by an audiologist, otologist, or neurologist.

When conducting a history and hearing examination, first determine how close to the patient to stand in order to be heard, understood, and still respect personal space. Territoriality is a strong factor among many elderly, especially in acute and extended care facilities, where patients may be wheelchair bound or bedridden with side rails posing natural barriers. Questions may have to be shortened, simplified, or reworded in the most common terms to achieve mutual understanding. Position yourself in easy view of the patient (this enhances lipreading) and speak directly toward him or her. Use slow and exaggerated speech. Lipreading may be more difficult for the older adult with cataracts or visual deficits. Speaking louder may make matters worse and speech discrimination more difficult. Maintain your voice in the lower frequency range, which is more likely to be heard. Shorten questions and keep the wording simple. If a patient has a hearing aid, check to see that it is being worn, is turned on, and the battery is still functional. If there is a language barrier, plan to have an interpreter, perhaps a family member, or give the patient a pencil and paper to write responses. Many people who have English as a second language can understand spoken and written English more than they can communicate by speaking. Speak directly to the patient, even though questions must be interpreted. Use expressiveness and gestures to enhance establishing rapport.

Clinical Pearl

Intervention: A good hearing aid can be made by placing the earpiece of the stethoscope into the patient's ears and talking into the diaphragm.

HISTORY AND INTERVIEW

A complete history of the symptoms the patient is experiencing and a quick assessment of the level of hearing loss and its effect on the person's ability to hear and verbally communicate should be done.

A hearing loss represents a change in amount, pattern, or interpretation of incoming stimuli as a result of physiologic or environmental disruptions. The patient's ability to hear directions can be determined by simply asking if he or she can hear your conversational level voice. Be alert to clues of communication problems. Some of the more common problem areas include a reluctance on the part of the patient to continue participating during interviews, lack of eye contact, inability to remember, answering questions or participating in conversation with inappropriate responses, short attention span, or signs of physical discomfort or fatigue. Persons with hearing deficits tend to apply selective concentration, hearing only what they want to hear and conserving their energy by ignoring what seems unimportant (listening can be fatiguing). Even mild hearing loss can considerably affect the patient's total well-being and lifestyle.

Evaluate the history of hearing loss, dizziness, vertigo, pain, or tinnitus with special attention to the onset. A self-administered questionnaire designed to detect emotional and social problems associated with impaired hearing can be administered.

RISK FACTORS

The older adult is not only faced with catabolic processes that cause hearing loss but also must contend with other contributing factors that lead to hearing impairment. Common among these are conditions producing high fevers, diabetes, syphilis, myxedema, traumatic injuries, and recurrent infections producing perforation or scarring of the eardrum. In addition, hearing loss has been reported as a result of exposure to environmental excessive noise, such as jets, guns, and construction and factory noise, and to ototoxic drugs, such as streptomycin, quinine, and salicylates.

PHYSICAL EXAMINATION

An acute unilateral complaint of hearing loss should alert the nurse that the condition is not related to the aging process. It may signify onset of acute illness, trauma, or lesions of the auditory nerve.

When performing the otologic exam on an older adult, consider the following:

- Place the largest speculum that will fit into the external canal on the otoscope.
- Straighten the ear canal by pulling upward and backward on the auricle. If pain occurs, it may indicate presence of otitis externa.
- Tilt the patient's head toward the opposite shoulder for ease of examination. This helps to compensate for the oblique direction of the ear canal.
- Note any cerumen (earwax) or hair follicles in the external canal. Earwax varies in color (brown to pale yellow), consistency (watery to hardened solid), and amount from person to person but is generally more solid in the older adult.
- Include visualization of the tympanic membrane eardrum.

Table 8-1	COLOR RELATED TO EARDRUM ABNORMALITY	
	Yellow/amber	Serum/fluid (serous otitis)
	Bluish	Blood behind the drum
	White/cotton-like growth	Infection (bacterial or fungal), purulence behind the eardrum
	Pink/red	Infection of the middle ear (myringitis)

The color of cerumen may be indicative of eardrum abnormalities. Table 8-1 highlights varying colors of earwax and specific conditions associated with them.

Tuning fork testing can be done to assess hearing and function of the eighth cranial nerve. If hearing is normal or if there is equal bilateral deafness, the tone will be heard equally in both ears. If the patient has sensorineural loss, the tone will be heard in the unimpaired ear. If conductive loss is present the tone will be heard better in the impaired ear. Rinne's test is used for testing bone versus air conduction. In normal hearing and sensorineural loss, the tone will be heard longer alongside of the ear (air conduction is greater than bone conduction). Patients who report hearing the tone equally well in both areas may have conductive and sensorineural (mixed) losses.

Hearing testing can be accomplished with an audiometer or on gross examination by speaking or discerning speech discrimination (Serra, 1988). Gross hearing can be determined by using the watch-tick test and standing behind the person while asking simple questions in a normal tone of voice. Don't ask yes or no questions, but rather, ask questions that are open ended, such as the day of the week or the condition of the weather. If the patient cannot see you, his or her ability to lip-read or read body language is obstructed. Speak slowly and vary the tone of your voice.

DIAGNOSTIC TESTS

The most important diagnostic test for detecting hearing problems is the audiogram. The audiogram consists of a sound stimulus (either a pure or musical tone or spoken word) that is used to determine the ability to hear and discriminate sounds. Other lab tests, such as scanning and neurologic screening exams, also may be performed to rule out any other problems. Table 8-2 lists the major causes of hearing loss and the tests used to evaluate these losses in the older adult.

NURSING DIAGNOSES

Nursing diagnoses for the older adult with hearing impairment must reflect the effect the deficit has on daily living and lifestyle and the influence on perception, behavior, and personality. Potential nursing diagnoses for a patient with a specific hearing problem include the following:

• Impaired Verbal Communication related to hearing impairment
• Impaired Social Interaction related to hearing deficit

Table 8-2	TYPES OF HEARING LOSS AND TESTS USED TO EVALUATE THEM	
	Conductive Loss Evaluation	Conductive Hearing Loss Tests
	Impacted earwax Edematous/infected external canals (otitis externa) Perforation of tympanic membranes Infection of the middle ear (otitis media) Otosclerosis	Otoscopic examination Audiometry Tuning fork testing
	Sensorineural Loss Evaluation	Sensorineural Loss Tests
	Presbycusis Ototoxicity (medications) Tumors of the auditory nerve	Audiometry Physical exam for eighth cranial nerve function History of medication use Tuning Fork testing
	Mixed Loss Evaluation	Mixed Loss Testing
	Tinnitus Otosclerosis	Audiometry Tuning fork testing

• Altered Thought Processes related to inability to evaluate reality resulting from a hearing deficit
• Diversional Activity Deficit related to loss of ability to perform usual favorite activities secondary to hearing deficit
• Impaired Home Maintenance Management related to hearing deficit
• Impaired Physical Mobility related to hearing impairment resulting from the aging process
• Self-Care Deficit related to hearing deficit
• Sensory or Perceptual Alterations related to hearing impairment resulting from the aging process
• High Risk for Injury related to lack of awareness of environmental hazards
• Body Image Disturbance related to loss of hearing function.

NURSING INTERVENTIONS

Communication with older adults with mild to moderate hearing loss may be difficult. Nurses, family members, and caretakers often forget the problem exists because it is not immediately self-evident. Encouraging families to assist the older adult's ability to communicate either with treatment or referral for a hearing aid can be gratifying for all concerned. It is important to determine the individual's actual deficits and capabilities and then work with him or her by maximizing strengths with visual cues, hearing aids, and body language. Teaching the family and patient appropriate interventions can improve their lives and self-esteem.

PATIENT AND FAMILY TEACHING

Patient and family education, as related to the degree of impairment, usually encourages compliance (Eliopoulos, 1992). The nurse should educate families that hearing loss is a threat to security and self-esteem. Families often need counseling and support in learning how to make listening situations optimal for the hearing-impaired older adult.

Use posters with pictures or manual signs for functional and everyday communication. When speaking, do not cover your mouth with your hands or turn your face away in the middle of a message. Give the patient every opportunity to read your body language as well as to hear. Emphasize nonverbal communication, such as facial expressions, eye contact, and gestures. Talk toward the best ear of the listener, and be certain the room lighting is adequate to allow the person to see your face clearly. Secure the attention of the person by facing the person, speaking his or her name, or touching him or her gently to show that you want to speak. Write out all important communication or instructions for the patient. This can also act as a reminder. Use a qualified sign language interpreter when available.

The family can assist with acquiring environmental aids, such as flashing lights or other visual alarms for telephones, the doorbell, alarm clocks, and signal bells (fire, burglar). Low-cost captioning for the television or an induction apparatus for the radio and television is also helpful. Teach the family some of the indicators of early hearing loss (listed below) so that early detection in other members is possible:

- Does the person seem inattentive, withdrawn, especially quiet, or inappropriately angered or irritated by others in the environment?
- Does the person stay away from social events, avoid learning new things in classes, complain of an inability to hear, or not understand directions?
- Does the person require frequent repetition of statements in order to comprehend? Can the person hear when being spoken to from another room?
- Does the person give inappropriate responses to questions or to the thought process of the conversation?
- Does the person have frequent ear infections or a family history of severe hearing loss?
- Does the person complain that his or her spouse has a hearing problem when it is evident that this is not the case?

HEARING AIDS

Evaluate the older adult for the possibility of a hearing aid. A hearing aid must fit and be worn to be effective. Many older adults remember the older models that functioned poorly. Significant improvements in engineering have made today's models superior in performance quality. The maintenance and care of a hearing aid is explained in the Patient Teaching Box. Hearing aids increase the ability to communicate with others but do not always restore hearing to normal sound quality. Hearing aids are made to be worn in several ways:

Patient Teaching Box
MAINTENANCE AND CARE OF A HEARING AID

Use the following guidelines to maintain and care for your hearing aid.

Strategies for compliance in using a hearing aid:

- Institute a breaking-in period after the initial purchase. Gradually increase the time you wear the hearing aid during the day. Wear it from two to three times a day for an hour in a controlled-volume setting (eg, listening to a radio, watching television, or talking with only one person in a quiet room).
- Encourage a family member or friend to attend sessions with the audiologist on the use of the aid.
- Wear the aid all the time during waking hours. The more accustomed you become to the amplified sound, the better you can use it for communication.
- Attend follow-up sessions after purchase of the aid to ask questions and receive advice on problems with use.
- Use speech reading to supplement auditory information in conversation.

(Modified for use from Staab, AS and Lyles, MF: Manual of Geriatric Nursing, Philadelphia: J. B. Lippincott, 1990, page 207.)

Maintenance and care of a hearing aid:

- Hearing a whistling sound means that the ear mold is not inserted correctly.
- Store the hearing aid in a dry, safe place.
- Clean the ear mold weekly with warm soapy water, and check for cracks or rough edges that may irritate the ears. Detach the ear mold from the hearing aid during cleaning.
- Replace ear molds every 2 to 3 years.
- Do not wear the hearing aid under the hair dryer or when using hair spray, because this will deteriorate the equipment.
- Insert the battery when the hearing aid is turned off.
- Always have an extra battery.
- Label the hearing aid with the owner's name to encourage return if misplaced or lost.

---

behind the ear, in the ear (resting in the ear canal), on the temple of a pair of eyeglasses, in a shirt pocket, or on a chest carrier. The body-worn aid is generally fitted only for persons with severe to profound hearing loss. Be certain that the patient and family have a clear understanding of the benefits and limitations of hearing aid use, before referring the patient for a hearing aid evaluation. If a hearing aid is acquired, the nurse should review strategies for maintaining and caring for the instrument as well as compliance issues.

HEALTH PROMOTION

Health promotion and disease detection are important to discover persons with hearing deficits before they withdraw from society and become isolated. Deafness can cause hostile or bitter attitudes from the spouse and significant others that are unconsciously directed toward the hearing-impaired person. The older adult should be counseled to have periodic audiometric examinations and prompt treatment of any ear condition, particularly infections. Trauma from exposure to environmental noise, such as from lawn mowers and tractors, can be prevented by wearing earplugs or sound-reducing devices. Teach the older adult to remove cerumen with irrigation of the external canal rather than with cotton-tipped applicators, keys, or hairpins, which may cause canal infection or perforation of the eardrum.

Specific referrals to the otologist or audiologist may be useful, particularly if a hearing device is needed. Hand-held voice amplifiers are useful for communication when the need is only for increased volume.

Cochlear implants (multichannel devices) are effective for older adults with clinical deafness. Candidates are carefully selected by an otologist and audiologist and require lengthy rehabilitation after surgical implantation. The criteria for selection are strict, but many adults have benefited from the device.

In long-term facilities where many hearing aids may be in use, soft chimes or other auditory cues other than loud bells may be used to announce special events, such as meals or activities. Some general suggestions for communicating with the institutionalized older adult are shown in Display 8-1.

Community support can be obtained from such groups as the National Hearing Aid Society, the American Speech and Hearing Association, and the National Association for the Deaf. Referrals to these agencies may be made directly by the nurse, patient, or family. Phone numbers for local chapters can be found in the yellow pages of the phone book.

Display 8-1
GENERAL SUGGESTIONS FOR COMMUNICATING WITH THE INSTITUTIONALIZED OLDER ADULT PATIENT

- Note on the intercom button and on the patient's chart that the patient has a hearing deficit.
- Provide accurate information on the most effective way to communicate with the patient.
- Use normal speech movements when talking, and avoid exaggerated lip movements.
- Never restrict both arms of deaf patients with ties or needles, because they depend on their hands for communication.
- Use charts, pictures, or models when explaining medicine and procedures. Be prepared to explain in several different ways.
- If the patient uses a hearing aid, always allow him or her to wear it.
- Provide written information. Nurses should use written statements or questions if necessary to clarify that communication is taking place.
- Use a qualified sign language interpreter whenever possible.
- Emphasize nonverbal communication, such as eye contact, facial expressions, and simple caring touches, and communicate within the personal zone of 1 to 4 ft, using gestures with verbal messages.
- Design a communication poster that fits individual needs and hang it on the wall near the patient's bed. Keep it simple, so that others, such as the nurse's aids and nurses, are more motivated to use it.

Adapted from Andrews and Wilson, The Deaf Adult in the Nursing Home, 1991 with permission.

Nursing Care Plan

FOR PATIENTS WITH HEARING IMPAIRMENT

Nursing Diagnosis: Sensory/Perceptual Alterations: Impaired Verbal Communication related to hearing deficit or hearing impairment.

Definition: A state in which the individual experiences or is at risk of experiencing a decreased ability to speak related to a change in the amount, pattern, or interpretation of auditory stimuli.

Assessment Findings:
1. Lethargy, withdrawal
2. Anxiety, confusion, irritability
3. Noncommunicativeness or inappropriate responses
4. Refusal to perform usual personal care behaviors
5. Increase in ritualistic behaviors
6. Fearfulness, paranoid tendencies
7. Impaired language due to reduced speech discrimination
8. Increased dependency characteristics
9. Inability to follow directions or participate during history interview
10. Lack of eye contact
11. Inability to remember, short attention span
12. Lightheadedness or vertigo
13. Report of spouse as having a hearing problem

Nursing Interventions with Selected Rationales:
1. Assess level of hearing loss and its effect on the capabilities of the individual to hear and communicate.
   Rationale: Reduce communication problems by maximizing the existing strengths with visual cues and body language. Be aware that older adults often hide their inability to hear.
2. When speaking with the patient, position yourself in easy view of the patient and speak directly towards him, slowly with exaggerated speech.
   Rationale: Maintain a lower varied tone to your voice to maximize communication by using vision in place of hearing.
3. Shorten sentences, keep the wording simple, and use expressiveness in facial and hand gestures.
   Rationale: Short simple sentences are more easily understood.
4. Keep background or extraneous noise to a minimum when teaching or talking.
   Rationale: Reduction in extraneous noise facilitates hearing.
5. Talk toward the best ear of the patient.
   Rationale: Hard-of-hearing patients will usually indicate by turning their best hearing ear toward the source of the sounds. Speaking toward this ear will facilitate sound wave transfer.
6. Ensure that room lighting is adequate.
   Rationale: Good lighting allows the patient to clearly see your face and lips.
7. Secure the patient's attention by gently touching them or speaking their name.
   Rationale: Attention of the listener will increase communication.
8. Examine the patient's ears.
   Rationale: Examine for cerumen impaction.

(continued)

Nursing Care Plan

FOR PATIENTS WITH HEARING IMPAIRMENT *(Continued)*

9. Remove cerumen with wax softeners such as commercial softeners or preparations, diluted peroxide water, or room temperature oils or irrigation.
   Rationale: Impacted cerumen is a natural blockage of sound waves.
10. Teach the caregiver/family how to perform an ear irrigation.
    Rationale: The caregiver can remove ear wax accumulation if properly taught the procedure.
11. In patients with frequent wax accumulation, advise them to use softeners once or twice monthly.
    Rationale: Frequent use of softeners will prevent impaction.
12. Write out all important communications or instructions.
    Rationale: Written instructions can be referred to by the patient and family if forgotten.
13. Teach the patient to wear earplugs or sound-reducing devices when mowing the lawn or using machinery that makes loud, vibrating noise (some older adults' hobbies include wood working, welding or sculpting, or lightweight construction).
    Rationale: Adequate noise protection may decrease further hearing impairment.
14. Acquire prompt treatment of all ear conditions, particularly infections.
    Rationale: Rapid treatment may avoid further hearing loss.
15. Caution against use of cotton-tipped applicators, keys, or hairpins to remove cerumen from the external canal.
    Rationale: Use of foreign objects to clean canals may cause trauma to the eardrum or canals.
16. Advise patients who get recurrent otitis externa during bathing, swimming, or hair washing to plug ear canals with cotton saturated with petroleum jelly or to wear ear plugs.
    Rationale: Ear plugs will protect eardrums and canals from spread of infections.
17. If a hearing aid is acquired, be certain that the person has the manual dexterity to use it, an understanding of the instrument, and the motivation to deal with adjusting to the use of the aid.
    Rationale: If the older adult doesn't feel adept with the hearing aid, they may not use it.
18. Be prepared to deal with the frustration of persons associated with the hearing-impaired older adult and to educate them in ways of more effective communication with the person.
    Rationale: Dealing with the hearing impaired can be very frustrating to the caregiver.
19. Evaluate the extent to which the person has projected his or her hearing loss onto others and the motivation for improvement of communciation skills.
    Rationale: Greater motivation will result in greater communication skills.
20. Provide the patient and family with counseling and support in learning how to make listening situations optimal for the hearing impaired person.
    Rationale: Understanding promotes better relationships.
21. Refer the family and patient to local, state, and national support groups for education, advice, and treatment.
    Rationale: Support groups are free of cost and are support for many problems encountered in dealing with hearing loss.

(continued)

Nursing Care Plan

FOR PATIENTS WITH HEARING IMPAIRMENT *(Continued)*

22. Install amplifiers on the telephone and flashing signals on doors and telephones for the severely hearing impaired patient.
    Rationale: These products assist the older adult by using the other senses to increase awareness.
23. Evaluate the patient's regimen for drugs whose toxic symptom is known to be tinnitus.
    Rationale: Tinnitus may be eliminated if the toxic drug is reduced in dosage or eliminated.
24. Encourage the patient to use a nighttime bedside radio or tape recorder.
    Rationale: A radio or tape recorder will provide an artificial source of ambient noise to mask the tinnitus.
25. Be aware that tinnitus can add to the patient's communication difficulties.
    Rationale: Tinnitus interferes with listening ability. Provide the patient with reassurance that tinnitus is a nonprogressive symptom and may disappear in time or may increase with fatigue or stress.

Desired Patient Outcomes/Discharge Criteria:

1. Patient communicates effectively with others.
2. Patient acquires a hearing aid that fits and functions to alleviate the hearing deficit.
3. Patient and family demonstrate ability to care and maintain the instrument.
4. Patient attends social functions and socializes with the family and community.
5. Patient is able to regain independence.
6. Family and patient comply with therapeutic approaches.

REFERENCES

Andrews, J. F., & Wilson, H. F. (1991). The deaf adult in the nursing home. *Geriatric Nursing, 12*(6), 279–283.

Christian, E., Dluhy, N, & O'Neill, R. (1989). Sounds of silence. *Journal of Gerontological Nursing, 15*, 11.

Eliopoulos, C. (1992). Sensory deficits. In C. Eliopoulos (Ed.), *Gerontological nursing* (2nd ed.), 267. Philadelphia: J. B. Lippincott.

Eliopoulos, C. (1993). Cognitive-perceptual functional health pattern. In C. Eliopoulos (Ed.), *A guide to the nursing of the aged* (p. 208). Baltimore: Williams & Wilkins.

Serra, K. W. (1988). Audiological assessment program. *Journal of Gerontological Nursing, 14*, 19.

Staab, A. S., & Lyles, M. F. (1990). Ear and nose disorders. In A. S. Staab & M. F. Lyles (Eds.), *Manual of geriatric nursing* (pp. 197–221). Glenview, ILL: Scott, Foresman, Little, Brown.

BIBLIOGRAPHY

Burgraf, V., & Stanly, M. (1989). *Nursing the elderly.* Philadelphia: Lippincott.

Matteson, M. A. (1988). Age-related changes in the special senses. In M. A. Matteson and E. McConnell (Eds.), *Gerontological Nursing* (pp. 318–322). Philadelphia: Saunders.

Smeltzer, C. D. (1993). Primary care screening and evaluation of hearing loss. *Nurse Practitioner, 18*(8), 50–55.

Zivic, R. C., & King, S. (1994). Cerumen-impaction management for clients of all ages. *Nurse Practitioner, 18*(3), 29–36.

C H A P T E R

Problems With Speaking and Swallowing

Objectives

1. Describe the physiologic changes of aging associated with speaking difficulties and swallowing problems.
2. Describe psychosocial issues of aging related to speaking and swallowing problems.
3. Identify steps in the nursing assessment of an older adult with speaking and swallowing problems.
4. List nursing diagnoses associated with speaking and swallowing problems.
5. Describe appropriate nursing interventions for the older adult with speaking and swallowing problems.

INTRODUCTION

THE ABILITY TO COMMUNICATE THOUGHTS, ideas, and feelings empowers an older adult to be a part of a community and to avoid isolation. It imparts dignity and independence while allowing a means for necessary socialization. In society, many communicative interactions involve the consumption of food and drink. There are strong emotional and social issues surrounding eating apart from nutritional and hydration concerns. For some, food represents love, and love exemplifies food. Problems with speaking can force the older adult to surrender independence and lead to feelings of frustration, anger, and isolation. Teaching families compensatory strategies may help them communicate on a functional level with their loved ones, thereby promoting independence, self-esteem, and socialization. Impaired swallowing may lead to diminished appetite, decreased motivation to eat, and depression. Because many social interactions revolve around food, the older adult may feel increasingly isolated. Loss of the ability to eat safely or the ability to communicate can have a devastating effect on the older adult's quality of life.

Staab, AS and Hodges, LC: ESSENTIALS OF GERONTOLOGICAL NURSING,
© 1996 J. B. Lippincott Company

NORMAL PHYSIOLOGIC CHANGES

Research into language capabilities suggests that there is a relationship between deterioration of language skills and the normal aging process, although there is considerable individual variability. Studies have shown that older adults perform more poorly than their younger counterparts on various language tasks, including comprehension, naming, definitions, and processing information. The most stable evidence regarding language changes among older adults concerns tasks that involve processing complex language, such as interpreting narratives and conversations.

Differences have also been shown in how older adults express themselves. Older adults use less abstract language. Grammar is usually simpler. They may violate rules of language, such as taking turns in conversation and allowing enough space between partners. Depending on the listener, the older speaker may take longer, start over more frequently, and use longer utterances. This may contribute to the inaccurate perception of senility and alter how the listener responds to the older speaker.

Neurologic changes impairing the sensorium may account for some of these changes. Differences in electroencephalogram measures, cerebral blood flow measures, and evoked response changes have been noted in older adults. An example of a neurologic change is loss of hearing acuity resulting from noise exposure or presbycusis, which can result in missing or misunderstanding conversation. Loss of visual acuity can affect the ability to tune in to body language and nonverbal language signals, such as facial expressions. The older adult may require a longer time to respond because processing time is lengthier. This may be due to decreased neurotransmitter production and fewer neurotransmitter binding sites in the brain.

Numerous physiologic and psychological changes may affect the older adult's ability to safely eat and drink. Loss of dentition, dental caries, and gum disease make chewing difficult. Decreased muscle tone and muscle mass as well as diminished motor control exacerbate chewing difficulties. Together these factors may preclude consumption of anything other than soft or pureed consistencies. This diminishes enjoyment and motivation to eat.

Neurologic changes associated with aging result in a number of sequelae that can impair swallowing function. Decline in olfactory (smell) and gustatory (taste) sensations may contribute to decreased appetite and poor motivation to eat. Decreased sensation in the mouth or pharynx may result in a delay in the initiation of the swallow reflex, thereby increasing the risk for aspiration.

Changes in the functioning of the upper gastrointestinal tract, including diminished or inefficient sphincter control (cricopharyngeal and gastroesophageal sphincter), poor esophageal motility, and reflux may limit the consistencies, amounts, and variety of foods an older adult may enjoy safely.

ABNORMAL PHYSIOLOGIC CHANGES

Cognitive changes can negatively affect communicative abilities. Memory loss can result in continuation of one theme or the inability to follow or maintain conversation. Attention deficits and disorientation result in confused, confabulatory (making up answers), and tangential (talking about a different topic) speech.

Aphasia is a language disorder characterized by difficulty in expressing or understanding language as a result of damage to the language centers of the brain (left hemisphere in most persons). This damage can result in speaking difficulty (expressive aphasia) and/or in understanding language (receptive aphasia).

Dysphagia is defined as a swallowing disorder characterized by difficulty in oral preparation for the swallow, or in moving material from the mouth to the stomach.

PSYCHOSOCIAL ISSUES

Speech and language deficits present significant self-care problems for the older adult. Many older adults live alone and have few people who are familiar with their habits and routines of self-care. They may be unable to make their needs and wishes known to caretakers or health care professionals.

Health promotion is affected by speech and language deficits, because the older adult may be unable to accurately describe symptoms to health professionals. Caretakers and health professionals may be unable to relate to the older adult who has a receptive language problem, because they may be unable to comprehend information presented by the nurse.

Human relationships are built on the ability to communicate. Therefore, speech and language problems may result in disruptions in relationships. When family members are unable to cope with communication problems, complete severance of relationships may occur. For some, the prospect of spending the remainder of their lives with someone who will be unable to communicate or has impaired ability to communicate is unacceptable.

Changes interfering with safe swallowing give rise to psychological reactions surrounding what had always been a normal and enjoyable routine of eating. Frequent choking episodes stemming from either delay in the swallow reflex or regurgitation of refluxed material may lead to fear or anxiety. Inability to handle certain consistencies may result in excessive time required to eat. Eating very slowly may create embarrassment and withdrawal. Chewing difficulty, decreased sensation, frequent choking and coughing episodes, and associated gastrointestinal problems all contribute to decreased appetite and motivation to eat. Difficulties in eating may lead to an underlying depression. The depression further diminishes motivation to eat, exacerbating the older person's risk for malnutrition and dehydration.

Swallowing difficulties have a significant effect on the patient's ability to perform self-care, especially feeding. Food and eating carry strong emotional significance, which may contribute to a sense of well-being, self-worth, and self-concept. In many patients, swallowing disorders accompany motor, sensory, and cognitive deficits. These may compound the feelings of dependency and inadequacy. When the patient can no longer consume those foods that have emotional significance because of the inability to swallow, he or she experiences a loss of a basic form of comfort. The consistency of foods allowed on the diet (eg, chopped) may be equated with baby food and contribute further to diminishing self-acceptance and feelings of inadequacy.

Food habits are affected by culture, socioeconomic factors, family traditions, preferences, and religious laws. Eating or dining generally occurs in a social environment. The patient with dysphagia who experiences retention of food in the mouth, choking, coughing, and drooling while eating, is often reluctant to eat in the presence of others, thereby missing the pleasure of social contact with friends and family. Social isolation may be experienced unless intervention is directed toward helping the patient to accept the swallowing disorder and to manage in a social situation.

NURSING ASSESSMENT

The patient and family should be questioned regarding problems with speech and language, cognition, and swallowing. The nurse can detect problems with speech rhythm and articulation during spontaneous conversation with the patient. Fluency, paraphrasing, word omissions, and misuse can also be detected during the interview.

The nurse also must be alert for swallowing difficulties in patients with altered levels of consciousness, severe confusion, and disorientation. The presence of a tracheostomy tube, recent extubation, severe dysarthria, and the absence of a gag reflex should alert the nurse to the potential for swallowing disorders and aspiration. The nurse should observe patients at high risk for swallowing disorders and promptly intervene to prevent complications, such as aspiration pneumonia with concomitant fever.

HISTORY AND INTERVIEW

Asking the patient to follow specific commands allows the nurse to assess the patient's comprehension of spoken language. The patient's understanding can be assessed by asking simple yes/no questions whose answers indicate that the patient comprehends what is being asked. Questions should be asked in such a way that their answers are absolute. For example, ask "Did you have eggs for breakfast?" rather than "Did you enjoy your breakfast this morning?" The patient may respond verbally, by nodding the head, or by pointing. If the patient is unable to verbalize, the nurse can assess the ability to point on request to specific objects in the room, pictures, and body parts. Nonverbal clues, such as looking at the named object, should be avoided.

 ▷ *Clinical Pearl*

Planning/Implementation: The degree to which a patient comprehends language is a critical factor in planning care.

To assess the relationship between cognition and language ability, the patient should be asked to repeat various letters, words, and sentences as well as numbers and series of numbers. To assess the ability to perform serial repetitions, the patient can be asked to name days of the week or months of the year, to count, or to recite simple poems and nursery rhymes. If the patient is unable to verbalize, assess the ability to sing familiar songs. Assess the patient's orientation and grasp of reality by asking biographic questions, and confirm the answers by comparing the person's responses with chart information or with family members. An older adult with speech and language problems and confusion may be very convincing in the confabulation of answers. Assess immediate, short-term, and long-term memory. Whatever the cause of aphasia/ dysphasia, the symptoms are the same and are due to an interruption in the neuronal circuits responsible for communication.

Diligent nursing assessment and observation are essential to discovering dysphagia. Initially, a patient or family member may report difficulty swallowing food and/or liquids. During the admission assessment, the nurse should question the patient and family regarding problems with chewing and swallowing or problems with certain food consistencies.

PHYSICAL EXAMINATION

The older adult's ability to comprehend and perform simple commands should be assessed. First, ask the patient to perform a simple task, such as "Stick out your tongue" or "Raise your right hand." To assess the patient's ability to perform progressively more complex commands, the nurse may use a series of directives, as shown below. This helps the nurse assess the degree to which a patient comprehends multiple directions.

- Step 1: "Pick up the coin."
- Step 2: "Pick up the coin and place it in the cup, and hand the cup to me."

The nurse should assess the patient's ability to name objects by showing various pictures of objects. If the patient is unable to name the object, he or she may be requested to select the correct name from a list of words. To determine the ability to retrieve specific words from memory, the nurse may request the patient to complete sentences. It is important for the nurse examiner to consider the patient's premorbid level of literacy so as not to interpret a physical problem as illiteracy. Specific commands and questions to assess speech and language ability are shown in Display 9-1.

Examine the oral cavity, noting loose teeth, sores in the mouth, facial droop or weakness, tongue deviation, and the amount and consistency of secretions. The gag and swallowing reflexes should be assessed. Inspect the oral cavity for residual food (Hickey, 1992). Request the patient to demonstrate a voluntary cough and observe for reflexive cough. Observe for choking, drooling, or coughing during or after eating or drinking. Assess the mental status of the patient, observing for distractibility, orientation, memory, and ability to follow instructions. In addition, note intelligibility of speech and quality of voice. Observe for gurgling and wet, hoarse, or breathy voice.

Patients who do not demonstrate adequate airway protection should not be given anything by mouth until cleared by the speech-language pathologist. A thorough examination by the speech-language pathologist should include an oral-facial examination (of facial structure and function), oral sensory and motor examination, and observation of the patient swallowing different consistencies. Further assessment might include evaluation of laryngeal function, including vocal quantity and resonance, assessment of cough reflex, and, if indicated, a video fluoroscopic examination or modified barium swallow to evaluate the mechanics of swallowing.

Display 9-1

SPEECH AND LANGUAGE SCREENING COMMANDS/QUESTIONS

Auditory Comprehension: Receptive Aphasia

- Instruct patient: "Close your eyes, keep them shut; now open them."
- Instruct patient: " Touch your ear, nose, elbow, knee."
- Hold up two objects and have patient discriminate between the two: have patient point to the brush, cup, comb, razor, washcloth, pencil, paper, toothpaste.
- Have patient point to items in room: window, door, chair, television, blanket
- Instruct patient to put the comb beside the brush
- Instruct patient to put the comb between the brush and the razor.

Speech: Expressive Aphasia

- Examiner holds up or points to object (pen, cup, watch, etc.) and asks, "What is this called?"
- Engage the patient in conversation. Ask what happened, where patient is, and why. Ask about family.
- Make note of orientation, sentence structure, and word-finding deficits.

Reading Comprehension: Receptive Aphasia

- Have patient match the following words to the objects (print each word on separate strips of paper): brush, comb, pencil, cup.
- Have the patient read the following sentences and mark, point to, or say yes or no (print sentences far apart, one at a time, using large, clear letters):
  - Are there 12 months in a year?   Yes   No
  - Is Christmas in June?   Yes   No
  - Does the sun rise in the east?   Yes   No
  - Do you tell time with a watch?   Yes   No

Writing: Expressive Aphasia

- Ask the patient to write the alphabet.
- Ask the patient to write his or her name and address.
- Ask the patient to copy simple words. (Examiner writes them first, one at a time.)
- Ask the patient to write words from dictation: woman, sun, top, place.

Speech Production: Dysarthria or Apraxia

- Ask the patient to imitate tongue protrusion, elevation, depression, and movement laterally. (Note drooling or swallowing difficulty.)
- Ask the patient to repeat rapidly the following sounds: pa, pa, pa; ta-ta-ta; ka, ka, ka; petticoat, petticoat, petticoat.
- Ask the patient to say the following words, either by reading them or repeating them after the examiner: cross, seven, Massachusetts, Methodist, Episcopal.

DIAGNOSTIC TESTS

Medical data that may aid in assessing the origin of communicative disorders include skull x-ray, electroencephalography, brain scan, computed tomography (CT), positron emission tomography (PET), magnetic resonance imaging (MRI), spinal tap, angiogram, and electrocardiogram.

Medical origins and diagnoses that predispose a patient to swallowing difficulties include cerebrovascular accident, head trauma (closed head injury), dementia, pneumonia (aspiration), and advanced age/malnutrition. Before initiation of any intervention, the patient should ideally undergo a through dysphagia evaluation, including x-ray and a study of swallowing (video fluoroscopy) by a speech-language pathologist.

NURSING DIAGNOSES

Nursing diagnoses can be related not only to the difficulty with speaking or swallowing but also to the alteration of body image. The following is a list of some selected nursing diagnoses based on a specific patient with speaking or swallowing difficulty:

- Body Image Disturbance related to speaking or swallowing disorder
- Impaired Verbal Communication related to effects of aphasia on expression or interpretation
- Personal Identity Disturbance related to speaking or swallowing disorder
- Altered Role Performance related to inability to speak or difficulty swallowing
- Self-Esteem Disturbance related to handicap
- Impaired Social Interaction related to speaking or swallowing disorder
- High Risk for Aspiration related to swallowing disorder
- Potential Sensory or Perceptual Alterations: Gustatory related to swelling disorder
- Impaired Swallowing related to mechanical impairment.

NURSING INTERVENTIONS

Nurses can greatly help patients and families adapt to life-altering changes resulting from impaired communication and swallowing by providing education, counseling, and emotional support. Nursing interventions assist the patient and family in coping with the numerous changes in their lives as a result of the underlying cause of the problem as well as the deficit itself.

PATIENT AND FAMILY TEACHING

The nurse should teach the patient and family about the communication problem, the prognosis, and resources available for recovery. For many families, a role change occurs, especially if the patient was the sole support of the family. The spouse may have to assume a new role of wage earner and household manager. Teach family members to seek ways to allow the patient to continue to feel valuable and valued and to contribute verbally and otherwise to the extent of their ability. Family members must be encouraged to foster the patient's independence and to continue to provide support as needed. In collaboration with the speech-language pathologist, teach families means to promote communication, including therapeutic communication, skills of acknowledgment, active listening, and "I" messages. See Display 9-2 for suggestions for working with the patient with speech and language problems.

For assisting the older patient with swallowing difficulties while eating, the nurse should teach basic nutritional information and the importance of a well-balanced diet in maintaining and promoting growth and repair of body tissue. To teach a patient to eat, the nurse must start with small amounts and

Display 9-2

STRATEGIES FOR PATIENTS WITH IMPAIRED SPEAKING (APHASIA)

Aphasia is a communication impairment characterized by a difficulty in expressing, a difficulty in understanding, or a combination of both.

1. By assessing abilities, identify a method the patient can use to communicate basic needs. Provide alternative methods of communication, such as paper and pencil, alphabet letters, hand signals, eye blinks, head nods, bell signals, and flash cards with pictures (glass of water, bedpan) or words depicting frequently used phrases ("Wet my lips," "Move my foot"). Encourage the patient to point, use gestures, and pantomime.
2. Create an atmosphere of acceptance and privacy and provide a nonrushed environment in which the patient can take his or her time talking and enunciating words carefully with good lip movements.
3. Promote communication by assessing the patient's frustration level and do not push beyond it. Estimate 30 seconds of passed time before providing the patient with the word he or she may be trying to find (except when the patient is frustrated or needs the request immediately, such as for a bedpan). Provide cues through pictures or gestures.
4. Listen and observe if the patient speaks slowly and rephrase the message aloud to validate it. Respond to all attempts at speech, even if they are unintelligible (eg, "I do not know what you are saying. Can you try to say it again?"). Ignore mistakes and profanity. Don't pretend you understand if you do not.
5. Verbally address the problem of frustration over inability to communicate, and explain that patience is needed for both the nurse and the person who is trying to talk. Maintain a calm, positive attitude, such as "I can understand you if we work at it." Maintain a sense of humor but allow for tears. For the patient who has a limited ability to talk, encourage writing letters or keeping a diary to vent feelings and share concerns, and provide alternative methods of self-expression, such as dancing/exercising/walking, writing/drawing/painting/coloring, humming/singing, or helping with tasks such as opening mail and choosing meals.
6. Promote comprehension by assessing hearing ability (use of functioning hearing aids), and assess ability to see (encourage the patient to wear his or her glasses).
7. Improve comprehension by speaking when the patient is ready to listen and gain attention with gentle touch on the arm and a verbal message of "Listen to me" or "I want to talk to you." Achieve eye contact, if possible.
8. Teach techniques to significant others by which to improve communications. Encourage the family to share feelings concerning communication problems. Explain the reasons for labile emotions.

progress slowly as the person learns to handle each step. The nurse may begin with ice chips, move to an eyedropper of water or juice, continue onward to small amounts of semisolid or pureed foods, then introduce a soft diet, and finally implement a regular diet. Avoid the use of straws by patients with swallowing difficulty, because they propel a large bolus into the oropharynx that the patient is unable to manage. Any limitations and rationale regarding liquids and food consistencies must be understood. If tube feedings are necessary, the caregivers must understand safe feeding techniques. They must be given a name and phone number of someone to call if problems arise. Health teaching should include instruction to the patient and family concerning treatment, rationale, and methods for implementation. Guidelines for care of the older adult with swallowing difficulties are presented in the Patient Teaching Box (see also Fig. 9-1).

RESOURCES

A team approach is best used in working with patients experiencing communication difficulties. A team may include the patient, family, nurse, speech-language pathologist, physical therapist, physician, and social worker. The nurse who has 24-hour access to the patient can facilitate a unified, organized approach to the recovery of speech.

Specific referrals to speech-language deficits and problems are indicated when significant swallowing or speech-language deficits or problems are encountered. An evaluation by an audiologist may be beneficial if decreased or impaired hearing is potentially contributing to the language problem. Evaluation by a neurologist, geriatrician, or social worker may be indicated to assist with the myriad of associated problems, such as social isolation or inability to return to or remain in a prior living arrangement. Consultation with a nutritionist is recommended to assist with nutritional assessment, diet modification, and planning. Appropriate resources are available, such as speech therapy, group therapy, counseling (individual or family), and/or psychiatric care. Community support and further information can be obtained from groups such as the American Heart Association, Easter Seals, stroke clubs, and local rehabilitation units.

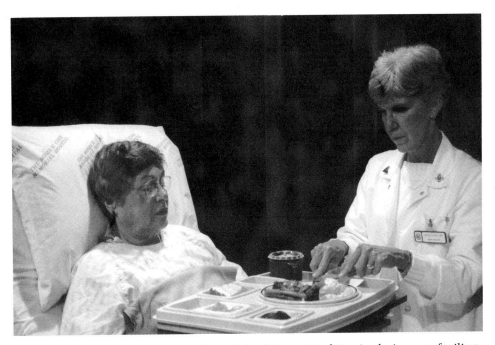

Figure 9-1. Patient is seated upright and food is cut into bite-sized pieces to facilitate swallowing.

Patient Teaching Box
CAREGIVER GUIDELINES FOR SWALLOWING DIFFICULTIES

Use the following guidelines when caring for an older adult with swallowing difficulties:

- Seat patient in an upright position (60 to 90 degrees) during meals and for 15 to 30 minutes after meals (in bed supported with pillows or upright in a chair).
- Avoid the use of straws because they propel excessive amounts of liquid too rapidly into the oropharynx, increasing the risk of aspiration.
- Watch patient for pocketing of food on weak side. Make sure the mouth is cleared frequently and rinsed before and after meals.
- Encourage patient to control the rate and amount of intake by taking small bites and sips.
- Thicken liquids if patient has difficulty with water and other thin liquids (commercially prepared substances for thickening are available).
- Instruct the patient to tuck chin or tilt head toward affected (weak) extremities to facilitate swallowing when initiation of swallowing is delayed.
- For patient with unilateral paralysis, instruct patient to turn head to weak side to prevent pooling of food or liquid in pharynx.
- Provide frequent oral care (before and after meals).
- Discontinue feeding if patient exhibits frequent coughing, choking, spikes of fever or becomes congested.
- Remember that just because a patient does not cough when swallowing does not mean that aspiration has not occurred.

SENSORY STIMULATION

Sensory stimulation is beneficial to the patient, especially that which involves interaction with another person or groups of persons. Activities involving all the senses appear to be more advantageous than visual or verbal stimulation alone. Memory or reminiscing activities give the older person an opportunity to use a greater variety of words and modes of communicating than standard reality orientation activities, which have been used traditionally.

The nurse must attempt to simplify all aspects of communication and introduce only one topic or idea at a time. Long sentences and complex words should be avoided. It is unnecessary to speak loudly unless the older adult's hearing is affected. Speak slowly and naturally. Avoid speaking in a patronizing tone or as if to a child. Introduce questions or ideas that require simple responses from a patient.

For the nurse to effectively communicate with the patient with aphasia or dysphasia, it is essential for the patient to be goal directed and to focus his or her full attention on the task. Generally, the nurse should be positioned directly in front of the patient. All environmental distractions should be eliminated. Focus on increasing the number and variety of responses from the patient rather than on correcting mistakes. Maintain a relaxed, unhurried attitude and, if possible, allow more time to care for the aphasic patient. Help the patient achieve a sense of accomplishment, not failure. Success breeds continued success in communicating.

ORAL HYGIENE

Because the patient has decreased sensation in the oral cavity and decreased awareness of the status of oral hygiene, the nurse must assume greater responsibility for assisting with oral hygiene to prevent oral complications, such as stomatitis and crusting of the oral mucosa and to promote comfort. The following are several strategies to promote healthy oral care:

- Remind the patient to clear the mouth frequently to remove pocketed food.
- Encourage cleaning the teeth and oral cavity with foam sticks or a soft toothbrush at least four times a day (after meals and at bedtime) and to rinse the mouth with water or normal saline solution afterward.
- Avoid mouthwashes containing alcohol, because they tend to have a drying effect on the oral mucosa.
- Use a lip moisturizer or lubricant to prevent drying and disruption of mucous membranes.

DIET AND NUTRITION

Health promotion is affected by the patient's inability to consume the food and nutrients essential for health maintenance. The nurse must focus on preventing dehydration, malnutrition, and pneumonia. The older adult who is unable to eat (swallow) his or her usual diet with adequate amounts of bulk may have increased difficulty with constipation, a major problem for many normal adults. Measures must be taken to promote adequate elimination.

The eating environment should be attractive, pleasant, and lack distractions. TV and radio should be eliminated to allow the patient to focus on the feeding session. Early on, isolate the patient to avoid embarrassment due to drooling, retained food in the mouth, and the need to provide constant verbal and visual cues to chew and swallow. Progress to allowing the patient to eat with a small group of patients for a time and then in a more populated environment. Ensure that cold foods are served cold and hot foods are served hot.

Nursing Care Plan

FOR A PATIENT WITH SWALLOWING DISORDERS

Nursing Diagnosis: Impaired Swallowing related to mechanical impairment of the mouth, muscle paralysis or paresis, or inability to participate in automatic eating behavior secondary to decreased cognition.

Definition: The state in which an individual has decreased mobility to voluntarily pass fluids and/or solid foods from the mouth to the stomach.

Assessment Findings:

1. Observed evidence of difficulty in swallowing and/or evidence of aspiration
2. Stasis of food in oral cavity
3. Facial weakness or asymmetry
4. Coughing, choking, drooling
5. Apraxia (ideational, constructional, or visual)
6. Wet, gurgly voice after swallowing

(continued)

Nursing Care Plan

FOR A PATIENT WITH SWALLOWING DISORDERS *(Continued)*

7. Excessive secretions
8. Prolonged eating time

Nursing Interventions with Selected Rationales:

1. Assess for causative or contributing factors, such as mechanical impairment of oropharyngeal structure, muscle paralysis, or paresis after a cerebrovascular accident
   Rationale: Factor identification aids in individualization of treatment plan.
2. Assist the individual with moving the bolus of food from the anterior to the posterior of mouth by placing food in the posterior mouth where swallowing can be ensured. Use a syringe with a short piece of tubing attached, a glossectomy spoon, and soft food such as gelatin, custard, or mashed potatoes.
   Rationale: Assistance with moving food reduces or eliminates the impairment.
3. Use products such as artificial saliva, papain tablets, or meat tenderizer made from papaya enzyme dissolved in the mouth 10 minutes before eating, and provide frequent mouth care and increase fluid intake.
   Rationale: These measures help prevent or decrease thick secretions.
4. Concentrate on solids rather than liquids. Give solids or liquids separately.
   Rationale: Liquids are generally less well tolerated.
5. Keep extraneous stimuli at a minimum while eating (eg, no television or radio, no verbal stimuli unless directed at task).
   Rationale: A calm relaxed environment enhances eating.
6. Instruct patient to hold breath while swallowing and to concentrate on the task.
   Rationale: Concentration improves awareness and controls swallowing.
7. Have patient sit up in a chair with neck slightly flexed and maintain upright position for 10 to 15 minutes after eating.
   Rationale: Proper positioning minimizes possibility of aspiration.
8. Observe for swallowing and check mouth for emptying. Avoid overloading mouth, because this decreases swallowing effectiveness.
   Rationale: Observation and inspection allows for evaluating patient's ability and prevents possibility of aspiration.
9. Have suction equipment available and functioning properly.
   Rationale: Prompt action, if aspiration occurs, can minimize its effect.
10. Keep patient focused on task by reinforcing any voluntary action and giving directions until finished swallowing each mouthful.
    Rationale: Focusing and reinforcement enhances the effectiveness of the patient's attempts at swallowing and reduces the possibility of aspiration.
11. Initiate health teaching and referrals to a speech pathologist and dietitian, as indicated.
    Rationale: Follow up on referrals promote compliance.

Note: If the above strategies are unsuccessful, consultation with physician may be necessary for alternative feeding techniques, such as parenteral nutrition.

Desired Patient Outcomes/Discharge Criteria:

1. The Patient will report improved ability to swallow.
2. The patient and/or family will:
   • Describe causative factors when known
   • Describe rationale and procedures for treatment
   • Demonstrate appropriate techniques for feeding and swallowing.

REFERENCES

Hickey, J. V. (1992). *The clinical practice of neurological and neurosurgical nursing.* Philadelphia: Lippincott.

BIBLIOGRAPHY

Bates, B. (1995). *A guide to physical examination* (6th ed.). Philadelphia: J. B. Lippincott.

Carpenito, L. J. (1993). *Nursing diagnosis: Application to clinical practice* (5th ed.). Philadelphia: J. B. Lippincott.

Conway-Rutkowski, B. L. (1982). *Carini and Owens' neurological and neurosurgical nursing.* St. Louis: Mosby.

Darley, F. L. (1982). *Aphasia.* Philadelphia: W. B. Saunders.

Davis, G., Albyn, M., & Wilcox, J. (1985). *Adult aphasia rehabilitation: Applied pragmatics.* San Diego: College-Hill Press.

Doenges, M., & Moorhouse, M. (1991). *Nurses' pocket guide: Nursing diagnoses with interventions.* Philadelphia: F.A. Davis.

Johns, D. F. (1985). *Clinical management of neurogenic communicative disorders.* Boston: Little, Brown.

Meehan, M. (1992). Nursing diagnoses: Potential for aspiration. *RN, 55*(1), 30–35.

Richter, J. E. (1992). A new common sense approach to dysphagia. *Patient Care, 26*(15), 87–101.

Rubin-Terrado, M., & Linkenheld, D. (1991). Don't choke on this: a swallowing assessment. *Geriatric Nursing, 12,* 6.

Snyder, M. (Ed.). (1991). *A guide to neurological and neurosurgical nursing.* New York: Wiley.

Vancura, B. J. (1993). A program to assist sensory-impaired patients. *Medsurg Nursing,* April (2), 131–-135.

Yen, P. K. (1991). When swallowing is a problem. *Geriatric Nursing, 12*(6), 313.

10

Problems With Drug Administration

Objectives

1. Explain the major age-related changes in pharmacokinetics and pharmaco-dynamics.
2. Plan strategies to counteract some common drug-induced illnesses in older adults.
3. Conduct a medication assessment teaching session with an older adult.
4. Develop a care plan to demonstrate appropriate interventions for administration of medications to an older adult.

INTRODUCTION

THE PROBLEMS THAT OLDER ADULTS HAVE with drug administration are complex and present a difficult management problem for nurses. Generally, older adults are more sensitive to drugs, experience prolonged drug effects, have more adverse reactions, have more difficulty understanding drug regimens, and take a larger number of pills. Diseases common to the older adult, psychosocial adaptations, and biologic aging changes affect pharmacokinetics and pharmacodynamics, making correlating the right medication for the right person for the right reason difficult. It is sometimes said in jest that all nurses do when caring for the older adult is "push pills." That is not an accurate portrayal of the nurse's role or the older adult's priorities, although dispensing medications is an important part of the nurse's role.

There are numerous issues related to the problems that the older adult has with drug administration. Along with their increasing numbers, older adults usually have a complex history marked by chronic illness, multiple medication regimens, and have a high risk for adverse drug reactions. Although older adults represent 12% of the total population, they purchase approximately 25% of prescription medications and 30% of over-the-counter medications

(Denham, 1990). Approximately 65% of older adults use over-the-counter medications (Oles, 1990). Studies show that older adults are more likely to self-medicate by using over-the-counter medications that are left over from previous illnesses and use drugs shared by friends (McConnell, 1988).

Older adults who are discharged home from the hospital are usually alone and are prescribed regimens that include three to eight medications (Chenitz, Salisbury, & Stone, 1990). The number of medications in a regimen is a safety issue, because studies show that older adults are likely to make errors in medication administration in addition to misusing and abusing drugs (Sidel et al., 1990). Because older adults are typically discharged home with the responsibility of self-care, including medication administration, they need preparation for assuming this responsibility.

To ensure the effective outcome of the older adult being able to self-manage the medication regimen, the nurse must use good assessment skills and understand the physiologic and psychosocial changes of aging. The nurse must feel comfortable administering the wide variety of medications used by this population. It is imperative that the nurse be well versed on the topic of medication administration when preparing older adults to self-administer their medications.

PHYSIOLOGIC CHANGES

It is important to understand the effect of the aging process and chronic illness on pharmacokinetics (a drug's alteration during absorption, distribution, metabolism, and excretion) and pharmacodynamics (the mechanism by which specific drug dosages produce specific biochemical and physiologic changes in the body). Pharmacokinetic factors, in addition to the drug dose, control the drug's concentration at the site of action, influencing the intensity of drug effects, both planned and unplanned.

Ingesting multiple drugs depends on a high level of kidney function for excretion. A decrease in general kidney function can lead to problems with metabolizing nephrotoxic medications, such as aminoglycoside antibiotics, nonsteroidal anti-inflammatory drugs, and contrast mediums used in x-ray procedures.

Attention to age-related changes in physiology that affect drug response is important in understanding pharmacokinetics and dynamic changes in the older population. The brain's mass, number of active cells, and blood flow decrease, while the protective mechanism of the blood–brain barrier becomes more permeable. This change leads to an increase in the number of central nervous system symptoms, such as confusion and disorientation, which is seen when older adults react negatively to medications in their regimen. With age, the range between the desired effect (therapeutic) and an adverse reaction narrows. Rigidity of the lens of the eye and an increase in the level of hearing loss affect the ability to understand instructions. The diminished ability to see pills and to read instructions on medication labels and on educational materials is common. Inability to hear instructions greatly affects the ability to follow a regimen and practice safe self-administration. These normal changes of aging are also related to trends of medication overdosing and underdosing. In the older adult, normal changes in the gastrointestinal tract can affect drug absorption. The most common changes include increased gastric pH level, decreased absorptive surface, decreased motility, and decreased gastric empty-ing. However, even with these apparent changes, absorption of most oral med-ications remains unaffected.

Body composition and blood flow to the vital organs affects the drug's dis-tribution throughout the body. In the older adult, normal aging changes result in reduced total body water and muscle mass and increased fat, which varies the effects on the kinetics of water-soluble and fat-soluble medications. An in-crease in body fat intensifies the potential for drug accumulation, which may lead to drug toxicity. Chronic disease states in the older adult have been asso-ciated with significantly lower levels of serum albumin, which negatively af-fects protein binding, resulting in changes in the blood levels of drugs.

The liver and kidneys are the primary organs responsible for breaking down (metabolism) and removing (excretion) most drugs from the body. A decrease in liver blood flow and/or diminished activity of the metabolizing capacity of the liver can adversely affect drug metabolism. Hepatic mass decreases with age, resulting in changes in liver function. Such factors as concurrent drug use, diet, illness, and alcohol and cigarette use affect a drug's elimination rate. The best documented alteration associated with old age is the reduction in elimination rate by the kidneys (Montamat, Cusack, & Vestal, 1989). Along with a decline in the creatinine clearance rate (measurement of filtration rate), there is a correlated decline in glomerular filtration and tubular secretion rates with aging. Because of changes in renal function, drugs that undergo complete or partial renal elimination have diminished clearance in the older adult. To complicate issues, these expected physical changes are further influenced by disease (see Table 10-1).

PSYCHOSOCIAL ISSUES

Psychosocial issues associated with medications include quality of life, life changes, self-esteem, social support, and mastery (Sheahan, Hendricks, & Coons, 1989). Self-esteem can be affected by having to take a number of med-ications. For example, the patient may not be able to do desired activities be-cause of the restraints of a medication regimen. In many cases, he or she may also need social support to comply with medication regimens, such as getting the prescription filled, taking the medication properly, renewing the prescrip-tion, or even going to the physician to obtain the prescription. Often, the older adult who is unable to perform these tasks is embarrassed to say so or to ask for help. Mastery of drug administration techniques is a challenge for the older adult and is a defining characteristic of an independently functioning older adult.

If advertisements imply that there is "a pill for every ill," the older adult seems especially prone to this sales tactic. This mind-set is especially prevalent in relation to use of over-the-counter medications. Studies show that 82% of older adults who live independently use over-the-counter medications (Shea-han, Hendricks, & Coons, 1989). Because advertisements are devised to sell products, most provide little quality information about the medicine being promoted. Many older adults consume these medications with little knowledge about their potential and actual effects. This misplaced faith may put older adults at risk for drug misuse and harmful medication effects.

Older adults are at high risk for not taking medications or not taking them

Table
10-1

ALTERED DRUG RESPONSES WITH THE AGING PROCESS

Age Related Changes	Effect of Change	Applicable Drugs
Absorption		
Reduced gastric acid	Rate of absorption may be delayed	Antibiotics
Increased pH (less acid)		Anticoagulants
Reduced gastrointestinal motility	Extent of absorption not affected	H₂ antagonists cimetidine rantidine
Prolonged gastric emptying		Calcium channel blockers
Distribution		
Decreased albumin sites	Significant changes in protein binding, leading to a higher level of unbound drug; therefore, more effect and faster metabolism and excretion	Highly protein-bound drugs
		Oral anticoagulants
		Oral hypoglycemics
		Calcium channel blockers
		Furosemide
		Nonsteroidal anti-inflammatory drugs
		Quinidine
		Phenytoin
Reduced cardiac output	Decreased perfusion of many bodily organs	
Impaired peripheral blood flow		
Increased percentage of body fat	Increasing proportion of body fat leads to increased ability to store fat-soluble drugs; also leads to accumulation of drugs and delayed excretion	Selected fat-soluble drugs
		Barbiturates
		Valium
		Phenothiazine
Decreased lean body mass	Decreased total body volume, leading to higher peak drug levels	Alcohol
		Morphine
Metabolism		
Decreased cardiac output and decreased perfusion of the liver	Decreased metabolism and delayed breakdown of drugs, leading to extended duration of action, accumulation, and toxicity	All drugs metabolized in the liver
Excretion		
Decreased renal blood flow	Decreased renal efficiency	Aminoglycoside antibiotics
	Decreased rate of elimination/increased duration of action	Cimetidine
Loss of functioning nephrons		Chlorpropamide
		Digoxin
	Increased danger of accumulation and toxicity	Procainamide

as prescribed. The most commonly reported reason the older adult fails to follow the prescription is the belief that the drug is not needed in the dose prescribed (Leirer, Morrow, Pariante, & Sheikh, 1988). This suggests that independent judgments are made on how to use the medication once the patient is at home. Special efforts should be made to promote the knowledgeable use of prescription and over-the-counter medications (Sheehan, Hendricks, & Coons, 1989).

Older adults frequently make some degree of error when taking their prescription medications (Santo-Novak & Edwards, 1989). Because they often have chronic illnesses and are often on long-term drug therapy, medical reevaluation may be infrequent (Schwertz & Buschmann, 1989). There is also an alarming trend for older adults to consult less often with their physicians concerning medication regimens (Cartwright, 1990). These conditions often contribute to the older adult's tendency toward multiple drug administration problems. Older adults who take more medications need more frequent reevaluation, supervision, and consultation.

NURSING ASSESSMENT

Understanding the importance of compliance problems and having the ability to assess for them is a necessary skill for the nurse. Begin by considering the patient's medical history relative to chronic illnesses, complex medication regimens in the treatment plan, and the patient's knowledge of medications and administration. Other factors placing the patient at risk for compliance problems include communication impairments, such as vision, hearing, and speech and language disorders. Be aware of the patient's opinion about the significance of the symptom that is being treated and his or her beliefs about the outcome of therapy.

HISTORY AND INTERVIEW

Collecting a medication history is the first step in gathering vital information concerning the older adults's level of understanding of medication use, disease process, symptoms of adverse reactions, financial constraints, and personal values affecting appropriate medication-taking behaviors. Some categories to include when assessing drug administration problems are as follows:

- Demographic data (age, sex, education, household size)
- Medical diagnoses
- Current medication (number and types of prescription and over-the-counter medications, home remedies, and medical devices)
- Technical problems with medication use (identifying and distinguishing different pills, opening medication bottles, reading medication labels, memory problems, awareness of potential interactions with food, and difficulty swallowing medication)
- Side effects and allergies (knowledge and ability to handle)
- Pharmacy services
- Source of medications (pharmacy, mail order)
- Physician interaction (how the interaction went and what information was received)
- Medication-taking behavior (use and misuse, responses to hypothetical sit-

uations, system used to take medications on schedule, and perceptions about medication taking)
• Alcohol use with medication.

During the assessment phase, correlating the older adults' medications with their disease processes will delineate the appropriateness of the regimen. The nurse should advocate that all unnecessary drugs be avoided. Evaluation of an inappropriate dosage amount can be a red flag for potential adverse drug reactions. The dosage amount may be a major determinant in an adverse response when first noticed by the patient or primary caregiver. Choice of medication form and assessment of packaging are easily addressed reasons for noncompliance. Assessment of the regimen should always include questions concerning the patient's use of memory and self-help aids.

Clinical Pearl

Intervention: If the patient has a problem with compliance because of the form of the medication or packaging, suggest using an alternative form, such as a liquid or a crushable tablet, and ask the pharmacist to replace childproof caps with regular caps (if appropriate).

Assessment of social and ethical issues should include questions about the cost of medications, attitudes and expectations about taking medications, the effect of medication on quality of life, and the perceived importance of each medication. Include prescription and over-the-counter medications in obtaining this part of the assessment.

Additional history information should address the following:

• Financial status
• Readiness, willingness, and ability to learn
• Values and attitudes about health perceptions and expectations
• Learning needs
• Available community resources and support systems
• Involvement in outside activities, social involvement, and dependency on care providers
• Receptivity to teaching, including physical condition, emotional state and maturity, intellectual status, learning goals and style, developmental level, stage of adaptation, self-esteem, life experiences, health and religious beliefs, sociocultural background and socioeconomic status, and support system

RISK FACTORS

Barriers to safe and correct self-administration of medications vary and constitute a major area of assessment. The older adult's vision, hearing, and memory; level of independence with activities of daily living; and available resources must be considered as potential risk factors (McConnell, 1988; Wright, 1991). Reading ability, reasoning ability, judgment, motivation, and fine motor coordination are also potential barriers. Manual dexterity is an important skill in the administration of medications. Assessment of these areas must be undertaken before implementation of a medication regimen to facilitate effective self-administration.

Assess for the presence of known-culprit drugs, which are highly associated with adverse drug reactions (eg, antibiotics, hormone-replacement drugs, steroids, anticonvulsants, anticoagulants, antiarthritics, sedative-hypnotics, and social drugs [caffeine, nicotine, marijuana, alcohol]).

Older adults most at risk for drug interactions include those older than age 75, women, and those with a diagnosis of acute illness, unstable disease, or kidney or liver dysfunction. Other factors include multiple drug use, long-term therapy, a history of noncompliance, or seeing more than one prescriber (multiple physicians or midlevel providers). Often, older adults have long-standing beliefs and attitudes concerning medication use. Many have preconceived notions about what medication can and cannot do for them. Some self-manage based on the belief "a pill for every ill" and "if one pill is good, two might be even better." The resulting polypharmacy is risky because of the increased risk of adverse drug interactions. Some older adults fear medications and do not even want to take aspirin. Lack of knowledge concerning medications is a common problem for older adults responsible for self-medication.

Alterations in pharmacokinetics and dynamics of aging place the older adult at great risk for harmful drug effects, drug interactions, and iatrogenic illnesses. The risk is greater when multiple drugs are used. It is therefore not surprising to find that iatrogenic illnesses and deaths due to drugs are more common among older than among younger adults (Denham, 1990).

Certain disease processes result in changes in the functioning of the renal, hepatic, and cardiovascular systems, thereby increasing the risk of problems with medication administration. Particular medications present an inherent iatrogenic risk. Evaluate each older adult's medication list for the inclusion of barbiturates, benzodiazepines, cimetidine, digoxin, heparin, iron preparations, levodopa, lithium carbonate, phenothiazines, phenytoin, propranolol, tricyclic antidepressants, and warfarin. Generally, these medications may have exaggerated and unexpected effects on the older adult. Many adverse effects are related to prolongation of half-life. Examples of this mechanism can be seen with barbiturates, benzodiazepine, digoxin, propranolol, and tricyclic antidepressants. In cases in which these medications are used, the dose may need to be reduced, the need for continued use must be reviewed frequently, and, in some cases, an alternate treatment may be necessary.

Other medications have undesired effects for various reasons, such as dopamine receptor supersensitivity, as is seen with phenothiazine, and an increased percentage of free drug leading to unreliable total serum levels, as is seen with phenytoin. Cimetidine may cause confusion and/or disorientation and should be avoided. Because of altered gastrointestinal absorption, iron preparations are not absorbed and may yield a poor response. The dose may need to be increased. Levodopa may cause blood pressure to drop, thereby increasing the risk of falls. The appropriate dose may be less than expected.

PHYSICAL ASSESSMENT

A comprehensive nursing physical assessment related to drug administration should include the following:

- Drug assessment, including over-the-counter medications, prior adverse drug reactions, and presence of unnecessary drugs

- Cardiac and kidney function evaluation
- Examination for other diagnoses that may affect absorption, distribution, metabolism, and excretion
- Functional status evaluation (vision, hearing, manual dexterity, and memory).

A review of systems is helpful in organizing data collection about any signs and/or symptoms that may affect medication administration. The data collected may suggest a side effect or an adverse reaction to a medication. Findings may suggest an aging change that would alter the way the medication would be administered or influence the older adult's ability to self-administer the medication.

If any signs or symptoms are found, further evaluation to determine the cause and effect of the problem is necessary. Questions to consider are, "Is this the onset of an acute process?" "Could this be a drug reaction, either side effect or adverse reaction?" and "Will this finding affect the older adult's ability to learn about and administer the medication?"

DIAGNOSTIC TESTS

Therapeutic drug monitoring is instrumental in helping maintain the older adult on the correct medication dosage. Plasma monitoring is helpful when the patient's medical situation is complex, such as when he or she is in the hospital or in a nursing home. Monitoring is seen frequently in patients with renal, hepatic, thyroid, and/or cardiovascular diseases. Results of monitoring can help clarify problems when there is an altered response. Poor response may be related to noncompliance, poor absorption, altered metabolism, or an unexpected resistance or sensitivity.

Correct dosage is necessary to get the most benefit and the least side effects from the medication. The correct dosage is based on the medication's therapeutic range (window). The range is important because if the level of medication rises above a certain point, chances of toxicity are greater; conversely, if the level is too low, the medication will not be effective. In the older adult, therapeutic response is even more important than in younger adults, because a standard dose may prove to be more toxic due to an aging metabolism or excretion capability. Drug-level monitoring is most helpful when this window is narrow, such as with digoxin, lithium, and theophylline. Monitoring is used often in reference to analgesics, antiarrhythmics, antibiotics, anticonvulsants, bronchodilators, and tricyclic antidepressants.

NURSING DIAGNOSES

Older adults, as a group, have more chronic illnesses than others managed by the use of medications. Because of this preexisting tendency toward multiple illnesses and the concurrent use of drugs, the health status of older adults often presents as a therapeutically complex picture. The following is a list of potential nursing diagnoses associated with older adult drug use:

- Altered Thought Processes related to drug interactions
- Constipation related to mobility reduction and dehydration
- Functional Incontinence related to drug effects

- High Risk for Injury related to orthostatic hypotension, dizziness, visual disturbances, impaired judgment, and sedation
- Noncompliance related to complex medication regimens
- Noncompliance related to side effects
- Noncompliance due to insufficient funds
- Noncompliance due to insufficient knowledge of medication regimen
- Knowledge Deficit related to drug administration regimen.

NURSING INTERVENTIONS

A creative nurse finds various ways to tailor a standard drug administration intervention for each older patient. The nurse's role in assisting the patient to overcome limitations related to medication knowledge and/or skill deficits is vital. The nurse uses many methods, including teaching, supporting, and providing a developmental environment, to effectively address these types of limitations. With older adults, learning is more effective if the nurse develops educational materials, sets aside teaching time, and sits down with the patient to educate him or her. Unfortunately, in today's fast-paced hospital setting, this approach is often impossible. Problems with medication administration often cannot be addressed until close to discharge, and then they are sometimes abbreviated or omitted. Therefore, nurses need to know ways to develop an efficient, reliable, realistic, and effective plan for patient medication education (Ruzicki, 1989).

PATIENT AND FAMILY EDUCATION

The nurse's role in evaluating the older adult's problems with drug administration begins with assisting and/or guiding the person in determining individual self-care demands or needs. This task is accomplished in several stages.

- Assess the older adult's ability to engage in the act of drug administration.
- Determine the presence of any limitation in ability to complete this act (deficits in knowledge and/or skill of drug administration).
- Assist the patient to formulate a plan that addresses these deficits.

The nurse's responsibilities lie in the areas of administering, teaching, collaborating, monitoring, and evaluating. The nurse's role in drug administration is usually limited to the acute care setting and involves little patient input. The nurse is mostly concerned with the five "rights"—patient, drug, dose, time, and route. During drug administration sessions, ask questions directed at evaluating the older adult's ability to perform drug administration tasks as he or she intends to do at home. This area of questioning can begin with "Tell me how taking your pills fits into your daily routine" and "Tell me what you know about this pill." Depending on the patient's answers during these sessions, positive behaviors and information can be reinforced, while inaccurate or incomplete behaviors and information can be addressed.

The nurse's responsibility for medication education is based on implementing a supportive strategy that assists the patient in overcoming limitations in knowledge and/or skill. To develop this strategy, the nurse must select the combination of methods that will most effectively aid the patient in addressing problems involved in drug administration. Development of this strategy is based on the awareness of three major factors that will affect potential development of problems with drug administration: the older adult's cognitive status, functional status, and health status. Goal setting and establishing outcome criteria for safe drug administration is a collaborative process between the nurse and the older adult. Efforts must be made to continuously evaluate the patient's abilities to engage in self-care practices that define safe drug administration (Kennedy, 1990). Some important approaches to be used with older adults are as follows:

- Include family members of the older adult's choosing.
- Use short, frequent teaching sessions.
- Check for memory deficits.
- Present one medication at a time.
- Associate medication administration with daily activities.
- When using written material, use large print and avoid glossy surfaces to increase readability.
- When planning written information, particularly drug calendars, avoid using green and blue inks together, because yellowing of the lens of the eye makes distinguishing the difference difficult.
- Use person's life experiences to deal with new situations, deal with the loss of health, relate to attitude about medication taking, and prepare for death.
- Allow for interruptions associated with hospital-related stress (sensory underload and overload, disorientation, sleep deprivation, and pain).
- Collaborate with physicians, pharmacists, and other health care professionals.

Important knowledge components to include in a teaching plan are the drug name, purpose, dosage, and form/appearance. The description should include the expected duration of treatment, administration schedule, storage instructions, and precautions. The older adult should be aware of the potential adverse reactions, actions to take if a dose is missed, evaluation of expiration date, and the need to always carry a list of medications (prescribed and over-the-counter). Other important components to include in a teaching plan are:

- Ability to read and comprehend medication label
- Ability to open pill bottle and the need and availability of childproof caps
- Proper storage techniques and the need to dispose medications older than 1 year and antibiotics older than 6 months
- Use of medication calendar or container to organize medications.

 ▷ *Clinical Pearl*

Intervention: Patient education may not always be the top priority because inadequate staffing and shortened hospital stays often force the nurse to make difficult decisions among many priorities in the overall work context. Nurses, therefore, need to be creative in their approaches to patient education.

The teaching plan is aimed at reducing drug administration problems for the older adult. The plan should be directed toward helping the adult prevent or detect adverse drug reactions during the earliest stages. A thorough assessment will delineate the older adult's level of intellectual ability, attitudes, interests, values, and physical/motor skills.

Adequate time for discussion, initial demonstration by the nurse, and practice and return demonstration by the older adult is essential. Not feeling rushed and having adequate time is an issue for the older adult when attempting to apply new information.

In most cases, the older adult patient will be able to be responsible for managing the medication regimen to some extent. Even so, planning for potential sources of support during periods of acute illness or unforeseen problems is suggested. Because of limited income, most older adults will benefit from a plan that considers the amount of money available for medication purchase.

Ensuring home medication compliance is a problem for most nurses. Because of the trend of increasing acuity levels and restrictive lengths of stay, it is typically a challenge to implement an effective medication education program focused on consistently reinforcing the patient's home-care ability. Although patient education regarding self-care issues, such as medication administration, has probably never matched the need, the advent of shorter hospital stays due to diagnosis-related groups (DRGs) and the nursing shortage have compounded the problem by lessening the time and personnel needed to address this need. Therefore, most older adults go home with inadequate knowledge and skills to cope with the complex task of managing their illnesses, especially through self-medication. Yet because older adults are at great risk for drug hazards, patient education and practice are critical needs for safe self-care for this segment of the population.

Unfortunately, no single strategy for teaching patients about their medication regimen may be effective. Strategies that may enhance self-care medication behaviors include the following:

- Evaluating a patient's comprehension of medication instructions
- Simplifying the medication schedule
- Providing a color-coded self-monitoring system
- Substituting generic drugs whenever possible.

When older adults are helped to gain relevant drug information and skills through individualized teaching strategies, they can make safe and effective medication decisions.

HEALTH PROMOTION

Nurses have a responsibility to collaborate with the prescribing physician, hospital and community pharmacist, and other caregivers involved in the older adult patient's drug administration practices. Each of these persons should know any pertinent data concerning actual or potential problems with drug administration for that older adult. The goal is to help the older adult to assimilate drug administration skills into his or her daily routine. The physician can be assisted by any knowledge that the nurse has about the patient and potential or real problems associated with drug administration. Both hospital and community pharmacists can act as watchdogs for drug interactions and for ways to improve the regimen and performance of individual medications. Pharmacists play an important and necessary role as a resource person to all of the collaborating parties. Caregivers can be involved in the collaboration process by being included in the appropriate assessment, education, and return demonstration sessions.

The goal of successful drug therapy is to treat the condition in accordance with the older adult's feelings about quality of life, based on mutually developed treatment objectives.

- Prevent adverse drug reactions related to drug errors by educating the older adult patient thoroughly
- Advocate the use of decreased drug doses and use of less toxic agents
- Make suggestions to the person prescribing the drugs for alternatives for drugs that cross the blood–brain barrier
- Intervene to promote the drug's beneficial effects and to minimize drug reactions
- Include large print on medication labels for those with visual impairments.

SAFETY PROMOTION

Monitoring the older adult's progress toward desired outcomes related to drug administration must be a continuous, systematic appraisal. The monitoring role is based on evaluation of desired results, untoward side effects, and adverse drug reactions. Judging patient responses directly or evaluating reports of response can help define areas of needed change in the regimen. The Patient Teaching Box provides helpful hints for safe self-drug administration.

Using an evaluation period will help the older adult identify effective strategies for avoiding drug administration problems. The nurse will benefit from an evaluation by noting any pitfalls to prevent recurrence of problems. Safe drug administration can be enhanced if the nurse monitors and evaluates the older adult patient as he or she administers medications during practice sessions before hospital discharge. Desired and unwanted drug effects and plasma drug levels can also be evaluated at this time.

Patient Teaching Box
APPROACHES TO SAFE SELF-DRUG ADMINISTRATION

Helpful Hints for Safe Self-Drug Administration:

- Inform all health care providers what medications are being taken, who prescribed them, and for what reason, condition, or disease. Carry a list of medications and over-the-counter drugs at all times.
- Keep all medications in a prominent place.
- Drink 8 oz of water with medications to promote drug absorption and to decrease the possibility of gastrointestinal adverse reactions.
- Use a drug calendar to reinforce any verbal instructions and as a visual reminder for home use. Take an ordinary calendar and write the medication and dosage on each day. Cross the day off after the drug is taken. Associate medication administration with daily activities.
- Use an egg carton instead of expensive drug compartment boxes to plan daily drug regimen.
- When using written instructions, use larger print, avoid glossy surfaces, and identify with colored labels or dots if needed.

PREVENTION AND DETECTION OF PROBLEMS

The nurse can prevent and/or detect problems related to drug administration by knowing the current trends and issues involved with aging and in caring for older adult patients. Some of these trends and issues include:

- Living with chronic illness and being involved in treatment plans, including hospitalization and complex drug therapies
- Living alone
- Dealing with functional decline
- Managing drug therapy independently
- Knowing pharmacokinetic and dynamic changes related to aging
- Recognizing adverse drug reactions
- Dealing with iatrogenic illness.

As a person's general status, including functional ability, changes due to aging and/or disease, so does the ability to take care of himself or herself independently. Ability to complete desired and required tasks is affected by age, diagnosis, educational background, financial situation, knowledge base, skills ability, cognition, functional ability, and social support (Orem, 1991).

Adverse drug reactions are two to seven times more likely for the older adult (Denham, 1990); 20% to 25% of hospital admissions for persons older than age 65 are secondary to adverse drug reactions (Schwertz & Buschmann, 1989). Adverse drug reactions are often mistaken for signs and symptoms of disease or, worse, for normal aging. Examples of this phenomenon are anticholinergic effects, episodes of depression, extrapyramidal symptoms, postural hypotension, and mismanagement of medication regimen, especially self-medicating with over-the-counter medications.

Preventing adverse drug reactions is a major goal in drug therapy of the older adult. Too often, a drug reaction can impair the older adult's functional status. In treatment plans, nondrug therapies are preferable. If a drug is needed, consideration of drug–drug, drug–alcohol, drug–disease, and drug–nutrition interactions are imperative (Lamy & Michocki, 1988). Because iatrogenic illness due to drugs results in increased morbidity and mortality in older adults (Denham, 1990), preventing the problems associated with drug administration is the ideal strategy. Patient education can provide an older adult with relevant knowledge and skills required to make informed and safe choices about drug consumption, thereby decreasing problems related to drug administration.

PATIENT COMPLIANCE

In every situation, when a new medication is prescribed, nursing interventions can have an impact on the effectiveness of the regimen. Factors that may explain why patients have difficulty complying with their medication regimens include complex prescriptions, presence of chronic illness, cognitive dysfunction (delirium and dementia), normal aging, lack of understanding of initial drug information given, inability to recall the information, and reluctance to ask for information. Recognizing these factors can enable the nurse to plan interventions for increasing the patient's requirements in relation to knowledge and skills.

Once a patient has been identified as being at risk for compliance problems, he or she should receive the necessary assistance to best prepare him or her for successfully dealing with this problem. A medication education teaching plan will probably be most effective if it includes the use of a drug calendar designed to delineate each drug and its administration schedule, practice sessions throughout hospitalization focusing on administering medications, and use of a pillbox (Gibson, 1989). Compliance is more likely when the information presented fits the needs and lifestyle of the older adult, because he or she will perceive the information as being meaningful and useful. Effective education promotes the older adult's informed choices, knowledge, and self-care behaviors in independent self-medication. Attention to the availability of adequate resources also affects compliance issues (Larrat, Taubman, & Willey, 1990). Some general principles to promote compliance include the following:

- Explain that there is no drug treatment to combat the aging process.
- Explain expected effects, possible side effects, and storage requirements.
- Have patients tell what they know about the prescriptions and over-the-counter medications that they are taking.
- Evaluate the patient's understanding of the treatment regimen, including nondrug therapy.
- Evaluate for the use or need for a memory aid.
- Encourage the use of one pharmacy.
- Discourage self-medication.
- Discourage the use of alcohol and concurrent use of any medications.
- Set mutual goals for safe medication administration.

Nurses must feel comfortable fostering older adults in the new role of health care consumer. Older adults must be assisted with understanding the importance of seeking periodic reevaluation and supervision of long-term drug therapies. The outcome of an effective teaching plan is a supportive strategy that assists the older adult in overcoming limitations in knowledge and skill.

Nursing Care Plan

FOR PATIENTS WITH DRUG ADMINISTRATION PROBLEMS

Nursing Diagnosis: Knowledge Deficit related to drug administration regimen.

Definition: The state in which an individual lacks specific knowledge or skills that affect ability to maintain health due to effects of aging, sensory deficits, language barrier, cognitive limitations, information misinterpretation, unfamiliarity with information resources, lack of interest in learning, lack of exposure or recall, denial of need to learn, lack of desire to learn, and inadequate economic resources. The problem may be one or any combination of the assessment factors.

Assessment Findings:
1. Relates problem with medication to nurse or other caregiver
2. Inaccurately uses terms related to drug administration, such as wrong drug name, action, route, or schedule

(continued)

Nursing Care Plan

FOR PATIENTS WITH DRUG ADMINISTRATION PROBLEMS *(Continued)*

3. Has knowledge and/or skill deficits and does not realize it
4. Is unable to explain therapeutic medication regimen
5. Repeatedly requests information on needed knowledge and/or skills
6. Fails to seek help or follow prescribed regimen
7. Displays inappropriate or exaggerated behaviors related to medication taking
8. Is unable to return performance of necessary knowledge/skills required to administer medications
9. Does not take medications

Nursing Interventions with Selected Rationales:

1. Teach patient about medication's purpose, correct dosage, common side effects, and administration instructions, including what to do if dose is missed.
   Rationale: Adequate knowledge of drug regimen is essential for health promotion, safety, and compliance.
2. Assist with setting up a medication calendar.
   Rationale: A medication calendar acts as a visual reminder, promoting safety and compliance.
3. Assist patient with reading and understanding information on medication labels.
   Rationale: The ability to read and understand label information prevents potential problems with drug administration.
4. Teach about proper storage and checking expiration date.
   Rationale: Proper storage and currentness of medication promote therapeutic drug action.
5. Teach about availability and use of non-childproof caps and organization containers.
   Rationale: Ease in opening containers and organization promote safe self-administration.
6. Inform of any dietary changes if necessary.
   Rationale: Dietary changes may be necessary to prevent food–drug interactions.
7. Encourage continued follow-up with health care provider.
   Rationale: Continued follow-up allows for evaluation of medication regimen and any changes necessary to prevent and/or minimize potential problems.
8. Include family members and other support persons in teaching sessions.
   Rationale: Including others in patient education encourages the patient and promotes compliance with therapy.

Desired Patient Outcomes/Discharge Criteria:

1. Patient verbalizes personal drug administration problems.
2. Patient uses suggestions that specifically address documented drug administration problems (sensory impairment, memory deficit, manual dexterity, financial difficulties, knowledge and/or skill deficits).
3. Patient effectively self-administers medications while dealing with acknowledged administration problems. Dependence on external human assistance is kept to a minimum.
4. Patient and necessary support system administer the regimen and can troubleshoot basic problems such as missing doses and expected side effects, and report adverse reactions.
5. Patient assimilates the medication regimen into the daily routine.

REFERENCES

Cartwright, A. (1990). Medicine taking by people aged 65 or more. *British Medical Bulletin, 46*(1), 63–76.

Chenitz, W. C., Salisbury, S., & Stone, J. T. (1990). Drug misuse and abuse in the elderly. *Issues in Mental Health Nursing, 11,* 1–15.

Denham, M. J. (1990). Adverse drug reactions. *British Medical Bulletin, 46*(1), 53–62.

Gibson, J. (1989). A new approach to better medication compliance. *Nursing 89, 5,* 49–51.

Kennedy, L. M. (1990). *The effectiveness of a self-care medication education protocol on the home medication behaviors of recently hospitalized elderly.* Unpublished doctoral dissertation, the University of Texas at Austin.

Lamy, P. O., & Michocki, R. J. (1988). Medication management. *Clinics in Geriatric Medicine, 4*(3), 623–638.

Larrat, E. P., Taubman A. H ., & Willey, C. (1990). Compliance-related problems in the ambulatory population. *American Pharmacy, NS30*(2), 18–23.

Leirer, V. O., Morrow, D. G., Pariante, G. M., & Sheikh, J. I. (1988). Elders' nonadherence, its assessment, and computer assisted instruction for the medication recall training. *Journal of the American Geriatrics Society, 36,* 877–884.

McConnell, E. S. (1988). Pharmacological considerations. In M. A. Matteson & E. S. McConnell (Eds.), *Gerontological nursing: Concepts and practice* (pp. 589–623). Philadelphia: W. B. Saunders.

Montamat, S. C., Cusack, B. J., & Vestal, R. E. (1989). Management of drug therapy in the elderly. *New England Journal of Medicine, 321*(5), 303–309.

Oles, K. S. (1990). Pharmacology. In A. Staab & M. Lyles (Eds.), *Manual of geriatric nursing* (pp. 111–119). Glenview, IL: Scott, Foreman/Little, Brown.

Orem, D. E. (1991). Self-care, self-care requisites, therapeutic self-care demand. In D. E. Orem (Ed.), *Nursing: Concepts of practice* (4th ed.) (pp. 117–145). St. Louis: Mosby–Year Book.

Ruzicki, D. A. (1989). Realistically meeting the educational needs of hospitalized acute and short-stay patients. *Nursing Clinics of North America, 24*(3), 629–635.

Santo-Novak, D., & Edwards, R. M. (1989). Rx: Take caution with drugs for elders. *Geriatric Nursing, 2,* 72–75.

Schwertz, D. W., & Buschmann, M. T. (1989). Pharmacogeriatrics. *Clinical Care Nursing Quarterly, 12*(1), 26–37.

Sheahan, S. L., Hendricks, J., & Coons, S. J. (1989). Drug misuse among the elderly: a covert problem. *Health Values, 13*(3), 22–29.

Sidel, V. W., Beizer, J. L., Lisi-Fazio, D., Kleinmann, K., Wenston J., Thomas, C., & Kelman, H. R. (1990). Controlled study of the impact of educational home visits by pharmacists to high-risk older patients. *Journal of Community Health, 15*(3), 163–174.

Wright, G. (1991). Geropharmacology: an individualized approach. *Journal of the American Academy of Nurse Practitioners, 3*(2), 85–89.

BIBLIOGRAPHY

Ansello, E. F. (1991). Aging issues for the year 2000. *Caring Magazine, 2,* 4–12.

Ignatavicius, D. D., & Baynre, M. V. (1991). Assessment of the urinary system. In *Medical surgical nursing: A nursing process approach* (pp. 1819). Philadelphia: W. B. Saunders.

Mahoney, D. F. (1994). Appropriateness of geriatric prescribing decisions made by nurse practitioners and physicians. *Image, Journal of Nursing Scholarship, 26*(10), 41–46.

Smeltzer, S. C., & Bare B. G. (1992). Biophysical and psychosocial concepts related to health and illness. In *Brunner and Suddarth's Textbook of medical surgical nursing* (pp. 186–189). Philadelphia: Lippincott.

Stilwel, J. E. (1988). Common health problems that threaten compliance in the elderly. *Topics in Geriatric Rehabilitation, 3*(3), 34–40.

Swift, C. G. (1990). Pharmacodynamics: changes in homeostatic mechanisms, receptor and target organ sensitivity in the elderly. *British Medical Bulletin, 46*(1), 36–52.

Tideiksaar, R. (1990). Principles of drug therapy in the elderly. *Physician Assistant, 2,* 29–46.

Tregaskis, B. F., & Stevenson, I. H. (1990). Pharmacokinetics in old age. *British Medical Bulletin, 46*(1), 9–21.

Problems With Nutrition

Objectives

1. List the physiologic changes of aging that affect nutritional status.
2. Describe the psychosocial changes of aging associated with changes in nutritional status.
3. Identify steps in the nursing assessment of a patient to screen and/or diagnose nutritional problems.
4. Discuss nutritional problems commonly seen in the older adult.
5. List nursing diagnoses associated with nutritional problems.
6. Design nursing interventions for the patient with nutrition-related problems.
7. Develop a nursing care plan for a patient with nutrition-related problems.

INTRODUCTION

NUTRITION PLAYS A VITAL ROLE IN THE GROWTH and development, health promotion and maintenance, disease prevention, and recovery of persons throughout the life span. The health status of the older adult is greatly influenced by lifelong nutritional practices established early in life as well as current practices, and both can affect activities of daily living and quality of life.

Nutrition is probably the most important single factor affecting the health of the older adult. Unfortunately, current nutritional practices of the older adult may be lifelong habits that are extremely difficult to change. Lifestyle has the greatest effect on nutrient intake (Kunkel, 1991), and the older adult may experience physiologic and/or psychological changes of aging that affect nutrition.

Malnutrition includes not only deficiencies of nutrients but also dehydration, undernutrition, nutritional imbalances, obesity, and the effects of alcohol abuse. Inappropriate dietary intake for conditions with nutritional implications and the presence of underlying physical or mental illness with treatable nutritional implications affect the quality of the older adult's life. In addition, nutritional status may deteriorate over time (Nutrition Screening Initiative,

1991). Protein–energy malnutrition among older adults has been identified in 59% of nursing home residents, 65% of hospitalized medical and surgical patients, and 22% of outpatients older than age 70 (Williams, 1993). The nurse with expertise can assist the older adult in attaining or maintaining optimal nutritional status in health and disease throughout life and in preventing malnutrition.

NORMAL PHYSIOLOGIC CHANGES

Physiologic changes associated with aging may cause changes in nutritional status of the older adult, or changes in nutritional status may cause physiologic changes. The maxim "You are what you eat from your head to your feet" is true, because most of the essential nutrients (carbohydrates, proteins, fats, vitamins, and minerals) cannot be produced by the body. These nutrients must come from an outside source to provide the body with essential materials for maintenance and repair, and then they must be absorbed, metabolized, and excreted to help the body maintain homeostasis.

As the body ages, several musculoskeletal changes take place. Body composition changes, resulting in decreased lean muscle mass (skeletal muscles diminish in size) and bone density and increased fat mass. The basal metabolic rate decreases because of decreased muscle mass, and the older adult requires less calories to keep the body functioning properly. Caloric requirements decrease to an average of 1,600 to 1,800 calories per day for women and 2,000 to 2,400 per day for men.

Increased cross-linking of collagen reduces tissue elasticity, thereby affecting functioning of musculoskeletal, cardiovascular, pulmonary, and renal system functioning. Cardiac output decreases and total peripheral resistance increases, resulting in lowered perfusion of nutrients and oxygen to all body tissues. Total lung capacity decreases, and the older adult relies more on diaphragm movements to expand and contract the lungs, hence increasing sensitivity to intra-abdominal pressure. For example, large meals or a slumped body position would increase intra-abdominal pressure and consequently prevent expansion of the lungs. The body loses the ability to clear wastes and concentrate urine decreases due to loss of kidney function, placing the older adult at an increased risk for fluid and electrolyte imbalance.

Because of changes in the senses (taste, smell, sight, and touch), the older adult may experience decreased sensory enjoyment of food and may be unable to differentiate foods that are too hot or cold, thus increasing the risk of oral mucosa damage. Poor sight or sense of touch may interfere with the older adult's ability to shop for food.

A lowered responsiveness to internal cues of hunger and thirst can contribute to older adults' inadequate intake of food and liquid, placing them at risk for dehydration, fluid and electrolyte imbalance, and nutrient deficiencies. Changes in the oral cavity make chewing and digesting food more difficult for the older adult. One half of the older adult population older than age 65 have no teeth, one fifth have periodontal disease, and only one third have a full set of teeth.

Oral health influences nutrient and fluid intake, breathing, self-esteem, self-concept, appearance, and communication. Good mouth and dental care is an essential component of health care for the older adult. Barriers to obtaining

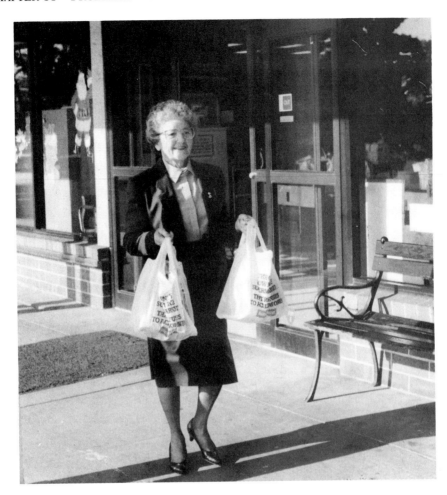

dental care may include negative attitudes related to preventive dental care, viewing loss of teeth as a normal part of the aging process, lack of dental insurance, and the cost of dental care. Because of other health problems, the older adult may not or cannot maintain optimal oral hygiene. Other common contributing factors include malnutrition, dehydration, high alcohol intake and tobacco use, trauma to the mouth (nasogastric tubes, ill-fitting dentures, sharp edges of teeth, improper use of cleaning devices), chemotherapeutic drugs with mucous membrane toxicity, radiation to head or neck, and immunosuppression.

Changes throughout the gastrointestinal tract related to aging greatly affect digestion. Salivary secretions decrease due to slowed functioning of the salivary glands, resulting in decreased taste, greater difficulty clearing food from the oral cavity, and more difficulty in swallowing foods. Decreased hydrochloric acid and gastric secretions in the stomach; reduced enzymes, absorptive surface, and villi height of the small intestine; and decreased motility of the large intestine make digestion and absorption of nutrients more difficult.

These physiologic changes may result in decreased food intake and impaired digestion and absorption of nutrients, especially vitamin B_{12}, iron, calcium, and zinc. The older adult may exhibit behavioral patterns that produce physiologic changes related to nutrition. For example, overuse of laxatives may contribute to reduced absorption of essential fat-soluble vitamins, such as vitamins A, D, E, and K. The nurse must avoid stereotyping the older adult and recognize that the degree of change is highly individualized.

ABNORMAL CHANGES

Approximately 85% of Americans older than age 65 suffer from one or more chronic diseases that may benefit from therapeutic nutrition intervention. Acute or chronic diseases often greatly affect the older person's appetite and diet. Disease-related symptoms, such as gastric distension, can lead to breathlessness or abdominal pain; gas, diarrhea, dysphagia (pain on swallowing), distortion of taste or smell, and nausea and/or vomiting usually decrease food intake.

Gastroesophageal reflux is a problem experienced by many older adults, and its prevalence increases with age. The lower esophageal sphincter is incompetent and, combined with a hiatal hernia, can lead to substernal burning and regurgitation of stomach contents. The older adult often reports heartburn and substernal chest pain. The symptoms occur most often 1 to 4 hours after meals. Reclining, belching, and increased intra-abdominal pressure aggravate the symptoms.

Forty-five percent of Americans older than age 65 use multiple prescription drugs. These medications can alter appetite, absorption, and metabolism of nutrients. Disease and medications can also contribute to impaired cognitive function. Confusion and memory loss may result in deficient or excessive food and nutrient supplement intake. A patient who is sedated or required to wear restraints may be compromised in the ability to obtain, prepare, and ingest food and fluids.

Severe psychological disturbances, such as psychotic depression, paranoia (the patient may believe the food is poisoned), and dementia (patient is unwilling to swallow or develops a gag reflex), can result in complete disinterest in food. In extreme cases, the older adult may stop eating altogether as a signal that life is not worth living and that he or she wishes to die (Roe, 1992).

PSYCHOSOCIAL ISSUES

The older adult faces psychosocial changes that may profoundly affect nutritional status, including changes in the living environment, the loss of a spouse, loved ones and friends, and altered socioeconomic status. The source and adequacy of income is most important to good nutrition. Forty-two percent of women and 17% of men older than age 65 have household incomes of less than $6,000 per year. Diminished or limited income may make it difficult for the older adult to budget enough for nutritious food or may lead to unhealthy food choices, such as overprocessed foods or foods high in sodium, fat, or empty calories. The older adult who has limited income may qualify for economic assistance and food programs. Some may have adequate income but choose to live in poverty because of fear of running out of resources.

The prevalence of depression is high for the older adult population. A large percentage of those older than age 65 live in institutional settings, where they find the food and/or environment to be unpleasant. Moving from a familiar environment to an unfamiliar one with strangers is often traumatic and can result in depression, causing overeating or lack of interest in food. The older adult may find the environment or food to be unappealing. Food aversion, antipathy to one or more foods, unwillingness to eat, or dislike of eating is more common in older adults, resulting in decreased food intake, which causes nutritional deficiencies (Roe, 1992). Food aversions can be caused by an unpleasant eating environment, thoughts, tastes, or smells of foods that evoke unpleasant memories, or association of foods with unpleasant qualities. Some institutional environments provide situations that provoke food aversions, such as unattractive, dirty, or noisy surroundings, unpleasant smells, room temperature extremes (room too cold or too hot), poor food service, monotonous, unattractive food, unfamiliar food, portions that are too large or too small, or foods too hot or too cold. Sometimes older adults can be disturbed by unpleasant company, such as noisy or very ill patients, and interferences at meals, such as interruptions to administer medications, procedures, or tests. Reports of malnutrition in institutionalized older persons range from 10% to 85% (Kerstetter, Holthausen, and Fritz, 1992).

Other changes in the older adult's environment could be loss of a spouse or companion. Thirty-three percent live alone, which may contribute to feelings of loneliness and depression, adversely affecting eating habits. Even if the older adult moves in with relatives, he or she might feel lonely and isolated while at home when others go off to work or school. Although adequate food may be prepared, these foods may be different from foods usually eaten, or feelings of depression and loneliness might cause loss of interest in eating. The older adult may skip meals rather than eat alone. Those who live alone at home might have difficulty in obtaining and preparing foods. The weather or fear of falling or being robbed may keep them from going to the supermarket.

Changes in physical appearance or health status as a process of aging may cause older adults to feel embarrassed, self-conscious, or depressed. These feelings may increase vulnerability to fad diets and supplements that claim to provide eternal youth and good health. Personal taste preferences, lifetime eating habits, and lack of socialization during meals may also influence psychological responses to food intake. Erroneous dietary beliefs may lead to inclusion or exclusion of certain foods or supplements. For example, an older adult may believe that milk is not needed in the adult diet; thus, unless other dairy foods are included, calcium and protein intake decreases. The older adult may take excessive vitamin and mineral supplements, which may lead to vitamin toxicity for fat-soluble vitamins.

Functional illiteracy is a major handicap for 50 million American adults. For the older adult unable to read, food shopping can be frustrating and embarrassing, often resulting in the inability to purchase nutritionally sound foods.

Cultural eating habits may have a profound effect on nutritional status. Many geographic, cultural, and ethnic groups have characteristic cooking and eating habits that influence consumption of foods and nutrients. For example, in the southeastern United States, high-fat, high-sodium foods are eaten daily by many older adults. Pork fat in the form of lard or bacon fat is used to fry meats and season starches and vegetables. Fat drippings from cooked meats are used to prepare gravies and sauces and are added to casseroles. Such a high fat intake in the daily diet adversely affects long-term health.

NURSING ASSESSMENT

Screening and assessment for nutritional risks and indicators should be a part of all health evaluations. The U.S. Preventive Services Task Force (1990) recommends that nutritional screening and diet counseling be a part of the health exam for the healthy older adult. For the ill older adult, good nutrition is vital to the healing process. Nutritional status should be evaluated at predetermined intervals and again when illnesses or new risk factors occur. Any deviation from optimal health increases the risk for poor nutrition.

Nutritional care is an essential component of quality nursing care. The nurse often works interdependently with other members of the health care team, such as with a registered dietitian or clinical nutritionist. Nurses may assess nutritional status for the following reasons:

- To identify nutritional problems related to health promotion, disease prevention, or treatment
- To identify self-care deficits related to nutrition
- To evaluate a patient's response to instruction or treatment
- To provide a baseline measurement for later evaluation of the patient's progress
- To provide an opportunity for the patient and/or caregiver to ask questions or to learn about nutrition and eating practices and their relationship to health.

The nurse spends more time with the patient than does any other health professional and is in a unique position to assess nutritional status. Nutritional status is as important a vital sign of overall health as is blood pressure or pulse rate. A history of food and fluid intake, socioeconomic status, and other factors affecting nutritional status are included. The physical examination along with anthropometric measurements and laboratory tests are used to identify existing clinical signs and symptoms of poor nutrition.

HISTORY AND INTERVIEW

Nutritional assessment is a multifaceted process that requires using many formats and forms for collecting nutritional data. When obtaining the nutritional history, the nurse needs to include questions that will elicit the following information:

- Patient's age and sex
- Patient/family information
  - Number and ages of persons in household
  - Race, ethnic, and cultural background
  - Religious affiliations that affect food
  - Educational level and reading ability
  - Financial status (money available for food)
  - Identification of person who purchases, prepares, and/or serves food
  - Recent changes in family
  - Motivation to eat balanced meals
- Environmental data
  - Place of residence, the living environment, and other factors affecting food availability (geography, climate)

- Daily activities, hobbies, and leisure activities
- Home and neighborhood facilities for purchasing, storing, preparing, and serving foods
- Health history
  - Recent changes in health, weight, and height
  - Recent changes in functional or mental/cognitive status
  - Recent attempts to change nutrient intake
  - Health habits affecting nutrient intake
  - Usual bowel and bladder habits
  - Use of medications, laxatives, and nutritional supplements affecting nutrition
  - Past and present exercise patterns
  - Health problems, handicaps, or surgery
  - Dental health
- Dietary history
  - Usual intake of foods and fluids (types and amounts)
  - Food preferences and aversions
  - Number, frequency, and time of meals and snacks
  - Appetite changes
  - Chewing or swallowing difficulties
  - Food allergies and symptoms
  - Problem foods that cause indigestion, gas, or diarrhea
  - Usual alcohol intake.

The history may reveal risk factors that suggest suboptimal nutritional status and the underlying cause of the nutritional problem. The nurse should complete a health history to identify potential and existing problems.

When completing the clinical history, also look for problems that may contribute to future nutritional problems, such as poorly fitting dentures or lack of dentures. It is much easier to prevent a nutritional problem than to cure one.

Question the older adult about oral comfort, chewing ability, dental habits, and attitudes toward oral care including:

- Problems chewing or swallowing foods
- Difficulty with soreness or bleeding in the mouth
- Bleeding gums
- Teeth that hurt, that are loose, or that are sensitive to hot or cold temperatures
- Dryness of mouth or tongue
- Last time dental care received
- Reasons for seeking dental care
- Dental hygiene routine (type, frequency, and equipment used)
- Use of dental floss
- Routine for care of dentures or bridges (if applicable)
- Concerns about oral care or dentition (Miller, 1990).

Remember to ask about prescription and nonprescription medications and nutritional supplements, and whether they are used routinely or occasionally. The Patient Teaching Box contains a screening form that can be used to identify warning signs for poor nutrition in the older adult. This form can be completed by the older adult or caretaker and could also be used with groups of persons to identify those who need more in-depth assessment.

Patient Teaching Box
DETERMINE YOUR NUTRITIONAL HEALTH: A SCREENING FOR THE OLDER ADULT

To determine your nutritional health score, do the following: Read the statement. Circle the number in the *Yes* column for those that apply to you. Add all the circled numbers.

	YES
I have an illness or condition that made me change the kind and/or amount of food I eat.	2
I eat fewer than 2 meals per day.	3
I eat few fruits or vegetables, or milk products.	2
I have 3 or more drinks of beer, liquor or wine almost every day.	2
I have tooth or mouth problems that make it hard for me to eat.	2
I don't always have enough money to buy the food I need.	4
I eat alone most of the time.	1
I take 3 or more different prescribed or over-the-counter drugs a day.	1
Without wanting to, I have lost or gained 10 pounds in the last 6 months.	2
I am not always physically able to shop, cook, and/or feed myself.	2
TOTAL SCORE	

Total your nutritional score. If it's

0–2   **Good!** Recheck your score in 6 months.

3–5   **You are at moderate nutritional risk.** See what can be done to improve your eating habits and lifestyle. Recheck your score in 3 months.

6+   **You are at high nutritional risk.** Bring this checklist next time you visit your nurse or doctor. Talk with him or her about the problems you have and ask for assistance to improve your nutritional health.

Remember these important points:

1. Be aware of any diseases or chronic condition or medication that causes you to change the way you eat.
2. Feeling sad, depressed, confused, or forgetful can cause changes in appetite, digestion, energy level, weight, and well-being.
3. Skipping meals, drinking alcohol, or eating too much can lead to poor health.
4. A healthy mouth, teeth, and gums are needed to eat. Be certain your dentures fit.
5. Investigate sharing finances and social contacts for meals, such as congregated meals and senior group meals. Being with people has a positive effect on morale and well-being.
6. Do not ignore losing or gaining a lot of weight.
7. Get help with shopping and buying and cooking food if you need it.

(Nutrition Screening Iniative, 1991)

Assessment of dietary intake, one component of a nutritional assessment, provides a baseline for determining whether the older adult's diet contains deficient or excessive amounts of calories or nutrients and determines whether intervention is needed. It also allows an opportunity for the patient or caregiver to voice dietary concerns.

The dietary assessment helps the nurse identify problems or potential problems related to food intake. One of the major contributors to nutritional problems in the older adult is decreased food intake, often the first sign of a potential nutritional problem. Lack of optimal food intake may have multiple causes. It is important to obtain information about foods consumed, the amount consumed, and the method of food preparation (eg, fried, broiled, steamed). Tools that may be used to obtain this information include a 24-hour food diary, dietary intake records (1-, 3-, or 7-day records), and a food frequency and diet history.

Probably the most frequently used method is the 24-hour food diary combined with the diet history. When using the 24-hour food diary, the nurse might associate activities with food intake and ask such questions as "When did you get up yesterday morning and when did you first eat?" "What did you eat?" "How much did you eat?" "How was the food prepared?" "Then, what did you do, and when did you eat again?" It is important to avoid labeling the meals as breakfast, lunch, or dinner unless the informant uses the label first.

The patient is also asked to differentiate between the amount served and the amount consumed, especially if the patient is institutionalized. It is important to determine if foods eaten in the past 24 hours are similar to usual intake. If hospitalized, food consumption in the hospital or nursing facility may be quite different from foods usually consumed at home.

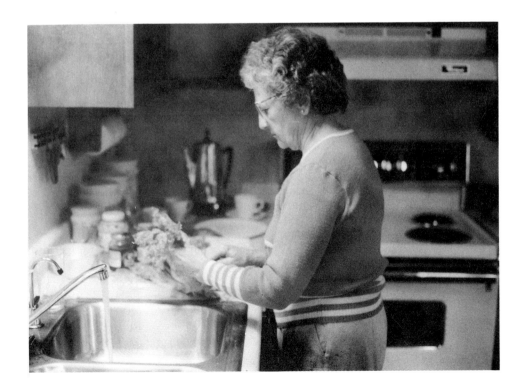

> ### *Clinical Pearl*
>
> *Assessment: To help the patient more accurately identify amounts consumed, the nurse can have various sizes of glasses, spoons, and food models and ask the patient to identify the size of the serving consumed.*

Once intake is recorded, it is compared with recommended daily intake using tools such as the *Food Guide Pyramid: A Guide to Daily Food Choices,* dietary guidelines for older adults, and *Recommended Daily Allowances* (National Research Council, 1989) for older adults (estimated by extrapolation from recommendations from younger adults [Ahmed, 1992]) (see Table 11-1).

The nurse also plays a major role in primary prevention of nutritional problems by screening for changes in dietary intake and helping the patient try to correct the inadequate intake before physical or biochemical changes occur. The nurse can use knowledge related to nutrition to provide anticipatory guidance to the older adult. Any change in the older adult's life can affect food intake.

Adequate hydration is essential for normal body functioning. Many older adults have decreased sensitivity to thirst, and with changes in mental status, they may forget to drink adequate fluids. Some older adults may restrict intake because of problems with incontinence or ambulating to the bathroom. Inadequate fluid intake may alter the body's metabolism of nutrients and medication and may lead to increased risk of infection and illness. Laboratory tests may be misinterpreted if the patient is not adequately hydrated and is not assessed for dehydration.

To assess fluid intake, the nurse should question the patient about the types and amount of fluid intake, identify any recent changes in intake and cause for changes, and compare actual intake to recommended intake. The nurse can calculate baseline requirements, making allowances for abnormal losses (such as drainage from a fistula or wound), deficits (dehydration from elevated temperature), or excesses (edema from congestive heart disease), and compare them with actual intake. Various methods are used to determine baseline fluid requirements; one formula used by health professionals is shown in Display 11-1.

Screening for income, education, and social activity can identify significant risk factors for nutritional problems. It is important to determine if the patient has adequate resources for food and food preparation and if he or she lives alone, is house bound, or is unable to or prefers not to spend money on food. It is also important to assess if the patient can read.

Older adults are more vulnerable to problems in the environment related to food safety. When assessing the older adult's environment, discuss food storage and sanitation.

Cultural eating habits may have a profound effect on nutritional status. An assessment of ethnic and cultural practices related to nutrition may identify risk factors for nutritional deficiencies or excesses. Certain food groups may be missing from the older adult's diet. For example, if the person practices vegetarianism, meat and milk products may be omitted from the diet; thus, obtaining adequate protein and calcium would be more difficult.

Table 11-1	RECOMMENDED DIETARY ALLOWANCES FOR THE OLDER ADULTS (51+ YEARS OLD)*	Men	Women
	Average Weight[†]	77 kg	65 kg
		170 lb	143 lb
	Average Height[†]	173 cm	160 cm
		68 in	63 in
	Calories age 51+	2,300	1900
	Calories per kg	30	30
	Protein	63 g	50 g
	Vitamin A (RE)[1]	1,000	800
	Vitamin D	5 µg	5 µg
	Vitamin E (α-TE)[2]	10 mg	8 mg
	Vitamin K	80 µg	65 µg
	Vitamin C	60 mg	60 mg
	Thiamin	1.2 mg	1.0 mg
	Riboflavin	1.4 mg	1.2 mg
	Niacin (NE)[3]	15 mg	13 mg
	Vitamin B_6	2.0 mg	1.6 mg
	Folate	200 µg	180 µg
	Vitamin B_{12}	2.0 µg	2.0 µg
	Calcium	800 mg	800 mg
	Phosphorus	800 mg	800 mg
	Magnesium	350 mg	280 mg
	Iron	10 mg	10 mg
	Zinc	15 mg	12 mg
	Iodine	150 µg	150 µg
	Selenium	70 µg	55 µg

*The allowances are intended to provide for individual variations among most healthy persons older than age 51 as they live in the United States under usual environmental stresses. Diets should be based on a variety of common foods to provide other nutrients for which human requirements have been less well defined.

[†]Weights and heights of reference adults are actual medians for the U.S. population of the designated age, as reported by National Health and Nutrition Examination Survey II. The use of these figures does not imply that the height-to-weight ratios are ideal.

[1]RE = retinol equivalents

[1]RE = 1 µg retinol or 6 µg β-carotene

[2]α-TE-α–tocopherol equivalent

1mg d-α-tocopherol = 1α-TE

[3]NE = niacin equivalent

[1]NE = 1 mg of niacin or 60 mg of dietary tryptophan

Adapted with permission *Recommended Daily Dietary Allowances 10th Edition.* Copyright 1989 by the National Academy of Sciences. Published by National Academy Press, Washington, DC.

RISK FACTORS

The nurse should be familiar with the following risk factors associated with poor nutritional status in older adults and the clinical indicators of poor nutrition used to identify those in need of nutritional counseling and/or interven-

Display 11-1
METHODS FOR DETERMINING FLUID REQUIREMENTS OF OLDER ADULTS

Use the following formula to determine oral or intravenous fluid requirements for the older adult. Keep in mind that if the patient has abnormal losses or excess fluid, adjustments should be made. If the patient's weight is recorded in pounds, convert it to kilograms by dividing the weight by 2.2.

Formula: 1500 mL + [15mL × {body weight in kilograms − 20}]
= Estimated Daily Fluid Needs

tions. The risk factors, if present, should be identified during the nursing assessment. The major risk factors are as follows:

- Inappropriate food intake related to meal/snack frequency; quantity/quality of foods or food groups; dietary modifications, whether self-imposed or prescribed; or alcohol abuse
- Poverty related to source and adequacy of income, which affects economic assistance from various programs and food expenditures and resources
- Social isolation related to support systems and/or living arrangements
- Dependency/disability related to functional status (performance of activities of daily living), disabling conditions, and/or inactivity/immobility
- Advanced age (80+)
- Acute/chronic diseases or conditions
- Chronic medication use related to prescribed or self-administered use (White, 1991)

PHYSICAL EXAMINATION

Physical signs and symptoms of poor nutrition provide vital evidence for a diagnosis of a nutritional problem. The physical examination can identify medical conditions that may cause poor nutrition or may identify poor nutrition that will lead to other medical problems. A review of systems is beneficial, because an abnormal sign may indicate the need for a more thorough examination.

Physical signs and symptoms can be a clue to poor nutrition, but they must be interpreted with caution, because the physical symptom may have multiple causes. For example, the presence of edema may indicate a protein deficiency, but it may also indicate inflammation, excessive sodium intake, congestive heart failure, or restrictive clothing. Table 11-2 lists some clinical signs of malnutrition.

Poor dentition is a common problem that contributes to poor nutrition in the older adult. Nursing assessment of the older adult includes physical examination of the lips, tongue, teeth, oral mucosa, and dentures/prosthetics.

Anthropometric measures are noninvasive methods for obtaining information about body stores of fat and muscle. Common measurements used to assess body composition include height, weight, skin-fold thickness, and arm and waist circumferences, which provide information about body size, weight, and proportions. Measurements of height and weight are easily obtained for ambulatory older adults, but for bedridden adults and those unable to stand, these measurements are more difficult and/or require special equipment. For those unable to stand, if the scale has a broad base, a chair of known weight

Table 11-2	CLINICAL SIGNS OF MALNUTRITION	
	Condition	Possible Nutritional Basis
	Emaciation	General malnutrition
	Orthopedic problems	Calcium or vitamin D deficiency
	Peripheral neuritis	Vitamin deficiency from alcohol abuse or diabetes mellitus
	Dermatitis	Pellagra secondary to chronic disease
	Night blindness	Vitamin A deficiency
	Redness of tongue	Macrocytic anemia resulting from deficiency of vitamin B_{12}, intrinsic factor, or folic acid
	Hemarthrosis and purpura	Ascorbic acid deficiency
	Folliculitis	Vitamin A deficiency
	Ascites and enlargement of liver	Protein deficiency

can be placed on the scale. For bedridden patients, a hoist scale or bed scale can be used. Measurements for all older adults may be difficult to interpret due to lack of data for comparison. Most available reference data are for the older white adult. Differences have been reported between younger black and white American adults, but little research has been done on anthropometric measurements in the older adult.

A height estimate can be calculated from knee height, and weight can be calculated using calf circumference, knee height, mid-arm circumference, and subscapular skin-fold thickness (Chumlea, Roche, and Mukherjee, 1984). Body composition can be evaluated using skin-fold thicknesses, mid-upper arm circumference, and mid-upper arm muscle circumference. Skin-fold thickness can be measured using Harpenden or Lange calipers or various plastic calipers. Measurements obtained are then compared with norms or standard tables. Measurement of a fold of skin and subcutaneous fat, usually in the triceps or subscapular areas, provides an indirect but well correlated estimate of total body fat.

A rough measure can be made by pinching a fat fold on the back of the arm or lower chest. A fold greater than 1 in. indicates probable obesity, and a fold smaller than $1/2$ in. indicates too little subcutaneous fat.

Measurements of mid-upper arm muscle circumference are only estimates, because the formula assumes that the arm is perfectly round and the thickness of the humerus is included. The measurement also is affected by sex, degree of obesity, and age. Fat is more easily compressed in females, the obese, and persons older than age 40. Norms for anthropometric measurements for nonwhites are not available. The nurse needs to use discretion in interpreting measurements in these persons. If the older patient is in a balanced state of nutrition, height, weight, skin-fold thickness, and body circumference should fall within norms on standard tables.

Body water, body fat, and bone density measurements can be done with special instrumentation. The nurse may be asked to assist with these measurements, or in some settings, the nurse receives special training and then completes these measurements. Once measurements are made, the measurements are compared with norms or standard tables to determine if abnormalities are present. Changes in body measurements over time should be carefully evaluated for an indication of nutritional problems. Errors in measurements and interobserver reliability are also potential problems. The trained health care professional frequently makes judgments about body weight such as "The patient is obese" or "The patient is underweight" without objective measurements. However, without actual measurements of body weight or fat, it is difficult to evaluate changes in the measurements. However, the measurements are of little value in evaluating nutritional status. Body fat measurements are better clinical indicators of overweight or underweight.

DIAGNOSTIC TESTS

Biochemical assessment uses hematologic and other laboratory tests to determine nutritional status. Laboratory tests are used to screen for nutritional problems and to confirm or refute diagnoses that are based on other assessment parameters. Laboratory test results for the older adult are more difficult to interpret because of age-related changes and lack of normal values for the older adult. In addition, there may be problems with collecting samples, such as 24-hour urine samples for the incontinent patient. Fluid and electrolyte imbalances or medications may alter the results. The more commonly used laboratory diagnostic tests for assessment of nutritional status are listed in Table 11-3.

Normal values and indications for use in the older adult are described in the Appendix. Albumin is the most useful and economic indicator of poor nutrition and protein malnutrition (Ferguson et al., 1993). Similarly, total cholesterol can indicate poor nutrition at both extremes. Levels below 150 mg/dL have been associated with increased mortality in nursing home populations

Table 11-3	LABORATORY (BIOCHEMICAL) TESTS USED TO EVALUATE THE NUTRITIONAL STATUS OF THE OLDER ADULT	
Protein	Serum albumin
	Serum transferrin
	Blood urea nitrogen
	Hemoglobin and hematocrit
	Creatinine-height Index
Immune function	Skin sensitivity tests
	Lymphocyte count
Lipids	Cholesterol and triglycerides
	Ketones
	Fecal fat
Carbohydrates	Blood or urine glucose
	Hemoglobin A1C
Vitamins and minerals	Prothombin time and blood clotting time
	Serum phosphate
	Alkaline phosphatase
	Serum levels of K, Mg, Ca, P, Cl
	Serum vitamin B_{12} and Shilling urinary vitamin B_{12}

Refer to Appendix I for ranges and nursing implications

(Ives, Bonino, Traven, & Kuller, 1993), and levels above 240 mg/dL have been identified as high risk by the National Cholesterol Education Program (Nutrition Screening Initiative, 1991). For most older adults, the more routine laboratory tests, such as hemoglobin or hematocrit, cholesterol, and glucose, along with anthropometric measurements, clinical history and physical examination, dietary analysis, and environmental and fluid assessment are sufficient to reveal those signs that point to nutritional problems.

If the focus of assessment is only on negative practices, the patient may feel hopeless and overwhelmed. As the nurse completes a nutritional assessment, he or she must focus on the positive aspects, thus helping the older patient and family member or caregiver to understand how good nutritional practices will promote improved health and well-being. For example, rather than focus on how much fried food is consumed and the high level of cholesterol, instead emphasize that reducing consumption of fried food will have a positive effect on blood cholesterol and reduce the risk of heart disease.

 Clinical Pearl

Assessment: Nutritional assessment components can be easily identified by remembering the "ABCDEF" method:

A nthropometric measurements: height, weight, skin-fold
B iochemical tests: lab tests such as cholesterol, albumin
C linical history and physical exam
D ietary analysis
E nvironmental assessment
F luid intake

NURSING DIAGNOSES

Once the assessment information is collected, it is analyzed and nutritional problems are identified. Nursing diagnoses related to nutrition include the following:

- Altered Nutrition: Less Than Body Requirements related to chewing or swallowing difficulties, anorexia resulting from chemical dependence, difficulty or inability to procure food
- Altered Nutrition: More Than Body Requirements related to increased intake from chemical or metabolic changes
- High Risk for Altered Nutrition: More Than Body Requirements related to family history of obesity
- Altered Health Maintenance related to intake in excess of metabolic requirements
- Ineffective Individual Coping related to increase in eating in response to stressors
- Altered Comfort related to chemotherapy as evidenced by nausea and vomiting
- Fluid Volume Deficit related to decreased oral intake or abnormal fluid loss

- Fluid Volume Excess related to excessive sodium/fluid intake
- Feeding Self-Care Deficit related to cognitive deficit paralysis
- Altered Oral Mucous Membrane related to dehydration or mechanical trauma from ill-fitting dentures.

NURSING INTERVENTIONS

The nurse plays a major role in assisting the older adult learning to manage nutritional problems and to monitor progress. Providing adequate nutrients and fluids in a pleasant environment and encouraging the family and the patient to take an active role in decision making about nutritional care is essential to good nutrition.

PATIENT AND FAMILY EDUCATION

Health teaching about good nutritional practices and about managing nutrition-related problems may be required after the nurse completes a nutritional assessment. The nurse should include the patient and family in developing individualized recommendations to incorporate into the patient's daily lifestyle. Always explain the rationale for the dietary changes along with the health benefits and risks. Discuss general diet principles, incorporating recommendations into the patient's usual eating habits with minimal changes. Identify suggestions for purchasing and preparing food. Use large lettering and write all instructions clearly. Teach them about oral hygiene and ways to cope with any limitations in performing oral hygiene measures. Actively assist the older adult in obtaining optimal nutritional status by educating him or her regarding nutrition and diet. Use the food guide pyramid on page 161 as a guide for suggestions.

Help the patient maintain a healthy lifestyle by providing the individualized guidelines listed in the Patient Teaching Box.

If gastric reflux is a problem, the nurse can instruct the patient in methods that assist in decreasing reflux, which include the following:

- If obese, lose weight to decrease intra-abdominal pressure.
- Avoid coughing, straining, bending, and other activities that increase intra-abdominal pressure.
- Avoid constrictive clothing, girdles, and abdominal supports.
- Modify food intake, such as fats, chocolates, excessive alcohol, and foods that irritate the stomach.
- Stop smoking.
- Avoid overeating and large meals.
- Sleep with the head of the bed elevated.
- Refrain from eating before reclining.
- Prevent constipation and avoid straining at stool.
- Obtain other treatments as necessary.

Antacids seem to be effective in 60% to 70% of persons with reflux (Burke & Walsh, 1992). The goal of therapy is to modify or reduce reflux. Muscle weakness and postural changes associated with aging can aggravate the problem. The patient and family should be instructed in positioning and antacid therapy.

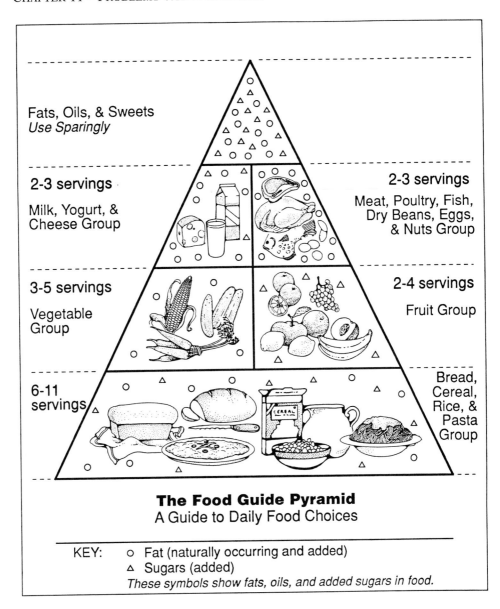

Fats, Oils, & Sweets
Use Sparingly

2-3 servings

Milk, Yogurt, & Cheese Group

2-3 servings

Meat, Poultry, Fish, Dry Beans, Eggs, & Nuts Group

3-5 servings

Vegetable Group

2-4 servings

Fruit Group

6-11 servings

Bread, Cereal, Rice, & Pasta Group

The Food Guide Pyramid
A Guide to Daily Food Choices

KEY: o Fat (naturally occurring and added)
        △ Sugars (added)
        These symbols show fats, oils, and added sugars in food.

ORAL HYGIENE AND MAINTENANCE

The goal of nursing care is to maintain or attain optimal oral health and oral comfort. The frequency of oral health maintenance will vary according to the patient's health status and self-care ability. All persons should have their teeth and mouths cleaned at least once after meals and at bedtime (Carpenito, 1993). A soft toothbrush with a nonabrasive toothpaste can be used to brush the teeth, tongue, and inner sides of cheeks. The mouth should be rinsed with water. The nurse may need to perform oral hygiene maintenance for institutionalized older patients or any patients unable to do it themselves and teach ways of coping with disabilities. For persons unable to tolerate brushing,

Patient Teaching Box
"YOUR HEALTHY DIET PLAN"

Instructions for _____ (patient's name) acquired from their ideas and nutritional assessment include:

Based on the information about your nutrition and eating habits that you shared with me and my findings during the physical exam, the following are some of the behaviors that are healthful: _____

_____

Behaviors that you and I have identified that are unhealthy include _____

_____

If you change these behaviors, you will decrease the risk of _____

_____

Is this something that you think you are interested in doing? _____

Foods that are recommended include _____

_____

The amounts include _____

_____

Foods that should be avoided include _____

_____

Recommendations should be incorporated into your usual eating habits with minimal change. Ways that you might change your eating habits include _____

What do you see that you will need to change? _____

Ways you can get the support you need to make these changes.

Suggestions for food purchasing and preparation:

A shopping list (unless patient institutionalized) with changes in food preparation and some recipes can be planned with patient (family) and attached to instructions.

One day's planned food intake can be attached to instructions

Potential problems and potential solutions include _____

_____

For questions contact _____

moist applicators may be used to swab the teeth and mouth, and the mouth may be irrigated with water. Lemon/glycerin swabs should be avoided when stomatitis is present. If the patient is unconscious or at risk for aspiration, place the person on his or her side and have suction equipment readily available to prevent aspiration. If needed, a tongue blade or bite block can be used to keep the mouth open.

The teeth should be flossed and the mouth inspected for lesions, sores, or excessive bleeding every 24 hours. Alcohol-containing mouthwashes should be avoided because of their drying effect. In addition, excessive use of hydrogen peroxide for mouth care should be avoided. If oral pain is present, an oral pain solution can be ordered by a physician or dentist (Carpenito, 1993).

Dentures and bridges should be removed and cleaned. The dentures should be brushed with a stiff, hard toothbrush and rinsed in cool water. Stains and odors can be removed from dentures by soaking them overnight in 8 oz of water and 1 teaspoon of laundry bleach (avoid bleach on any appliance with metal). Hard deposits can be removed by soaking dentures in white (not brown) vinegar overnight. If commercial liquid denture cleaners are used, brushing is still required (Carpenito, 1993). Leaving dentures out for prolonged periods results in changes in gum structure and a poor fit and thus should be avoided.

FLUID INTAKE

Nursing actions to help the older adult increase oral fluid intake and prevent dehydration include developing a plan for obtaining and drinking needed fluids, with input from the patient and/or caregiver. The plan should be specific as to the amount and type of fluid offered at specific times. Setting a goal for short time intervals, such as 2- or 3-hour intervals rather than 8-hour shifts and involving the patient and/or caregiver in recording or monitoring the amount consumed is essential to ensure compliance. If the patient is prohibited from eating or drinking because of scheduled procedures, the goal must be modified to compensate for lack of fluid intake during the prohibited time. Certain foods and fluids, such as coffee and alcohol, have a diuretic effect, and additional fluid intake may be required to compensate for fluid loss through diuresis. It is most important that the patient be placed in an appropriate sitting position while drinking to avoid choking and/or aspiration. If dehydration develops, normal fluid–electrolyte balance should be returned as safely as possible. If adequate fluid intake by mouth is not possible, parenteral fluids may be necessary. Careful monitoring of intake and output along with electrolyte levels and urine osmolality is essential.

The nurse can play a major role in assisting the older patient to learn to manage nutritional problems as well as to monitor progress. General guidelines for maintaining health and preventing disease are outlined in Display 11-2.

ALTERNATE FEEDING METHODS

Nurses play a major role in ensuring that older adults are adequately nourished, especially in long-term care. They have major responsibility for providing enteral feedings and parenteral nutrition. The choice of feeding method and formula is determined by the patient's physical condition.

For persons unable or unwilling to eat adequate foods and fluids, alternative routes for getting nutrients into the body may be necessary. Enteral feed-

Display 11-2
DIETARY GUIDELINES FOR HEALTH AND DISEASE PREVENTION

- Maintain physical activity.
- Maintain healthy weight.
- Maintain a varied and nutrient-dense diet.
- Maintain adequate fluid intake.
- Maintain protein intake at moderate levels.
- Increase intake of starches and other complex carbohydrates.
- Reduce total fat intake to ≤ 30% of kilocalories. Reduce saturated fat intake to ≤ 10% of kilocalories and cholesterol intake to <300 mg/day.
- Limit dietary sodium intake to 2 to 5 g.
- Maintain an optimal intake of calcium, fluoride, and magnesium.
- Limit alcoholic beverages to ≤ 1 oz of pure alcohol in a single day.
- Maintain eating as a social activity.
- Use dietary supplements only if clinically indicated.
- Identify eating problems and develop a plan for addressing problem areas.
- Practice prevention of nutrition problems, especially for high-risk groups.

(Horwath, C. *Nutrition and the older adult.* Princeton: Continuing Education Center, Inc., 1991)

ings deliver a liquid diet by mouth or tube, commonly called "tube feeding," into a functioning or partially functioning gastrointestinal tract. Often, if the person is able to eat but is unable to consume adequate amounts of nutrients, oral enteral feedings can be used to supplement intake. Parenteral nutrition is a special feeding method using peripheral or central veins to achieve necessary nutritional support when the normal gastrointestinal route cannot be used. Tube feedings and parenteral nutrition have become increasingly common to help the older adult, who is unable to be fed orally, obtain essential nutrients. Enteral nutrition may be indicated in the following situations:

- Admitting diagnosis of malnutrition or undernutrition
- Five to 7 days of oral intake of 50% or less
- Severe protein–energy malnutrition (neoplasm, inflammation, trauma, burns, chemotherapy, radiation)
- Coma or depressed mental status
- Unintentional weight loss of more than 10% of usual body weight in 6 months
- Unplanned weight loss of 5% in 1 month or less
- Severe pressure sores (Stage III or IV)
- Neurologic or psychiatric disorders (often resulting in dysphagia)
- Chronic aspiration
- Abnormality of gastrointestinal tract (pancreatitis, fistula, short-bowel syndrome, malabsorption, inflammatory bowel disease)

For enteral feedings to be effective, the older patient must be able to digest and absorb foods normally. Enteral feeding preserves intestinal integrity and can be done economically. A variety of formulas are available, ranging from blended baby foods to elemental formulas. Special care should be taken to satisfy the psychological and social needs as well as the physical needs of the patient who is tube fed. Although nutrition can be maintained, the religious, social, and cultural aspects of eating are denied. The food no longer looks, tastes, or smells familiar. Involvement of the patient and/or caretaker may be helpful.

If an oral supplement is not appropriate, tube feedings may be ordered. The tube may be inserted nonsurgically through the mouth or nose, such as a nasogastric, orogastric, or nasoduodenal tube, or surgically or endoscopically through an opening into the gastrointestinal tract, such as in esophagostomy, gastrostomy, jejunostomy, or percutaneous endoscopic jejunostomy.

Three different methods for delivering tube feedings are available: bolus, continuous drip, and cyclic. Bolus feeding is convenient. Usually, 240 to 400 mL of the feeding is administered over a short period by gravity drip over 30 to 45 minutes. This method of feeding allows the person to move about the environment and participate in activities; however, intolerance problems and risk of aspiration, especially when tubes are inserted through the mouth and nose, are greater than with other methods. When using the bolus method, gastric residual should be monitored carefully to avoid complications.

The continuous drip method involves a feeding pump or gravity delivering the feeding over 24 hours. This method reduces the possibility of pulmonary aspiration and complications of intolerance and is associated with smaller residual volumes. With the continuous drip method, the older adult has limited mobility, and the nurse must routinely check gastric residual. If intake is interrupted for an hour or more, adjustments to compensate for lost calories must be made.

If the older adult needs a dietary supplement, is in a transitional stage from tube to oral feedings, or is in active rehabilitation and tube feeding is interrupted for long intervals, the cyclic method of feeding is indicated. This feeding method allows flexibility for delivering the feedings at night or at specified times during the day.

When administering a tube feeding by any method, the nurse should be aware of the following:

- Formula (commercial name)
- Number of calories per 24 hours
- Volume to be given for 24 hours and strength of formula
- Frequency of feedings per 24 hours
- Volume of water in addition to the prepared formulas
- Site of entry for tube feeding (nasogastric, percutaneous endoscopic jejunostomy, gastrostomy, jejunostomy)
- Method of administration (bolus, pump, drip, gravity).

Significant complications can occur with tube feedings. The nurse plays a vital role in monitoring and preventing complications, the most common and deadly of which is aspiration (Table 11-4). In one study, aspiration occurred in up to 56% of patients (Henderson, 1991). To help prevent aspiration, placement of the tube and gastric residual must be routinely checked before feeding, the patient should be positioned at a 45-degree angle, and suction equipment must be available. Nausea, vomiting, and diarrhea from tube feedings can usually be minimized, because these usually stem from rapid feeding rates (Bockus, 1991). Fluid and electrolyte imbalances and hyperglycemia are common in tube-fed patients. Skin care around the surgically or endoscopically inserted feeding tube site and oral hygiene for all tubes used are essential to prevent complications. The goal is to provide essential nutrients and fluids safely and effectively in the most acceptable manner with as few complications as possible.

If enteral nutrition is not appropriate or inadequate to meet the patient's needs, parenteral nutrition may be necessary. Parenteral nutrition may be
(text continues on page 168)

Table 11-4

ENTERAL TUBE FEEDING COMPLICATIONS AND PROBLEM SOLVING

Problem	Cause	Prevention/Treatment
Mechanical complications		
Aspiration pneumonia	Delayed gastric emptying, gastroparesis	Reduce infusion rate.
		Select isotonic or lower-fat formula.
		Administer formula at room temperature.
		Regularly check gastric residuals.
	Gastroesophageal reflux	Use small-bore feeding tubes to minimize compromise of lower esophageal sphincter.
	Diminished gag reflex	Keep head of bed elevated 45 degrees during and after feeding.
		Initially and regularly check tube placement.
		Feed into duodenum or jejunum, especially for high-risk patients.
Pharyngeal irritation, otitis	Prolonged intubation with large-bore NG tubes	Use small-bore feeding tubes whenever possible.
Nasolabial, esophageal, and mucosal irritation and erosion	Prolonged intubation with large-bore NG tubes	Use smaller caliber feeding tubes made of biocompatible materials.
	Use of rubber or plastic	Tape feeding tube properly to avoid placing pressure on the nostril. Consider gastrostomy or jejunostomy sites for long-term feeding.
Irritation and leakage at ostomy site	Drainage of digestive juices from stoma site	Attention to skin and stoma care. Use gastrostomy tubes with retention devices to maintain proper tube placement.
Tube lumen obstruction	Thickened formula residue	Irrigate feeding tube frequently with clear water. Avoid instilling medications into feeding tubes. Irrigate tubes with clear water before and after delivering medications and formula.
	Formation of insoluble formula-medication complexes	
GI complications		
Diarrhea	Low-residue intolerance (lack of bulk)	Select fiber-supplemented formula.
	Rapid formula administration	Initiate feedings at low rate.
		Temporarily decrease rate.
	Hyperosmolar formula	Reduce rate of administration.
		Select isotonic formula or dilute formula concentration and gradually increase strength.
	Bolus feeding using syringe force	Reduce rate of administration.
		Select alternate method of administration.
	Hypoalbuminemia	Use elemental diet, or parenteral nutrition until absorptive capacity of small intestine is restored.

(continued)

Table 11-4

ENTERAL TUBE FEEDING COMPLICATIONS AND PROBLEM SOLVING
(Continued)

Problem	Cause	Prevention/Treatment
GI complications (continued)		
	Lactose intolerance	Select lactose-free formula (most commercial formulas are lactose-free).
	Fat malabsorption	Select low-fat formula.
	Microbial contamination	Use good handling and administration techniques.
	Rapid GI transit time	Select fiber-supplemented formula.
	Prolonged antibiotic treatment or other drug therapy	Review medication profile and eliminate causative agent, if possible.
		Repopulate normal gut flora with commercial lactobacillus.
Cramping, gas, abdominal distension	Nutrient malabsorption	Select formula that restricts offending nutrients.
	Rapid intermittent administration of refrigerated formula	Administer formula by continuous method.
		Administer formula at room temperature.
	Intermittent feeding using syringe force	Reduce rate of administration.
		Select alternate method of administration.
Nausea and vomiting	Rapid formula administration	Initiate feedings at low rate and gradually advance to desired rate.
	Gastric retention	Temporarily decrease rate.
		Select isotonic formula.
		Reduce rate of administration.
		Use half-strength formula.
		Select low-fat formula.
		Consider need for change in feeding route (eg, feed into duodenum or jejunum).
Constipation	Inadequate fluid intake	Supplement fluid intake.
	Insufficient bulk	Select fiber-supplemented formula.
	Inactivity	Encourage ambulation, if possible.
Metabolic complications		
Dehydration	Inadequate intake or excessive losses	Supplemental fluid intake.
		Monitor fluid intake and output.
Overhydration	Rapid refeeding	Reduce rate of administration, especially in patients with severe malnutrition or major organ failure.
	Excessive fluid intake	Monitor fluid intake and output and patient condition.

(continued)

Table 11-4

ENTERAL TUBE FEEDING COMPLICATIONS AND PROBLEM SOLVING (Continued)

Problem	Cause	Prevention/Treatment
Metabolic complications (continued)		
Hyperglycemia	Inadequate insulin production for the amount of formula being given	Initiate feedings at low rate.
		Monitor serum and urine glucose.
	Stress	Use oral hypoglycemic agents or insulin if necessary.
Hypernatremia	Inadequate fluid intake or excessive losses	Supplemental fluid intake.
		Monitor fluid intake and output.
Hyponatremia	Inadequate intake	Supplement sodium intake.
	Fluid overload	Restrict fluids.
	Inappropriate antidiuretic hormone secretion syndrome	Use diuretics, if necessary.
	Excessive GI fluid losses	Replace with fluids of similar composition.
Hypophosphatemia	Aggressive refeeding of malnourished residents	Monitor serum levels.
	Insulin therapy	Replenish phosphorus levels before refeeding.
Hypercapnia	Excessive carbohydrate loads given residents with respiratory dysfunction and CO_2 retention	Select low-carbohydrate, high-fat formula.
Hypokalemia	Aggressive refeeding of malnourished resident	Monitor serum levels.
		Provide adequate potassium.
Hyperkalemia	Excessive potassium intake	Reduce potassium intake.
	Decreased excretion	Monitor serum levels.

administered through a peripheral vein for those patients requiring short-term therapy and fewer than 2,500 calories per day (peripheral parenteral nutrition) or through a central vein for those patients requiring long-term therapy and a caloric intake of up to 4,000 calories per day (total parenteral nutrition).

Total parenteral nutrition is used to maintain or restore fluid and electrolyte balance, prevent deterioration and achieve homeostasis, and provide minimum protein and caloric requirements. Total parenteral nutrition is indicated in the following situations:

- Abnormality of the gastrointestinal tract (massive small bowel resection)
- Ingestion of food is impossible (obstruction)
- Intractable diarrhea or vomiting
- Impaired digestion and absorption, such as malabsorption, radiation enteritis, or ulcerative colitis

- Trauma to the gut, such as short-bowel syndrome, or edema due to severe malnutrition
- Receipt of high-dose chemotherapy, radiation, and/or bone marrow transplantation (American Dietetic Association, 1992)

When parenteral nutrition is administered, the infusion must be monitored closely. Equipment, such as tubings and filters, needs to be changed according to the institution's or agency's policy. Strict monitoring and care of the insertion site is essential. Fluid and electrolyte balance and intake and output should be assessed frequently. When an alternative feeding route becomes available, total parenteral nutrition should be gradually discontinued.

WEIGHT MANAGEMENT

Obesity is the most common nutritional problem in the United States, and the prevalence of obesity in older adults is 25% to 52% (Kunkel, 1991). Obesity usually occurs before age 75, is more prevalent in women than in men, and is associated with functional impairments and increased health risks. With aging, the basal metabolic rate decreases, and energy expenditure usually decreases; thus, food (caloric) intake must decrease accordingly to prevent overweight and obesity. Healthy eating habits and regular exercise throughout life are the best prevention. Treatment of obesity by strict dieting is seldom preferred, and unless the older adult is committed to permanent changes in eating and/or exercise, cyclic weight loss may do more harm than good.

In providing nursing care for the morbidly obese (persons weighing more than twice their ideal body weight), the nurse must rethink the routine. Special equipment may be necessary. In planning for the patient's admission, the nurse may want to check equipment specifications or check with the hospital's engineering department before using a piece of equipment on a morbidly obese older adult. Side rails, trapeze bars, and wheelchairs may break under excessive weight (Brentin & Sieh, 1991). In assessing the obese patient, the blood pressure cuff must be the appropriate size for the person's arm. If the cuff is too small, the reading may be falsely high and the tissue of the arm may be damaged. A thigh cuff may be the best option. Once techniques that work are identified, document them on the patient's chart so that everyone uses the same techniques.

Drug therapy and intravenous therapy may need to be adjusted for the obese adult. Many drug doses are based on weight and body water. Other drugs have an affinity for adipose tissue. Intramuscular injections given with the standard $1^1/2$-in. needle may be intra-adipose injections. Because blood flow to adipose tissue is sluggish, absorption may be delayed and duration of action prolonged. Cutaneous skin patches may work ineffectively in obese patients, because cutaneous tissue is not as well perfused. For intravenous therapy, a longer intravenous catheter may be necessary, because the veins may be more deeply embedded, making it more difficult to locate veins and start the intravenous therapy. Once started, edema at the intravenous site may be more difficult to detect (Brentin & Sieh, 1991).

For the obese older patient, bed rest may increase complications, especially related to respiration, circulation, and skin integrity. The older obese adult who is bedridden is at increased risk for hypoventilation, venous thrombosis, and skin breakdown. Aggressive skin care, semi-Fowler's position, and mobility decrease these risks.

Nursing Care Plan

FOR A PATIENT WITH POOR NUTRITION

Nursing Diagnosis: Altered Nutrition: Less Than Body Requirements related to changes in ingestion and digestion of food.

Definition: A state in which an individual who is not on nothing-by-mouth (NPO) status experiences or is at risk for experiencing reduced body weight related to inadequate intake or digestion of food.

Assessment Findings:
1. Inadequate food intake: less than recommended with loss of weight
2. Increased metabolic needs in excess of intake with weight loss
3. Body weight 10% to 20% or more below ideal weight for height and frame
4. Triceps skin folds, mid-arm circumference and mid-arm muscle circumference less than 60% of standard (Carpenito, 1993)
5. Decreased serum albumin or pre-albumin level and decreased serum transferrin level or iron-binding capacity
6. Poor muscle tone or muscle weakness
7. Diarrhea/hyperactive bowel sounds
8. Sore, inflamed buccal cavity
9. Nausea, vomiting, or (reported) gastrointestinal pain

Nursing Interventions with Selected Rationales:
1. Complete nutritional assessment and evaluate extent/degree of deficit.
   Rationale: Nutritional assessment provides a baseline for future assessments.
2. Assess causative/contributing factors to help determine plan of care.
   Rationale: Identification of factors aids in developing appropriate strategies.
3. Establish dietary plan and identify behavioral changes.
   Rationale: A dietary plan helps provide goal-directed activities and behavioral changes and helps ensure compliance and enhances success.
4. Monitor food and fluid intake/parenteral fluids/electrolytes, as ordered.
   Rationale: Continued monitoring prevents complications and allows for adjustments as necessary.
5. Monitor lab reports and report abnormal values.
   Rationale: Lab values provide an early indication of progress or deterioration.
6. Involve patient, caregiver, and family in plan and in teaching/supporting behavioral change.
   Rationale: Patient and family involvement helps to ensure compliance.
7. Reinforce medical interventions by explaining and clarifying for patient and family.
   Rationale: Knowledge of interventions promotes adherence to therapeutic regimen.
8. Determine food preferences and provide them within limitations of treatment plan.
   Rationale: Individualization to include patient preferences enhances possiblity of success.
9. Assist patient to determine and avoid foods that cause intolerance or increase gastric motility.
   Rationale: Determining problematic foods helps eliminate possible causative factors interfering with eating.

(continued)

Nursing Care Plan

FOR A PATIENT WITH POOR NUTRITION *(Continued)*

10. Promote socialization and a pleasant, relaxed environment for eating: minimize unpleasant procedures, odors, and sights (before meals and snacks) that may have a negative effect on food consumption.
    Rationale: A calm, pleasant atmosphere enhances meal time.
11. Assist or provide oral care and hand/face care before/after meals and as needed.
    Rationale: Oral care keeps the mouth clean and moist and helps with enhancing taste; hygiene allows the patient to feel refreshed, comfortable, and prepared for eating.
12. Review drug regimen and side effects for effects on food intake.
    Rationale: Certain medications can interfere with nutrient absorption.
13. Assist patient in obtaining resources or assistance with eating/obtaining foods.
    Rationale: Appropriate resources and assistance help promote adequate intake.
14. Offer smaller amounts of foods more frequently.
    Rationale: Small, frequent feedings prevent feelings of fullness and gastric distension and minimize discomfort associated with eating.
15. Consult with dietitian, physical therapist, or psychologist, as indicated.
    Rationale: Consultation with other health care professionals can assist in addressing specific problems interfering with nutrition.

Desired Patient Outcomes/Discharge Criteria:

1. Patient's weight loss stabilizes and/or gradually increases.
2. Patient can verbalize understanding of causative factors and necessary interventions.
3. Patient can demonstrate behaviors and management techniques necessary to manage problem (if medical condition is incurable) or to correct problem.

REFERENCES

Ahmed, F. (1992). Effect of nutrition on the health of the elderly. *Journal of American Dietetic Association, 92*(9), 1102–1108.

American Dietetic Association. (1992). *Nutrition care in nursing facilities* (2nd ed.). Chicago: Author.

Bockus, S. (1991). Troubleshooting your tube feedings. *American Journal Nursing, 91*(5), 24–30.

Brentin, L., & Sieh, A. (1991). Caring for the morbidly obese. *American Journal Nursing, 91*(8), 40–43.

Burke, M., & Walsh, M. (1992). *Gerontologic nursing care of frail elderly.* St. Louis: Mosby–Year Book.

Carpenito, L. J. (1993). *Nursing diagnosis application to clinical practice* (5th ed.). Philadelphia: J. B. Lippincott.

Chumlea, W. C., Roiche, A. F., & Mukherjee, D. (1984). *Nutritional assessment of the elderly through anthropometry.* Columbus, OH: Ross Laboratories.

Ferguson, R. P., O'Connor, P., Crabtree, B., Batchelor, A., Metchell, J., & Coppola, D. (1993). Serum albumin and prealbumin as predictors of clinical outcomes of hospitalized elderly nursing home residents. *Journal of the American Geriatrics Society, 41*, 545–549.

Henderson, C. T. (1991). Safe and effective tube feeding of bedridden elderly. *Geriatrics, 46*(8), 56–66.

Horwath, C. C. (1991). *Nutrition and the older adult.* Princeton: Continuing Education Center, Inc.

Ives, D. G., Bonino, P., Traven, N. D., & Kuller, L. H. (1993). Morbidity and morality in rural community-dwelling elderly with low total serum cholesterol. *Journal of Gerontology, 48,* M103–M107.

Kerstetter, J. E., Holthausen, B. A., & Fritz, P. A. (1992). Malnutrition in the institutionalized older adult. *Journal of American Dietetic Association, 92*(9), 1109–1116.

Kunkel, M. B. (1991). Nutrition and aging. In E. M. Baines (Ed.), *Perspectives on gerontological nursing* (pp. 323–335). Newberry Park, CA: Sage Publications.

Miller, C. A. (1990). *Nursing care of older adults: Theory and practice.* Glenview, IL: Scott, Foresman.

National Research Council, Food and Nutrition Board. (1989). *Recommended dietary allowances* (10th ed.). Washington, DC: National Academy Press.

Nutrition Screening Initiative. (1991). *Nutrition screening manual for professional caring for older America.* Washington, DC: Greer, Margolis, Mitchell, Grinwald.

Roe, D. A. (1992). *Geriatric nutrition* (3rd ed.). Englewood Cliffs, NJ: Prentice Hall.

U.S. Preventive Services Task Force. (1989). *Guide to clinical preventive services.* Baltimore: Williams & Wilkins.

White, J. V. (1991). Risk factors for poor nutritional status in older Americans. *American Family Physician, 44,* 2087–2097.

Williams, S. R. (1993) *Nutrition and diet therapy.* St. Louis: Mosby.

BIBLIOGRAPHY

Collensworth, R. E., & Boyle, K. (1989). Nutritional assessment of the elderly. *Journal of Gerontological Nursing, 15*(12), 17–21.

Durant, D. (1992). Food safety and nutrition concerns for the elderly who live alone. *Food and Nutrition News, 64*(4), 27–29.

Frisancho, A. R. (1981). New norms of upper limb fat and muscle areas for assessment of nutritional status. *American Journal of Clinical Nutrition, 34,* 2542.

Hoffman, N. B. (1991). Dehydration in the elderly: Insidious and manageable. *Geriatrics, 46*(6), 35–38.

Horwath, C. C. (1991). Nutrition goals for older adults: A review. *Gerontologist, 31,* 811–821.

Jenkins, C. H. (1988). *Nutrition and the older adult.* Princeton, NJ: Continuing Professional Education Center, Inc.

Jenkins, C. H., & Edlund, B. (1992). Nutritional assessment. In J. P. Bellack & B. J. Edlund (Eds.), *Nursing assessment and diagnosis* (2nd ed.). Boston: Jones and Bartlett.

12

Problems With Sleep, Rest, and Consciousness

Objectives

1. Identify physiologic changes of aging related to sleep, rest, and consciousness.
2. Describe how psychosocial changes of aging may relate to sleep, rest, and consciousness.
3. Identify steps in the nursing assessment of an older adult experiencing a problem with sleep, rest, or consciousness.
4. Describe the effects of common medications on the sleep/wake cycle in older adults.
5. List common sleep problems in the older adult.
6. Describe potential problems related to unconsciousness in the older adult.
7. Develop a nursing plan of care for an older adult experiencing a problem with sleep, rest, or consciousness.

INTRODUCTION

CHANGES IN SLEEP, REST, AND CONSCIOUSNESS often affect one's lifestyle and interfere with the ability to maintain control of many important functions. Some problems, such as insomnia or decreased ability to rest, may develop so gradually that older adults and their families are not aware of the extent of changes that have occurred over time. Other problems may occur suddenly, such as loss of consciousness with a stroke, that require quick adaptation to profound losses. With all problems of sleep, rest, and consciousness, professional nursing expertise can help both older adults and their families to understand the nature of the problem and to develop effective management strategies.

Staab, AS and Hodges, LC: ESSENTIALS OF GERONTOLOGICAL NURSING,
© 1996 J. B. Lippincott Company

Sleep is defined as a natural periodic interruption of consciousness in which body functions are restored. A normal night's sleep involves cycling back and forth among various stages of sleep. There are two types of sleep. The first type, nonrapid eye movement (NREM) sleep, includes two light and two deep sleep stages. As individuals progress through these stages, they experience deeper sleep. The second type of sleep, rapid eye movement (REM) sleep, is a deep sleep associated with dreaming.

In the older adult, the patterns of sleep are altered. There is an increase in the quantity of light sleep (Stages 1 and 2) and a decrease in the quantity of deep sleep (Stages 3 and 4). These deeper stages of sleep are considered to be necessary for physical restoration of body functions.

NORMAL PHYSIOLOGIC CHANGES

A wide variety of physiologic changes can affect sleep, rest, and consciousness. These changes are most evident in the nervous system. A person's state of consciousness is closely related to the interaction of the brain's cerebral hemisphere and the central gray matter of the upper brain stem. For the hemispheres to function normally in maintaining consciousness, there must be arousal or activation of the cerebral cells.

Aging brings about physiologic changes in the nervous system that can affect activation of cerebral cells. The number of neurons begins to decrease in middle age, followed by a steady decline in efficiency of the nervous system. Both sensory and motor aspects of the central nervous system may be altered. The effective function of neurotransmitters, essential for smooth communication within the nervous system, gradually declines with aging, thus altering processes related to onset and maintenance of sleep. Peripheral nerves also degenerate, leading to decreased sensory and motor conduction velocities. The changes in the older adult's nervous system create a need for greater intensity of stimuli to elicit responses and may result in slower responses to stimuli.

Sensory changes, such as visual impairment, may reduce sensitivity to external cues of lightness and darkness that prompt sleep patterns. In the older adult, circadian rhythm changes occur, which may affect heart rate, body temperature, volume of urine secreted, and excretion of urinary potassium.

These physiologic changes often result in altered sleep and rest patterns, but there is great variability among older adults. Sleep disturbances tend to increase with each decade and affect more than one third of those older than age 75. Most older adults do not have 8 hours of uninterrupted sleep. They may require a longer period of time to fall asleep and may awaken more frequently and earlier in the morning. Some older adults may experience no Stage 4 sleep. They may have shorter periods of REM sleep, which is considered essential for efficient brain functioning.

The older adult tires more easily and requires a longer period of restorative time after an activity. A lack of rest may lead to a lowered energy level, causing one to refrain from previously enjoyable activities. In addition, older adults require more time to adjust to changes in the normal sleep/wake pattern. This is important to consider when they are ill, hospitalized, or enter a nursing home.

ABNORMAL PHYSIOLOGIC CHANGES

Sleep disorders, such as sleep apnea, periodic limb movement, and restless legs syndrome, occur frequently in the older adult. In addition, older adults with dementia often have disturbed sleep/rest patterns.

SLEEP APNEA

Sleep apnea is thought to occur in as many as one third of older adults and is diagnosed as a lack of air flow out of the nose and mouth lasting more than 10 seconds (Mitchell, 1988). A diagnosis of sleep apnea means that during hours of nighttime sleep, there are at least 30 episodes of apnea, observed during NREM and REM sleep. These periods of apnea may occur as many as 300 times during a night and last as long as 120 seconds each.

Sleep apnea is 15 times more common in men than in women and is often associated with obesity and certain physical characteristics, such as a short, thick neck. It is common in persons with chronic obstructive lung disease. Sleep apnea is also frequently found in patients with Alzheimer's disease. Persons with sleep apnea may complain of sleepiness during the day because of interrupted sleep during the night. They may not realize that they are experiencing apnea, because many of the apneic periods are brief, and they may not awaken. Often the person observing the patient's sleep may be the one to notice the characteristic loud snorting sound that occurs when pressure, which has built up in the blocked airway, is suddenly cleared. If untreated, sleep apnea can cause life-threatening cardiovascular and respiratory complications.

PERIODIC LIMB MOVEMENT

The sleep disorder of periodic limb movement, often referred to as nocturnal myoclonus, is characterized by repetitive leg contractions occurring as often as every 30 seconds. The contractions occur in clusters lasting 5 to 60 minutes, and they may cause fragmentation of sleep and insomnia. No definite cause is known for this condition, but it occurs often with diabetes, renal disease, withdrawal from some sleeping medications, and excessive intake of caffeine or alcohol.

 Clinical Pearl

Assessment: A clue that a patient has periodic limb movement is the complaint of a sleep partner of being kicked at night. The characteristic jumping movements of the patient's legs at night may awaken the partner but not the patient.

RESTLESS LEGS

Restless legs syndrome is a sleep disorder in which the older adult experiences an extremely uncomfortable creeping, crawling, and wormlike sensation deep in the leg muscles. There is an almost uncontrollable urge to move the legs, stand, and walk. These sensations usually occur as the patient is drowsy, either while sitting in a chair for long periods of time or in bed while trying to fall asleep. The restless legs sensations often occur during sleep, causing the patient to awaken. The cycles are often repeated many times during a night, causing severe disturbance of sleep patterns. Total sleep time may be drastically reduced, with some nights of almost complete wakefulness.

SLEEP/REST DISTURBANCES RELATED TO DEMENTIA

Older adults who have symptoms of dementia, including those with Alzheimer's disease, often experience disturbances in the sleep/wake pattern. These persons present a special challenge to their caregivers, who must identify creative strategies for management of problems related to sleep and rest. Significant changes in the sleep/wake pattern may occur in early stages of dementia, before decreased cognitive functioning is evident. These changes include increased NREM sleep, decreased REM sleep, decreased deep sleep, and increased prevalence of sleep apnea. Persons with dementia may be spastically disoriented when awakening at night and need to have extra security measures implemented. Insomnia and wandering that occur at night with these older adults are important factors in a family's decision to seek institutional placement for the patient, and the family needs a great deal of support throughout this decision-making process.

DECREASING LEVELS OF CONSCIOUSNESS

There are many conditions representing a continuum of decreased levels of consciousness, from mildly decreased alertness to a comatose state. A disorder such as a slow-growing intracranial tumor can cause a gradually reduced level of consciousness. A decrease in level of consciousness can occur rapidly with a head injury after a fall, such as with a subdural hematoma. Bleeding or swelling of tissues within the cranial cavity can lead to rapid loss of consciousness and the need for emergency medical treatment to reverse the increasing intracranial pressure. Early recognition and intervention can prevent permanent brain damage. Brain infarction, hypoxia, hypoglycemia, and drug toxicity are other causes of loss of consciousness.

A common condition in the older adult that can cause rapid loss of consciousness is cerebrovascular accident, more commonly referred to as stroke. Although the incidence of stroke has decreased in recent years, it is the second leading cause of death for persons older than age 75 and remains an important problem for the older adult.

PSYCHOSOCIAL ISSUES

Changes in living style and personal relationships can affect the older adult's response to the environment. Anxiety and depression are common and may affect sleep/rest patterns, resulting in isolation from previous social activities. In turn, changes in meaningful daily routines can affect long-standing sleep behaviors. With the death of a spouse, the older adult may be faced with the strangeness of sleeping alone in a bed that had been shared with a partner for many years. The resulting emotional stress can cause disturbed sleep.

Frequent arousals from sleep may cause older persons to worry that they are not sleeping enough, even when the actual decrease in their total sleep time is minimal. Because napping during daytime hours may increase, it is important that this behavior is not perceived as laziness.

When older adults encounter stressful situations, they may require more time to return to baseline levels of emotional stability than younger persons. In addition, the older adult's perceptions of rest and comfort may change. A lowered energy level may lead to a perception of decreased comfort, resulting in increased aggressiveness and irritability.

NURSING ASSESSMENT

Most older adults do not seek out health professionals specifically for problems with sleep or rest. These problems may have developed so gradually that the older adult and the family have accepted them as normal.

In assessing the sleep and rest patterns of the older adult, the nurse should not use norms for young people. What is normal for one patient may not be for another. It is important to be aware that disturbed sleep and rest may lead to behavior and personality changes. The older adult deprived of sleep and rest may become irritable, depressed, confused, or disoriented.

HISTORY AND INTERVIEW

A sleep history is essential for effective assessment of changes in the sleep/rest pattern. If the older adult cannot provide this information, a family member or close friend should be interviewed. Table 12-1 shows one format for taking a sleep history. This method of organizing information in the sleep history helps to ensure a complete assessment of sleep and rest by using the acronym REST: R = review of perceptions; E = evaluation of related factors; S = sleep disorders; and T = typical daytime and nighttime routines.

Diet, tobacco, caffeine, and many medications may cause insomnia, daytime drowsiness, agitation, confusion, delirium, or drug dependence in the older adult. It is important to elicit information about the patient's prescription and over-the-counter medication use. Emotional stress, chronic disease, and depression are causes to be considered (Table 12-2).

It is important to recognize that the arousal component of consciousness may be reflected not only in problems of sleep and rest, but also in the condition of unconsciousness. Changes in the level of consciousness may occur rapidly and require quick and accurate assessment by the nurse. If the patient cannot respond appropriately to questions, it is important to obtain information from friends or family related to recent changes in the patient's level of consciousness.

The nurse should elicit information related to conditions that may alter consciousness, such as head injury, intracranial tumors, infectious diseases of the central nervous system, hypoglycemia, hyperglycemia, alcoholism, and stroke. The older adult should be questioned about any events in which level of awareness was altered. Transient ischemic attacks may have occurred without the person seeking medical attention. Important factors to explore in the history are periods of lethargy, drowsiness, confusion, disorientation, dizziness, headaches, and amnesia. Episodes in which the older adult had difficulty maintaining attention and concentration on a task are important to identify as well as periods of transient weakness or paralysis.

(text continues on page 180)

Table 12-1

SLEEP HISTORY

Interview the patient or family about the following factors:

Review of perceptions related to the problem
  Describe the sleep problem (in patient's own words).
  How long has the problem existed?
  How has the sleep pattern changed?
  When does the problem occur?
  What improves the sleep problem?
  What makes it harder to sleep?
  How serious is this problem to you?

Evaluation of related factors
  Describe typical eating patterns for a 24-hour period.
  Is alcohol used?
  Is smoking a factor?
  What medications are taken?
  Are any medications used to promote sleep?
  Is there evidence of depression or anxiety?
  Are there any chronic illnesses?
  Is there pain or discomfort during the day or night?
  Are there fears during the day or night?
  Are any specific factors related to the problem (eg, change in living quarters, change in
      eating habits, mental or physical changes, illnesses)?

Sleep disorders
  Is there snoring during sleep?
  Do legs jerk at night or during the day?
  Are there crawling, restless feelings in the legs that result in a need to stand up and
      walk?
  Do you feel sleepy during the daytime?

Typical daytime and nighttime routines
  Describe typical daytime activities.
      How has this sleep problem changed usual routines?
      Are there naps during the day? How often, how long, and when?
  Describe a typical night's sleep. Include:
      Where sleep occurs
      What is eaten or drunk 1 hour before bedtime
      Bedtime
      Bedtime routines
      How long it takes to fall asleep
      Number of awakenings
      Length of time awake at night
      Activities when awakened
      Strategies for falling back asleep
      Total number of hours of sleep
      Awakening time in morning

Table **12-2**	**MEDICATIONS AFFECTING THE SLEEP/WAKE CYCLE**

Category	Potential Effects

Benzodiazepines
    Examples: Dalmane, Serax, Halcion,
        Valium
	Increased onset of sleep
	Decreased deep sleep
	Suppressed rapid eye movement (REM)
	Residual daytime sleepiness
	Dizziness

Nonbenzodiazepines
    Example: BuSpar
	Less effective in patients recently on
	    benzodiazepines
	4–6 weeks needed for maximum effectiveness

Narcotics
    Examples: Demerol, Morphine,
        Codeine
	Suppressed REM
	Suppressed cerebral oxygenation
	Insomnia
	Unusual dreams
	Daytime drowsiness

Barbiturates Examples: Seconal, Nembutal	Increased onset of sleep Decreased deep sleep Suppressed REM Rapid tolerance
Alcohol	Suppressed REM Early and frequent wakening Apnea
Tranquilizers Examples: Equanil, Atarax, Vistaril	Daytime drowsiness Short-term memory loss
Antipsychotics Examples: Thorazine, Haldol	Daytime drowsiness Short-term memory loss Confusion Impaired attention
Antidepressants Example: Tofranil	Suppressed REM Increased tiredness

Stimulants
    Examples: Dexedrine, caffeine.
        theophylline
	Delayed sleep onset
	Increased wakefulness
	Decreased deep sleep
	Decreased total sleep

Antihistamines Examples: Benadryl, Benylin	Daytime drowsiness Confusion, delirium

(continued)

Table 12-2

MEDICATIONS AFFECTING THE SLEEP/WAKE CYCLE *(Continued)*

Category	Potential Effects

Antihypertensives
  Diuretics
  Examples: Diuril, Esidrix, Lasix
	Frequent awakenings to void if given late in the day

Beta Blockers Examples: Inderal, Aldomet, Catapres	Insomnia, nightmares Daytime sleepiness Insomnia Suppressed REM Fragmented sleep

Cardiovascular Drugs
  Digoxin
  Norpace
	Drowsiness, nightmares
	Confusion
	Short-term memory loss

PHYSICAL EXAMINATION

The physical examination includes a review of systems for identifying changes in the older adult's behavior that suggest disturbances with sleep or rest. A neurologic exam may reveal such disturbances as nystagmus (rapid, involuntary movement of the eyeball), hand tremor, ptosis (drooping of the eyelid), increased sensitivity to pain, and masklike facial expressions that may be related to sleep deprivation. Other symptoms identified by a review of systems include fatigue, decreased alertness, listlessness, decreased ability to concentrate, diminished motor skills, agitation, restlessness, and irritability.

The response to general stimuli in the environment and to specific verbal stimuli should be assessed during the physical exam. The older adult may have difficulty following instructions during the examination due to presence of sensory impairments. The nurse should observe if the person responds to noises, movement of objects in the room, and especially to specific questions or commands. In making this assessment, it is important to consider the effect of possible decreased levels of vision and hearing in the older adult.

In addition to determining the amount and type of stimulus, the nurse should note the nature of the older adult's response to the stimulus:

• Does the head or body move toward or away from a stimulus?
• Do eyes follow a moving object in the room?
• Do eyes open in response to a command?
• Does the patient verbalize appropriately?

Determining the exact nature of response to a stimulus is important in assessing changing levels of consciousness. The minimum assessment goal is to differentiate between three levels of consciousness:

• Alert and able to follow commands
• Awake and opens eyes but unable to follow commands

• Comatose: unable to open eyes, verbalize intelligibly, or follow verbal commands

Various methods and tools for describing level of consciousness are available and help detect subtle changes in neurologic status. Measurement tools such as the Glasgow Coma Scale (Table 12-3) should be used to assess more specific degrees of arousability.

Cranial nerve responses should be tested. Reflex responses to stimuli should be evaluated. Painful stimuli should not be used except when there is no response to auditory stimuli or nonpainful tactile stimuli. When any kind of stimuli are applied, the nurse should observe and record patient responses, such as withdrawal of an extremity from the stimulus, movement of the head or body toward the stimulus, opening of the eyes, verbalization, or more complex responses, such as obeying commands.

The physical exam should also include testing of sensory position sense, proprioception, cerebellar function, and gait. Abnormal movements of the extremities and signs of meningeal irritation, such as neck stiffness, should be evaluated.

DIAGNOSTIC TESTS

For definitive diagnosis of a chronic sleep disorder, a polysomnogram (continuous recording of an electroencephalogram and an electro-oculogram to monitor the sleep stages during an all-night sleeping period) is done. Ventilation, heart rate, respiratory effort, and gas exchange are also monitored.

Table 12-3

GLASGOW COMA SCALE

Behavior	Observation	Score
Opens eyes	Spontaneously	4
	To verbal stimulus	3
	To pain stimulus	2
	Not at all	1
Best verbal response	Oriented	5
	Confused	4
	Inappropriate words	3
	Incomprehensible sounds	2
	None	1
Best motor response	Obeys commands	6
	Localizes	5
	Flexion withdrawal	4
	Abnormal flexion	3
	Abnormal extension	2
	None	1

Scale used to assess specific degrees of arousability—a decrease in the score indicates a decreasing level of consciousness.
Maximum score 15: Awake and alert
Minimum score 3: Coma

Adapted from Mitchell, P. H. (1988). Consciousness: An overview. In Mitchell, Hodges, Muwaswes, & Wallecst (Ed.), *AANN'S Neuroscience Nursing* (pp. 57–66). Norwalk, CT: Appleton & Lange.

NURSING DIAGNOSES

In formulating a plan of care for a patient with problems with sleep, rest, and consciousness, the following nursing diagnoses should be considered:

- High Risk for Injury related to repeated awakening at night and confusion
- Impaired Verbal Communication related to decreased level of consciousness
- Altered Thought Processes related to inadequate sleep or decreased level of consciousness
- Impaired Physical Mobility related to cerebrovascular accident
- Sensory or Perceptual Alterations related to neurologic disorder or insomnia
- Self-Care Deficit, Bathing/Hygiene, Feeding, Dressing/Grooming, Toileting related to decreased level of consciousness or insomnia
- Body Image Disturbance related to neurologic disorder or sleep apnea
- Sleep Pattern Disturbance related to pain, hospitalization

NURSING INTERVENTIONS

Once a careful nursing assessment has been made, the nurse must identify interventions that support functional abilities, prevent further injury or dysfunction, and correct or minimize any effects of disabilities.

It is important to recognize that there are wide variations in individual sleep patterns of older adults. If the older adult has adapted to a sleep pattern that may seem unusual but is not compromising daily life activities, interventions may not be needed.

PATIENT AND FAMILY EDUCATION

The nurse can teach older adults and their families how to monitor subtle changes in sleep patterns, such as by using a sleep diary (see the Patient Teaching Box). Monitoring changes in patterns can help to determine which factors serve to enhance sleep and which act as barriers to sleep. Careful evaluation of changes may help to establish that an older adult who spends considerable time awake in bed may still be receiving an adequate amount of sleep.

Many older adults do have sleep patterns that are disruptive to their lives and to those of their families. For these persons, patient and family teaching can be helpful. Information about sleep changes that occur with aging can help persons plan effective strategies for adapting to their problems. The nurse can help the patient and family understand that sleep habits are deeply ingrained and that patience is needed to change long-standing sleep routines.

Patients with persistent sleep problems experience many sleepless nights and need much emotional support to help them adjust to their seriously altered sleep/wake patterns. Frequent sleep disruptions may leave them drowsy during the day, and nurses should educate them about the potential for injury if they should fall asleep while smoking, driving, or engaging in other activities that require alert levels of consciousness. Family members, who may stay awake at night to ensure the safety of the older adult who "walks the floor" at night, need to recognize the need for their own sleep. The nurse can be instru-

Patient or Family Teaching Box
SLEEP DIARY

Instruct the patient or family as follows:

Write down your activities for a 24-hour period. Do this for at least 7 days. Examples of some usual activities are given below. Add others that you think might be related to the amount of sleep and rest you get during a day.

Day _____ of diary

ACTIVITY   **TIME**

Morning wake-up time
Naps
Bedtime
Breakfast
Lunch
Dinner
Snacks
Alcohol
Smoking
Physical exercise (write the type of exercise)
Reading
Watching TV
Talking with friends or family
Activities outside of the home
Activities 1 hour before bedtime

How did you feel today?

Rested?
Tired?
Sleepy?
Bored?
Depressed?
Stressed?
Fearful?
Did you have any pain?
Were you uncomfortable? What type of discomfort?
Length of time before falling asleep
Number of times awoke during night
Length of time awake during night
Activities when awake at night

mental in helping family members identify realistic strategies for providing for their own much-needed sleep.

A patient with decreased level of consciousness is not fully alert to the potential for injury. The nurse ensures a safe environment for the patient by teaching family members to recognize the potential for falls, burns, and other injuries. Family members can be taught ways to safety-proof the home to prevent such injuries.

The sudden decrease in consciousness that comes with a transient ischemic attack or stroke is frightening, especially because the symptoms may recur and cause further injury. Older adults and their families need to be educated about the major risk factors in occurrence of strokes. The nurse can help the older adult to understand the rationale for preventive measures, such as the anticoagulant nature of aspirin, and to identify strategies, such as a healthful diet and regular exercise program, for promoting a healthy lifestyle that will decrease risk factors for stroke.

ENVIRONMENTAL MODIFICATION

In exploring the patient's perceptions about sleep and rest, it is important to identify ways to promote self-care and to explain how changes in behavior can promote health. Transient sleep disturbances that have existed less than 3 weeks are likely due to situational factors. The nurse can help the patient and family modify their environment to minimize sleep disturbances. The older adult may be getting too much environmental stimulation, such as with persistent noise of a television, or too little stimulation, such as when isolated in a room of the home away from other family members. Whenever possible, the older adult should be included in planning natural adaptations of the environment.

When awakened during the night, older adults need to be cautious in arising from bed. Slowed neurovascular reflexes that occur with aging can lead to postural hypotension and dizziness with sudden position changes. Older adults may be confused on awakening, forgetting temporarily where they are, and may become frightened. Changes in visual acuity may contribute to confusion. A night-light in the bedroom helps to promote mental and physical security. Placement of familiar belongings, such as a favorite quilt or picture, in the bedroom can help to provide visual cues for reorientation.

Clinical Pearl

Intervention: An older adult awakening frequently during the night may develop a pattern of going to the bathroom with each awakening. It may be useful to repattern these awakenings by going to the bathroom after the first awakening, but trying to fall back asleep without getting up at the second awakening. Breaking the pattern by alternating the times one actually follows the urge to go to the bathroom may help to decrease the amount of time awakened at night.

PROMOTION OF FUNCTIONAL ABILITIES

Older adults and family members may focus on deficits and overlook the patient's functional abilities. Whenever possible, the nurse should plan interventions that encourage the older adult's self-care abilities. Consulting with other health care professionals, such as with a physical, occupational, or speech therapist, can help promote the older adult's independence. The nurse can be instrumental in coaching the older adult to perform such activities as prescribed exercises, speech therapy, and adaptations to activities of daily living.

NURSE AS SUPPORTER

The nurse can help older adults and their families to understand the nature of the problem, cope with losses imposed by the problem, and implement creative strategies that allow the older adult to maintain as normal and satisfying a life as possible.

SLEEP PROMOTION

Establishment of pleasant bedtime routines can promote sleep. The older adult may find it helpful to keep only sleep-related activities in the bedroom. Regular times for going to bed and arising should be developed to meet individual needs. A greater sensitivity to cold may lead to a need to wear socks while sleeping and to use an extra blanket. Quiet activities, such as pleasant reading, listening to music, meditating, or praying, during the hour before bedtime can help to promote sleep (Fig. 12-1).

Involvement of the older adult in meaningful daytime and early evening activities can lead to physical and mental satisfaction that makes a period of sleep seem welcome. Regular, moderate physical exercise appears to increase deep sleep and duration of sleep. Exercise increases blood flow in the brain and thus may promote sleep by helping to restore normal body rhythms. Intense physical or mental exercise, however, should not be undertaken in the hours directly before bedtime.

When moved from their usual sleeping environment to a hospital or nursing

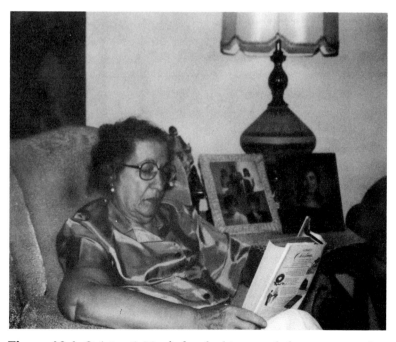

Figure 12-1. Quiet activities before bedtime can help to promote sleep.

home, most older adults experience some disruption of sleep. They may be fearful of the strange environment and hesitant to volunteer information about their usual bedtime routines.

The institutional environment may lack light and dark cues to promote sleep. In addition, lack of mobility, changes in routine activities, bright lights, strange noises, and frequent awakenings for nursing procedures interfere with normal sleep and rest. The nurse should attempt to make the patient as comfortable as possible in the new environment, offering encouragement to maintain as many routine sleep habits as possible. Efforts should be made to group routine nursing procedures to avoid unnecessary awakening of the patient. The nurse should explain tests, procedures, and other factors related to the patient's illness to diminish anxiety that may interfere with restful sleep.

After an acute illness or surgery, the nurse should encourage early ambulation and resumption of usual daily routines. Frequent position changes and back rubs can promote comfort. It is difficult for the nurse caring for the older adult in the hospital or nursing home to know whether to administer an as-needed sleep medication. Thus, the patient's sleep history as well as knowledge regarding effects of the medication on sleep patterns is critical in decisions related to administering these medications.

The nurse needs to be alert for problems of sleep disorders in the hospitalized older adult. Because standing and walking are often the only ways to relieve the sensations of restless legs, these persons may spend many hours at night walking when they are at home. Nurses need to recognize the potential need for these patients to walk at night in the hospital and should provide an environment that ensures the older adult's safety when walking. The use of bed-length side rails and restraints should be avoided, because they can contribute to serious injuries. Patients may fall and injure themselves when attempting to get out of restraints or crawl over side rails to walk off the restless legs sensation.

DIET AND NUTRITION

Adjustment of the diet can be helpful in promoting sleep. Stimulants such as caffeine and nicotine should be avoided. Large meals, especially in the evening, can lead to sleep disruption and should be avoided. Alcohol should be avoided at bedtime, because although it may hasten falling asleep, it often leads to fragmented sleep, causing a decrease in total sleep time. Decreased blood sugar levels during the night may result in awakening with feelings of hunger; a light snack may help the person to fall back asleep.

Decreasing the amount of fluids ingested after supper combined with emptying the bladder before going to bed can help to decrease the disruption of sleep caused by the urge to void.

Clinical Pearl

Intervention: A bedtime snack of warm milk, which contains tryptophan, a natural sedative, may be beneficial in promoting sleep.

MEDICATION ADMINISTRATION

Some physical discomforts, such as pain, incontinence, coughing, and leg cramps, may cause problems with sleep. The nurse can help the older adult and family understand the relationship of these discomforts to sleep disturbance. Careful timing of the older adult's medications, such as giving pain medication before bedtime, can ease physical discomforts and enhance quality of sleep and rest. Patients and their families should understand the peak times of such medications as laxatives and diuretics so that administration can be timed to avoid sleep disruption (see Table 12-2).

If sleeplessness persists despite the adjustment of psychosocial and environmental factors or if the older adult is undergoing a temporary stressful experience, medications such as nonbenzodiazepine hypnotics may be tried. Short-acting benzodiazepines (lorazepam, oxazepam, temazepam, triazolam) may be helpful when used cautiously. The older adult should limit these medications to three to four times a week during the trial period. Barbiturates should be avoided, and over-the-counter sleep medications should be used only with medical supervision. Older adults need lower doses of these medications than do younger adults, and their response to medications must be monitored carefully by the nurse and family members, especially in relation to excessive drowsiness, confusion, increased excitability, hostility, vision disturbances, and hallucinations.

A variety of medications may be used for the patient with decreased level of consciousness. Medication may be given to prevent seizures and minimize the potential for clot formation. If cerebral edema is present, osmolar diuretic therapy may be instituted to decrease intracranial pressure and prevent herniation of the brain stem. If hypertension is present, antihypertensive medications may be given.

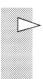

Clinical Pearl

Planning: Many older adults, feeling deprived of sleep, turn to prescription and over-the-counter sleep medications. These medications, however, may actually contribute to deterioration of sleep quality in the older adult and, if possible, should be avoided.

It is important that older adults and their caregivers maintain careful communication with the primary physician regarding all medications. Many older adults see a variety of specialists, each of whom may be unaware of medications prescribed by another. Polypharmacy, a situation in which many medications are prescribed, is a common cause of adverse drug reactions in the elderly. The nurse along with the primary physician can help older adults maintain a current list of all medications.

Nursing Care Plan

FOR PATIENTS WITH SLEEP PATTERN DISTURBANCE

Nursing Diagnosis: Sleep Pattern Disturbance related to pain, response to hospitalization, and nocturia.

Definition: A state in which the individual experiences sleep disruption causing interference with fulfillment of biologic and emotional needs.

Assessment Findings:
1. Complaints of difficulty falling asleep
2. Complaints of difficulty remaining asleep
3. Complaints of fatigue on awakening
4. Dozing frequently during the day
5. Depression

Nursing Interventions with Selected Rationales:
1. Review patient's perceptions related to the problem: history of problem, how it has changed since hospitalization, what makes it better, what makes it worse.
   Rationale: Patient's perceptions of problems and changes in problem can help to isolate important factors causing problem.
2. Evaluate factors related to the problem: smoking, timing of medications, effects of illness, presence of pain, fluid intake and output.
   Rationale: Patient may be unaware of factors that are exacerbating problem during hospitalization.
3. Rule out likelihood of sleep disorder: evaluate for periods of apnea, jerking of legs, and complaints related to restless legs.
   Rationale: Sleep disorders may gradually worsen, and patient may not be aware of a sleep disorder until hospitalization exacerbates the problem.
4. Identify patient's typical daytime and nighttime routines at home: Have patient describe how hospitalization has changed daytime and bedtime activities.
   Rationale: Altering the hospital environment to allow for resuming some routine daytime and bedtime activities can help to establish more stable sleep/ rest patterns.
5. Develop schedule for administration of analgesic that allows for patient decision making regarding dose and frequency of administration.
   Rationale: Pain can be controlled to meet patient's need for comfort, thus promoting sleep/rest.
6. Discuss with physician and patient various possibilities for increasing the amount of exercise while in the hospital.
   Rationale: Lack of exercise can increase joint stiffness and decrease ability to gain needed sleep/rest.
7. Discuss with patient the need for social stimulation and help patient plan visiting sessions to enhance sleep/rest.
   Rationale: Too much or too little social stimulation can detract from quality of sleep/rest.
8. Plan for naps at regular times during the day.
   Rationale: Sleep disruptions at night may increase the need for sleep during the day.
9. Evaluate need for and timing of fluids.
   Rationale: Decreasing the amount of fluid ingested before bedtime can decrease awakenings triggered by the need to void during the night.

(continued)

Nursing Care Plan

FOR PATIENTS WITH SLEEP PATTERN DISTURBANCE *(Continued)*

10. Plan for sleep/rest needs after discharge. Discuss with patient, spouse, or other family members some measures to promote sleep/rest in the home environment.
    Rationale: Knowledge of factors interfering with sleep/rest can promote self-care related to the problem.

Desired Patient Outcomes/Discharge Criteria:

1. Patient will describe factors, including physiologic, psychosocial, and environmental factors, related to the problem.
2. Patient will assist in controlling factors in a hospital environment to promote sleep/rest.
3. Patient will identify measures to implement at home to enhance sleep/rest.
4. Patient will differentiate between temporary sleep/rest disturbances and a potential sleep disorder and identify resources for exploring future problems related to sleep/rest.

REFERENCES

Mitchell, P. H. (1988). Consciousness: An overview. In Mitchell, Hodges, Muwaswes, & Wallecst (Ed.), *AANN'S Neuroscience Nursing* (pp. 57–66). Norwalk, CT: Appleton & Lange.

BIBLIOGRAPHY

Bootzin, R. R., & Perlis, M. (1992). Nonpharmacologic treatment of insomnia. *Journal of Clinical Psychiatry, 53*(Suppl 6), 37–41.

Cadiux, R. J. (1993). Geriatric psychopharmacology. *Postgraduate Medicine, 93*(4), 281–301.

Gall, K., Petersen, T., & Riesch, S. K. (1990). Night life: Nocturnal behavior patterns among hospitalized elderly. *Journal of Gerontological Nursing, 16*(10), 31–37.

Horne, L. A. (1991). No more wakeful nights: Helping elderly people to sleep properly. *Professional Nurse, 6*(7), 383–385.

Jelinski, M. A., & Fettig, M. (1993, July/August). Sleep patterns of home or hospitalized Alzheimer's disease patients. *American Journal of Alzheimer's Care and Related Disorders and Research*, 36–39.

Jensen, D. P., & Herr, K. A. (1993). Sleeplessness. *Nursing Clinics of North America, 28*(2), 385–405.

Locsin, R. C. (1989). Sleeplessness among the elderly. *Rehabilitation Nursing, 13*(6), 340–341.

Monane, M. (1992). Insomnia in the elderly. *Journal of Clinical Psychiatry, 53*(Suppl 6), 23–28.

Pollak, C. P., Perlick, Linsner, J. P., Wenston, J., & Hsieh, F. (1990). Sleep problems in the community elderly as predictors of death and nursing home placement. *Journal of Community Health, 15*(2), 123–135.

Shapiro, C. M., (1993). Impact and epidemiology of sleep disorders. *British Medical Journal, 306*, 1604–1607.

Swift, C. G., & Shapiro, C. M. (1993). Sleep and sleep problems in elderly people. *British Medical Journal, 306*, 1468–1471.

Problems With Skin, Hair, and Nails

Objectives

1. Compare and contrast age-related changes in the skin, hair, and nails.
2. Delineate the risk factors that influence the status of the skin in older adults.
3. Identify steps in the nursing assessment of the skin, hair, and nails of older adults.
4. Discuss nursing interventions useful in treating skin, hair, and nail disorders.
5. Develop a nursing care plan for an older adult with a pressure ulcer.

INTRODUCTION

THROUGH THE EYES OF A YOUTH-ORIENTED society, age-related changes in the skin, hair, and nails outwardly distinguish the young from the old. This recognition generates positive attitudes toward older adults in many cultures. However, in American society, negative responses frequently cause psychosocial discomfort and isolation among this age group. Gerontophobia (fear of growing old) often leads persons to use medications, cosmetics, and various treatments to try to camouflage these apparent signs of aging. For example, in the United States alone, more than $10 billion is spent on cosmetics in an attempt to prevent, reverse, or retard aging of the skin, hair, and nails (Gilchrest, 1986).

Skin, hair, and nail disorders are common in the older age group. Older adults often experience multiple skin disorders along with hair and nail problems, many of which can be prevented. Most are treatable without hospitalization; however, others, such as pressure sores or skin ulcerations, may require extended hospitalizations. Furthermore, they cause the patient prolonged discomfort, emotional trauma, and are a great economic cost both to the individual and to society (Gilchrest, 1986).

Some skin conditions, such as pruritus (itchy skin) and herpes zoster, may indicate systemic disease. Differential diagnosis of skin lesions in older adults is often difficult, because lesions are less identifiable than in the young. Therefore, a biopsy is recommended as the most definitive method of diagnosis. Because of changes in the immune system of older adults, they are more likely to develop infections from wounds, healing is slower, and acute disorders become chronic more rapidly (Balin, 1990).

Nurses play a key role in preventing and detecting many skin, hair, and nail disorders by regularly assessing the skin and appendages, referring the patient to a physician, and through effective nursing intervention. They can prevent the need for long-term care by preventing skin breakdown and promptly treating pressure ulcers and other lesions. Intelligent problem solving and knowledge of the latest prevention and treatment modes are necessary. Health teaching for the older adult and family helps to ensure continued health as well as contributes to overall satisfaction and fulfillment.

NORMAL PHYSIOLOGIC CHANGES

Epidermal cellular turnover decreases with age, resulting in a slower rate of healing and a greater likelihood of secondary infections developing after trauma. With aging, the thickness of the epidermis remains unchanged in sun-protected areas but atrophies in exposed areas of the body. A decreased number of melanocytes impairs the skin's protection from ultraviolet rays, thereby increasing the risk of skin cancer. A decreased number of Langerhans' cells also may account for a diminished skin immune response and a greater likelihood of the development of skin tumors and fungal or viral infections (Gilchrest, 1986).

The loss of about 20% of dermal thickness with age accounts for the thin, almost translucent quality of skin seen in many older adults. With aging, elastin fibers thicken and fragment while the vascular bed, collagen layer, and fibroblasts diminish (Fenske & Lober, 1990). Wrinkles develop with dermis atrophy, reduction of subcutaneous fat, and changes in the elastic network. Thinning of vascular walls accounts for the older adult's tendency to bruise easily. Susceptibility to skin-tear type injuries results from collagen fibers that have less elasticity when stressed. Blister formation is more likely to occur (Balin, 1990). Because of a decrease in subcutaneous tissue and the capillary network, the older adult is more prone to hypothermia or hyperthermia. Because foreign material clearance is decreased, older adults are more prone to extended allergic effects, reduced resolution of blisters, and delayed or masked treatment responses (Richey, Richey, & Fenske, 1988) (Table 13-1).

Age-related changes in the epidermis and dermis result in dry, leathery skin, inflammation, wrinkles, dyspigmentation, broken blood vessels, nodules, and premalignant lesions. With aging, there is atrophy of the subcutaneous tissue, especially in the face, hands, and legs. The abdomen tends to show fat cell accumulation, especially around the waist in men and on the thighs in women, without an increase in caloric intake. Chronic foot problems, such as corns, calluses, ulcerations, and pain, are also thought to be due to tissue atrophy (Fenske & Lober, 1990; Miller, 1995).

The cutaneous end organs are responsible for the sensations of touch, pressure, and vibration. With aging, pacinian and Meissner's corpuscles of the peripheral nervous system decrease in number, resulting in diminished sensations. Implications for older adults include difficulties with ambulation and manipulation of objects and the potential for traumatic injury, especially

Table 13-1	STRUCTURAL CHANGES ASSOCIATED WITH AGING OF THE SKIN	
	Structural Changes	Clinical Correlates
	Epidermis	
	Flattened dermo-epidermal junction	Shear-type injuries, increased blistering
	Decreased melanocytes	Uneven tanning, less barrier to ultraviolet light, actinically induced neoplasms
	Decreased Langerhans' cells	Neoplastic permissiveness, decreased contact dermatitis
	Cytoarchitectural disarray	Tendency to neoplasia
	Dermis	
	Great tensile strength	Less "give" under stress
	Elastic fiber changes	Lax skin, wrinkles
	Dermal ground substance changes	Decreased dermal clearance, prolonged contact dermatitis
	Decreased vascularity	Pale skin, increased risk for hypothermia/hyperthermia
	Decreased density	Poor insulation
	Appendages	
	Decreased function/number of sweat glands	Decreased sweating response, dry skin, less body odor
	Sebaceous gland hyperplasia	Small, yellow papules over face, forehead; comedones, cysts
	Nail changes	Soft, fragile, easily torn, dull
	Onychogryphosis	Shoe discomfort, fungal opportunistic infection
	Hair changes, loss of melanocytes	Hair graying
	Vellus hair changes to terminal hair	Bristle hair in ears, in nose in men, and on lip in women
	Decreased innervation	Susceptibility to burns, injury; decreased ability to perform fine maneuvers

From Fenske, N. A., & Lober, C. W. (1990). Skin changes of aging: Pathological implications. *Geriatrics, 45,* 30, reprinted with permission

burns. Nerves responsible for pain perception show little evidence of change with age (Balin, 1990).

The number of sebaceous glands in the older adult remains about the same, but the glands get larger and the sebum output decreases. Sun exposure causes hyperplasia of these glands with possible blackhead or cyst formation. Eccrine glands decrease in number and function, resulting in decreased perspiration and risk of hyperthermia. Older adults have a less distinct body odor because of decreased secretory function and accumulation of lipofuscin in the apocrine glands (see Table 13-1).

Age-related changes reflected in the hair are graying, hair loss, androgenetic alopecia (baldness), and an increase in facial hair in women. An estimated 50% of the population has gray hair by age 50 (Ebersole & Hess, 1994). Scalp hair tends to gray more rapidly than body hair as a result of melanocyte loss from the hair bulbs. Atrophy of the hair follicles causes balding. Beginning at the front temporal area in men as early as in their 20s, most men have some balding by the latter decades of life. Hair tends to become thinner for women in the vertex and frontal regions and finer and thinner in the pleural region. Some older adults' hair even turns shades of yellow or yellowish green, some of which may be due to smoking. Coarse terminal hairs tend to grow on the chin and upper lip of women and on the ears of men, making it difficult to cut. Both men and women experience diminishing amounts of hair on the legs and in the axillary and pubic regions. Loss of hair may contribute to the older person's feeling of being cold and create a greater susceptibility to trauma. Change in hair color and loss of hair alters the older adult's self-image and may influence self-concept. Hair-coloring products, wigs, or cosmetic surgery are used by many older adults (Miller, 1995).

With aging, the nail plates become thinner, yellowish or white, and duller. Longitudinal striations become more visible, with ridging and beading along the nail plate. The crescent-shaped lunula gradually disappears. Nail growth slows with age; fingernails grow more rapidly than toenails. Nails also become more brittle, with a greater tendency to split. Toenails usually grow thicker and hard, often due to fungal infections. Other times, they become misshapen, causing soft tissue irritation and infection. Because of these changes, trimming the nails, wearing shoes, and walking may become difficult for the older person (Goldfarb, Ellis, & Voorhees, 1990). See Table 13-1 for structural changes associated with aging of the skin.

ABNORMAL PHYSIOLOGIC CHANGES

Common skin disorders affecting older adults' medical treatment and nursing care are listed in Table 13-2 (see p. 206). The nurse should become familiar with these by linking the descriptions of the various lesions to pictures. Differential diagnosis and treatment is best left to a physician. The nurse's role in physical assessment is vital, however, in initial identification of skin disorders.

PRURITUS

Pruritus, or itching skin, is more prevalent in cold-weather climates. It is annoying to the person and should not be overlooked as a trivial complaint. Although it may be the result of dry skin, there are other causes, such as an allergic reaction, urticaria, scabies, or lice. Patients in long-term-care facilities are sometimes exposed to scabies, which presents a major nursing challenge. Itching at times becomes so severe that scratching draws blood. The itch sometimes interrupts sleep and causes depression and even suicide. Pruritus may be symptomatic of systemic diseases such as renal, malignant, hematologic, endocrine, hepatobiliary, psychogenic, or symptomatic of drug use (Boswell, 1989; Duncan & Fenske, 1990).

SKIN INFECTIONS

Impaired immunity in older adults increases the vulnerability to infections, especially those of the integumentary, genitourinary, and gastrointestinal systems. Skin infections include those commonly seen in a pressure ulcer, herpes zoster, scabies, herpes simplex, and cellulitis. Not only are these costly to the individual and society, but at times they cause sepsis and death. The incidence of nosocomial infections, those acquired in an institution such as a hospital or long-term-care facility, is twice as great for persons older than age 70 than for those 20 to 40 years old. Most of these infections are caused by organisms found in the patient's skin, nasopharynx, or perineum. Food and water, defective hand washing, or infestation by visitors or staff may also incite infection (Stolley & Buckwalter, 1991).

PRESSURE ULCERS

Pressure ulcers present an awesome challenge to nurses who care for older adults. Most pressure ulcers can be prevented; however, factors present in the health care system often inhibit optimal attention to prevention. These include:

- Lack of knowledge concerning the latest methods of pressure ulcer prevention
- Failure to use and accurately interpret a valid pressure ulcer risk assessment
- Use of only one or inappropriate pressure ulcer prevention program on a consistent basis
- Lack of staff to administer prescribed treatments
- Inadequate funds

Pressure ulcers result when tissues are deprived of oxygen and nutrients. Waste products are not removed and cells die. Causes are many, but the most predominant cause is prolonged pressure, usually over the bony prominences. The areas at greatest risk for breakdown are the elbows, heels, sacrum, coccyx, scapulae, iliac crests, greater tuberosities, and lateral and medial malleoli. On the surface, a pressure ulcer may appear small, yet most often the underlying subcutaneous and muscular tissues are damaged as well.

Shearing forces all contribute to pressure sore development. Other factors include poor nutrition and poor hydration. Adequate protein and carbohydrate intake, plus minerals and vitamins, especially vitamins A and C, are necessary. Weight loss decreases subcutaneous tissue and increases the likelihood of pressure ulcer formation. Other disease states, such as diabetes, altered mental status, anemia, cardiovascular disease, hypoxia, and musculoskeletal disabilities, place persons at risk. Age-related changes in the dermis and the epidermis, decreased sensory perception, chronic health problems, and multiple health problems also predispose the older adult to pressure ulcer formation (Burd et al.; 1992; Mulder & Albert, 1990).

PSYCHOSOCIAL ISSUES

Skin disorders occur more often in older adults who are depressed, physically ill, or debilitated, perhaps because they neglect to or are unable to adequately care for the skin and appendages properly. Age-related skin, hair, and nail changes, especially those apparent to others, may influence the older person's self-image and self-confidence. How a person looks may contribute greatly to a positive self-concept and often dictates the level of social interaction with others. Older adults who show signs of aging, the presence of skin disorders, or the inability to care for themselves may receive negative reactions from others, both socially and professionally. Our society is so preoccupied with a youthful appearance that billions of dollars are spent annually on cosmetics, hair coloring, and cosmetic surgery to alter physical appearance. There are nonsurgical options, such as retinoic acid (Retin-A), chemical peels, dermabrasion, collagen injections, and surgical options, such as a face-lift, liposuction, and fat transplantation (Fenske & Albers, 1990). Most of these treatments are effective for varying periods of time and can greatly enhance the lives of older persons who choose to use them.

NURSING ASSESSMENT

Each time the nurse completes an assessment on the older adult, a thorough skin and appendage assessment is essential. Much of the history and examination can be conducted while assessing other parts of the body.

HISTORY AND INTERVIEW

Through a history and physical assessment, the nurse can determine the potential for and the existence of skin, hair, and nail problems. Early detection is the key to preventing and caring for most skin, hair, and nail disorders.

When conducting an initial assessment on any older adult, the nurse should ask the following questions:

- Do you have or have you had any of the following skin problems?:
  - Rashes
  - Moles (color changes, bleeding)
  - Bruising
  - Swelling
  - Itching
  - Sores that do not heal
  - Hair loss
  - Infection around nails
  - Traumatic injuries
  - Skin breakdown
  - Visible veins
- Are you currently being treated for any health problems? If so, do any of these prevent you from caring for your body, hair, or nails?
- Are you receiving any treatments for these health problems?
- Are you taking any medications from the doctor or over the counter? List medications, dosages, and regimen.
- Have you ever had any reaction to medications? List and describe them.
- What types and amount of food do you eat daily?
- How much and what kind of fluid do you drink daily?
- Do you drink alcohol? How much? Frequency?
- Have you had any skin problems? Describe them and the treatment given.
- Have you had any skin trauma, such as radiation or chemical exposure?
- Do you have any problems with your hair or nails?
- Are you able to cut your fingernails and toenails?
- How many hours are you exposed to the sun daily?
- Do you use a sunscreen? What sun protection factor is it?
- Have you ever had allergic reactions to insects or plants?
- How often do you take a bath or shower?
- What type of soap do you use?
- Are you able to bathe yourself? If not, who helps you?
- Do you use any skin creams, medications, or cosmetics? What are they?

RISK FACTORS

Skin conditions develop from both intrinsic (within the body) and extrinsic (outside the body) causes and are categorized as inflammatory, infectious, benign, premalignant, and malignant. Intrinsic factors result from one's genetic makeup or are due to chronologic aging, whereas extrinsic factors are those arising from outside of the individual and from the environment. Both significantly influence the skin status; however, extrinsic factors are more likely to be prevented and treated. The nurse should be familiar with intrinsic and extrinsic risk factors for skin, hair, and nail problems.

▷ Clinical Pearl

Assessment: Skin turgor is not always a precise indicator of hydration in older adults because of normal aging changes.

Intrinsic Factors. Each person is born with a unique genetic makeup. Genes dictate sex, race, hormonal balance, rate of aging, and propensity for disease. Because of genetic makeup, some individuals show signs of aging, such as wrinkles, baldness, or premature graying, earlier than others. Inherited skin color dictates sensitivity to ultraviolet rays and susceptibility to skin cancer. People with darker skin, which contains more melanin, are less sensitive to ultraviolet rays than are those with fair hair and blue eyes (Fitzpatrick, 1989).

Extrinsic Risk Factors. An extrinsic risk factor for skin, hair, and nail problems is habitual sun exposure. Ultraviolet rays cause damage to the epidermis and dermis and result in premature aging (photoaging) on exposed areas of the body and predispose older adults to skin cancer. Exposure to the sun causes malignant melanomas, one of the fastest growing types of cancer. Climatic conditions, such as heat, cold, dry air, wind, and high humidity are risk factors. Dry air lessens skin hydration, while hot, humid air potentiates excoriation of adjacent skin surfaces. Radiation therapy and chemotherapy, systemic diseases, elevated body temperatures, and impaired oxygen transport all increase the likelihood of skin, hair, and nail disorders. Malnourished older adults, especially those with a negative nitrogen balance, lack of vitamins and mineral, and fluid deficits, are predisposed to skin breakdown and pressure ulcers. Skin disorders can be caused by ingestion of certain medications, such as corticosteroids, which may cause hyperpigmentation or hypopigmentation and increased hair growth on the face and body; penicillin, streptomycin, and chlorpromazine, which may cause skin rashes; and antipsychotic medications, which cause photosensitivity. External prostheses, such as eyeglasses and braces, can cause skin irritation. Bedridden, incontinent persons are particularly prone to pressure ulcers, as are persons with depression or dementia, who are less likely to care for their skin properly. Socioeconomic lifestyle patterns and cultural hygiene practices may contradict healthy skin practices.

PHYSICAL EXAMINATION

The physical examination should include inspection and palpation of the skin. Irwin (1991) stressed the need to be aware of special techniques in assessing persons with various skin colors. Nurses should consistently observe patients for identification of skin disorders. The nurse records the size, color, location, and pattern of disorders or lesions and any drainage or bleeding. Careful inspection should be given to sun-exposed skin or that which has been chronically irritated. Although older adults tend to heal well, the process is slower. During the physical examination, the nurse considers the following questions:

- What color is the skin?
- Is there any variation in skin pigmentation?
- Are there signs of vascularity, such as bruising, bleeding, petechia, or ecchymosis?
- Are there signs of exposure to the sun?
- What is the temperature of the skin? Feel with the backs of your hands and compare parts of the body.
- Are there signs of dryness, oiliness, or sweating?
- What is the turgor of the skin? Use a skin area protected from the sun, such as the abdomen.
- Are there any areas of swelling? Describe the degree.
- Are there any scars? Describe the scars.
- Are there any wounds that will not heal? Describe size, location, appearance, depth, exudate, or bleeding.
- Are there any bruises? Look for signs of abuse or falling.
- Are there any lesions? Are they local or generalized? Where are they located?
- What type, color, size, and shape are they?
- What type of border does it have?
- What is the symmetry?
- Is there any drainage from the lesion?
- Is there any body odor?
- What is the color, shape, length, and condition of the nails and surrounding tissue?
- What is the color, texture, quantity, and distribution of the hair?
- What is the condition of the scalp?

When conducting the physical examination, the nurse should consider the following psychosocial and environmental components:

- Are there any signs of mental illness, such as dementia or depression?
- Is the clothing clean and sufficient for the weather?
- What are the financial resources?
- What is the condition of the home?
- Are there adequate facilities for bathing?
- Who lives in the house with the patient?
- Is there a caregiver to assist the patient with skin, hair, and nail care?

DIAGNOSTIC TESTS

On admission to any health service, nursing assessment should include a total body skin assessment and a review of serum, urine, and any additional diagnostic tests for abnormal results. Those persons at risk should be assessed for their potential for pressure ulcer formation. The Braden scale (Display 13-1) is one of the best such scales because of its established validity. It is composed of six subscales: sensory perception, moisture, activity, mobility, nutrition, and friction and shear. Scores range from very high (no risk) to very low (greater risk) (Bergstrom, Braden, Laguzza, & Holman, 1987). The Braden scale can be used initially and regularly to determine the progress of the disease. Ratings of pressure ulcers for formation and treatment are determined by stage, as shown in Figure 13-1. It is important to examine the surrounding tissues for
(text continues on page 201)

Display 13-1
BRADEN SCALE FOR PREDICTING PRESSURE SORE RISK

Patient's Name _____   Evaluator's Name _____   Date of Assessment _____

Sensory Perception Ability to respond meaningfully to pressure-related discomfort	**1. Completely Limited:** Unresponsive (does not moan, flinch, or grasp) to painful stimuli, due to diminished level of consciousness or sedation. OR limited ability to feel pain over most of body surface.	**2. Very Limited:** Responds only to painful stimuli. Cannot communicate discomfort except by moaning or restlessness. OR has a sensory impairment that limits the ability to feel pain or discomfort over 1/2 of body.	**3. Slightly Limited:** Responds to verbal commands, but cannot always communicate discomfort or need to be turned. OR has some sensory impairment that limits ability to feel pain or discomfort in 1 or 2 extremities.	**4. No Impairment:** Responds to verbal commands. Has no sensory deficit that would limit ability to feel or voice pain or discomfort.
Moisture Degree to which skin is exposed to moisture	**1. Constantly Moist:** Skin is kept moist almost constantly by perspiration, urine, etc. Dampness is detected every time patient is moved or turned.	**2. Very Moist:** Skin is often, but not always, moist. Linen must be changed at least once a shift.	**3. Occasionally Moist:** Skin is occasionally moist, requiring an extra linen change approximately once a day.	**4. Rarely Moist:** Skin is usually dry, linen only requires changing at routine intervals.
Activity Degree of physical activity	**1. Bedfast:** Confined to bed	**2. Chairfast:** Ability to walk severely limited or nonexistent. Cannot bear own weight and/or must be assisted into chair or wheelchair.	**3. Walks Occasionally:** Walks occasionally during day, but for very short distances, with or without assistance. Spends majority of each shift in bed or chair.	**4. Walks Frequently:** Walks outside the room at least twice a day and inside room at least once every 2 hours during waking hours.

	1	2	3	4
Mobility Ability to change and control body position	**1. Completely Immobile:** Does not make even slight changes in body or extremity position without assistance.	**2. Very Limited:** Makes occasional slight changes in body or extremity position but unable to make frequent or significant changes independently.	**3. Slightly Limited:** Makes frequent though slight changes in body or extremity position independently.	**4. No Limitations:** Makes major and frequent changes in position without assistance.
Nutrition Usual food intake pattern	**1. Very Poor:** Never eats a complete meal. Rarely eats more than 1/3 of any food offered. Eats 2 servings or less of protein (meat or dairy products) per day. Takes fluids poorly. Does not take a liquid dietary supplement. OR is NPO and/or maintained on clear liquids or IVs for more than 5 days.	**2. Probably Inadequate:** Rarely eats a complete meal and generally eats only about 1/2 of any food offered. Protein intake includes only 3 servings of meat or dairy products per day. Occasionally will take a dietary supplement. OR receives less than optimum amount of liquid diet or tube feeding.	**3. Adequate:** Eats over half of most meals. Eats a total of 4 servings of protein (meat, dairy products) each day. Occasionally will refuse a meal, but will usually take a supplement if offered. OR is on a tube feeding or TPN regimen which probably meets most of nutritional needs.	**4. Excellent:** Eats most of every meal. Never refuses a meal. Usually eats a total of 4 or more servings of meat and dairy products. Occasionally eats between meals. Does not require supplementation.
Friction and Shear	**1. Problem:** Requires moderate to maximum assistance in moving. Complete lifting without sliding against sheets is impossible. Frequently slides down in bed or chair, requiring frequent repositioning with maximum assistance. Spasticity, contractures or agitation leads to almost constant friction.	**2. Potential Problem:** Moves feebly or requires minimum assistance. During a move skin probably slides to some extent against sheets, chair, restraints, or other devices. Maintains relatively good position in chair or bed most of the time but occasionally slides down.	**3. No Apparent Problem:** Moves in bed and in chair independently and has sufficient muscle strength to lift up completely during move. Maintains good position in bed or chair at all times.	

Total Score

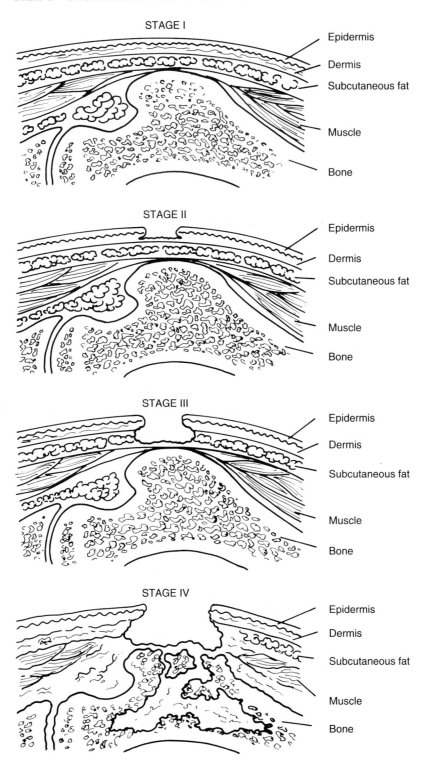

Figure 13-1. Classification of pressure ulcers.

ischemia, induration, and inflammation, because their presence suggests the outcome of the ulcer treatment.

NURSING DIAGNOSES

Based on the complete assessment of the older adult, common nursing diagnoses associated with the problems of the skin, hair, and nails include the following:

- Impaired Tissue Integrity related to skin lesions/pressure ulcers
- High Risk for Infection related to pruritus and scratching
- Body Image Disturbance related to skin rash
- Sleep Pattern Disturbance related to pain and itching
- Altered Nutrition: Less Than Body Requirements related to anxiety or depression
- Body Image Disturbance related to hair loss from therapy
- Impaired Tissue Integrity related to injury to toenails
- Powerlessness related to escalating bills from hospitalization for pressure ulcers

NURSING INTERVENTIONS

Nurses must thoroughly assess each situation or abnormality of the skin, hair, and nails; outline the hazards for the patient and family; and use appropriate interventions to promote optimal healing. Nursing interventions should address prevention, treatment cost, and treatment effectiveness.

PATIENT AND FAMILY EDUCATION

Nurses can promote healing in patients by teaching energy-saving interventions through environmental modifications, such as maintaining a comfortable room temperature. The nurse needs to teach energy-saving techniques for daily care and provide an environment conducive to adequate rest and sleep. Healing is promoted by providing adequate food and fluid intake; maintaining an exercise regimen; ensuring that the patient correctly takes prescribed medications; avoiding nosocomial infections; helping to maintain clear, dry skin; and teaching improved health habits, such as those listed in the Patient Teaching Box. The family needs to be taught to eliminate environmental hazards that may cause trauma to the skin through burns, falls, or injury.

Additionally, the patient and family should receive the following instructions:

- Reduce psychosocial stress by providing a supportive environment, which will also promote healing.
- Keep all skin surfaces clean by using a mild soap, rinsing well with water, and patting dry. Apply an emollient on the skin.
- Use cornstarch on skin areas that rub together.
- Maintain a toileting schedule and check adult briefs or the bed every 2 hours to prevent skin irritation from urine and feces. Wash, rinse, and immediately dry skin soiled with urine, feces, or perspiration.
- Use protective pressure prevention mattresses or other types of protective skin products, such as sheepskin, heel protectors, and pillows to prevent pressure areas.

Patient Teaching Box
CARE OF SKIN, HAIR, AND NAILS

Use the following strategies to instruct the patient and family in the care of skin, hair, and nails:

- Inspect the skin frequently for lesions, ulcers, bruises, cracks, changes in color, swelling, and numbness.
- Eat a well-balanced diet, including foods rich in vitamins A and D.
- Drink about eight glasses of water each day and maintain humidity in the home by using a humidifier if necessary.
- Exercise daily (active or passive) to promote circulation.
- Avoid round garters or constrictive clothing.
- Avoid using heating pads or hot-water bottles.
- Limit the time in the sun, avoiding the hours 10 AM to 3 PM. Apply a sunscreen with sun protection factor 15 or greater. Wear a large-brimmed hat and cotton clothing that covers the body or use an umbrella.
- Bathe about three times a week with water about 100° F. Use superfatted soaps, such as Dove, or plain water. Rinse well and pat dry. Bath oils help to lubricate the skin, but great care should be taken if used in a bath or shower because of the potential danger of falling. They are best applied after a bath.
- Lubricate the skin with an emollient immediately after bathing, while the skin is warm and moist. Lubrication can be repeated several times a day if the skin is dry or itchy or if living in a cold climate.
- Wash hair and scalp thoroughly at least weekly.
- Soak toenails and fingernails in warm water, cut nails straight across, and apply emollient to feet and dry. Seek help from a beautician or podiatrist if unable to cut own nails.
- Wash clothes and bedding in a mild detergent and use a fabric softener.

The American Cancer Society recommends a monthly skin self-examination plus a skin examination by a physician every 3 years for persons older than age 20 and every year for those older than age 40. If discovered early, most skin lesions are curable and present no threat to life. The patient and family should be instructed in the correct method for a skin self-examination (Fig. 13-2).

SKIN INTEGRITY

In developing a treatment regimen for the prevention of pressure sores, the nurse must always consider the risk factors related to ulcer formation and healing, because ulceration depends greatly on the patient's physiologic and psychological state (Mulder & Albert, 1990). The skin must be assessed for unusual lesions, irritations, or breaks. Bedridden patients should be assessed daily, particularly for skin over bony prominences.

 Clinical Pearl

Intervention: To prevent shear and friction skin tears, avoid pulling patients up in bed, which would involve sliding the skin against the sheets; instead use a pull sheet (draw sheet) and an overhead trapeze.

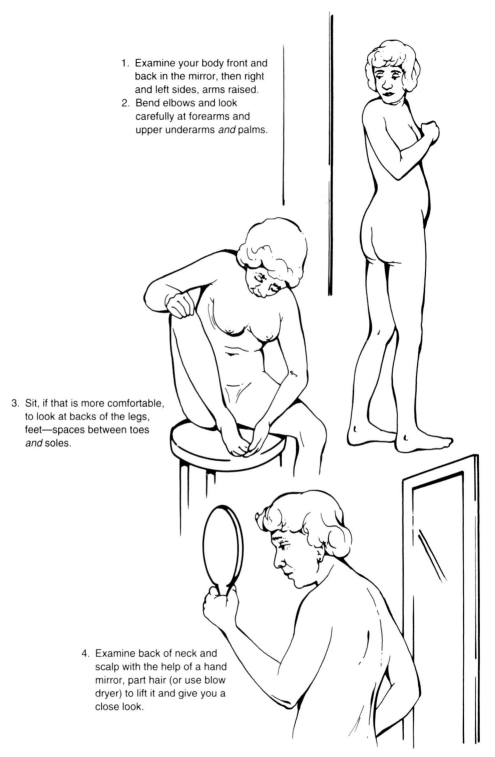

1. Examine your body front and back in the mirror, then right and left sides, arms raised.
2. Bend elbows and look carefully at forearms and upper underarms *and* palms.

3. Sit, if that is more comfortable, to look at backs of the legs, feet—spaces between toes *and* soles.

4. Examine back of neck and scalp with the help of a hand mirror, part hair (or use blow dryer) to lift it and give you a close look.

Figure 13-2. Skin self-examination. (Adapted with permission from American Cancer Society.)

Suggested treatment modalities of pressure sores include various types of dressings and dressing materials, irrigation of the ulcer with normal saline solution, electrical stimulation, surgical debridement, surgical repair, and the use of various pressure-reduction mattresses and devices. Attention must be given to fluid and nutritional support as well as to treatment of infection or anemia. More conventional treatment methods, such as topical antibiotic ointments, heat lamps, massaging around pressure sores, and use of various other irrigants, are ineffective, and some are even harmful. A multimodal approach to prevention and treatment of pressure ulcers is essential, because a single method is never sufficient to ensure ulcer healing.

LIFESTYLE CHANGES

Various lifestyle changes and a multidisciplinary team approach to the treatment of skin problems or a pressure sore are essential, because many body systems are involved. The patient and family's psychosocial needs are very important. Because skin problems, such as pressure sores, are disfiguring, the patient's self-concept and ability to perform activities of daily living, work, and necessary social interactions may be affected. Heavy financial obligations weigh on the family, who may even be responsible for prolonged caregiving responsibilities. Some patients may require extended care in a long-term-care facility, which is costly and difficult for the patient and family. Discharge planning, patient and family teaching, and referral to community resources are essential in the management of these patients. Prevention of and care for patients with pressure sores demands knowledge, creative nursing, and commitment to an effective treatment regimen.

Nursing Care Plan

FOR A PATIENT WITH IMPAIRED TISSUE INTEGRITY

Nursing Diagnosis: Impaired Tissue Integrity related to skin breakdown (pressure ulcer).

Definition: Redness or opening in the skin involving any or all of the following tissues: epidermis, dermis, hypodermis, muscle, or bone caused by pressure; chemical or physical trauma resulting in decreased blood, oxygen, or nutrition to tissue and lack of waste product removal, resulting in death to cells and infection.

Assessment Findings:
1. Reddened skin over bony prominences
2. Blister formation of skin
3. Presence of skin tear or ulcer formation

Nursing Interventions with Selected Rationales:
1. Assess skin status daily, especially over bony prominences.
   Rationale: Daily assessment provides a baseline for future assessments and early identification of problems.

(continued)

Nursing Care Plan

FOR A PATIENT WITH IMPAIRED TISSUE INTEGRITY *(Continued)*

2. Maintain the patient on a well-balanced diet, especially rich in vitamins A and C plus food supplements for adequate nutrition.
   Rationale: A well-balanced diet supports skin healing.
3. Assess fluid intake and maintain patient on about 2000 mL per day.
   Rationale: Adequate hydration maintains tissues and helps with tissue healing.
4. Encourage activity and daily exercise, or if wheelchair or bedridden, change patient's position every 2 hours.
   Rationale: Position changes increase blood flow to all areas and help prevent skin breakdown.
5. If skin breakdown does occur, avoid using a heat lamp.
   Rationale: Heat promotes excessive drying; if used consistently, it may even retard wound healing.
6. Arrange for patient's bedding and clothing to be washed in mild soap and rinsed well.
   Rationale: Washing with mild soap and rinsing well helps to avoid skin irritation.
7. Monitor progress of pressure sore daily or bi-weekly using a skin care documentation record.
   Rationale: Consistent documentation ensures communication of improvement or deterioration to all health care team members.
8. Change a soiled pressure sore dressing immediately. Wash ulcer with a mild soap and water, rinse well, and pat dry. Apply new dressing. Keep ulcer free from soiling by urine and feces.
   Rationale: Rapid intervention promotes healing and prevents further breakdown.
9. Assist in the debridement process using irrigation, wet-to-dry dressings, and enzymatic agents to promote healing. Do not use enzymatic agents if necrotic tissue is present.
   Rationale: Debridement removes any dead tissues, cleanses the area, and allows for new tissue growth.

Desired Patient Outcomes/Discharge Criteria:

1. Patient and family will comply with prescribed therapeutic regimen.
2. Patient's skin will be intact and free of any signs of skin disruptions, ulcer, or infection.
3. Patient is free of pain and discomfort.
4. Patient is able to return to functioning socially with people in the community.

Table 13-2

COMMON SKIN CONDITIONS OF OLDER ADULTS

Noninflammatory, Inflammatory, and Infections

Lesion	Appearance	Treatment strategies	Nursing intervention
Xerosis (dry skin)	Dry white scale; flaky, especially in lower legs; causes itching (pruritus)	1. Avoid irritants such as alkaline soaps. 2. Use skin emollients.	1. Use superfatted soaps. 2. Increase fluid intake to 2000 mL daily. 3. Increase room humidity. 4. Moisturize skin. 5. Limit total body bathing; do so in water with an oil. 6. Use sunscreens. 7. Wear soft, nonconstricting clothing.
Solar elastosis (photo aging)	Wrinkled; rough; leathery; yellow, red, brown, or flesh-colored plaques or papules. Pigmentation irregular.	1. Sunscreen, sun protection factor 15–25 2. Avoid sun on skin. 3. Biopsy 4. Cryosurgery	1. Instruction on use of sunscreens, sun protection factor 15–25 2. Avoid being outside 11 AM–3 PM 3. Wear protective clothing. 4. Wear hat, use umbrella.
Seborrheic dermatitis	Primary lesion has erythema, white scale, or yellow greasy scale on scalp, ears, side of nose, and around eyebrows	1. 1% hydrocortisone cream 2. Antifungal agents 3. Systemic antibiotics for secondary infection	1. Antiseborrheic shampoo. 2. Keep clean and dry. 3. Apply topical medications

Acne rosacea	Acneiform papules or pustules. Chronic inflammatory hyperplasia of the sebaceous glands, especially on midface, forehead, or chin	1. Topical
		    a. erythromycin
		    b. clindamycin
		    c. sulfur
		    d. corticosteroids, mild
		    e. Retin-A
			1. Apply topical ointment and teach patient.
			2. Caution patient to avoid stimuli that cause vasodilation, such as drugs, hot liquids, highly seasoned foods, and alcohol

Contact dermatitis	Erythematous, vesicular eruptions; pruritic, crusting, scaly skin on skin exposed to irritant or allergic contact	1. Discover and remove irritant 2. Cortisone cream in severe cases 3. Oral antihistamines 4. Corticosteroids	1. Use care not to use alkaline soaps or astringents. 2. Keep sheet away from contact with allergen.
Acrochordons (skin tags)	Pendunculated pink to brown papules on neck, trunk, axilla, or near eye	1. Removal by scissor excision 2. Electrocautery	1. Avoid tight clothing causing chronic irritation. 2. If in an area that is chronically irritated, encourage patient to have it removed.

(continued)

Table 13-2

COMMON SKIN CONDITIONS OF OLDER ADULTS *(Continued)*

Noninflammatory, Inflammatory, and Infections

Lesion	Appearance	Treatment strategies	Nursing intervention
Stasis dermatitis	Common involvement in lower leg varacosities, erythema, variable edema, reddish brown puncta. Eczematous eruptions. Ulcerations and infection may develop, sometimes from scratching	1. Avoid long periods of sitting or standing. Elevate leg; Apply stockings immediately on arising. 2. Apply corticosteroid cream or take drug orally if oozing or blistering. Soaks: Burow's solution 2.5% 3. Oral antibiotics (erythromycin) 4. Occlusive dressings 5. If systemic cause, Unna's boot.	1. Keep leg elevated. 2. Apply support hose. 3. Administer antibiotics or antiinflammatory drugs. 4. Soak area with Burow's solution. 5. Apply topical ointment. 6. Monitor progress.
Stasis/venous ulcers	Common involvement of lower extremities, venous ulcers, painless, epidermal, and dermal. Skin layers and subcutaneous tissues may be involved with surrounding skin pigmented brown, hair loss, atrophy, scaling. Ulcer bed is cyanotic, bleeds easily.	1. Dressing or Unna's pastel boot. Elevate leg. 2. Cleansing and debridement 3. Treat infection with antibiotics 4. Compression stockings if arterial blood flow is sufficient 5. Fibrinolytic therapy 6. Large ulcers may need skin grafting or bypass surgery 7. Venous and arterial studies 8. Doppler ultrasound 9. Topical, antibiotics, corticosteroids	1. Teach how to elevate affected leg above right atrium level; keep patient as active as possible. 2. Teach patient to purchase correct elastic stockings and how to use them. 3. Apply dressings and ulcer care as prescribed. 4. Avoid clothing that is constrictive. 5. Use emollient on dry skin. 6. Encourage not to traumatize leg.
Arterial ulcers	Pale, cold leg with trophic changes, ulcer with scant granulation tissue. Edges seem infarcted and sloughing on foot, toes, heel or distal leg, due to chronic arterial occlusion. Claudication and pain at rest, continuous, even severe	1. Bed rest 2. Avoid trauma to extremities 3. Buerger-Allen exercises 4. Stop smoking 5. Vasodilator and adrenergic medications 6. Arterial studies 7. Doppler ultrasound	1. Check skin color, temperature. 2. Assess peripheral pulses. 3. Prevent chilling. 4. Avoid constrictive clothing. 5. Encourage well-balanced diet. 6. Teach patient to report any infection.
Herpes zoster shingles	Vesicles grouped with reddened base in a bandlike distribution along person's dermatome. Does not cross midline.	1. Wet compresses 2. Calamine lotion 3. Topical steroids 4. Oral steroids 5. Antiviral medications 6. Analgesics	1. Apply compresses. 2. Apply steroids and calamine lotion. 3. Administer oral steroids. 4. Administer analgesics. 5. Psychological support.

(continued)

Table 13-2

COMMON SKIN CONDITIONS OF OLDER ADULTS *(Continued)*

Noninflammatory, Inflammatory, and Infections

Lesion	Appearance	Treatment strategies	Nursing intervention
Per Lèche/ angular cheilitis	Inflammation at corner of mouth. Tenderness, fissuring, maceration	1. Antifungal 2. Antibacterial 3. Steroid three times/ day 4. Evaluation of teeth by dentist, because it may be due to jaw regression or dentures that do not fit.	1. Apply ointment ordered. 2. If inflammation continues, consult dentist.

Actinic keratosis	Reddened area that gradually becomes rough, turns to yellowish crust or scale. Precursor of squamous cell cancer on face and hands (sun-exposed areas)	1. Cauterization
		2. Surgical removal
		3. Cryosurgery
		4. Topical chemotherapy
		  a. 5-fluorouracil
		  b. Fluoroplex 1%
		  c. Efudex 2% or 5%
			1. Encourage patient to use sunscreen–sun protection factor 15–25.
			2. Discourage being in sun between 11 AM and 3 PM.
			3. Wear hat, use umbrella, wear protective cotton clothing.
			4. Observe postoperatively for infection and healing.
			5. Teach patient how to use topical medication.

Lentigo maligna	Hyperpigmented macule with border that is irregular on sun-exposed area. May turn malignant.	1. Surgical excision	1. Encourage patient to use precaustions against ultraviolet rays. 2. Assess skin, refer to dermatologist if suspicious lesion. 3. Observe postoperatively for infection and healing.
Leuko-plakia	Slightly raised white translucent to dense opaque lesion with or without ulcer formation	1. 5-Fluorouracil cream 2. Surgical excision 3. Electrosurgery 4. Cryosurgery 5. Accutane	1. Teach regular inspection of oral mucosa, lips, and vulva. 2. Encourage to stop smoking. 3. Seek dental care for any oral area chronically irritated.
Basal cell carcinoma	Pearly, small, translucent nodules with telangiectasis. Areas of induration; superficial ulcer atrophy with crust often found on the face and back of hand	1. Curettage, electro-desiccation 2. Surgical excision 3. Cryosurgery 4. Radiation therapy 5. Topical chemotherapy 6. Mohs' chemosurgery	1. Encourage patient to seek medical follow-up every month for 6 months after lesion removal. 2. Assess skin, refer to dermatologist. 3. Postelectrosurgery wound should remain open without antibiotics or dressings. 4. Encourage patient to use precautions against ultraviolet rays.

(continued)

Table 13-2	COMMON SKIN CONDITIONS OF OLDER ADULTS *(Continued)*			
	Noninflammatory, Inflammatory, and Infections			
	Lesion	*Appearance*	*Treatment strategies*	*Nursing intervention*
	Squamous cell carcinoma	Shallow ulcer with an elevated, wide, indurated border and scaling. Bleeds easily.	1. Electrodissection 2. Curettage 3. Lymph node dissection if advanced 4. Radiation therapy 5. Isotretinoin 6. 5-Fluorouracil cream	1. Assess and refer to physician if suspicious lesion. 2. Observe postoperatively for infection and healing. 3. Dress wounds as necessary. 4. Encourage patient to use precautions against ultraviolet rays.
	Malignant melanoma	Asymmetric, irregular borders and pigment with shades of tan, brown, and black	1. Surgical excision may be wide and deep 2. Lymph node dissection 3. Chemotherapy 4. Radiotherapy 5. Electrodesiccation and curettage 6. Careful follow-up for metastases	1. Assess patient for suspicious lesions; refer to physician. 2. Preoperative and postoperative care, observe for infection and healing. 3. Psychological support. 4. Special nursing related to side effects of chemotherapy and radiation therapy.

Data from Chenitz, Stone & Salesbury, 1990; Fitzpatrick, 1989; Goldfarb, Ellis & Voorhees, 1990; Smoller & Smoller, 1992; Staab & Lyles, 1990.

REFERENCES

American Cancer Society. (1985). *Why you should know about melanoma.* New York: Author.

Balin, A. K. (1990). Aging of human skin. In W. R. Hazzard, R. Andres, E. L. Bierman, & J. P. Blass (Eds.), *Principles of geriatric medicine and gerontology* (2nd ed.) (pp. 383–412). New York: McGraw-Hill.

Bergstrom, W., Braden, B. J., Laguzza, A., & Holman, V. (1987). The Braden scale for predicting pressure sore risk. *Nursing Research, 36*(4), 205–210.

Boswell, G. V. (1989). Pruritus. In M. J. Pathy & P. Finucnae (Eds.), *Geriatric medicine* (pp. 288–296). New York: Springer-Verlag.

Burd, C., Langemo, D., Olson, B., Hanson, D., Hunter, S., & Sauvage, T. (1992). Skin problems: Epidemiology of pressure ulcers in a skilled care facility. *Journal of Gerontological Nursing, 18,* 29–39.

Chenitz, W. C., Stone, J. T., & Salesbury, S. A. (1991). *Clinical gerontological nursing,* Philadelphia: W. B. Saunders.

Duncan, W. C., & Fenske, N. A. (1990). Cutaneous signs of internal disease in the elderly. *Geriatrics, 45*(8), 24–29.

Ebersole, R., & Hess, P. (1994). *Toward healthy aging: Human needs and nursing response* (4th ed.). St. Louis: Mosby.

Fenske, N. A., & Albers, S. W. (1990). Cosmetic modalities for aging skin: What to tell patients. *Geriatrics, 45*(9), 59–67.

Fenske, N. A., & Lober, C. W. (1990). Skin changes of aging: Pathological implications. *Geriatrics, 45*(3), 27–32.

Fitzpatrick, J. E. (1989). Common inflammatory skin diseases in the elderly. *Geriatrics, 44*(7), 40–47.

Gilchrest, B. A. (1986). Dermatologic disorders in the elderly. In I. Rossman (Ed.), *Clinical geriatrics* (3rd ed.) (pp. 375–387). Philadelphia: J. B. Lippincott.

Goldfarb, M. T., Ellis, E. N., & Voorhees, J. J. (1990). Dermatology. In C. Cassell, D. E. Riesenberg, L. B. Sorensen, & J. R. Walsh (Eds.), *Geriatric medicine* (2nd ed.) (pp. 383–393). New York: Springer-Verlag.

Irwin, M. J. (1991). Assessing color changes for dark-skinned patients. *Advancing Clinical Care,* *6*(6), 8–10.

Miller, C. A. (1995). *Nursing care of older adults: Theory and practice* (2nd ed.). Philadelphia: J. B. Lippincott.

Mulder, G. D., & Albert, S. F. (1990). Skin problems associated with pressure. In R. W. Schrier (Ed.), *Geriatric medicine* (pp. 149–155). Philadelphia: W. B. Saunders.

Richey, M. L., Richey, H. K., & Fenske, N. A. (1988). Age-related skin changes: Development and clinical meaning. *Geriatrics, 43*(4), 49–64.

Smoller, J., & Smoller, B. R. (1992). Skin malignancies in the elderly. *Journal of Gerontological Nursing, 18*(5), 19–23.

Staab, A., & Lyles, M. (1990). *Manual of geriatric nursing.* Glenview, IL: Little, Brown

Stolley, J. M., & Buckwalter, K. C. (1991). Iatrogenesis in the elderly: Nosocomial infections. *Journal of Gerontological Nursing, 14*(9), 30–34.

BIBLIOGRAPHY

Bates, B. (1995). *A guide to physical examination* (6th ed.). Philadelphia: J. B. Lippincott.

Eliopoulos, C. (1993). *Gerontological nursing.* Philadelphia: J. B. Lippincott.

Goodridge, D. M. (1993). Pressure ulcer risk assessment tools: What's new for gerontological nurses. *Journal of Gerontological Nursing, 19,* 23–27.

Habif, T. A. (1990). *Clinical dermatology: A color guide to diagnosis and therapy* (2nd ed.). St. Louis: Mosby.

Jones, P. L., & Millman, A. (1990). Wound healing with the aged patient. In B. M. Beaver & D. M. Cooper (Eds.), *Nursing clinics of North America* (pp. 263–277). Philadelphia: W. B. Saunders.

Kurban, R. S., & Kurban, A. K. (1993). Common skin disorders: Diagnosis and treatment. *Geriatrics, 48,* 30–42.

Maklebust, J., & Sieggreen, M. (1991). *Pressure ulcers: Guidelines for prevention and nursing management.* West Dundee, IL: S.N. Publications.

McKenry, L. M., & Salerno, E. (1992). *Mosby's pharmacology in nursing.* St. Louis: Mosby.

National Pressure Ulcer Advisory Panel. (1989). *Pressure ulcers: Incidence, economics, risk assessment.* Consensus Development Conference Statement. West Dundee, IL: S.N. Publications.

Needham, J. F. (1993). *Gerontological nursing: A restorative approach.* Albany, NY: Delmar.

Pariser, D. M., & Phillips, P. K. (1994). Basal cell carcinoma: When to treat it yourself, and when to refer. *Geriatrics, 49*(3), 39–44.

Perez, E. D. (1993). Pressure ulcers: Updated guidelines. *Geriatrics, 48,* 39–44.

Rogers-Seidl, F. F. (1991). *Geriatric nursing care plans.* St. Louis: Mosby.

Stone, J. T. (1991). Pressure sores. In W. C. Chenitz, J. T. Stone, & S. A. Salesbury (Eds.), *Clinical gerontological nursing: A guide to advanced practice,* Philadelphia: W. B. Saunders.

White, M. W., Karam, S., & Cowell, B. (1994). Skin tears in frail elders: A practical approach to prevention. *Geriatric Nursing, 15*(2), 95–99.

14

Problems With Circulation

Objectives

1. Distinguish the cardiovascular changes due to the aging process from those resulting from pathophysiology associated with disease.
2. Incorporate physiologic symptoms and psychosocial needs of older adults into a plan of nursing care.
3. Relate family and support system needs to a plan of nursing care.
4. Design patient and family interventions that control lifestyle risk factors for cardiovascular disease.
5. Develop teaching plans that prepare the patient and family for incorporating medications and lifestyle changes into activities of daily living.

INTRODUCTION

AS THE AGE AND NUMBER OF OLDER ADULTS increase, so does the incidence of problems with the heart and circulation. Heart and blood vessel disease is the major cause of disability and death in older adults (Wenger, 1990). Older adults present a special nursing challenge, because they may respond to heart, blood vessel, and circulation problems by slowing down and decreasing activities. Retirement occurs about the same time that many older adults begin to experience circulation problems. The more sedentary lifestyles and decreased activity levels accompanying retirement allow adaptation to circulation changes. In addition, older adults may not report symptoms because they believe that these are normal aging experiences. There are also many lifestyle risk factors that influence development of problems with circulation. For all of these reasons, the older adult with heart, blood vessel, and circulation problems is a challenge for the nurse. Special nursing assessment and nursing interventions are needed to plan care for the older adult with circulation problems.

Changes occurring in the circulatory system are due to normal aging, lifestyle risk factors, and disease processes. With more sophisticated diagnostic techniques and larger cross-cultural research samples of older adults, we

Staab, AS and Hodges, LC: ESSENTIALS OF GERONTOLOGICAL NURSING,
© 1996 J. B. Lippincott Company

may find that many circulatory changes are determined more by lifestyle and environment than by aging and disease (Miller, 1995). Even with circulation changes, older adults may not experience functional problems. Some age-related changes, however, do affect circulation and many begin in the arteries.

NORMAL PHYSIOLOGIC CHANGES

Normal physiologic aging in the arteries includes arterial thickening and fibrosis, an increase of collagen fibers, a decrease in elastic fibers, and an increase of calcium deposits. The arteries become increasingly rigid and tortuous. These normal physiologic changes can result in increased peripheral resistance to blood flow; reduced blood flow to all organs, especially the kidneys; increased blood pressure with widening pulse pressure; and decreased baroreceptor sensitivity. Clinically, these changes result in a more forceful pulse, increased systolic blood pressure, and postural hypotension. In addition, most older adults have some atherosclerosis. Therefore, it may be difficult to separate normal physiologic changes associated with aging from those resulting from disease (Wilson & Smith, 1992). Capillaries become thicker and stiffer, impeding the exchange of nutrients and oxygen at the tissue level.

The normal loss of elasticity and stiffer arteries resulting from aging creates an increased resistance to blood flow. By the age of 80, there is a 50% decrease in the ability of the arteries to stretch (Christ & Hohlock, 1988). The aorta becomes progressively rigid, thus the heart has to work harder to circulate the blood, the systolic blood pressure rises, and the left ventricle may become enlarged. This loss of elasticity and inability to stretch makes arteries unable to respond to the increased oxygen need that occurs with strong emotion and/or exercise. This further contributes to circulation problems.

Likewise, to compensate for periods of high blood pressure, the baroreceptor mechanisms lower heart rate. Baroreceptors, a major blood pressure regulating mechanism, show the age-related changes of thickening and stiffening. These changes can lead to a drop in blood pressure with sudden position changes, resulting in a greater risk of falls and injuries.

Heart muscles stiffen and the heart valves become thick and rigid. The mitral and aortic valves are affected most often because of the high pressure gradients within the heart. The heart then has to work harder to pump blood. The resistance of the aorta causes the left ventricle to become stiff, less pliable, and larger as it pumps against the added pressure caused by aortic elasticity loss. The left ventricle may become 25% thicker (Christ & Hohlock, 1988). Although the resting cardiac output is unchanged, there is a drop in cardiac output with exercise, which affects blood flow to the organs. The brain, coronary arteries, and kidneys receive less blood in older adults than in younger adults. Decreased blood flow to the brain increases the risk for dizziness and confusion. Decrease in blood flow to the coronary arteries decreases availability of oxygen for the heart. This leads to a decreased ability of the heart to respond to exercise and stress.

With aging, fibrous tissue increases in the sinoatrial node and pacemaker cells diminish, resulting in rate and rhythm changes. In general, the heart rate slows with age. Although the resting heart rate is unchanged, it can no longer rise as much with exercise (Buike & Walsh, 1992; Miller, 1995). In addition, tachycardia is poorly tolerated, because the heart needs more time between beats to recover. These changes can result in electrocardiogram (ECG) changes and a decreased ability of the heart to respond to stress, emotions, fever, exercise, and drugs. Sudden emotional and physical stressors can lead to arrhythmias, which can cause heart failure and even death (Malasanos, Barkauskas, & Stoltenberg-Allen, 1990).

ABNORMAL PHYSIOLOGIC CHANGES

Older adults with circulation problems experience a variety of conditions and medical diagnoses. Some of the problems are due to normal physiologic aging (postural hypotension and hypertension) and some to disease processes (congestive heart failure [[CHF]). In addition, arterial obstruction can be caused by a thrombus, with gradual development of symptoms or an embolus (floating clot) with sudden onset of symptoms. Myocardial infarction (MI) and cerebral vascular accident (CVA) are examples of sudden obstruction of an artery. One cause of thrombus and embolus formation is atherosclerosis, a common circulation problem that contributes to many circulation problems in older adults.

ATHEROSCLEROSIS

Most older adults have some degree of atherosclerosis, making it difficult to separate the normal physiologic changes due to aging from those due to the disease process. Atherosclerosis begins with fatty streaks on the inner surface of the artery, which progress to fibrous plaque. This plaque is composed primarily of fat. The artery gradually becomes calcified, thrombosed, and rigid. The disease process may develop over a period of years, because 50% of the artery must be occluded before symptoms develop. This reduction in the size of the arteries creates barriers for oxygen exchange in the tissues, resulting in tissue hypoxia (lack of oxygen) and pain.

Atherosclerosis is a systemic disease and can occur anywhere in the body. It is the most common cause of coronary artery disease, peripheral arterial disease, and CVA.

POSTURAL HYPOTENSION

Postural hypotension is another common condition of older adults that can be a significant problem. Postural, or orthostatic, hypotension is not a disease process but a lowering of the blood pressure that results from sudden position changes thought to affect the baroreceptor reflex. Other causes of postural hypotension are disorders in the nervous system, circulation problems, medications (Harrell, 1988), hypovolemia, adrenal insufficiency, and physical deconditioning. Hypertension at any age reduces baroreceptor sensitivity (Miller, 1995) and increases the incidence of postural hypotension.

Systolic blood pressure readings that drop 20 mm Hg or more when moving to an upright position are diagnostic for postural hypotension. The higher the resting blood pressure, the greater the blood pressure fall when the person stands (Buike & Walsh, 1992). Postural hypotension may be greater in the morning, because blood volume tends to be lower and dehydration higher on awakening (Carpenito, 1993). Standing for long periods leads to pooling of blood in the lower extremities due to flabby muscles and venous insufficiency. The decrease in cerebral blood flow is exacerbated by tachycardia, bradycardia, arrhythmias, any activity that initiates Valsalva's maneuver (coughing, straining, lifting), volume depletion with dehydration, and prolonged bed rest.

HYPERTENSION

Hypertension is a common circulatory disease and a risk factor for the older adult. In general, blood pressure increases gradually between 30 and 70 years of age. Specifically, the diastolic pressure increases gradually until men are in their 50s and women in their 60s. The systolic blood pressure increases more in women and to a greater degree than the diastolic pressure. There is a slight decrease in systolic and diastolic blood pressure in both men and women in their 70s (Miller, 1995). Hypertension increases the rate of atherosclerosis, increases the work of the heart, and can lead to heart failure. Blood pressure over 160/95 mm Hg doubles the risk of death in men and increases mortality in women (Harrell, 1988). Hypertension also increases morbidity. Increased diastolic pressure causes changes in the kidney, heart, and retina. Untreated hypertension can lead to complete loss of kidney function and blindness. Increased systolic pressure also causes memory problems and loss of ability to concentrate due to either the high systolic pressure or the medications used to treat the hypertension. The diagnosis of hypertension is based on systolic blood pressure readings above 160 mm Hg and diastolic readings above 90 mm Hg on three different occasions.

Besides the normal physiologic changes in older adults, risk factors for hypertension include age, presence of diabetes and obesity, and non–health related habits. Pathologic conditions that contribute to hypertension include severe anemia, renal artery stenosis, hormonal changes in the renin-angiotensin system, and tumors of the adrenal gland.

The signs and symptoms of hypertension vary widely, from having no symptoms to memory loss, epistaxis (nosebleeds), slow tremors, and nausea and vomiting. The treatment goal is always to lower blood pressure gradually. To avoid syncope and falls associated with hypertension, treatment generally consists of dietary sodium reduction, an exercise program, medication, and smoking cessation, when appropriate.

PERIPHERAL ARTERIAL DISEASE

Peripheral arterial disease results when the arteries are unable to supply the tissues with adequate blood and oxygen. It can have a gradual onset or a sudden onset. Gradual onset is caused by a buildup of atherosclerosis in the arteries or by the vascular changes brought on by diabetes. Sudden onset is caused by any condition that leads to a sudden occlusion of the arteries, such as thrombus, embolus, or trauma.

The two types of peripheral arterial disease are chronic and acute. Arteriosclerosis obliterans (chronic) is the most common type of peripheral arterial disease in older adults. It occurs gradually as the arteries, usually the femoral, popliteal, and tibial, become stiff and inelastic from the buildup of arteriosclerosis. With exercise, which requires a larger supply of oxygen to the tissues, the sclerotic vessels are unable to dilate and increase oxygen supply to meet the demand. Postural changes and extreme temperature changes, especially exposure to cold, also can cause symptoms (Yurick, Spier, Robb, Ebert, & Magnussen, 1989). Exposure to cold causes the arteries to constrict, decreasing blood and oxygen supply to the tissues. Intermittent claudication is especially common in smokers (Buike & Walsh, 1992). Smoking one cigarette causes vasoconstriction for up to an hour (Bright & Georgi, 1992). Symptoms include a charley horse or leg muscle cramp and a dull, aching pain in the buttocks, calf, or thigh that diminishes with rest. The pain is caused by lack of oxygen (hypoxia) to the tissues. Additional symptoms include tightness, burning, and fatigue. At night, when the legs and feet are level with the heart, arterial blood flow is more compromised, resulting in night pain. Night pain or pain at rest is indicative of severe arterial insufficiency (Bright & Georgi, 1992). Untreated, intermittent claudication can result in extremity ulceration, gangrene, infection, tissue necrosis, and limb loss. This is especially true for patients with diabetes (Buike & Walsh, 1992). Additional findings include absent or weak pedal pulses, absent leg and toe hair, and thin, shiny, taut, dry, and/or scaly skin.

Acute arterial insufficiency occurs with a sudden onset of pain due to arterial blockage, frequently from a clot that cuts off the blood supply. Serious tissue damage can develop quickly, so immediate medical care is indicated. Patients with atrial fibrillation; those who have undergone invasive arteriography or vascular surgery; and those with lacerated, severed, or compressed arteries are at additional risk for developing acute arterial insufficiency. The symptoms of acute arterial insufficiency depend on the size and location of the obstruction. They begin suddenly with burning or aching pain below the level of the occlusion. Moving the extremities increases the pain. There may be numbness, pallor, coldness, weakness, and paresthesia. Pulses may be weak or absent. Capillary refill is absent, and the toes become progressively blue as the blood supply is diminished. The treatment goal is to prevent ischemic damage and the development of complications, such as ulcers and gangrene.

MYOCARDIAL INFARCTION

Myocardial infarction (MI) is ischemia and necrosis of the myocardium that occurs when the blood flow through one or more coronary arteries is occluded. Persons older than age 70 have a mortality rate twice as high as for younger persons (Christ & Hohlock, 1988). The age-related changes along with the risk factors predispose older adults to MI. An acute MI may occur without the older adult experiencing pain. In addition, physical exertion and even eating a large meal are risk factors for precipitating an MI in this age group.

The symptoms of MI in older adults may be subtle. Chest pain is less common as a presenting symptom in an older adult having an MI. The classic symptoms of crushing substernal pain radiating down the arms and diaphoresis are rare in those older than age 75 (Sequeira & Cannon, 1990). Dyspnea is the most common symptom of MI in those older than age 85 (Sequeira & Cannon, 1990). Other clinical signs and symptoms are acute confusion, palpitations, worsening heart failure, syncope, stroke, dizziness, and acute renal failure. Subtle changes requiring careful assessment include excessive fatigue, altered mental status, unusual behaviors, and changes in eating patterns (Wenger, 1990). ECG changes may observed, but they can be challenging to interpret if preexisting cardiac disease is present. Laboratory results after MI can be confusing, because older adults have less lean body mass, which influences the CPK and creatinine levels (Wenger, 1990).

Older adults are at additional risk for silent MI, which can result in **sudden** death caused by arrhythmias resulting from the myocardial damage. More of the complications of MI, such as serious arrhythmias, congestive heart failure (CHF), cardiogenic shock, and cardiac rupture, are common in this age group (Christ & Hohlock, 1988). MI may also lead to progressive renal failure. As people age, they experience high morbidity and mortality from atherosclerotic coronary heart disease. Coronary heart disease causes more than two thirds of all cardiac deaths in older adults (Wenger, 1990). All chest pain in the older adult signals the need for careful assessment, because even minor chest pain, especially if accompanied by dyspnea on exertion, may indicate an MI (Yurick et al., 1989).

ARRHYTHMIAS

Age-related heart changes increase the susceptibility of the older adult to arrhythmias. Ventricular premature complexes are present in most adults who are older than age 80 (Wenger, 1990). In addition to the physiologic changes caused by the thickening around the sinoatrial node and internodal tracts, low cardiac output caused by low blood volume can lead to arrhythmias. Eating a large meal, which diverts blood from the heart, and dehydration, which causes low blood volume, can cause arrhythmias. Anything that results in a greater oxygen demand for the myocardium, such as exercise or stress, can cause arrhythmias. Hypokalemia (low potassium level) from diuretic therapy, digitalis toxicity, systemic infections with fever, or significant blood loss can cause arrhythmias. Arrhythmias also occur in acute conditions, such as MI, pulmonary emboli, and CHF (Buike & Walsh, 1992). The most common cause of arrhythmias in older adults is hypertensive heart disease. Regardless of the cause, arrhythmias are serious in older adults, because they have a decreased tolerance due to less cardiac output.

Arrhythmias can result from or precipitate an MI. Thrombus and embolus formation may result from the irregular heartbeats. Because the heart is unable to pump enough blood through the coronary arteries, angina may be present. Syncope and transient ischemic attacks can occur from decreased cardiac output, leading to diminished blood flow to the brain. This increases the risks for falls and accidents. Arrhythmias may precipitate CHF, be life-threatening, and lead to sudden death.

Atrial fibrillation is the most common arrhythmia. Many older adults with atrial fibrillation have no symptoms as long as the heart rate does not exceed 90 beats/minute and there is adequate ventricular filling. In addition to the signs and symptoms of the pathologic conditions such as MI, CHF, and pulmonary emboli, other less obvious symptoms that occur from the compromised circulation and resulting oxygen deficit are changes in mentation, personality, and behavior. The nurse must be exquisitely sensitive to subtle changes in patients with arrhythmias, because they may be difficult to identify. A slight change in appetite or behavior alerts the nurse to assess further. Because stress increases catecholamine stimulation of the heart, modification of the environment may be needed. The treatment goal is to reinstate cardiac rhythm and to decrease formation of emboli from the pooling blood.

ANGINA

Angina pectoris may result from an MI, or it may be due to atherosclerotic lesions in the coronary arteries. It is the most common cause of death and hospitalization among older adults (Newman & Smith, 1991). Angina, chest pain caused by lack of oxygen to the heart muscle, results when the coronary arteries are unable to dilate due to atherosclerosis or aging changes, thereby increasing the amount of oxygen needed by the myocardium. There is no damage to the myocardium, because angina does not result in tissue necrosis. Angina is diagnosed by the history of pain, the physical assessment, and an ECG during the attack. Stable angina occurs as a predictable pattern, such as with increased physical activity, with severe emotional stress, with environmental temperature extremes, and after eating a big meal, at which time blood is diverted to the digestive system. Other conditions, such as anemia and hyperthyroidism, can cause anginal symptoms. Angina becomes unstable when the symptoms occur in an unpredictable pattern and/or there is a change in the frequency and duration of symptoms. Angina caused by coronary artery spasm is called Prinzmetal's angina. It is easily differentiated because the pain usually occurs at night and awakens the person.

The symptoms of angina include pain lasting 10 minutes or less. The symptoms may be described on a continuum from pressure and discomfort to feelings of suffocation or a crushing sensation. Shortness of breath, extreme fatigue, or even syncope may indicate angina in older adults (Esberger & Hughes, 1989). The treatment goal is to reduce pain with medication and to determine the extent and degree of coronary artery occlusion with cardiac catheterization. When a severe blockage occurs, cardiac bypass surgery may improve the quality of life.

 ### Clinical Pearl

Assessment: It is important to remember when assessing for anginal pain that older adults may have an increased tolerance to pain and decreased activity levels, and they may compensate by slowing down activity levels.

CONGESTIVE HEART FAILURE

CHF occurs more frequently in older adults. It is the most common diagnosis for hospitalized adults older than age 65 (Letterer, Carew, Reid, & Woods, 1992). CHF can result from the tissue necrosis of MI and after cardiac bypass surgery. Noncardiac causes of CHF in older adults include pneumonia, hyperthyroidism, fever, and anemia. CHF occurs when the myocardium is forced to pump blood against an area of greater pressure. In left-sided heart failure, the heart is unable to pump blood out of the left side of the heart, so fluid builds up in the lungs. The first symptom may be overwhelming fatigue, thus it is important to assess carefully when older adults complain of fatigue or when their activity level changes drastically. Another covert symptom is two-pillow orthopnea. Patients may forget to report this, because it is insidious and they may not identify it as a symptom. Other signs and symptoms include dyspnea on exertion and a dry, hacking cough that progresses to a productive cough with white, clear mucus and then to the pink, frothy mucus typical of pulmonary edema. The heart rate increases as the heart attempts to pump blood, the pulse is bounding, there may be heart sound changes on auscultation, and the patient will have crackles (also called rales). Crackles produce the same sound that rolling a lock of hair near the ear produces and indicates air passing through moisture in the small air passages.

Right-sided heart failure is due to pulmonary hypertension and/or progression of left-sided heart failure. The first symptoms may be swelling in the feet and ankles, which progresses to pitting edema and swelling in the legs. At night, the patient may experience nocturia because the fluid is reabsorbed and the feet are elevated (Esberger & Hughes, 1989). As the condition worsens, the edema will be present in the mornings. An increase in systemic fluids leads to increased pressure in the renal tubules, causing sodium to be retained, thus increasing the edema and CHF. The patient eventually experiences anorexia because the blood pools in the abdomen. This is accompanied by hepatomegaly and ascites. The treatment includes diuretics and digoxin.

PSYCHOSOCIAL ISSUES

Older adults are dealing with multiple lifestyle changes, environmental changes, and losses. These stressors can increase the release of catecholamines, which, in turn, increase the work of the heart. Unresolved grief may render older adults unable to cope with additional losses. Identifying and modifying stressors can support older adults in dealing with past and present stressors. Significant others and members of the patient's support system may need information and support for themselves to increase support for the older adult.

NURSING ASSESSMENT

Nursing assessment of the older adult with circulatory problems presents special nursing challenges. Many of the symptoms are atypical, subtle, and unusual. For example, mental changes may be the first symptom of CHF. Fatigue, dyspnea, digestion, and mental and behavioral changes may indicate angina or MI. The absence of chest pain does not mean that coronary artery disease is absent (Wenger, 1990). Therefore, any complaints of upper trunk discomfort should be taken seriously and assessed carefully.

HISTORY AND INTERVIEW

A careful and detailed nursing history reveals essential information. A description of daily activities and how they have changed in the last 5 years provides information about beginning symptoms or lifestyle alterations used to accommodate physical changes. Information needs to be specific. For example, how far can you walk without being tired or having pain? Past and present exercise habits and participation in sports activities will provide information regarding lifetime activity levels. Low activity levels can indicate circulatory problems, so determine how far the patient can walk without shortness of breath, dyspnea, fatigue, or pain.

A thorough diet history includes a 24-hour recall to identify intake of high sodium (use of canned vegetables, bouillon cubes, processed foods) or fat (frequent red meat, fried foods), adequate calories, and nutrients. Determine the amount of alcohol consumed by counting the number of ounces drunk per day. Ask patients to list all medications and over-the-counter drugs that they are taking. If they are smokers, determine the number of cigarettes per day and the length of time they have been smoking.

A specific history of physical problems includes describing any chest pain, breathing problems (use of pillows at night, respirations after climbing stairs), special heart problems (palpitations, flutters, pounding, skipped or extra beats, racing), weight gain, and swelling in feet, ankles, legs, shoulders, or arms. Ask, "What has your doctor told you about your heart?" Assessment also includes identifying any sleep problems; symptoms of high levels of anxiety, such as dry mouth or feelings of nervousness or irritability; and palpitations, muscle tension, or extreme fatigue. Sensitive and careful assessment is required to determine if there is use of negative coping strategies, such as excessive sleeping, use of drugs and alcohol, and feelings of helplessness and hopelessness. It can be difficult to differentiate between psychosocial problems and circulation problems, because fatigue and palpitations are common to both. It is very important to ask patients how they perceive the situation. Asking how long they have had these problems and how they have coped with them in the past provides important information for both assessment and interventions. Because confusion and forgetfulness accompany both psychosocial problems and circulation problems, it is important to interview the family and interpersonal support group.

RISK FACTORS

Investigate the family history and risk factors to determine if there is a family history of circulatory problems, such as MI, CVA, hypertension, or diabetes. Uncontrollable risk factors for developing circulation problems are age, sex, diabetes, and hereditary predisposition. Risk factors that can be controlled are smoking, hypertension, obesity, dietary habits, hyperlipidemia, a sedentary lifestyle, and a stressful lifestyle.

PHYSICAL EXAMINATION

Physical assessment includes height, weight, and blood pressure readings. Check blood pressure in both arms while the patient is lying down, sitting, and standing. See Display 14-1 for the proper procedure for the older adult.

Careful and consistent assessment of blood pressure is needed to avoid false-high readings and unnecessary treatment (Cooper, 1992). All pulses should be checked: apical, brachial, radial, femoral, popliteal, dorsalis pedis, and posterior tibialis. The jugular vein should be assessed for venous distension. Auscultation should be done on the carotid arteries and on the arteries in the lower extremities to identify bruits, the sounds heard when blood goes through an obstructed artery. Auscultation of the heart and chest should be done to identify abnormal heart sounds, rhythms, and breath sounds. Identify any tachypnea or crackles.

Inspection of the skin should be done to identify color, edema, and atrophy (shiny, thin skin). Assess the older adult in a room with natural light and warm temperature, and provide privacy. Fluorescent lighting and shivering may interfere with skin assessment and give false data. Compare the right side to the left side. Palpate the skin to determine if the temperature is the same in both arms and both legs. Assess sensation and motor function (Buike & Walsh, 1992). Check capillary refill in extremities. Observe the legs in the dependent position. With arterial insufficiency, the legs will have a red discoloration in this position and will remain red for longer than 15 seconds (Bright & Georgi, 1992).

Display 14-1

GUIDELINES FOR THE ASSESSMENT OF BLOOD PRESSURE IN THE OLDER ADULT

Preparation for blood pressure assessment in older adults:
- Explain procedure and reasons for blood pressure check.
- Place patient in warm, quiet environment.
- Do not measure blood pressure until at least 1 hour postprandial.
- Provide an opportunity for relaxation before assessment.

Method of taking blood pressure:
- Be sure that the cuff is the right size for the patient.
- Take blood pressure **in both arms** while patient is lying, sitting, and standing.
- Support arm and have sphygmomanometer at heart level.
- Inflate cuff to 20 to 30 mm Hg higher than systolic pressure.
- The first sound that is heard is the systolic pressure reading.
- The last sound that is heard is the diastolic pressure reading.

Findings:
- The normal diastolic pressure between lying and standing is plus or minus 10 mm Hg.
- Three separate readings on different days are needed to diagnose hypertension.

DIAGNOSTIC TESTS

Review laboratory results for information about serum electrolytes, renal and hepatic function, cardiac enzymes, and white blood cell count. The ECG is a noninvasive test that determines cardiac function and presence or absence of arrhythmias. Continuous information of cardiac functioning is obtained by having patients wear a Holter monitor (used to determine arrhythmias that may be causing clinical symptoms but that occur periodically or with routine activity) for 1 day or longer. A stress test (an ECG done while exercising) should be explained to the patient as a carefully controlled and monitored test used to evaluate the coronary arteries. Angiograms and cardiac catheterization may be done to visualize the patency of the coronary arteries and assess the heart valves and the circulatory system. It is imperative that older adults be well hydrated before taking the test to prevent acute renal failure.

NURSING DIAGNOSES

Older adults with circulatory problems may experience a symptom, such as fatigue, that has more than one origin. Therefore, the nursing diagnosis must be specific. There are numerous nursing diagnoses for older adults with circulatory problems, including the following:

- Activity Intolerance related to pain in lower legs with exertion
- Activity Intolerance related to impaired oxygenation for activities of daily living resulting from decreased circulation to the heart muscle
- Fatigue related to low hemoglobin or poor perfusion
- High Risk for Fluid Volume Deficit related to increased output secondary to diuretics

- High Risk for Fluid Volume Excess related to decreased cardiac pumping ability
- High Risk for Injury related to poor cerebral perfusion secondary to postural hypotension
- Knowledge Deficit related to new medication and lifestyle changes
- Pain related to poor circulation in the lower extremities or poor perfusion of the myocardium
- Sexual Dysfunction related to antihypertensive medication
- Social Isolation related to frequent urination resulting from diuretic therapy
- Altered Thought Processes related to poor cerebral perfusion

NURSING INTERVENTIONS

Nursing care for patients with circulation problems is challenging. Circulation problems affect multiple body systems and all lifestyle activities. In addition, prevention and rehabilitation are major components of a health plan. Sensitivity to the psychosocial needs of older adults increases the ability of the nurse to gather data and plan interventions specific to patients and their families. Nursing care outcomes depend on the ability of the nurse to communicate with older adults, involve patients and families in planning care, and determine appropriate and realistic goals and follow-up on a continuing basis. Long-term relationships with older adults, when possible, increase their sense of security and feeling of being cared about. The rewards for the nurse include a sense of having made a difference in the life of patients and their families.

Circulation problems can cause sudden, life-threatening events, such as an MI or CVA, potentially precipitating a need for life support interventions ranging from feeding tubes to ventilators. Decisions regarding the use of these interventions should be made before the event occurs. Advanced directives and durable power of attorney need to be addressed with each older adult experiencing circulatory problems. Older adults, their significant others, and members of their support system need information and an opportunity to discuss the issues with an objective person in order to make an informed decision.

MEDICATION ADMINISTRATION

Older adults with circulatory problems take multiple medications. Because they often have less lean body mass, low fluid reserve, slower metabolism, and decreased renal and hepatic function, titration of dose and assessment of response is very important. Assess laboratory data for renal and kidney function and signs of dehydration. In addition, diminished eyesight and a tendency toward forgetfulness suggest that teaching and devising methods to separate doses is essential. The most common medications for circulation problems are digoxin, nitrates, beta blockers, and calcium channel blockers (Table 14-1).

Clinical Pearl

Intervention: A lower dose of nitroglycerin may be indicated for older adults, because loss of baroreceptor activity increases the tendency for postural hypotension.

Table 14-1   DRUG, NURSING IMPLICATIONS, SIDE EFFECTS, AND TEACHING

Drug (uses)	Nursing Implications	Side Effects	Teaching

Digoxin (congestive heart failure, arrythmias)	Check apical pulse for full minute
	Notify physician if >100 or <60
	Monitor serum potassium level
	Monitor respirations
	Weigh daily
	Monitor intake and output
	Monitor neck vein distention
	Use with caution in older adults
	Assess liver and kidney function
		Nausea, vomiting, diarrhea, headache, weakness, fatigue, irregular or slow pulse	Take pulse before taking medication
			Weigh daily
			Report to physician if:
			  5-lb gain
			  Pulse >100 or <60
			  Visual problems: yellow-green haze or halo
			  Loss of appetite
			  Nausea/vomiting/diarrhea
			  Headache
			  Weakness/fatigue
			  Irregular or slow pulse
			  Change in heart rhythm
			  Blurred or dimmed/double vision or blind spots
			  Mood alterations

Nitroglycerin (sublingual) (to relax and dilate blood vessels)	Monitor antihypertensives Monitor blood pressure Monitor dosage (lower dosage needed with increased age to avoid toxicity)	Headache, dizziness, weakness, nausea/vomiting, hypersensitivity, orthostatic hypotension	Place tablet under the tongue and do not swallow Slight burning sensation means tablet potent Discard tablets with no burning sensation Remove tablet if pain stops Take in sitting position; change positions slowly Keep bottle with a few tablets close at hand Do not attach to body Store in original, airtight, dark container Remove cotton and do not replace Check expiration date

Drug	Nursing Considerations	Side Effects	Patient Teaching
Oral nitroglycerin	Same	Same	Assure it is not addicting Take before or with experience of angina Take before activity May take one tablet every 5–10 minutes × 3 tablets Seek medical attention for pain >15 minutes
Nitroglycerin patch	Avoid getting on fingers Remind to get up slowly	Same	Take with full glass of water Take 1 hour before or 2 hours after meals Avoid alcohol, which may increase vasodilation Remove previous patch before applying Wash and dry area Put new patch in clean, dry area without hair Do not place patch over irritated skin Do not wear near microwave oven
Lingual spray	Do not inhale Wait 10 seconds before swallowing		Release spray under tongue
Beta blockers (hypertension, angina, arrhythmias)	Monitor heart rate closely Do not give to diabetics Check pulse Do not give with asthma	Fatigue, lethargy, bradycardia, hypotension, nausea, vomiting, diarrhea, fever	Report any of the following: Unexplained bruising or bleeding Fever or sore throat Severe or persistent drowsiness Severe depression or long-lasting "blues" Discuss potential for sexual dysfunction
Calcium channel blockers (arrhythmias, angina, hypertension)	Take pulse daily Provide good mouth care Check liver enzymes Give carefully with beta blockers and antihypertensives	Headaches, constipation, hypotension	Caution person not to stop taking drug suddenly Report any of the following: Change of 10 beats or pulse rate <50 Right upper quadrant pain Jaundice, color of stool, malaise

PATIENT AND FAMILY EDUCATION

Teaching may be the most important nursing intervention for patients with circulatory problems. Major lifestyle changes are generally required to decrease the continued formation of atherosclerosis and to build up collateral circulation in the heart and extremities. Including patients and their families in the planning is essential for their following the therapeutic plan. It is a challenge for the nurse to present this information in such a way that is acceptable to patients and families, because many older adults may be experiencing no overt symptoms and have difficulty understanding the need for changes. It is essential to emphasize the preventative aspects of these changes. Patient education is needed concerning dietary changes, weight loss, smoking cessation techniques, exercise programs, stress management, medications, and cardiac rehabilitation programs.

Patients taking cardiac medication and their families need specific instructions about the frequency of medications, when and how to take the medications, and use of over-the-counter medications. The Patient Teaching Box gives some specific instructions.

Weight Management. Patients and families need instruction about diet and ways to modify diet in terms of fat and sodium. Include the dietitian in planning an individualized diet program based on what patients eat, what they will and will not eat, and the resources available for purchasing, storing, and

---

Patient Teaching Box
FOR OLDER ADULTS TAKING CARDIAC DRUGS

- Take drug at approximately the same time each day.
- Do not skip a dose.
- Do not double a dose.
- Take with a meal or food.
- Keep appointments to have blood levels checked.
- Do not take over-the-counter drugs without consulting your doctor.
- Decrease alcohol consumption.
- Stop smoking.
- Take pulse daily.
- Report any weight gain greater than 2 lb per week.

If the drug being taken is a **nitrate:**
Learn how to take *sublingual nitroglycerin*

- Place tablet under the tongue and do not swallow.
  A slight burning sensation indicates tablet is potent.
  Discard tablets when there is no burning sensation.
  Remove tablet if pain stops and tablet not dissolved.
  A dry mouth can inhibit absorption.
- Take in sitting position
  If taken when supine, there is an increase in venous side effects.
  If taken when standing, there is an increase for postural hypotension.
- Keep bottle with a few tablets close at hand but not attached to the body, because body heat can decompose them.
  Keep in original, airtight, dark container in cool place.
  Remove cotton and do not replace.

preparing food. Because adequate nutritional intake is so important for older adults, creativity is needed to plan meals that meet dietary requirements and that patients will eat. The diet must not be so drastic that patients either do not adhere to the diet or decrease their intake. Modify the diet according to normal habits.

Weight loss for overweight older adults is important. Blood pressure can be lowered if overweight older adults will lose weight and incorporate other lifestyle changes (smoking cessation and an exercise program). A support program, either a support group or specific support interventions by family, can increase the ability to meet weight loss goals. The prescribed diets for patients with problems with circulation also include the following instructions:

- Rest before meals
- Avoid heavy meals
- Eat several small meals per day rather than three large ones
- Limit alcohol to 2 oz/day
- Do not add salt at the table; instead, use other food seasonings
- Avoid preserved foods (eg, ham, bacon)
- Avoid prepackaged, dehydrated foods that are high in sodium
- Use frozen, not canned, vegetables
- Limit dietary fat to 15% of calories
- Decrease or avoid caffeine
- Limit cholesterol to 300 mg/day

 Clinical Pearl

Intervention: It is better for the older adult to lose weight slowly, because weight loss can increase fats in the blood, thereby contributing to an increase in atherosclerosis.

Lifestyle Changes. Individual exercise programs for older adults are needed. Patients who have never exercised regularly need education about exercise benefits, specific plans, and support with follow-up to evaluate the plan. Including patients in the planning is essential if they are to follow the exercise regimen. The exercise program is planned to avoid excessive fatigue, limit injuries, and maintain functional abilities. It is important to teach patients to begin exercise with warm-up exercises and to end with cool-down exercises to prevent complications.

In addition to exercise programs, older adults need teaching about activities that increase safety, such as changing positions slowly, sitting on the side of the bed before standing, standing a few moments before walking, avoiding prolonged standing or sitting, avoiding stooping, using assistive devices for picking up articles on the floor, and exercising regularly. Additional instructions include avoiding hot baths, because they can cause vasodilation and hypotension as blood vessels dilate and blood pools. Valsalva's maneuver increases cardiac strain, so patients should be taught to avoid constipation and lifting heavy articles. Frequent, small meals are better, because eating a large meal diverts blood to the stomach and increases the chance of hypotension. Elastic stockings may increase circulation and decrease pooling. Patients should be taught when and how to apply and remove them. Additional interventions include prevention of dehydration with adequate fluid intake and some fluid intake before going to bed.

Nicotine stimulates catecholamine release, which increases heart rate and causes vasoconstriction of the coronary arteries. Smokers also have higher levels of carbon monoxide in their blood, which decreases the availability of oxygen for delivery to the myocardium. This information, given to patients with an attitude that they have a choice, may facilitate some change.

Although smoking is a controllable risk factor, many patients are reluctant or unable to stop smoking. A great deal of creativity and listening is required to find a way to help patients stop smoking. There are programs and support groups to help with smoking cessation. Contracts between the patient and nurse or patient and family are sometimes helpful. Agreement to decrease the number of cigarettes smoked per day may be the very best that the patient can accomplish. Although not ideal, this is a beginning.

Special supportive nursing care is needed by older adults for them to make needed lifestyle changes. It is a nursing challenge to motivate the patient and family to incorporate the drastic changes in lifestyle needed to ensure better health. A family conference may uncover problems and identify additional resources. Because there is a hereditary factor in the development of circulation problems and because early interventions are needed, the family conference provides an opportunity to teach them about risk factors and lifestyle modifications. The younger the person is when lifestyle changes are made, the better the chances for decreasing and/or postponing circulation problems. The family may need guidance to become a support system for the patient. In addition, it is difficult to change eating habits and almost impossible if the one who is doing the cooking does not understand the new diet or will not change meal preparation style. Therefore, the understanding and cooperation of each family member is important for interventions to be successful.

Referral to a program on cardiopulmonary resuscitation can be helpful in lowering family members' anxiety and feelings of helplessness. Teach them what to look for and when to call the physician and how to manage the emergency medical system, and help them prepare an emergency information file to take to the hospital. The emergency information file includes the name of the patient's physician; a medical history; the names, dosage, and times of all medications; insurance and/or Medicare numbers; and the names of family members to notify. This information is updated as needed and kept in a designated place known to all who stay with the older adult.

CARDIAC REHABILITATION

Older adults have a keen desire to remain independent. This desire is excellent motivation for them to participate in cardiac rehabilitation. The goals of rehabilitation include but are not limited to preserving and maintaining functional abilities, increasing strength and coordination, limiting or preventing anxiety and depression, and increasing and/or maintaining mental functioning. It is extremely important to include the family or members of the support system in the rehabilitation process, because some of the disease processes decrease oxygen to the brain and lead to confusion. Under stress, the older adult may be unable to retain new information. Family members or the patient's support system can reinforce information as needed. Group classes may be especially helpful to older adults, because there is an opportunity to share life experiences and suggestions for interventions (Harrell, 1988).

Cardiac rehabilitation is contingent on the nature of the problem, other illnesses, and the physiologic response of the patient (Anderson, 1991). Physical training in cardiac rehabilitation often begins in the hospital. Because bed rest leads to the development of additional problems, patients are usually given bathroom privileges if they can tolerate the activity. Ambulation is begun as soon as possible. While the patient is in the hospital, the nurse assesses exercise tolerance with frequent checks of heart and respiratory rates and skin color. Additional assessment includes a subjective evaluation. It is important that patients not be pushed beyond endurance, because this is more harmful than helpful.

Many hospitals have cardiac rehabilitation programs that patients join after a period of recuperation at home. Participation in these programs is determined by the patient's need and ability to participate. It is important for the nurse to teach patients the importance of exercise and to help them develop exercise programs. Collaboration with the physician is needed to determine the ideal exercise program. Generally, walking and swimming are good exercises. Patients should avoid exercise until at least 2 hours after eating.

COMMUNITY RESOURCES

The number of community services needed by the patient to return home after hospitalization can range from home oxygen to home health care aides, from bedside commodes to community transportation systems, and from Meals On Wheels to a "buddy" call each day. It is important for the nurse to become familiar with the resources in the community, be aware of the benefits of Medicare and Medicaid, and feel comfortable coordinating the multidisciplinary team in the hospital, from the social worker to the occupational therapist. Many communities have special programs for older adults that provide communication within easy reach in times of emergency (Johnson, Adams, & Bigely, 1992). This not only provides safety for the patient but also contributes to a sense of security.

Nursing Care Plan

FOR THE PATIENT WITH ORTHOSTATIC HYPOTENSION

Nursing Diagnosis: High Risk for Injury related to sudden fall in blood pressure as evidenced by dizziness, syncope, lightheadedness, or falls.

Definition: The state in which an individual is at risk for harm because of a perceptual or physiologic deficit, lack of awareness, or maturational age.

Assessment Findings:
1. Complaints of blurred vision with position changes.
2. Complaints of dizziness or "swimming in the head" with position changes.
3. Experiences of syncope or blackouts with or without falls or injury.
4. Experiences of changes after eating a large meal, taking diuretics, or taking a hot bath/shower or in extremely hot weather.

(continued)

Nursing Care Plan

FOR THE PATIENT WITH ORTHOSTATIC HYPOTENSION *(Continued)*

Nursing Interventions with Selected Rationales:

1. Avoid sudden position changes; assist patient to sit on side of bed for several minutes before standing, then to stand for several minutes before walking.
   Rationale: Sudden position changes prevent sudden loss of cerebral perfusion.
2. Encourage the patient to begin walking every day and to increase the distance walked on a regular basis.
   Rationale: Walking on a regular basis improves stamina and endurance and enhances collateral circulation.
3. Determine regular elimination pattern and ensure adequate fluid intake, dietary fiber, and roughage.
   Rationale: Adequate dietary intake helps prevent constipation and Valsalva's maneuver. Adequate fluid intake prevents dehydration leading to orthostatic hypotension.
4. Remove elastic stockings twice a day and change daily.
   Rationale: Removal of elastic stocking allows for assessment and cleaning of the lower extremities.
5. Do not bend or stoop.
   Rationale: Baroreceptors are unable to accommodate sudden changes in blood pressure.
6. Do not lift heavy objects that might institute Valsalva's maneuver.
   Rationale: Valsalva's maneuver increases cardiac workload.
7. Avoid hot baths and direct sunlight.
   Rationale: Heat promotes vasodilation.
8. Eat small, frequent meals rather than one large meal.
   Rationale: Small meals minimize the rapid shifting of blood to the digestive system.
9. Don't sit or stand for long periods of time. Do "pedal pumps" every hour. Encourage rocking in a rocking chair.
   Rationale: Activity assists with peripheral blood return and prevents pooling of blood in the lower extremities.

Desired Patient Outcomes/Discharge Criteria:

1. Patient verbalizes what contributes to postural hypotension.
2. Patient verbalizes and/or performs appropriate interventions to prevent postural hypotension.
3. Patient demonstrates how to rise from lying to sitting to standing.
4. Patient verbalizes the safety measures to make in the home to prevent injury.

REFERENCES

Anderson, J. M. (1991). Rehabilitating elderly cardiac patients. *Rehabilitation Medicine Adding Life to Years* [Special issue]. *154*, 573–578.

Bright, L. D., & Georgi, S. (1992). Is it arterial or venous? *American Journal of Nursing, 92*(9), 34–43.

Buike, M. M. & Walsh, M. B. (1992). *Gerontological nursing: Care of the frail elderly.* St. Louis: Mosby.

Carpenito, L. J. (1993). *Nursing diagnosis application to clinical practice* (5th ed.). Philadelphia: J. B. Lippincott.

Christ, M. A., & Hohlock, F. J. (1988). *Gerontologic nursing: A study and learning tool.* Spring-house, PA: Springhouse.

Cooper, K. M. (1992). Measuring blood pressure the right way. *Nursing 92, 22*(4), 75.

Esberger, K. K., & Hughes, S. T. (1989). *Nursing care of the aged.* Norwalk, CT: Appleton and Lange.

Harrell, J. S. (1988). Age-related changes in the cardiovascular system. In M. A. Matteson & E. S. McConnell (Eds.), *Gerontological nursing: Concepts and practice* (pp. 193–217). Philadelphia: W. B. Saunders.

Johnson, J., Adams, K., & Bigely, M. D. (1992). Cardiovascular function. In C. M. M. Buike & M. B. Walsh (Eds.), *Gerontological nursing care of the frail elderly.* St. Louis: Mosby.

Letterer, R. A., Carew, B., Reid, M., & Woods, P. (1992). Learning to live with congestive heart failure. *Nursing 92, 22*(5), 34–41.

Malasanos, L., Barkauskas, V., & Stoltenberg-Allen, K. (1990). *Health assessment.* St. Louis: Mosby.

Miller, C. A. (1995). *Nursing care of older adults.* Philadelphia: J. B. Lippincott.

Newman, D. K., & Smith, D. A. J. (1991). *Geriatric care plans.* Springhouse, PA: Springhouse.

Sequeira, M. K., & Cannon, L. A. (1990). Intervention in acute myocardial infarction. In G. Bosker, G. R. Schwartz, J. S. Jones, & M. Sequeira (Eds.), *Geriatric emergency medicine* (pp. 163–187). St. Louis: Mosby.

Wenger, N. D. (1990). Cardiovascular disease. In C. K. Cassel, D. E. Riesenberg, L. B. Sorensen, & J. R. Walsh (Eds.), *Geriatric medicine* (2nd ed.). New York: Springer-Verlag.

Wilson, D. D., & Smith, C. E. (1992) Nursing assessment cardiovascular system. In S. M. Lewis & I. C. Collier (Eds.), *Medical-surgical nursing assessment and management of clinical problems* (pp. 715–737). St. Louis: Mosby.

Yurick, A. G., Spier, B. E., Robb, S. S., Ebert, N. J., & Magnussen, M. H. (1989). *The aged person and the nursing process* (3rd ed.). Norwalk, CT: Appleton & Lange.

BIBLIOGRAPHY

Aaronson, I., Carlon Wolfe, W., & Schoener, S. (1991). Pressures that fall on rising; Ways to control postural hypotension. *Geriatric Nursing, 12*(3), 67.

Anderson, F. D. & Maloney, J. P. (1994). Taking blood pressure correctly, it's no off the cuff matter. *Nursing 94 24*(11), 34–44.

Baer, C. L., & Williams, B. R. (1988). *Clinical pharmacology and nursing.* Springhouse, PA: Springhouse.

Bushnel, F. K. L. (1992), Self-care teaching for congestive heart failure patients. *Journal of Gerontological Nursing, 18*(10), 27–32.

Clark, J. B., Queener, S. F., & Karb, V. B. (1994). *Pharmacological basis of nursing practice* (4th ed.). St. Louis: Mosby.

Flack, J. M., Woolley, A., Essenge, P. & Grimm, R. H. (1992). A rational approach to hypertension treatment in the older adult. *Geriatrics, 47*(11), 24–38.

Lazar, E. J., Lazar, J. M., & Frishman, W. (1992). Angina pectoris and silent ischemia in the elderly: A management update. *Geriatrics, 47*(7), 24–36.

Matzdoff, A. C., & Green, D. (1992). Deep vein thrombosis and pulmonary embolism: Prevention, diagnosis, and treatment. *Geriatrics, 47*(8), 48–63.

Miller, C. A. (1991). Calcium channel blockers to counter hypertension. *Geriatric Nursing, 12*(5), 259–260.

Miller, C. A. (1993). Congestive heart failure: Old and new drugs. *Geriatric Nursing, 14*(4), 223–224.

Miller, K. M. (1993). Nursing strategies for patients with silent myocardial ischemia. *Critical Care Nursing, 12*(5), 256–262.

Miller, M. M. (1994). Current trends in the primary care management of chronic congestive heart failure. *Nurse Practitioner, 19*(5), 64–70.

Morgan, S. (1993). Effects of age on cardiovascular functioning. *Geriatric Nursing, 14*(5), 249–251.

Newbern, V. (1991). Cautionary tales on using beta blockers. *Geriatric Nursing, 12*(3), 119–122.

Petrocitch, M., Vogt, T. M., & Berge, K. G. (1992). Isolated systolic hypertension: Lowering the risk of stroke in older patients. *Geriatrics, 47*(3), 30–38.

Yakawich, M. (1992). What you should know about administering nitrates. *Nursing 92, 22*(9), 53–55.

15

Problems With Respiratory Function

Objectives

1. List the physiologic changes of aging associated with the lungs and thorax.
2. Contrast chronic and acute respiratory problems in the older adult.
3. Describe the psychological changes of aging related to respiratory problems.
4. Identify steps in the nursing assessment of an older adult with respiratory problems.
5. List nursing diagnoses associated with respiratory problems.
6. Design nursing interventions for the older adult with chronic obstructive pulmonary disease.
7. Develop a nursing care plan for an older adult with ineffective airway clearance.

INTRODUCTION

THE RESPIRATORY SYSTEM, AS WITH ALL ORGAN systems of the human body, experiences physiologic and functional changes due to the aging process. Because the lungs function less efficiently with age, the goal of nursing care is to assist the older adult to adapt to the gradual normal changes of aging, to differentiate between normal aging changes and pathologic conditions, and to identify and promote strategies to maintain the highest level of independent function for the patient.

Age-related changes that affect pulmonary function place the older adult at risk for respiratory problems. Skeletal changes that result in curvature of the spine (kyphosis) can interfere with normal breathing mechanics, resulting in decreased mobility and physical activity. Stress, both physical and emotional, which can be tolerated in the younger adult, can cause fatigue and dyspnea in the older adult as a result of age-related changes in the respiratory system. The

Staab, AS and Hodges, LC: ESSENTIALS OF GERONTOLOGICAL NURSING,
© 1996 J. B. Lippincott Company

combination of respiratory and immune system changes increases the risk of pneumonia and influenza.

NORMAL PHYSIOLOGIC CHANGES

Musculoskeletal changes include an increase in the anteroposterior diameter of the chest wall due to elevation of the ribs and flattening of the diaphragm. Combined with calcification of costal cartilage, this reduces mobility of the ribs and promotes only partial contraction of the inspiratory muscles. Kyphosis, which normally develops as one ages, is often exaggerated by osteoporosis and vertebral collapse. This structural change can limit breathing capacity.

As a person ages, other musculoskeletal physiologic changes lead to a progressive decline in lung function. Combined with a reduction in respiratory muscle strength, increased rib stiffness, and loss of collagen, the elastic fibers within the alveolar walls (terminal bronchioli) lose inward elastic recoil. This produces a collapse of the small conducting airways, varying alveolar ventilation, and air trapping. The amount of air that can be expired after maximal inspiration is decreased as a result of these age-related changes (Hazzard, 1994). This causes a decreased forced vital capacity and maximal expiratory flow rate with an increased residual volume.

There also is a decline in the ability of pulmonary gases to move from alveoli to blood (diffusion capacity). This reduced diffusion capacity is due to loss of surface area of the alveolar-capillary membrane and the resulting differences in ventilation and/or blood flow.

Other normal changes associated with aging include reduced cough efficiency and decreased ciliary activity in the bronchial lining. These changes result in less efficient clearing of mucus and foreign material, which contribute to infection. The increased dead space at the lung base associated with structural changes in the chest contributes to decreased ventilation. Although ventilatory capacity decreases only a small fraction yearly, its cumulative effect over a lifetime makes the older adult more vulnerable to respiratory disease. These normal changes can mimic many of the pathologic changes found in persons with chronic airflow obstruction, but the changes due to aging do not result in elevations of blood carbon dioxide and bicarbonate. The differences are only quantitative. Whenever the older adult experiences a decrease in mobility or functioning, these factors must be considered. Decreased mobility or functioning can result in retention of secretions and altered chest expansion, making the patient more susceptible to infection and reduced ventilation.

ABNORMAL PHYSIOLOGIC CHANGES

Aging persons experience declines in lung function that are only partially due to the aging process. Decades of exposure to environmental pollutants, including cigarette smoke, in conjunction with changes in the mouth, nose, and other organs and metabolic factors all contribute to diminished lung function. Changes in the respiratory muscle, diaphragm, diffusion of alveoli and capillaries, and respiratory center can result in such problems as sleep apnea syndrome, obstructive and restrictive lung diseases, asthma, tuberculosis, pneumonia, and influenza. Respiratory infections can be mild, self-limiting disease processes of brief duration or can include lower tract infections involving viruses or bacteria in the lung.

SLEEP APNEA SYNDROME

Sleep apnea syndrome in the older adult is defined as a cessation of airflow at the level of the nostrils and mouth lasting for at least 10 seconds and exceeding eight episodes per hour of sleep. It results in arterial blood desaturation, sleep disruption, and daytime somnolence. There are three types of apnea:

- Central apnea, in which the inspiratory (central nervous system) drive ceases, as evidenced by the lack of diaphragmatic and intercostal muscle activity
- Obstructive apnea, in which intermittent closure of the upper airway prevents airflow despite inspiratory muscle contractions
- Mixed apnea (a combination of central and obstructive apnea), in which, initially, the inspiratory drive ceases, followed by its resumption without airflow due to upper airway obstruction (Farzan & Sattar, 1992)

Most older adults with sleep apnea experience the mixed type, are overweight, and frequently complain of excessive daytime sleepiness, nocturnal insomnia, tiredness, and headache on awakening in the morning. Snoring, restlessness, and abnormal motor activities during sleep are often reported by the spouse. Alcohol and sedatives increase the incidence of apnea.

CHRONIC LUNG PROBLEMS

Chronic lung conditions can cause restriction of lung expansion (restrictive lung disease) or cause obstruction or resistance to airflow (obstructive lung disease). Restrictive pulmonary conditions include fibrosis, sarcoidosis, and musculoskeletal conditions such as kyphoscoliosis and ankylosing spondylitis. Obstructive pulmonary conditions include emphysema, bronchitis, and asthma. Because all of these conditions alter the normal rate of airflow into and out of the lungs, the patient's need for oxygen is greatly increased. Patients with these conditions compensate for this need for oxygen with rapid, shallow breathing patterns due to inadequate lung expansion in the case of restrictive diseases or with slow, deep breathing patterns due to narrowed lumens and fluids in the respiratory tree in the case of obstructive conditions.

CHRONIC OBSTRUCTIVE PULMONARY DISEASE

The terms chronic bronchitis, emphysema, and chronic obstructive pulmonary disease (COPD) are often used interchangeably. Bronchitis, an infection of the bronchi, is clinically diagnosed as chronic bronchitis when there is a daily cough producing sputum for at least 3 months of the year for 2 consecutive years in the absence of other diseases that produce this finding. Emphysema has been redefined as a condition of the lung that affects the terminal alveoli by distension or rupture and loss of elasticity, which interferes with expiration. These conditions are characterized by a reduced airway lumen caused by marked mucosal thickening and increased airway compliance from destruction of the reduced lumen from tenacious mucus. Destruction of alveolar walls in emphysema reduces the capillary bed and, thus, decreases the pulmonary gas exchange surface. Older adults who experience a combination of chronic bronchitis and emphysema often have a long history of smoking. The continuation of smoking encourages progression of both conditions.

Functional changes occurring with obstructive lung disease include interference with transfer of carbon dioxide and oxygen between blood and alveolar air due to the destruction of lung tissues. There is an increased resistance to airflow during inspiration and expiration from injury and inflammation of bronchial tubes and an increased lung compliance from lung tissue damage. In obstructive lung disease, there is decreased muscle strength with ineffective action of the diaphragm and respiratory muscles. Functionally, breathing requires more work as the person ages. The diminished efficiency of breathing and reserve capacity results in a reduced tolerance for exercise and stress and a diminished ability to sustain work.

ASTHMA

Asthma, a condition resulting from spasmodic contractions of the bronchi, is characterized by spasms of shortness of breath and wheezing. A reversible, acute disease, asthma is caused by narrowing or constriction of the bronchi from irritating materials, such as pollens and cigarette smoke, with the cause of the reaction to the stimuli often unknown. Viral infections, exposure to cigarette smoke, air pollution, temperature changes, the taking of aspirin and other prostaglandin inhibitors, and emotional factors may precipitate attacks. Older adults who develop asthma in adulthood do not have a seasonal pattern to their illness, but the attacks are often preceded by a respiratory tract infection, usually viral. This type of asthma is often concomitant with chronic bronchitis and emphysema. The older adult responds clinically in much the same manner as the younger adult during an asthmatic attack. They present with dyspnea, expiratory wheezing, coughing, fatigue, and rhinorrhea, progressing to inspiratory wheezing and sputum production. Treatment is aimed at reduction of bronchospasm and increased pulmonary ventilation by assessment and removal of stimuli that are initiating the allergic response.

TUBERCULOSIS

Tuberculosis is one of the oldest diseases known. Poverty, overpopulation, and malnutrition characterize the environment in which tuberculosis is most prevalent. Worldwide, morbidity reaches approximately 20 million active cases annually. Developing third world countries are more affected than developed areas. The prime organ target of infection is generally the lungs. To develop the disease, an individual, unprotected by immune mechanisms, must have close and sustained exposure in an environment heavily laden with droplet nuclei (Schlossberg, 1988).

Increased morbidity of tuberculosis in the older adult in the United States shows a dramatic shift. Without segregating for ethnicity, older adults have the highest case rate of all age groups. Symptoms of tuberculosis in the older adult do not vary from those of younger patients and include cough with or without hemoptysis, weakness, shortness of breath, weight loss, and a low-grade fever, particularly in the evening. Older adults generally demonstrate disability and a failure to thrive.

PNEUMONIA

Pneumonia is defined as inflammation of lung tissue. In older adults, the causative agent is often bacterial, such as streptococcal pneumonia, but influenzal pneumonia (viral) is also a common source. Pneumonia can be fatal in the frail older adult. It is the most common cause of death in centenarians (Abrass, Besdine, Butler, Rowe, & Solomon, 1990). Because pneumonia is so often encountered in the frail elderly, especially in long-term-care facilities, nursing care can have far-reaching effects on the outcome. The older adult is at particular risk for pneumonia due to decreased immune response (immunosenescence), reduced pulmonary function associated with aging, the presence of complicating conditions such as COPD, and increased gram-negative pharyngeal colonization. The characteristic signs of pneumonia include fever, cough, and shortness of breath. Bacterial pneumonia has a more rapid onset, with thick sputum production varying in color from yellow to rust, indicating the presence of bacteria. Viral pneumonia generally has a more insidious onset—a dry, hacking cough with little or no sputum production. Pneumonia in the older adult can present atypically with confusion, lethargy, general malaise, or a combination of these signs. Fever, cough, and sputum production may be minimal or absent. Because the older adult usually has underlying chronic disease, these symptoms may be mistaken for exacerbation of already existing conditions. Aspiration pneumonia is a significant complication of swallowing difficulties, the use of feeding tubes, and life in an institutional setting. Of the bacterial pneumococcal pneumonia cases that occur each year, overall mortality can be as high as 50% despite the use of an antimicrobial. For the older adult at high risk, prophylactic treatment with penicillin is most important.

INFLUENZA

Influenza is generally a self-limiting disease of brief duration, but it can be a significant health risk in older adults, particularly if they have other chronic diseases, such as diabetes, or heart or lung disease. Older adults in institutions can be protected from infection by medication (amantadine) or isolation from visitors during the flu season. Influenza can be fatal despite antibiotics and high-tech therapy. Most cases of influenza are viral but can include mycoplasmas and Group A streptococcus. Symptoms include a history of exposure, nonproductive or productive cough, headaches, myalgias, low-grade fever, and general malaise.

PSYCHOSOCIAL ISSUES

Although chronic illness is not a certainty for older patients, statistics show that most older patients do have chronic conditions. Older patients experiencing chronic respiratory illness and the resulting disability can often develop psychosocial problems related to their loss of independence and personal control. In addition, the decreased respiratory reserve potential of the older adult often prolongs the acute illness recovery time, placing the patient at further risk for exacerbation of chronic conditions. This can increase the patient's anxiety, helplessness, immobility, and dependency. Lifestyle changes are often necessary to cope with chronic illness, placing the older adult at higher risk for altered self-concept, increased dependency on others, and, possibly, social isolation. As the physical disability increases, families must take over such tasks as home maintenance and housecleaning, causing the patient to feel a decreased sense of pride in performing these tasks and diminished self-esteem.

Problems related to respiratory function produce anxiety. Actual or anticipated dyspnea increases this anxiety. The older adult may feel more secure if the nurse or family member stays in close proximity. Threats to independence, personal control, self-determination, and well-being are areas of concern for the older adult. The person's response to illness and his or her strive for independence and personal determination play an important role in coping and adapting positively to the chronic respiratory problem. Having a strong social network can diminish the problems associated with social isolation when altered respiratory function limits activities.

NURSING ASSESSMENT

The nursing assessment of the respiratory system of the older adult should include history pertinent to the presenting respiratory problem and physical assessment of the lungs and thorax and of any system relative to the presenting problem.

HISTORY AND INTERVIEW

Data collection in the history should focus on areas related to the respiratory problem, with differentiation of normal changes and pathologic findings. The nurse should thoroughly analyze any significant respiratory symptom by questioning and documenting the onset of the symptom; characteristics of the symptom; the patient's course since the onset, including treatment and response; and a review of systems pertinent to the symptom. Functional activity must be assessed periodically during the course of ongoing respiratory problems and be compared with the baseline activity level of the older adult. Figure 15-1 is an example of an assessment tool that demonstrates baseline and current functional levels.

RISK FACTORS

Cigarette smoking is a significant contributor to pulmonary disease in both the young and old. In nonsmokers without respiratory disease, ventilatory function begins to decline beginning at age 25 to 35 and drops about 25 mL annually. In smokers, this drop can increase to 100 mL or more annually, and those at higher rates of decline are at greater risk for disease. Airways and lung parenchyma are extensively damaged by cigarette smoking. With prolonged smoking, the small airways are further damaged. Changes include fibrosis of the airways with narrowing, squamous cell changes, increased muscle mass, plugging of the lumen by mucus and inflammatory cells, and presence of a reduced number of airways. In cigarette smokers, clinically evidenced lung disease usually results from a sustained loss of ventilatory function beyond that associated with aging alone (Cherniack, 1991).

Air pollution has presented concerns to health care providers and environmentalists since the turn of the century, with the concentration of industry in heavily populated areas and dramatic increases in the number of automobiles.

	Baseline Activity Level	Current Status
Eating		
Hygiene		
Dressing		
Ambulation		
Home Maintenance		
Toileting		

Codes: Level 0: Independent
        Level I: Requires use of device (specify)
        Level II: Requires help of person
        Level III: Requires help of person and device (specify)
        Level IV: Totally dependent

Figure 15-1. Assessment of baseline activity level

Long-term exposure to noxious air pollutants combined with respiratory disease puts the older adult at high risk for morbidity and mortality.

Surgery and trauma increases the metabolic response due to inflammation in the anatomic (surgical) areas affected, leaving the previously normal systems, such as the lungs and urinary tract, vulnerable to infection. Preoperative pulmonary function of the older adult plays a significant role in the postoperative respiratory response. Abdominal plus thoracic surgery produces predictable alterations in pulmonary function postoperatively. Vital capacity is reduced 50% to 75% within 72 hours. This occurs gradually over 12 to 18 hours postoperatively. At 12 hours after surgery, the ventilatory reserve is significantly less than immediately after surgery. This reserve gradually improves unless complications occur, ranging from atelectasis to ventilatory failure.

The older adult with cardiac problems is at increased risk when pulmonary problems occur, because pulmonary dysfunction has adverse effects on the cardiac system. When hypoxia and hypoxic vasoconstriction become severe along with severe reduction in the cross-sectional area of the capillary bed, pulmonary hypertension develops. Pulmonary hypertension is associated with muscular hypertrophy and intimal changes of the pulmonary arteries. Pulmonary hypertension causes secondary changes in the right heart. Chronic hypoxia results in fixed pulmonary hypertension and cor pulmonale (Cherniack, 1991).

PHYSICAL EXAMINATION

In preparation for the physical exam, the older adult should be in a sitting position with the anterior and posterior chest exposed. The exam includes complete observation, palpation, percussion, and auscultation of the thorax and lungs. When auscultating the lungs of the older adult, begin at the base and progress to the apex, alternating from left to right. The patient is often limited in the amount of deep breathing he or she can do before tiring. The patient also uses accessory respiratory muscles and has a reduced diaphragmatic excursion. Older adults often exhibit diminished breath sounds and some chronic, mild adventitial sounds in their normal lung findings. Assure the patient that the gown sufficiently covers the body, so that he or she feels comfortable and not embarrassed. The nurse should make certain that the older patient's feelings regarding modesty and privacy are respected.

Because of the fragility of the older adult who develops respiratory problems, there is an increased vulnerability to mental status changes, thus evaluation of mental status should be a priority. Metabolic imbalance, hypoxia, and sensitivity to drug therapy are common causes of confusion in the older adult. Presence of a baseline cognitive deficit should be established on the first encounter with the older adult or on admission. If present, it should be documented. A delirium from hypoxia or metabolic imbalance should be suspected in the older adult with an acute respiratory problem who exhibits confusion.

 Clinical Pearl

Assessment: For the older adult who exhibits confusion, a mini mental status examination should be performed to evaluate the need for psychological referral.

DIAGNOSTIC TESTS

Radiologic studies, such as the chest x-ray and computerized tomography of the chest, demonstrate lung markings and heart size. Pulmonary function tests show the lung volumes and flow rates. Arterial blood gases show the amount of oxygen exchange and saturation by the blood. Other studies may include electrocardiogram, sputum evaluation, and a variety of blood tests, including a complete blood count.

The tuberculin skin test is the diagnostic measure used to identify persons infected with tuberculosis. The Centers for Disease Control and Prevention revised the standards for interpreting the skin test to include not only those who are infected but those who are at high risk of becoming infected and could benefit from preventive therapy (see Display 15-1). These new standards will help eliminate false-positive and false-negative results.

A sputum specimen for smear and culture for tuberculosis is the most reliable method to confirm active disease. If tuberculosis is suspected, the sputum is a difficult test to pursue with the older adult because of the inability to acquire a sputum specimen without an invasive procedure, such as bronchoscopy.

NURSING DIAGNOSES

Based on the history and physical findings, common nursing diagnoses associated with respiratory function in the older adult can be identified. These may include the following:

- Ineffective Breathing Pattern related to lower respiratory infection
- Ineffective Airway Clearance related to tenacious secretions and COPD
- Impaired Gas Exchange related to imbalance of ventilation perfusion mechanisms

Display 15-1
INTERPRETATION OF A POSITIVE TUBERCULIN SKIN TEST

1. An induration ≥ 5 mm in population who are likely to be infected with tuberculosis. This population includes:
   Recent close contact with tuberculosis
   Chest x-rays consistent with tuberculosis
   Immunosuppressed persons, especially human immunodeficiency virus–positive
2. An induration ≥ 10 mm (not in the above group) who have additional risk factors for development of tuberculosis. This population includes:
   Foreign-born persons from countries with high tuberculosis prevalence
   Intravenous drug users
   Homeless persons
   Nursing home residents
   Correctional institutional residents
   Person with other diseases associated with a high risk of tuberculosis
3. An induration ≥ 15 mm (not in the above groups). This population includes all others.

Adapted from Bass, J. B. (1990). Tuberculin test, preventive therapy and elimination of tuberculosis. *American Review of Respiratory Disease, 141*(4), 812–813.

- Impaired Physical Mobility related to decreased endurance and strength
- High Risk for Infection related to COPD, postsurgical condition
- Anxiety related to diagnosis of lung cancer

NURSING INTERVENTIONS

Nursing interventions focus on educating the older adult and the family about the disease process and the importance of compliance with drug therapy. Teaching may include the side effects of medications, techniques for manipulating mechanical bronchodilators, breathing exercises and coughing techniques to help clear airways, and helping patients cope with the long-term effects of chronic respiratory diseases and disability.

PATIENT AND FAMILY EDUCATION

Much of the nursing care related to respiratory problems involves patient education regarding the disease/disorder process and how it will affect the patient's functional abilities. The patient will need instruction in special precautions and prevention techniques, education on diet and medications and their side effects and what to do when side effects occur, and specific instruction in pulmonary toileting, which includes coughing and deep-breathing techniques.

The nurse must be knowledgeable about these disease processes and how they affect the physiologic and mental functioning of the older adult. The nurse must be alert for signs of more serious respiratory complications and often must educate the older adult to those signs as well. Hospitalized patients may need oxygen therapy or maintenance of patency of chest tubes or nasogastric tubes. A large portion of nursing care of the older adult with respiratory problems should include patient education on how to adequately live within the constraints of chronic disease.

DIET INSTRUCTIONS

Teaching the older adult about diet should include an assessment for signs and symptoms of malnutrition. Persons with respiratory problems often demonstrate excessive weight loss due to the following:

- Increased work of breathing requiring increased caloric intake to maintain weight
- A feeling of satiety with small amounts of food because of congestion of abdominal contents by the flattened diaphragm
- Dyspnea that interferes with eating
- Decreased appetite secondary to chronic sputum production
- Gastric irritation associated with bronchodilators and steroids

The older adult should be encouraged to eat more frequent, small meals and to select foods high in protein and calories with vitamin supplementation. Food supplements between meals, such as milk shakes, peanut butter or cheese crackers, fortified liquid drinks, creamed soups, nuts, and dried fruits, provide an excellent source of protein and calories.

Treatments for acute respiratory problems can include adequate hydration orally or intravenously to decrease tenacity of secretions and make them easier to expectorate, oxygen therapy to enhance breathing, bed rest, isolation, medication, and pulmonary rehabilitation to assist return to optimal function.

MEDICATION ADMINISTRATION

The major drug treatments for the older adult with respiratory problems include theophylline preparations, corticosteroids, antihistamines, isoproterenol, and cromolyn sodium. The major medications used for tuberculosis are rifampin, isoniazid, and ethambutol. Nurses should monitor specifically for gastric distress and liver and retinal toxicity. All of these drugs have significant toxic effects in older adults and must be monitored carefully. Many older adults experience toxicity when their dosages are within the range considered normal for adults.

Use of Inhalers. Inhaled bronchodilators are preferable to oral administration of medications for the older adult because of increased local efficiency, lower incidence of side effects, and more rapid onset of action. Many older adults have difficulty in using the inhaler-type medications because of reduced finger/hand dexterity, joint stiffness or arthritic hands, decreased sensation, or inability to read the fine print on instructions. Sometimes this can be overcome by using a pacer device such as a "rotohaler" or "dishaler," or changing to dry powder. These decrease aerosol deposition in the mouth and oropharynx and increase deposition in more peripheral airways (Dow & Holgate, 1990).

The accurate use of the metered-dose inhaler may include special adapters that can be placed on the apparatus to ease the use for the older adult with arthritic hands or fingers or peripheral neuropathy. For those with poor vision, step-by-step instruction with return demonstration can give the patient an increased sense of confidence in using the inhaler. Recent breath-activated metered-dose inhalers have been introduced, which assist in solving some of these problems of the older adult. The Patient Teaching Box explains the correct methods of use for the metered-dose inhalers.

Bronchodilators most commonly used are the inhaled beta$_2$-adrenoceptor agonists, such as salbutamol, terbutaline, and fenoterol. The therapeutic response occurs within a few minutes. The metered-dose inhaler is the preferred choice of therapy, because the medication action is local rather than systemic. This reduces the risk of systemic side effects, such as tremors, tachycardia, and hypokalemia. These side effects occur more frequently with use of nebulized or oral therapy due to the higher systemic circulating concentrations achieved. Nebulized therapy is reserved for acute problems or for older adults who cannot cope with metered-dose inhaler or dry powder devices or who did not respond to maintenance therapy. Inhaled corticosteroids are often prescribed as prophylactic agents in conjunction with inhaled bronchodilators. Commonly used steroids include beclomethasone, dipropionate, and betamethasone. Because steroids suppress the inflammatory response within the airways, this therapy is often used for older adults who require bronchodilators daily. Oral corticosteroids are prescribed when adequate control is not achieved with inhaled bronchodilators, corticosteroids, or oral bronchodilators (Dow & Holgate, 1990).

Older adults should rinse out the mouth and oropharynx with water after treatment to reduce the risk of oropharyngeal candidiasis, a side effect of corticosteroid therapy occurring in more than 10% of older adults. Because older adults may be taking multiple medications, Dow and Holgate (1990) suggested that all patients taking steroids should carry written information on the specific medication, dose, and how long treated. This information can be presented to any new care provider encountered to avoid adverse drug interactions when new medications are introduced, possibly preventing complications during acute illness or emotional stress when the older adult forgets or is unable to inform the care provider regarding all medications being taken.

Patient Teaching Box
INSTRUCTIONS FOR USING A METERED-DOSE INHALER

1. Shake inhaler to mix contents.
2. Inhale through nose, then slowly breathe out completely.
3. Hold unit 1 to 2 in. outside of open mouth (or use spacer device), and breathe out slowly and naturally.
4. Place mouthpiece in mouth.
5. Activate device by pressing down on inhaler while simultaneously inhaling slowly and deeply. Breathe in air from around the mouthpiece while inhaling.
6. Hold breath for 5 to 10 seconds.
7. Exhale through nose.
8. Rest at least 2 minutes (or according to manufacturer's instructions).
9. Repeat as ordered.
10. Rinse mouth with water and swallow.

Caution: Some asthmatic older adults may experience bronchoconstriction after using an inhaler. If you experience chest tightness after using an inhaler, you may be reacting to the propellant gases used to deliver the medication and should report this to your doctor or pharmacist immediately.

Anticholinergic agents, such as ipratropium bromide, are used mainly to inhibit vagal bronchospasm and as adjunct therapy in the treatment of airway disease. These drugs are less potent but can have a greater duration of bronchodilation than the inhaled beta$_2$-adrenoceptor agents with some patients. Many older adults can be relieved of airway obstruction with a prophylactic regimen, regular follow-up, and clear, concise education on the principles, techniques, and importance of compliance to therapy.

Mucolytic drugs decrease the viscosity and tenaciousness of mucus and facilitate mucociliary clearance. The oral iodide preparations affect airway disease through their anti-allergic and anti-inflammatory actions and through the stimulation of mucus secretions and ciliary action. Iodine provides action as an expectorant by stimulating the vagal gastropulmonary reflex. Guaifenesin is a commonly used expectorant that acts similarly to the iodides.

PREVENTION AND EARLY DETECTION

There are no cures for many of the respiratory diseases, but compliance and positive lifestyle changes can result in a longer, more comfortable life. Prevention is the strongest and most cost-effective approach to respiratory disease. The nurse can be instrumental in helping the older adult to adapt to the physical and emotional constraints of chronic pulmonary problems in tandem with a multidisciplinary team approach. Other members of the team may include the physician, respiratory therapist, exercise physiologist, social worker, and occupational therapist. The patient and family should be provided with respiratory-related health information, such as pollution indexes, techniques for avoiding exposure to a secondary infection, home humidification techniques, and community support groups. Leisure activities, food preferences, and lifestyle should be evaluated for problem areas. The patient and family should understand that a change in health status must be reported to the nurse or physician.

Prevention and early detection of tuberculosis are key elements of treatment, as is aggressive antibiotic therapy for treatment of persons already infected. Treatment for the disease generally includes drug therapy and rest. The Centers for Disease Control designed a strategic plan for eliminating tuberculosis in the United States that requires adequate therapy of all cases of active disease; prevention of new cases of tuberculosis by treating those who are currently infected but not diseased; and prevention of infection of persons who are not currently infected (Bass, 1990).

Older adults, many of whom live in institutional environments, are prime targets for infection. The nurse plays a key role in early detection and preventive measures. In institutions where large numbers of older adults are living together, such as nursing homes, nurses are responsible for surveillance to control the spread of tuberculosis (Display 15-2).

Older adults with chronic diseases are highly vulnerable to pneumonia. Severity increases with age. Prophylactic treatment for prevention is very important in the care of the older adult. Nursing interventions for pneumonia and influenza include education on vaccine immunization, appropriate diet, exercise, and a stress-reduced environment as adjunct therapy. Avoidance of large crowds during epidemics reduces the chances of contact with the causative agent. Important measures to implement include pulmonary toileting (deep-breathing exercises) on a regular basis to keep airways patent, frequent position changes when in bed, adequate hydration, and gradual resump-

Display 15-2

RECOMMENDED SURVEILLANCE TO CONTROL TUBERCULOSIS FOR INSTITUTIONALIZED OLDER ADULTS

The Centers for Disease Control and Prevention has developed specific guidelines to use to control tuberculosis.

Tuberculin skin testing (5 U) on all admissions, unless known to test positive.

Use of two-step method to identify reactors whose reaction has waned with time.

Testing all employed personnel.

Chest x-ray for all reactors.

Recording of all tests (negative and positive) in a standardized area of medical records for easy access of information.

Annual examination of all reactors (chest-x-ray or physical examination and/or sputum culture).

Resting all nonreactors whenever spread of tuberculosis is suspected and annually.

tion of physical activity, with emphasis on being out of bed as soon as possible. Concurrent with medical therapies, nursing care emphasizes the nutritional and hydration needs to maintain fluid balance and avoid nutritional deficiency. Bed rest increases the risk of decubiti, contractures, constipation, and depression. Nursing care should focus on all systems during the acute phase of treatment to prevent the long-term affects and disabilities that can develop quickly in the older adult.

Clinical Pearl

Intervention: Advise older adults, particularly those with respiratory problems, to avoid large crowds during infectious disease epidemics.

Aspiration pneumonia, one of the most common routes of pathogens to reach the lower respiratory tract in the older adult, is associated with conditions that compromise consciousness or cause dysphagia, such as stroke. Patients whose consciousness or gag reflexes are compromised are at high risk for aspiration pneumonia. If indicated, the older adult should be placed on aspiration precautions: elevate the head of the bed, check proper positioning of feeding tubes, and instruct patient not to eat during coughing episodes. Anyone coming in contact with the patient, including family, friends, and caregivers, should be made aware of the problem and interventions.

Nasal, gastrostomy, or jejunostomy tube feedings are often the selected nutritional therapy for older adults with swallowing problems, especially if complicated by the potential for malnutrition. Small-bore, weighted nasogastric tubes are associated with fewer respiratory infections, compared with the more commonly used large-bore, Levin-type feeding tubes. The reasons cited most frequently are greater patient comfort, less frequent tube displacement, and decreased risk of aspiration pneumonia. The older adult who is unable to manage fluids in the esophagus as a result of gastric reflux is managed with a jejunostomy feeding tube instead of the usual gastrostomy tube. Thus the stomach is bypassed to prevent aspiration pneumonia.

IMMUNIZATIONS

Older adults, especially those with chronic heart and lung disease, are at high risk of contacting influenza, which can be prevented or reduced in severity by immunization and chemoprophylaxis (American Thoracic Society, 1994). The pneumococcal vaccine is given once, with revaccination after 6 years only for older, very-high-risk persons. The influenza vaccine should be given annually to all older adults unless contraindicated. When the influenza vaccine is contraindicated, such as in patients with egg allergy or a prior reaction from the vaccine, amantadine can be used to decrease the risk of infection or to assist to ameliorate the disease process. It may be administered for up to 90 days in cases of repeated exposures. Older adults with immunosuppressive illness can benefit from both therapies—influenza vaccine and oral amantadine. When the older adult has been known to be exposed to influenza A, amantadine can be given and continued as a prophylactic measure.

OXYGEN THERAPY

Some older adults with severe disease may require supplemental individual-dose oxygen therapy to increase exercise tolerance, improve mental status, and reduce pulmonary and cardiac complications. Humidified oxygen is generally administered by nasal cannula or mask. Nasal cannula is best used if the patient requires therapy during meals. The nurse should teach the family and patient about how to clean the equipment as well as precautions against smoking in the household. Medicare reimburses for continuous oxygen therapy if blood gases demonstrate low oxygen saturation during exercise and sleep or evidence of cor pulmonale.

REHABILITATION PROGRAMS

The nurse should encourage participation in rehabilitation programs, because there are known benefits for the older adult with chronic lung problems despite the severity of disease. Knowledge of program location, both in the community and in the institution, can facilitate this participation. The success of the program depends on the patient and family's motivation and active involvement.

The basic premise of rehabilitation is to assist the older adult to reach the highest level of independence possible within the constraints of his or her disability. The challenge is to maintain the individuality and autonomy of the older adult during the rehabilitation process. Pulmonary rehabilitation programs should focus on the overall well-being of the patient, with emphasis on improving or restoring functioning within the patient's environment, improving quality of life, increasing exercise tolerance, encouraging more independence, increasing self-esteem, and reducing the need for hospitalization. Older adults who are not candidates include those with a psychiatric illness, with severe disease without pulmonary reserve, or with unstable heart disease. Pulmonary rehabilitation teams are multidisciplinary and include a respiratory therapist, physician, physical and occupational therapist, dietitian, pharmacist, psychologist or psychiatrist, and exercise physiologist.

Education will help the older adult to develop strategies to maintain patency and clearance of airways, avoid irritating environments, and establish breathing exercises that will increase or maintain respiratory endurance. Knowledge of appropriate diet, medication, and infection prevention are important components of educational programs on respiratory illness. Outcome measures used to evaluate rehabilitation programs include exercise endurance and increased duration of symptom-free periods.

Rehabilitation outcomes can be conflicting. Often the disease process appears unaltered, yet the human and social factors are demonstrated by an improved sense of well-being, comfort, and maintenance of functional independence. Outcomes can be compromised by other chronic disease conditions. These outcomes can dictate the amount of physical participation in which older adults can engage.

Nursing Care Plan

FOR OLDER ADULTS WITH RESPIRATORY PROBLEMS

Nursing Diagnosis: Ineffective Airway Clearance related to pulmonary congestion.

Definition: A state in which an individual is unable to clear secretions or obstructions from the respiratory tract to maintain airway patency.

Assessment Findings:
1. Abnormal breath sounds: rales, rhonchi, wheezes
2. Change in respiratory rate, depth
3. Cough with or without sputum production
4. Cyanosis
5. Dyspnea

Nursing Interventions with Selected Rationales:
1. Assess for changes from baseline in breath sounds, such as presence of rales, rhonchi, and wheezes.
   Rationale: Changes from baseline can indicate a deterioration in patient status. Frail elderly can decompensate quickly with an acute episodic respiratory problem.
2. Assess for signs of anxiety secondary to airway blockage or hypoxia.
   Rationale: Anxiety can further impair respiratory function.
3. Instruct patient and family in disease process and medication therapy.
   Rationale: Knowledge of the disease and medications improves compliance.
4. Assess for adverse effects of medications, such as tremors, tachycardia, and fatigue.
   Rationale: Prompt assessment can identify adverse effects quickly and allow for rapid interventions.

(continued)

Nursing Care Plan

FOR OLDER ADULTS WITH RESPIRATORY PROBLEMS *(Continued)*

5. Encourange coughing and deep breathing every 2 to 4 hours. Suction if necessary.
   Rationale: Coughing and deep breathing help to clear airways, and suctioning removes sputum that the patient is unable to expectorate.
6. Administer steroid therapy in combination with bronchodilators.
   Rationale: Steroid therapy suppresses inflammatory process within the airways allows for sputum production to be cleared, and decreases bronchospasm.

Desired Patient Outcomes/Discharge Criteria:

1. Older adult is able to raise sputum.
2. Sputum is clear and patient is afebrile.
3. Older adult is back to baseline functional and physical activity.
4. Older adult and family know the signs and symptoms to report to physician if they recur.
5. Older adult and family understand medication schedule and side effects.

REFERENCES

Abrass, I. B., Besdine, R. W., Butler, R. N., Rowe, J. W., & Solomon, D. H. (1990). *The Merck manual of geriatrics*. Rahway, NJ: Merck.

American Thoracic Society. (1990). Prevention of influenza and pneumonia. *American Review of Respiratory Disease, 142*(2), 487–488.

Bass, J. B. (1990). Tuberculin test, preventive therapy and elimination of tuberculosis. *American Review of Respiratory Disease, 141*(4), 812–813.

Cherniack, N. S. (1991). *Chronic obstructive pulmonary disease*. Philadelphia: W. B. Saunders.

Dow, L., & Holgate, S. T. (1990). Assessment and treatment of obstructive airway disease in the elderly. *British Medical Bulletin, 46*(1), 230–245.

Farzan, S. & Farzan, D. (1992). *A concise handbook of respiratory disease* (3rd ed.). New York: Appleton and Lange.

Schlossberg, D. (Ed.). (1988). *Tuberculosis* (2nd ed.). New York: Springer-Verlag.

BIBLIOGRAPHY

American Thoracic Society. (1962). Definitions and classifications of chronic bronchitis, asthma and pulmonary emphysema. *American Review of Respiratory Disease, 85*(5), 762.

Bass, J. B., Farrer, L. S., Hopewell, P. C., O'Brien, R., Jacobs, R. F., Rubin, F., Anider, D. E., & Thornton, G. (1994). Treatment of tuberculoses and tuberculosis infection in adults and children. American Thoracic Society and the Centers for Disease Control and Prevention. *American Journal of Respiratory and Critical Care Medicine, 149*(5), 1359–1374.

Blair, K. A. (1990). Aging: Physiological aspects and clinical implications. *Nurse Practitioner, 15*(2): 14–16, 18, 26–28.

Brown, R. B. (1993). Community-acquired pneumonia: Diagnosis and therapy of older adults. *Geriatrics, 48*(2), 43–50.

Cogen, R., Weinryb, J. N. (1988). Aspiration pneumonia in nursing home patients fed via gastrostomy tubes. *American Journal of Gastroenterology, 84*(12), 1509–1512.

Emery, C. F., Leatherman, N. E., Bueker, E. J., & McIntyre, N. R. (1991). Psychological outcomes of a pulmonary rehabilitation program. *Chest, 100*(3), 613–617.

Eubanks, D. H., & Bone, R. C. (1990). *Comprehensive respiratory care* (2nd ed.). St. Louis: Mosby.

Fink, G., Kaye, C., Sulkes, J., Gabbay, U., & Spitzer, S.A. (1994). Effects of theophylline on exercise performance in patients with severe chronic obstructive pulmonary disease. *Thorax, 49,* 332–334.

Gordon, M. (1991). *Nursing diagnosis: Process and application.* St Louis: Mosby–Year Book.

Griffith, D., & Idell, S. (1993). Approach to adult respiratory distress syndrome and respiratory failure in elderly patients. *Clinical Chest Medicine, 14*(3), 571–582.

Hazzard, W. R., Andres, R., Bierman, E., Blass, S. P. (1994). *Principles of geriatric medicine and gerontology* (3rd ed.). New York: McGraw-Hill.

Hurwicz, M., & Berkanovic, E. (1991). Care seeking for musculoskeletal and respiratory episodes in a Medicare population. *Medical Care, 29*(11), 1130–1145.

Johannsen, J. M. (1994). Chronic obstructive pulmonary disease: Current comprehensive care for emphysema and bronchitis. *Nurse Practitioner, 19*(1), 59–67.

Maas, M., Buckwalter, K., & Hardy, M. (1991). *Nursing diagnosis and interventions for the elderly.* Reading, MA: Addison-Wesley.

Marrie, T. J. (1993). Mycoplasma pneumonia requiring hospitalization, with emphasis on infection in the elderly. *Archives of Internal Medicine, 153*(4), 488–494.

Miller, C. A. (1995). *Nursing care of older adults: Theory and practice* (2nd ed.). Philadelphia: J.B. Lippincott.

Niederman, M. S., Clemente, P. H., Feinan, Feinsilver, S. H., Robinson, D. A. Ilowite, J. D., & Bernstein, M. G. (1991). Benefits of a multidisciplinary pulmonary rehabilitation program: Improvements are independent of lung function. *Chest, 99*(4), 798–804.

O'Donnell, D. E., Webb, K. A., & McGuire, M. A. (1993). Older patients with COPD: Benefits of exercise training. *Geriatrics, 48*(1), 59–62, 65–66.

Pfitzenmeyer, P., Brondel, L., d'Athis, P., Lacroix, S., Didier, J., & Gaudent, M. (1993). Lung function in advanced age: Study of ambulatory subjects aged over 75 years. *Gerontology, 35*(5), 257–275.

Ruben, F. L. (1993). Viral pneumonias: The increasing importance of a high index of suspicion. *Postgraduate Medicine,* 57–60, 63–64.

Schols, A. M. W. J., Mosteri, R., Soeters, P. B., & Wouters, E. S. (1991). Body composition and exercise performance in patients with chronic obstructive pulmonary disease. *Thorax, 46*(10), 695-699.

Schrier, R. W. (1990). *Geriatric medicine.* Philadelphia: W. B. Saunders.

Shapiro, I. (1990). *Clinical applications of respiratory care* (4th ed.). St. Louis: Mosby.

Stead, W. W., & Dutt, A. K. (1989). Tuberculosis in the elderly. *Seminars in Respiratory Infections, 4*(3), 189–197.

16

Problems With Tissue Oxygenation

Objectives

1. List some physiologic changes of aging related to tissue oxygenation.
2. Describe a typical assessment for an older adult with a problem with tissue oxygenation.
3. List nursing diagnoses appropriate for the older adult with problems with tissue oxygenation.
4. Identify nursing interventions for an older adult with problems with tissue oxygenation.
5. Develop a nursing care plan for a patient with altered tissue perfusion.

INTRODUCTION

THE OLDER ADULT MAY EXHIBIT PROBLEMS with tissue oxygenation caused by alteration in blood cell functioning, impaired venous return, and malignant disorders of the hematopoietic system. A reduction in oxygen-carrying capability because of decreased production or increased destruction of red blood cells, such as in anemias, affects tissue oxygenation. Many older adults experience problems with tissue oxygenation related to impaired venous return.

The older adult is at higher risk for developing malignant disorders of the hematopoietic system, such as chronic lymphocytic leukemia, polycythemia vera, and multiple myeloma. The incidence of these disorders peaks after 60 years of age. The problems with tissue oxygenation from chronic lymphocytic leukemia and multiple myeloma are a result of bone marrow failure. In polycythemia vera and secondary polycythemia, the abnormal increase in cells contributes to episodes of thrombosis, thereby interfering with tissue oxygenation.

Staab, AS and Hodges, LC: ESSENTIALS OF GERONTOLOGICAL NURSING,
© 1996 J. B. Lippincott Company

NORMAL PHYSIOLOGIC CHANGES

The basal rate of blood cell production does not seem to be altered by the aging process, however, there is a reduction in the capacity to respond to increased demand. During periods of stress, the older adult may present with alterations in tissue oxygenation because of an inability to respond to an increased demand for red blood cell production. The amount of space in the bone marrow occupied by blood cell tissue declines. Production of red blood cells is ineffective, and incorporation of iron into the red blood cells is impaired. Although there is a slight decrease in hemoglobin and hematocrit levels, hemoglobin levels less than 12 G/dL are considered below normal for both sexes.

In the older adult, there is a slight decrease in the number of platelets. The fibrinogen levels and factors V, VII, and VIII of coagulant activities demonstrate a mild increase. Major problems occurring with hemostasis result from an increased susceptibility of vessels to rupture and damaged endothelial surfaces because of aging. The erythrocyte sedimentation rate is increased. A higher range for fibrinogen and globulins occurs, while the range for albumin drops. Functional blood volume is reduced in response to decreased muscle mass and decreased metabolic rate. Hypoxia contributes to the reduced capacity to redistribute blood flow.

Changes associated with aging occur in the immune system. There is a decreased ability to respond to unfamiliar antigens because of the aging of the thymus gland. The decline in the functioning of the immune system results in an increased incidence of infection.

ABNORMAL PHYSIOLOGIC CHANGES

Problems with oxygenation are found when there is an increased hemoglobin concentration, possibly complicated by a chronic disease. Decreased red blood cell production, a disruption in venous circulation to the tissues, or a malignancy can result in abnormal changes in the older adult.

ANEMIAS

Inadequate iron results in iron deficiency anemia, characterized by a reduced hemoglobin concentration. Tissue hypoxia occurs because of inadequate oxygen delivery. Inadequate iron is available to form the heme component of hemoglobin.

Inadequate iron intake is rarely the cause of anemia. Insufficient protein intake, characterized by changes in serum albumin and transferrin levels, is strongly correlated with anemia (Lipschitz, 1994). These dietary inadequacies can be attributed to financial constraints of living on a fixed income, impaired mobility, and lack of transportation. These contribute to poor access to fresh foods and vegetables, lack of understanding of nutritional needs, impaired dentition, or disinterest in eating because of depression or living alone. The older adult can experience decreased iron absorption secondary to a subtotal gastrectomy or achlorhydria.

Problems with tissue oxygenation are often found with chronic diseases, such as inflammatory disorders, chronic renal disease, and malignancies.

Shortening of red blood cell life, changes in iron metabolism, and decreased production of red blood cells are seen. The most common chronic inflammatory state in which problems with oxygenation occur is rheumatoid arthritis. The chief problem in the chronic inflammatory state is a decreased compensatory bone marrow response. There is sufficient iron stored within the marrow, but its release from the reticuloendothelial cells is inhibited, resulting in low iron levels within the plasma.

In chronic renal disease, there is decreased red blood cell production because of an insufficient bone marrow response. This is thought to be related to sufficient erythropoietin production by the diseased kidney and/or low- and middle-molecular-weight substances that inhibit erythropoiesis. Hemolysis occurs, resulting in a shortened red blood cell life span. There is concomitant blood loss during dialysis and from frequent laboratory sampling. Depletion of iron stores from blood loss can be exacerbated by insufficient nutritional replacement. Additionally, there is fibrosis of the bone marrow in response to increased parathormone levels precipitated by the chronically low serum calcium levels.

Vitamin B_{12} Deficiency
A deficiency in vitamin B_{12} because of some interference with secretion of the intrinsic factor results in megaloblastic anemia. A megaloblast is a large, abnormal red blood cell with an easily destroyed cell membrane. Pernicious anemia usually results from malabsorption of vitamin B_{12}. Intrinsic factor is secreted by the gastric parietal cells and binds with vitamin B_{12}, promoting its absorption in the ileum. Without intrinsic factor, oral vitamin B_{12} cannot be absorbed. Because vitamin B_{12} is found in foods of animal origin, its deficiency, megaloblastic anemia, can be found in strict vegetarians.

Folic Acid Deficiency
A deficiency in folic acid also results in megaloblastic anemia. Impaired absorption of folate or inadequate dietary ingestion may result in folate deficiency. Folic acid is found in citrus fruits and green leafy vegetables. Chronic alcoholism and malabsorption syndromes impair folic acid absorption, producing folate deficiency.

VENOUS THROMBOSIS

Disruptions of circulation and tissue oxygenation can result from venous thrombosis. The obstruction in venous blood return leads to edema and impaired arterial blood flow with subsequent reduction in tissue oxygenation. Older adults have a higher incidence of thromboembolitic disease because they experience more disease states and conditions, such as hip fractures and stroke, in which deep vein thrombosis is a complication.

MALIGNANT DISORDERS

Advancing periods of malignant disorders are characterized by anemia and infections. Chronic lymphocytic leukemia, the most common leukemia found in older adults, is characterized by an increase in lymphocytes.

Multiple myeloma, most commonly seen in persons older than age 60, is a malignant disease resulting from proliferation of plasma cells. Anemia hypercalcemia and bone involvement are frequently present. Bone involvement often occurs, causing pathologic fractures in bone already weakened from osteoporosis.

Polycythemia vera, a myeloproliferative disorder seen primarily in the older adult, is characterized by increased numbers of erythrocytes, leukocytes, and platelets. It may be secondary to chronic anoxia, such as in older adult smokers with high carbon monoxide levels. There is an increase in blood viscosity and blood volume, resulting in the sludging of blood in tissues and organs. There is an increased incidence of thrombotic complications. The thrombosis produces problems with oxygenation.

PSYCHOSOCIAL ISSUES

One primary psychosocial change that occurs in the older adult with tissue oxygenation problems is confusion. Disorientation to time and place is an early sign of hypoxia. The older patient who is confused because of hypoxia may have difficulty following commands.

The older adult with activity intolerance related to inadequate oxygenation may become frustrated with the spacing of activities required to accomplish simple tasks. The patient may become frustrated and depressed. For the patient who must live with activity intolerance, a lifestyle adjustment may be needed. Those older adults who are diagnosed with chronic lymphocytic leukemia or multiple myeloma may experience grieving.

NURSING ASSESSMENT

Assessment of the older adult with problems of tissue oxygenation includes identifying several possible subjective symptoms, a thorough physical exam, and diagnostic studies.

HISTORY AND INTERVIEW

It is important to detect if the older patient is experiencing fatigue or weakness. Questions should focus on the patient's activity level and any changes that have occurred. These symptoms might be masked by a compensatory decrease in physical activity. The older adult may attribute a decrease in energy level to growing old. Family members, a good source of information, should be asked about any confusion that the patient may have exhibited. It must be ascertained if the patient has experienced syncope, dizziness, or falls. Questions about medical conditions and all medication taken, including prescribed and over-the-counter drugs, are significant. Gastrointestinal bleeding is the most common cause of iron deficiency anemia in the older adult. The nurse should ask the patient about using the following drugs: aspirin, alcohol, steroids, and nonsteroidal anti-inflammatory drugs.

The patient should be questioned about dietary intake, and the nurse should note if inadequate nutritional intake is involved. The older patient with vitamin B_{12} deficiency will present with many symptoms of iron deficiency anemia. The patient should be questioned about parasthesias of the extremities (abnormal sensations, such as numbness, burning, or pricking) or memory disturbances. Family members may identify mental changes ranging from depression and mood fluctuations to psychosis. The older patient with multiple myeloma often complains of back pain.

> *Clinical Pearl*
>
> *Assessment: Chronic constipation and a tendency to bundle up when others feel warm are often considered normal aging changes for the older adult. These complaints can also be signs of anemia.*

RISK FACTORS

A variety of factors have been identified that contribute to problems with tissue oxygenation. Iron deficiency anemia can be related to such factors as ulcers, esophageal varices, and colonic diverticula and tumors causing blood loss. Inadequate iron and protein intake also have been associated with iron deficiency anemia. Vegetarianism, surgeries such as total gastrectomy, and diseases of the terminal ileum have been associated with vitamin B_{12} deficiency. Chronic alcoholism, malabsorption syndromes, and certain drugs have been associated with folic acid deficiency. Any condition that promotes venous stasis, endothelial vessel damage, or hypercoagulability can predispose a patient to venous thrombosis and interfere with tissue oxygenation.

PHYSICAL EXAMINATION

During the physical examination, note if the patient presents with dyspnea. Vital signs should be monitored and any tachycardia should be noted. Conjunctivae and mucous membranes should be inspected for pallor. Nail beds should be inspected for concave malformations. A mild reduction of hemoglobin level in the older adult may exacerbate symptoms of existing disease. Some examples are an increase in anginal attacks or worsening of congestive heart failure. Symptoms would be manifested earlier than in a young adult because of the physiologic changes of aging. Muscle strength sensations and gait should be assessed. With vitamin B_{12} deficiency, muscle weakness and ataxia (incoordination of voluntary movements) may be present. Vibratory and proprioceptive sensations may be altered. Further assessment might reveal a yellow pall or and tongue atrophy with flattening of papillae. The older adult with folate deficiency presents with the same assessment findings as those with vitamin B_{12} deficiency without the neurologic deficits. If thrombophlebitis is suspected, neurovascular examinations of the extremities should be done. Patients may be asymptomatic but may complain of mild to moderate calf pain. The affected extremity should be palpated for an increase in skin temperature, swelling, and tenderness over the involved vein (groin or axilla). Dorsiflexion of the foot may elicit calf pain, called Homans' sign. Palpation of the calf muscle is more likely to elicit discomfort associated with deep vein thrombosis.

DIAGNOSTIC TESTS

For the older adult with possible iron or folate deficiency, the following laboratory studies may be ordered: hemoglobin, red blood cell count (indicates serum iron or folate levels), transferrin saturation, and total iron-binding capacity.

Venography, impedance plethysmography, and Doppler ultrasound are some of the diagnostic studies that may be performed on the older adult with possible thrombophlebitis. Partial thromboplastin times and prothrombin times will be used to monitor the effectiveness of anticoagulant therapy.

A Schilling test is frequently ordered for the older adult with possible pernicious anemia. The Schilling test, an indirect test of intrinsic factor deficiency, uses a 24-hour urine specimen to evaluate the ability to absorb vitamin B_{12} tagged with cobalt from the gastrointestinal tract. A fasting state of 12 hours is required (water is allowed). An oral dose of radioactive vitamin B_{12} is given. One hour later, an intramuscular injection of vitamin B_{12} is given to saturate the liver and serum binding sites. This allows any radioactive vitamin B_{12} absorbed from the gastrointestinal tract to be excreted in the urine. After the injection, the patient may eat and drink. The test requires a 24-hour urine specimen. A healthy person will absorb and excrete more than 8% of the administered radioactive vitamin B_{12}. In pernicious anemia, less than 8% will be excreted in the urine. If absorption of radioactive vitamin B_{12} is low, the test is repeated with the addition of an oral dose of intrinsic factor to rule out malabsorption problems. If there is then a rise in the excretion of radioactive vitamin B_{12}, then the problem is a lack of intrinsic factor, suggesting pernicious anemia. (Fischbach, 1992).

Diagnostic studies ordered for the older adult with a possible malignant disorder include a complete blood count and bone marrow aspiration. For the older patient with multiple myeloma, the following additional studies may be done: serum protein electrophoresis, immunoelectrophoresis, serum electrolytes, urinalysis, and bone x-ray.

NURSING DIAGNOSES

Many nursing diagnoses are appropriate for the older patient with oxygenation problems. Potential nursing diagnoses for the older adult include the following:

- Altered Nutrition: Less Than Body Requirements related to inadequate food/nutrient intake
- Altered Oral Mucous Membranes related to mucosal atrophy, stomatitis
- (High Risk for or Actual) Altered Peripheral Tissue Perfusion related to venous stasis, endothelial damage, and/or hypercoagulability
- High Risk for Activity Intolerance related to inadequate tissue oxygenation
- High Risk for Infection related to altered immune status secondary to disease process and/or chemotherapy
- High Risk for Altered Health Maintenance related to insufficient knowledge of disease management, anticoagulant therapy, chemotherapy, and/or radiation therapy
- Powerlessness related to inability to control disease progression/treatment
- Fatigue related to chronic decreased hemoglobin levels
- High Risk for Injury related to decreased cerebral tissue perfusion

NURSING INTERVENTIONS

The origins of the tissue oxygenation problems related to anemia in the older adult are primarily the result of gastrointestinal blood loss, insufficient protein intake, inadequate absorption, and the anemia of chronic diseases. Nursing interventions should be directed toward patient education regarding the origin and management of the anemia.

PATIENT AND FAMILY EDUCATION

The older adult with insufficient protein or iron intake needs dietary instruction on foods high in iron and/or protein. For example, heme iron contained in meats enhances the absorption of nonheme iron in other foods. Both should be combined in a meal. Vitamin C and citric acid increase the solubility of iron in the duodenum and should be included with the meal. It is particularly important for the vegetarian to include an excellent source of vitamin C with every meal. If iron supplements are ordered, inform the patient that the stool will turn black when taking ferrous sulfate. When possible, ferrous sulfate should be taken on an empty stomach, because taking it with food inhibits absorption. However, decreased absorption may be necessary to avoid gastric irritation. Warn the patient of the probability of constipation secondary to iron treatment and provide instructions for its management.

▷ Clinical Pearl

Intervention: Tannic acid, which is found in tea, inhibits absorption of nonheme iron (inorganic). Nurses should instruct patients with iron-deficiency anemia that tea should not be drunk with or shortly after meals to facilitate iron absorption.

For the older adult with folate deficiency, instruct him or her not to overcook vegetables, because this can destroy folic acid. Include vitamin C with foods high in folic acid, because it helps convert folic acid to its active form. Encourage the patient to eat raw vegetables and fruits.

For the older adult with oxygenation problems related to multiple myeloma, encourage the patient to participate in weight-bearing exercise to promote reabsorption of calcium. Warn the patient that assistance may be required during movement and ambulation because of the potential for pathologic fractures. Instruct the patient to drink plenty of fluids, because adequate hydration is essential to offset dangers of hypercalcemia and hyperuricemia. If nausea and vomiting are a problem, antiemetics may be necessary.

The increased incidence of thromboembolitic disease in older adults occurs because of the disease states that put them at risk for deep vein thrombosis. Education about risk factors, hydration, and activity can help prevent the development of deep vein thrombosis.

If the patient is receiving radiation therapy or medication therapy, such as anticoagulants or chemotherapy, specific instructions are needed to prevent further problems and maintain health (see the Patient Teaching Box).

ORAL HYGIENE MOUTH CARE

Special oral hygiene, such as for patients with stomatitis, includes flossing between teeth with waxed floss unless painful and using a soft toothbrush (further softened in hot water before brushing). Commercial mouthwashes containing alcohol should be avoided. If dentition is a problem, encourage the patient to see the dentist. If chemotherapy is used, thick saliva with a lowered Ph level often occurs. Rinsing the mouth with sodium bicarbonate and a saline mixture or hydrogen peroxide and saline or water will help alleviate the prob-

---

Patient Teaching Box
HEALTH MAINTENANCE

Follow these guidelines for health maintenance if you are receiving an anticoagulant, radiation, and/or chemotherapy:

• Use electric razors for shaving.
• Maintain skin integrity by avoiding injury and lubricating dry skin with lotions containing lanolin. Use caution in brushing teeth. Use a soft toothbrush.
• Avoid intake of aspirin, all nonsteroidal anti-inflammatory agents, and alcohol (acute abuse), which will enhance the effect of oral anticoagulants.
• Watch for petechiae (bruising) or bleeding and seek medical help.
• Keep all follow-up appointments for blood work. Blood work must be done to monitor the effects of oral anticoagulants.
• Wear a Medic-Alert bracelet or necklace.
• Avoid excessive intake of foods high in vitamin K, such as tomatoes; dark green, leafy vegetables; onions; bananas, and fish, because they will counteract oral anticoagulants.
• Maintain adequate hydration to facilitate maintenance of soft stool, integrity of mucous membranes, and adequate kidney function.
• Because of depressed immunity with radiation and chemotherapy, avoid crowds when there is a high incidence of upper respiratory infections; monitor temperature daily.
• Wash hands frequently to prevent infection.

---

lem. The lips should be kept moist and the mouth should be inspected for candida infections (pearly white patches). Mycostatin may be ordered to prevent and treat candida infections. A local analgesic (viscous lidocaine 2%) might be necessary 30 minutes before eating if oral pain interferes with intake. Maintenance of optimal nutritional status is important. Foods that are easy to swallow, not too dry, and will not traumatize painful areas of the mouth and gums should be eaten.

PAIN MANAGEMENT

Some older adults with oxygenation problems may experience pain related to their disease process. They should be encouraged to use prescribed pain control medication and evaluate its effectiveness. The older patient and the family should be involved in pain management techniques. Stress-management techniques, such as relaxation therapy, imagery, and medication are important adjunctive therapies in the management of pain. The use of distraction, such as conversation, reading, watching television, listening to radio, and playing games, is often helpful.

CONSULTATIONS AND REFERRALS

Consultations and referrals can be made when appropriate. Most older adults with problems with tissue oxygenation will need referral to a dietitian, social services, and a home health care worker. Specific referrals also may include the following:

• If the patient is an alcoholic, refer to Alcoholics Anonymous.
• If the patient has leukemia, refer to the Leukemia Society of America.
• If the patient has a malignancy, refer to the American Cancer Society.
• If nutritional intake is a problem, refer to Meals On Wheels.

Nursing Care Plan

FOR PATIENTS WITH TISSUE OXYGENATION PROBLEMS

Nursing Diagnosis: Altered Peripheral Tissue Perfusion related to venous stasis, endothelial damage, and/or hypercoagulability.

Definition: A state in which an individual experiences or is at risk of experiencing inadequate oxygenation and nutrition at the peripheral cellular level.

Assessment Findings:

1. Unilateral edema
2. Venous distension
3. Mild to moderate pain in calf or thigh
4. Calf pain or dorsiflexion of foot (Homans' sign)
5. Palpation of calf muscle elicits discomfort
6. Cyanosis

Nursing Interventions with Selected Rationales:

1. Educate patient and family about prevention of venous stasis.
   Rationale: Knowledge about preventive measures decreases the risk of problems developing.
2. Maintain adequate hydration.
   Rationale: Adequate hydration prevents fluid volume deficit.
3. Caution against prolonged sitting, standing, or lying in one position: encourage patient to elevate legs when sitting.
   Rationale: Circulation and venous return is enhanced by movement and elevation of lower extremities.
4. Warn patient not to cross legs at knees or ankles.
   Rationale: Crossing the legs interferes with venous return and promotes venous stasis.
5. Encourage the patient to walk several times a day; if ambulation is difficult, encourage passive or active leg exercises.
   Rationale: Exercise enchances circulation and promotes venous return.
6. Apply elastic stockings. Instruct patient not to wear restrictive clothing, such as tight shorts, pants, or girdles. Warn against wearing knee-high hose, thigh-high hose, or garters that have tight constrictive bands.
   Rationale: Elastic stockings provide graduated pressure, enhancing venous return. Restrictive garments interfere with venous return, promoting venous stasis.
7. If patient is on bed rest and at risk for thrombosis, elevate the foot of the bed on blocks.
   Rationale: Elevation of the foot of the bed encourages venous return.

Desired Patient Outcomes/Discharge Criteria:

1. Patient will identify risk factors for the development of thrombophlebitis.
2. Patient will identify necessary lifestyle changes.

REFERENCES

Bushnell, F. K. L. (1992). A guide to primary care of iron-deficiency anemia. *Nurse Practitioner,* *17,* 68-74.

Carpenito, L. J. (1993). *Handbook of nursing diagnosis.* Philadelphia: J. B. Lippincott.

Fischbach, F. T. (1992). *A manual of laboratory and diagnostic tests.* Philadelphia: J. B. Lippincott.

Fong, L. A. (1991). Balancing anticoagulant therapy. *Geriatric Nursing, 12*(1), 15–17.

Linker, C. A.(1994). Blood, In L. M. Tierney, S. J. McPhee, & M. A. Papadakis (Eds.), *Current medical diagnosis and treatment* (pp. 415–466). Norwalk, CT: Appleton & Lange.

Lipschitz, D. A. (1994). Anemia in the elderly. In W. R. Hazzard, R. Andres, E. L. Burman, & J. P. Blass (Eds.), *Principles of geriatric medicine and gerontology* (pp. 662–668). New York: McGraw-Hill.

Miller, C. A. (1993). Infections, resistant microbes, and older adults. *Geriatric Nursing, 14*(1), 55–56.

Miller, C. A. (1993). Update on warfarin: Special considerations for the elderly. *Geriatric Nursing, 14*(3), 167–168.

Scrimshaw, N. S. (1991). Iron deficiency. *Scientific American,265,* 46–52.

Snyder, C. S. (1990). Hematologic disorders. In A. S. Staab & M. F. Lyles (Eds.), *Manual of geriatric nursing* (pp. 357–388). Glenview, IL: Scott, Foresman Little Brown.

Strohl, R. A. (1992). The elderly patient receiving radiation therapy: Treatment sequelae and nursing care. *Geriatric Nursing, 13*(3), 153–156.

Yen, P. K. (1993). Nurses estimate elderly malnutrition. *Geriatric Nursing, 14*(6), 327–328.

Problems With Endocrine Function

Objectives

1. Describe the physiology of aging as it relates to target endocrine glands for diabetes, thyroid dysfunction, and osteoporosis.
2. Identify the abnormal changes associated with endocrine dysfunction.
3. Discuss the psychosocial changes associated with endocrine dysfunction.
4. Outline pertinent aspects of the history and physical assessment for a patient with diabetes, thyroid dysfunction, and osteoporosis.
5. Develop a nursing care plan and a teaching plan for the patient with diabetes, thyroid dysfunction, and osteoporosis.

INTRODUCTION

ENDOCRINE SYSTEM FUNCTIONING ARISES primarily from the hypothalamus, the pituitary gland, and the various target organs in which hormones are manufactured and controlled through feedback mechanisms. The major hormonal disturbances seen in the older adult are those associated with insulin production by the beta cells in the islets of Langerhans and its use in the body; the production of thyroid hormone by the thyroid gland and its metabolic clearance rate; and the loss of estrogen production by the ovaries. These hormone disturbances are manifested in commonly seen endocrine disorders in the older adult, such as diabetes mellitus, hyperthyroidism, hypothyroidism, and osteoporosis. These endocrine disturbances affect other body systems and can greatly affect the older person's quality of life. Often they disguise themselves as normal age-related changes or chronic diseases, making identification difficult. The signs and symptoms related to these problems are often different from those seen in the classic presentation in young and middle-age adults and often are not recognized until late in the disease course.

Staab, AS and Hodges, LC: ESSENTIALS OF GERONTOLOGICAL NURSING,
© 1996 J. B. Lippincott Company

The nurse plays a major role in helping to monitor for early detection and prevention and in providing information necessary to maintain a functional and productive lifestyle in older patients suffering from problems with endocrine function. Thorough nursing assessment and care planning can diminish the severity of these problems and enable the patient to make lifestyle adjustments necessary to preserve body function.

NORMAL PHYSIOLOGIC CHANGES

The basal metabolic rate may decline, and there may be diminished function of the pancreas and pituitary, thyroid, and adrenal glands. There is a progressive decrease in sensitivity to negative feedback control of hormones.

Compared with younger adults, the older adult has a reduced basal metabolic rate due to the decrease of muscle mass associated with aging. If the decrease of muscle mass is accounted for when calculating the basal metabolic rate, then the actual rate of metabolism is the same. Changes in the osmoregulatory center in the hypothalamus result in older adults having a diminished perception of thirst.

The pituitary gland exhibits little change with aging. Although there is progressively decreasing sensitivity of the hypothalamus and pituitary to negative feedback control, there are no actual changes in levels of corticotropin, growth hormone, thyrotropin, or basal or corticotropin-stimulated plasma cortisol. The adrenal cortex does experience alterations in responsiveness due to aging and also due to stress, such as from infections, trauma, or surgery (Staab & Lyles, 1990). There is a glandular decline in the gland's hormonal output.

There may be diminished function of the pancreas and the pituitary, thyroid, and adrenal glands. Reduced hormone production in other glands is also a normal result of aging. Cessation of estrogen and progesterone secretion by the ovaries causes the onset of menopause. Testosterone secretion declines slowly as the male ages. There is a decline in glucose tolerance, and the thyroid gland atrophies with age, causing reduced gland weight, follicular size, and colloid decrease with intrafollicular connective tissues increase. Age in itself does not affect serum levels of free thyroxine (T_4) or thyroid-stimulating hormone, although to balance normal reductions in basal metabolic rate, the older adult may experience a slight decline in thyroid-stimulating hormone production, T_4 synthesis, and thyroid activity. The metabolic clearance of thyroid hormone is decreased in the older adult, with normal feedback mechanisms preserving normal thyroid function.

There is a delayed and insufficient release of insulin from the beta cells of the pancreas in the older adult. In addition, there is believed to be a decreased sensitivity to cumulating insulin. The older adult's ability to metabolize glucose is reduced, and sudden concentrations of glucose cause higher and more prolonged hyperglycemia.

The aging process affects the body's ability to absorb calcium from the intestinal tract. Physiologically, the bones serve as the body's major storehouse of calcium. When the serum calcium level is too low, parathyroid hormone is secreted by the parathyroid gland, stimulating the release of calcium from the bones. Parathyroid hormone increases the removal of calcium from the body by stimulating osteoclastic bone resorption and increasing renal retention and intestinal absorption of calcium (Madison, 1989).

ABNORMAL PHYSIOLOGIC CHANGES

The most commonly seen abnormal physiologic changes that affect the older adult's endocrine function are those associated with the development of diabetes, hypothyroidism and hyperthyroidism, and osteoporosis.

DIABETES

It is estimated that 18.5% of the older adult population has diabetes, or almost one in every five people age 65 to 74 years. When impaired glucose tolerance is also considered, almost 40% of this age group has some impairment of glucose function (Harris, 1990). Most cases of diabetes in older adults are type II, or non–insulin dependent diabetes mellitus. This results primarily from insulin resistance rather than lack of insulin. The fasting glucose level increases due to a decrease in insulin production of the islets of Langerhans by about 6% per decade (Staab & Lyles, 1990). The major cause of increased glucose levels in older adults is peripheral insulin resistance, caused mainly by a postreceptor defect, although the actual number of insulin receptors may also be decreased (Morley & Kaiser, 1990). The beta cells in the islets are less sensitive to increased blood glucose levels, thus prolonging insulin release. Some older adults are unable to adequately inhibit glucose production in the liver. Aging has been associated with the deposition of amyloid, called amylin, in the islets of Langerhans. Amylin is released along with insulin from the pancreas, inhibits insulin-induced liver glycogenolysis, and blocks the effect of insulin on fat cells. Amylin probably plays a role in the cause of type II diabetes mellitus in older adults, along with other factors, such as obesity and decreased physical activity (Morley & Kaiser, 1990).

HYPOTHYROIDISM AND HYPERTHYROIDISM

Thyroid disorders, commonly seen in the older adult, are often signaled by changes in energy levels. Because the thyroid gland and its hormones regulate metabolic processes, many of the problems can be traced to alterations in thyroid function—either diminished (hypothyroidism) or elevated (hyperthyroidism) levels. Many of the signs and symptoms of hypothyroidism resemble those of the normal aging process and are therefore frequently missed. To prevent this, many clinicians advocate a yearly laboratory screening for thyroid function. Hyperthyroidism is more commonly being seen in the older adult population. Graves' disease is the most frequent cause of thyrotoxicosis in all age categories, but the number of cases of toxic multinodular goiter is also increasing (Cooper, 1990).

OSTEOPOROSIS

Osteoporosis, although not typically considered an endocrine disorder, is a major health problem associated with the reduction of estrogen production, along with changes associated with the effects of aging on bone. Osteoporosis is characterized by an excess of bone reabsorption over bone formation, leading to fractures resulting from minimal or no trauma. There are several types of osteoporosis, generally divided into primary osteoporosis and secondary osteoporosis. Primary osteoporosis consists of bone loss that results from the loss of estrogen at menopause and the aging process. Bone loss primarily occurs in the first 5 years after menopause.

Primary osteoporosis is categorized as type I or type II. Type I osteoporosis is postmenopausal and is therefore confined to women. Trabecular (cancellous) bone, found mostly in vertebrae, the pelvis, and other flat bones, is primarily affected, with commonly seen crush fractures of the vertebrae and Colles' fractures of the forearm. Type II osteoporosis is seen in both men and women and results in a loss of both trabecular and cortical (compact) bone. This condition is primarily found in the shafts of the long skeletal bones, with fractures including those of the proximal femur and vertebral wedge.

PSYCHOSOCIAL ISSUES

The psychosocial functioning of the patient may be affected by normal and abnormal changes related to endocrine function. Diabetes necessitates many lifestyle changes, such as changes in eating and other habits that have been acquired over many years. Depression is frequently seen in persons with thyroid disease, related to fatigue and changes in energy levels. In women, decreased estrogen levels reduces vaginal lubrication and may cause discomfort and sexual dysfunction. The pain associated with compression and other fractures resulting from osteoporosis can mean a significant change in functional status, which can lead to the onset of depression. Emotionally, the older patient must come to terms with changes involved with these problems and may require help with lifestyle adjustments.

NURSING ASSESSMENT FOR THE PERSON WITH DIABETES

The assessment of diabetes in the older adult is best accomplished with an in-depth history, physical assessment of various body systems, and diagnostic tests that principally involve the blood and urine.

HISTORY AND INTERVIEW

It is important to obtain a complete health history from an older patient who is suspected of being diabetic. Table 17-1 lists several questions the nurse can ask the patient, along with rationales. Although most of the significant information is presented in the history, physical assessment of the patient will elicit other clues.

PHYSICAL EXAMINATION

Blood pressure should be taken in both arms while the patient is lying, sitting, and standing. Because hypertension, common in patients with diabetes, can lead to myocardial infarction, stroke, and congestive heart failure, especially with elevated glucose levels, the traditional cardiac exam should be performed (Morley & Kaiser, 1990). The exam should include auscultation for bruits in the neck and estimation of heart size by either palpation of the point of maximal impulse in the apex or referral for a chest x-ray. All peripheral pulses

Table 17-1	**HISTORICAL INFORMATION TO BE OBTAINED FOR THE OLDER ADULT WITH DIABETES**

Question	Rationale
Are you feeling fatigued?	In hyperglycemia, insulin is not being used properly to get glucose into the cells to be converted to energy.
Have you lost weight recently?	Although the three cardinal symptoms of
Do you constantly feel hungry?	diabetes polyuria, polydipsia, and polyphagia are sometimes diminished in degree or not present, their presence should always be elicited.
Do you always feel thirsty?	Thirst may be a sign of dehydration signaling a passive hyperglycemic state and possible hyperosmolarity.
Have you had any numbness, pain, or tingling in the extremities?	These may signal peripheral neuropathy.
Do you have any family history of diabetes, especially in late life?	Diabetes tends to run in families.
Have you noticed any visual changes?	Increased blood sugar levels may cause blurring of vision.
Do you find yourself urinating frequently?	Urinary frequency may be due to osmotic diuresis of hyperglycemia (may be mistaken for a prostate problem, urinary tract infection, incontinence, or a consequence of diuretic therapy).
Have you had any seizures?	These may be a signal of hyperosmolarity due
Changes in your mental status?	to hyperglycemia.
Have you noticed any skin itching or new onset of a rash?	These may be secondary to uncontrolled diabetes.
Do you have any foot or skin ulcers?	Foot or skin ulcers frequently require more time for healing in persons with diabetes due to compromised circulation.
Do you wake up at night to urinate? If so, does it interfere with your sleep pattern?	Osmotic diuresis is caused by hyperglycemia.
Have you noticed that you fall more frequently?	Visual changes are associated with diabetes.
Do you have a history of high blood pressure?	Patients with diabetes often are at higher risk for cardiovascular problems.
Do you ever notice that your mouth is dry?	Dry mouth may be a symptom of hyperglycemia or impending hyperosmolarity.

should be checked, and temperature, color, and capillary refill time in the extremities should be noted.

Patients with diabetes are prone, with increasing longevity of the disease, to develop peripheral neuropathy, one of the leading complications of diabetes. Due to the insidious nature of the disease, many persons with type II diabetes already have neuropathy present when they are diagnosed. The neurologic exam should include testing for muscle strength, deep tendon reflexes, light touch, vibratory sensation, and position sense in the first and second toes. Inability to perceive 3-mm movements in the second toe suggests sensory loss (Riddle, 1990).

Ocular problems, such as glaucoma, cataracts, neuropathies, and transient refractive changes, tied to fluctuations in blood glucose levels, are more common in patients with diabetes than in the general population (Hector, Burton, & Lerner, 1987). Because appropriate assessment of the diabetic eye is difficult, a referral to an ophthalmologist for a yearly exam is appropriate. However, a visual acuity examination can easily be done by the nurse at least once yearly to screen for any new gross changes in vision. The most important task is to identify diabetes early in the older adult by being alert to symptoms and screening in suspicious cases. Existing retinal damage caused by uncontrolled hypertension can be prevented by regular blood pressure checks, with referral as necessary for treatment.

The patient's feet should be examined initially and at every office visit. The stockings or socks should be completely removed. Inspection of the feet should alert the nurse for lacerations, reddened areas, fungal infections, deformities such as diabetic claw toe, edema, and cracking. Other common foot problems are bunions, ingrown toenails, overgrown toenails, and corns and calluses. These older patients should be referred to a podiatrist. The dorsalis pedis and posterior tibial pulses are palpated bilaterally, and capillary refill time should be determined. The type of footwear the patient has on and whether proper socks or stockings are worn should be noted. Any abnormalities of gait should be noted, especially uneven weight-bearing, because these may aggravate foot problems.

Another area to be examined includes the genitourinary system. Symptoms such as vaginal itching, incontinence, or polyuria should be noted.

DIAGNOSTIC TESTS

The primary test in diabetes in the older adult is the plasma blood glucose test. The older patient may need to be referred for a test, but the nurse can do a fasting finger stick glucose sample. If the plasma glucose level is above 140 mg/dL after an overnight fast on at least two occasions, or if the 2-hour postprandial glucose level is above 200 on two occasions, this is considered diagnostic for diabetes. Glucose tolerance testing is rarely done in the older patient except to determine the exact renal threshold for glucosuria.

A dipstick analysis, which tests primarily for urinary red blood cells, proteinuria, and other potential causes of renal deterioration, should be performed. Serum blood urea nitrogen, creatinine, and electrolyte levels are important barometers of hydration status and renal function.

NURSING DIAGNOSES

Nursing diagnoses for the older adult with diabetes reflect the effect of the disease on multiple body systems and on the patient's lifestyle. Potential diagnoses for a patient with diabetes include the following:

- High Risk for Injury related to decreased tactile sensation, diminished visual acuity, and hypoglycemia

- Altered Comfort related to insulin injections, capillary blood glucose testing, and diabetic peripheral neuropathy
- Anxiety/Fear (individual, family) related to diagnosis of diabetes, potential complications, and self-care regimens
- Altered Nutrition: More Than Body Requirements related to intake in excess of need, lack of knowledge, and ineffective coping
- High Risk for Altered Health Maintenance related to insufficient knowledge of exchange diet, foot care, self-monitoring of blood glucose, and medications.

NURSING INTERVENTIONS

Diabetes in the older adult offers the nurse many opportunities for patient and family education, disease prevention through screening, and monitoring to prevent complications. Interventions in the older adult may be difficult because they may require alterations in long-standing lifestyle behaviors.

PATIENT AND FAMILY TEACHING

The principles of dietary modification, medication compliance, and exercise are all issues for which the patient will need to be responsible. The nursing concept of patient and/or family education enables the patient or caregiver to assume this task.

The nurse will need to explain diabetes, the relationship of blood glucose with the hormone insulin, diet, exercise, and the effects of illness or infection. The patient needs to know the symptoms of hyperglycemia and hypoglycemia and the time of the day this is most likely to occur, especially if on medication. The various target organs of diabetes should be reviewed, and the complications of diabetes, such as retinopathy, neuropathy, hypertension, peripheral vascular disease, and nephropathy, should be well understood by the patient.

Older people often have foot problems due to skin changes and decreased circulation. For those patients with diabetes, neuropathy is an insidious process and can indirectly lead to trauma or deformities of the foot from altered gait and infections. The Patient Teaching Box on foot care lists principles that should be reviewed with the patient or caregiver. For those patients with foot lesions or in need of routine foot care, a referral should be made to a podiatrist.

NUTRITION AND DIET THERAPY

There is considerable controversy over use of the strict dietary therapy for older adults with diabetes that is recommended for younger patients. The optimal diabetic diet for the older adult is one that is suitable for the patient's lifestyle and affords the best metabolic control. It is well known that there is a strong association between obesity and the onset of non–insulin dependent diabetes mellitus. Weight loss is generally the initial treatment for these patients, because even a moderate weight reduction may return the blood glucose level to within normal range. The physician or dietitian will prescribe the diet for the patient, hopefully taking into account the patient's food preferences, ethnic background, other medical problems, financial resources, and support system.

The nurse should be aware of the dietary plan given to the patient by the

Patient Teaching Box
FOOT CARE

- Visually inspect the feet and shoes daily.
- Wear footwear that provides adequate width; even weight distribution over sole of foot; a rounded, fairly high toe box; a removable padded insole with energy-absorbing properties; and soft uppers. Make sure the footwear is comfortable (Lypsky, Percoraro, & Ahroni, 1990).
- Wear nonconstricting hosiery (no knee-high hose).
- Dry feet thoroughly, especially between the toes.
- Cut toenails straight across; this should preferably be done by a medical professional.
- Moisturize skin, except between the toes, with an emollient.
- Wear cotton or wool socks daily.
- Avoid walking barefoot.
- Seek medical attention at the first signs of redness, swelling, infection, discomfort, or minor foot injuries.
- Wash hands before and after wound care, if any wounds are present.

physician or dietitian. Dietary instruction should emphasize keeping the diet simple yet flexible while incorporating changes slowly. The patient should understand the connection between diet and blood glucose levels. The patient and family should monitor weight closely. Teach the family that hypoglycemic episodes may stem from omission of meals and incorrect administration of insulin due to poor eyesight, poor coordination, and forgetting that a dose had been taken or a second dose had been administered. Instruct them to call the physician when experiencing an illness that makes the patient anorexic and decreases food intake. A home visit allows follow-up regarding menu suitability, meal preparation, and monitoring of actual intake.

BLOOD GLUCOSE MONITORING

Blood glucose monitoring is useful for all older adults with diabetes who are able to correctly learn the procedure. It helps the patient learn the relationship between diet, exercise, medication, and blood glucose level. The older patient with visual impairment may have difficulty reading the color indicators on the strip, but the digital numbers on the electronic meter can usually be read with ease. Medicare will help with payment for the meter and supplies if they are purchased during the course of a hospitalization.

Clinical Pearl

Assessment: When performing finger stick blood test, prick the finger with a lancet deeply enough so that little additional pressure is necessary to form a dropped sample. If in an effort to get the blood to drop, the finger is squeezed too much, there will be too much serum in the sample to obtain an accurate reading.

MEDICATION ADMINISTRATION

Because most older adults with diabetes have non–insulin dependent diabetes mellitus, some patients may have their blood glucose level adequately controlled by diet therapy alone. If the blood glucose is consistently above 250 mg/dL on dietary treatment, then medication, either oral hypoglycemics or insulin, is initiated. It is important to keep in mind that some older adults may have had diabetes for several years and are at high risk for developing end-organ complications. The medications used in diabetes—the sulfonureas and insulin—are generally used in this age group just as they are in the younger population. However, other factors, such as polypharmacy, malnutrition, and other chronic illnesses, must be considered, because these patients require careful supervision and are more sensitive to certain side effects (Peters & Davidson, 1990). Specific information regarding caring for the older adult who is taking oral sulfonurea medication is provided in Display 17-1.

Although most older patients with diabetes are non–insulin dependent, some patients whose blood glucose is not adequately controlled by oral agents may require insulin therapy. Most older patients can have their blood glucose level controlled by a single dose of an intermediate acting agent, such as NPH or lente, but some require more aggressive management. Insulin, usually regular, may be needed in acute situations such as infections and during and after surgery. Because the risks of hypoglycemia are greater in the elderly, the nurse must be vigilant in monitoring for symptoms. Those with altered sensorium, who may not be able to promptly recognize and get treatment for these symptoms, need special attention. Underlying cardiovascular disease, present in many older adults with diabetes, makes hypoglycemia potentially more dangerous. Uncontrolled hyperglycemia leads to dehydration and possible nonketotic hyperosmolar coma, which has significant mortality. Control of blood

---

Display 17-1

SULFONUREA: ORAL MEDICATIONS

Listed below is helpful information for the nurse caring for the older adult taking oral sulfonurea medication:

- Sulfonureas act only for patients who have some endogenous insulin secretion in the pancreas, because these drugs increase serum insulin levels.
- Strong evidence exists that these agents potentiate the action of insulin.
- Primary side effects are gastrointestinal (anorexia, heartburn, nausea, occastional vomiting, flatulence) and dermatologic. A reaction can be caused with ingestion of sulfonureas and alcohol, especially chlorpropamide.
- Anorexia and malnutrition, common in the elderly, can cause the hypoglycemic effect of these drugs to be accentuated.
- Alcohol, beta-blockers, coumadin, phenylbutazone, nonsteroidal anti-inflammatory agents, and sulfonamides can potentiate the effects of sulfonureas.
- Thiazides, furosemide, corticosteroids, phenytoin, beta-blockers, and alcohol can antagonize action.
- Chlorpropamide should not be used in the elderly because of its long half-life and duration of action.

glucose levels, which prevents symptoms of hyperglycemia, is thought to be sufficient treatment in the older adult population.

Some major points to consider in educating the older patient on insulin therapy are the type, dose, and action of the insulin ordered; proper injection technique and rotation of body sites; signs, symptoms, and management of hypoglycemia and hyperglycemia; and instructions on calling the physician if food intake is reduced or illness occurs. Many innovative products on the market can make it easier for the patient to self-administer insulin.

NURSING ASSESSMENT FOR THYROID PROBLEMS

Older adults experiencing thyroid dysfunction may present with few of the classic symptoms found in younger age groups. The nurse is in a key position to assess the patient for problems through carefully eliciting information in the health history, completing a physical examination, and reviewing pertinent laboratory findings.

HISTORY

When suspicions are raised about thyroid disease in the older adult, the nurse should be familiar with common symptoms found in this population. Table 17-2 lists the symptoms that the nurse should be alert for when gathering the older adult's history. It is important to be aware that the signs and symptoms associated with hypothyroidism resemble those of normal aging and that the symptoms of thyrotoxicosis in the older adult at times are masked. Those patients with masked or apathetic thyrotoxicosis present with depression, lethargy, weakness, and cachexia (Cooper, 1990). Patients who present with palpitations, worsening angina, symptoms of congestive heart failure, or atrial fibrillation should be referred to a physician for screening of thyroid disease. The

Table 17-2	SUBJECTIVE SYMPTOMS OF THYROID DYSFUNCTION	
	Hypothyroidism	Hyperthyroidism
	Decreased tolerance to cold	Agitation
	Lethargy	Confusion
	Constipation	Unexplained weight loss
	Fatigue	Nervousness
	Memory loss	Palpitations
	Decreased hearing	Tremulousness
	Loss of muscle, weakness	Anorexia
	Pain and stiffness in joints	Constipation
	Nasal stuffiness	Angina
		Increased cold tolerance
		Decreased heat tolerance

nurse should focus on questions about the onset, duration, and relief measures, if any.

PHYSICAL EXAMINATION

In examining the patient for thyroid dysfunction, the nurse should check several body systems. Table 17-3 outlines systems to examine and the possible findings in thyroid disease. It is important to note that in hyperthyroidism the classic sign of exophthalmos is present in less than 10% of older adults, but lid lag and lid retraction are seen in approximately one third of affected patients (Cooper, 1990). When examining the thyroid, note the size, shape, and consistency of the gland, and identify any nodules or tenderness. Nodules are found more commonly in older adults. If the thyroid gland is enlarged, listen over the lateral lobes to detect a bruit (Bates, 1987).

Table 17-3

OBJECTIVE SIGNS OFTEN SEEN ON ASSESSMENT OF THE OLDER ADULT WITH THYROID DISEASE

	Hypothyroidism	Hyperthyroidism
Vital Signs	Increased blood pressure Decreased body temperature Bradycardia	—
General	Pitting or nonpitting edema of the face and legs Prominent lips and nostrils Husky, weak voice	—
Weight	Gain Loss (if patient has decreased appetite)	—
Skin	Coarse, dry, thickened lifeless; dry hair	Warm, damp, fine, smooth
Eyes	Sparse eyebrows with loss of outer one-third margin	Exophthalmos, lid lag, lid retraction
Cardiovascular	Tachyarrhythmias may be present	Tachycardia or atrial fibrillation
Neurologic	Delayed recovery phase of deep tendon reflexes, especially ankle jerk, positional vertigo, cerebellar ataxia, gait disturbances, peripheral neuropathy on sensory exam	Tremors of tongue or hands
Lab data		
Thyroxine (T_4) or T_4 index	Low	Elevated
Thyroid-stimulating hormone	Elevated	—
Triiodothyromine	—	Elevated

> ### ▷ *Clinical Pearl*
>
> *Assessment: Although the assessment of the thyroid gland is important, the nurse must keep in mind that 20% to 30% of hyperthyroid older adults will have a gland that is nonpalpable, which makes laboratory data important in making the diagnosis.*

DIAGNOSTIC TESTS

Laboratory evaluation for thyroid disease can be more complicated in older patients. A low serum T_4 or free T_4 index with elevation of the serum thyroid-stimulating hormone is usually seen in hypothyroidism, but severe illness and the resultant recovery phase can impact on these values. The average patient with hyperthyroidism usually has an elevated T_4 level, free T_4 index, and tri-iodothyronine level. Radioactive iodine uptake tests may be ordered by the physician to confirm a suspected case. New ultrasensitive thyroid-stimulating hormone assays are now being used in borderline cases to help establish a diagnosis of hyperthyroidism.

NURSING DIAGNOSES

Once thyroid disease has been diagnosed and the patient is being treated, the nurse plays a major role in ensuring the compliance of the patient with treatment and monitoring for side effects of thyroid medications. Some nursing diagnoses that could apply to the older adult with a thyroid dysfunction include the following.

HYPOTHYROIDISM

- Altered Nutrition: More than body requirements related to intake greater than metabolic needs secondary to slow metabolic rate
- Constipation related to decreased peristalsis secondary to decreased metabolic rate and decreased physical activity
- Impaired Skin Integrity related to edema and dryness secondary to decreased metabolic rate and decreased physical activity
- Altered Comfort related to cold intolerance secondary to decreased metabolic rate.

HYPERTHYROIDISM

- Altered Nutrition: Less than body requirements related to intake less than metabolic needs secondary to excessive metabolic rate
- Activity Intolerance related to fatigue and exhaustion secondary to excessive metabolic rate
- Diarrhea related to increased peristalsis secondary to excessive metabolic rate
- Altered Comfort related to heat intolerance and profuse diaphoresis
- Activity Intolerance related to excessive thyroid hormone.

NURSING INTERVENTIONS

Thyroid dysfunction in the older adult offers the nurse opportunities to teach the patient and family appropriate drug therapy and monitoring techniques to prevent complications.

NUTRITION AND DIET THERAPY

The nurse must first evaluate the patient's diet to determine whether the patient is receiving the proper balance of food groups and calories. An eating plan that takes into consideration needs for weight gain or loss is devised and monitored by the nurse on a frequent basis. This is especially important with the patient who is receiving replacement thyroid hormone, because the patient's metabolic rate is likely to increase, thus increasing the need for additional calories. Patients who need increased calories may benefit from nutritional supplements as well as increased calories with food. The nurse may wish to consult a dietitian before selecting a supplement. Those patients with constipation should be encouraged to eat a high-fiber diet and drink adequate amounts of water, usually six to eight glasses daily. Following a regular toileting schedule for bowel evaluation can also be helpful.

COMFORT MEASURES

Older adults frequently have dry skin, as a result of the aging process and also of hypothyroidism. If the patient is edematous, frequent position changes are necessary to prevent sores from developing. The feet and legs should be elevated above the hip level when seated to facilitate lymphatic drainage and should be inspected frequently for signs of venous stasis, ulcers, and skin breakdown. Skin dryness can be alleviated by using emollients and drinking adequate fluids. For patients who are cold intolerant, the nurse can survey the home environment and assess the patient's resources for adequate clothing and warmth. Referrals may need to be made to social service agencies, who can assist older adults with inadequate housing, heating, or clothing. For hyperthyroid patients with heat intolerance and profuse sweating, the nurse can instruct the patient in using clothing made of natural fabric and taking frequent short baths in tepid water. Partial bathing followed by application of talcum or cornstarch can keep the patient feeling dry. A few patients may have exophthalmos, and the nurse must remind them to be diligent about applying lubricating drops or ointments, especially at night. An eye shield may be needed to keep the eyelids closed sufficiently.

MEDICATION ADMINISTRATION

Older adults with hypothyroidism will be taking replacement thyroid hormone. The nurse needs to provide information regarding the exact name of the thyroid preparation, dosage schedule, side effects, and purpose of the medications along with explaining the need for periodic laboratory testing for thyroid function, usually at least yearly. The physician adjusts the hormone level slowly to give the feedback mechanism time to respond appropriately and to avoid overstressing the cardiovascular system. If needed, the patient can be instructed on how to take his or her pulse and measure blood pressure. Hyperthyroid patients will need instruction about antithyroid medications, dosage and side effects, and the need for conscientious follow-up, because some patients develop symptoms of hypothyroidism.

NURSING ASSESSMENT FOR OSTEOPOROSIS

To appropriately assess the older adult for problems related to osteoporosis, a careful history, physical exam, and review of diagnostic tests results are necessary.

HISTORY

The patient may present with an initial complaint of severe pain at the site of involvement (usually the spine, hip, or wrist), which may occur after only minimal trauma or during everyday activities, such as making a bed. The nurse should ask the patient what was her maximum height, at what age menopause occurred, and whether it occurred naturally or was a result of an oophorectomy. The use of estrogen-replacement therapy and length of time treated should be ascertained. The nurse also needs to ask the patient about dietary calcium intake or calcium supplementation. Postmenopausal women need 1,500 mg of elemental calcium daily. Information about the use of vitamin D supplements or thiazide diuretics is also useful, because vitamin D facilitates calcium absorption from a small bowel, and thiazide diuretics can reduce urinary excretion of calcium.

RISK FACTORS

Risk factors associated with osteoporosis include advanced age, female sex, white race, thin frame, low bone mass, previous bone fracture, bilateral oophorectomy, chronic corticosteroid use, more than two alcoholic beverages per day, and dementia (Lindsay, 1989).

PHYSICAL EXAMINATION

In the physical assessment of the patient with osteoporosis, the areas that should be examined include height and back inspection. The patient's current height is measured, then height lost with aging is calculated. To calculate height loss, use the recall method of subtracting the current height from the patient's recall of maximum height or use the arm span method of subtracting current height from the arm span measurement. The back is inspected for kyphosis or kyphoscoliosis of the dorsal spine. Equal leg length is assessed by measuring the creases behind the knee to see if they meet or by inspecting the hips for unequal height. Wrists are assessed for pain with range of motion.

DIAGNOSTIC TESTS

Bone density testing allows the physician to make an unequivocal assessment of a patient's risk of osteoporosis. A relatively low-risk test called dual energy x-ray absorptiometry measures bone density and bone and bone mineral content in the peripheral and axial skeleton. The information received from the test is more precise than the older single-photon absorptiometry, which measures cortical bone in long bones, or dual-photon absorptiometry, which measures cortical and trabecular bone in the spine and hip. Quantitative computed tomography scans, which directly assess bone volume, provide separate analyses of bone mineral content and bone density in trabecular and cortical bone (Carr, Dawson-Hughes, & Ettinger, 1993). The nurse can explain these tests to the patient and their role in the determination of the diagnosis.

NURSING DIAGNOSES

Older patients with osteoporosis experience pain due to compression or other types of fractures and changes in mobility and body image. A few nursing diagnoses for the nurse to consider in these patients are as follows:

- Pain related to muscle spasm and fractures
- Altered Nutrition: Less Than Body Requirements related to inadequate dietary intake of calcium, protein, and vitamin D
- Impaired Physical Mobility related to limited range of motion secondary to skeletal changes
- Fear related to unpredictable nature of the condition.

NURSING INTERVENTIONS

The nurse plays a major role in the care of the older adult who has osteoporosis. Key among the interventions to be included in a plan of care are patient teaching, assistance in obtaining an appropriate and nutritious diet, and measures for prevention of the disease.

PATIENT AND FAMILY TEACHING

Osteoporosis, like diabetes, presents an excellent opportunity for the nurse to provide patient education for primary prevention. This can start many years before, especially for women beginning to experience menopause. The major areas to be covered in patient instruction include an explanation of the disease itself, pain management, dietary and/or supplementary calcium replacements, and safety measures, such as proper lifting and carrying techniques, to reduce the possibility of falling, and body mechanics for activities of daily living, such as housekeeping and hygiene. The older adult with osteoporosis may need a home safety evaluation to check for loose area rugs, stray cords, or need for assistive devices, such as bath benches or rails. Area rugs and stray cords should be removed. The nurse should also encourage the patient to do weight-bearing exercise, because it stimulates osteoblast function. Walking can be done by almost everyone and is less stressful on the joints, but other forms of exercise, such as bicycling, jogging, dancing, and tennis are also good weight-bearing activities. Swimming provides good exercise for those persons who may already have established disease.

NUTRITION AND DIET THERAPY

Women, especially postmenopausal women, need to obtain sufficient calcium for bone formation. Elemental calcium of 1,200 to 1,500 mg are needed daily by this group. Dietary sources include dairy products, especially milk and cheese, and leafy green vegetables. For those who are lactose intolerant or do not like milk or other dairy sources, supplements such as calcium tablets may be necessary. An assessment of the patient's current dietary intake of elemental calcium must be completed before recommending a supplement. Calcium supplements should be inexpensive, safe, and well tolerated. Some patients complain of flatulence, bloating, and constipation. Taking the supplement at bedtime promotes absorption and may lessen these side effects. Nurses should also counsel patients that excessive ingestion of protein and caffeine increases calcium excretion by the kidney, that cigarette smoking stimulates osteoclasts and deceases endogenous estrogen production, and that foods high in phosphorous, such as snack foods and sodas, may lead to calcium loss if consumed excessively.

PREVENTION

The key to improvement in the amount of pain and suffering caused by osteoporosis is prevention. Research is being done to find more therapies for prevention and treatment of this problem. Medications such as etidronate (Didronel), calcitonin (human) (Cibacalcin), and calcitonin (salmon) (Calcimar, Miacalcin) and low-dose estrogen replacement are being used to prevent osteoporosis, further deformity, and fracture. More and more people are becoming aware of this disease and are taking advantage of diet, exercise, and medication to prevent or stop further bone loss.

Nursing Care Plan

FOR THE PATIENT WITH HYPERTHYROIDISM

Nursing Diagnosis: Activity Intolerance, related to excessive thyroid hormone.

Definition: A reduction of one's physiologic capacity to endure activities to the degree desired or required because of an overproduction of thyroid hormone, usually due to Graves' disease or toxic single or multinodular goiter.

Assessment Findings:
1. Depression, lethargy, weakness, cachexia (masked hyperthyroidism)
2. Unexplained weight loss, nervousness, palpitations
3. Heat intolerance
4. Anorexia
5. Worsening angina
6. Possible atrial fibrillation
7. Possible exophthalmos

Nursing Interventions with Selected Rationale:
1. Provide patient education about disease process, treatment, and possible complications (hypothyroidism, atrial fibrillation).
   Rationale: Adequate knowledge helps promote compliance.
2. Instruct patient/caregiver about dosage and side effects of antithyroid medication.
   Rationale: Knowledge of drug therapy promotes compliance and ensures follow-up, should a problem arise.

(continued)

Nursing Care Plan

FOR THE PATIENT WITH HYPERTHYROIDISM *(Continued)*

3. Assess the patient's nutritional status and plan for additional intake if needed.
   Rationale: Adequate nutritional intake provides energy for activities.
4. Ensure periods of adequate rest for the patient.
   Rationale: Rest periods allow the patient to balance energy expenditures.
5. Teach patient to provide adequate eye lubrication, such as instillation of ointment if exophthalmos is present.
   Rationale: Lubrication prevents excessive drying.
6. Instruct pateint to wear clothing made of natural fabric, bathe for short periods in tepid water, and use cornstarch or talcum if heat intolerant.
   Rationale: Natural fabrics allow for heat evaporation, use of tepid water prevents additional overheating, and cornstarch and talcum absorb perspiration from heat intolerance and also promote a cool feeling and prevent irritation.

Patient Outcomes:

1. Patient rendered euthyroid.
2. Any atrial fibrillation that may develop is converted to normal sinus rhythm.
3. Patient/caregiver understands and complies with dosage, purpose, and side effects of therapy.
4. Patient does not experience any complications of the disease.

REFERENCES

Bates, B. (1987). *A guide to physical examination and history taking* (4th ed.). Philadelphia: J.B. Lippincott.

Carr, B. R., Dawson-Hughes, B., & Ettinger, B. (1993). A real world approach to osteoporosis. *Patient Care, 27*(8), 31–56.

Cooper, D. S. (1990). Thyroid disorders. In C. Cassel, D. Reisenberg, L. Sorensen, & J. Walsh. *Geriatric medicine* (2nd ed.) (pp. 239–255). New York: Springer-Verlag.

Gambert, S. R., & Escher, J. E. (1988). Atypical presentation of endocrine disorders in the elderly. *Geriatrics, 43*(7), 69–78.

Harris, M. I. (1990). Epidemiology of diabetes mellitus among the elderly in the United States. *Clinics in Geriatric Medicine, 6*(4), 703–719.

Hector, M., Burton, S., & Lerner, B. (1987). Diabetic retinopathy: Recommendations for primary care management. *Geriatrics, 42*(12), 51–60.

Lindsay, R. B. (1989). Osteoporosis: An updated approach to prevention and management. *Geriatrics, 44*(1), 45–54.

Lypsky, B. A., Percoraro, R. E., & Ahroni, J. H. (1990). Foot ulceration and infections in elderly diabetics. *Clinics in Geriatric Medicine, 6*(4), 747–769.

Madison, S. (1989). How to reduce the risk of postmenopausal osteoporosis. *Journal of Gerontological Nursing, 15*(9), 2–24.

Morley, J. E., & Kaiser, F. E. (1990). Unique aspects of diabetes mellitus in the elderly. *Clinics in Geriatric Medicine, 6*(4), 693–703.

Peters, A. L., & Davidson, M. B. (1990). Use of sulfonurea agents in older diabetic patients. *Clinics in Geriatric Medicine, 6*(4), 903–921.

Riddle, M. C. (1990). Diabetic neuropathies in the elderly: Management update. *Geriatrics, 45*(9), 32–36.

Staab, A. S., & Lyles, M. (1990). *Manual of geriatric nursing.* Glenview, IL: Scott, Foresman/Little, Brown.

BIBLIOGRAPHY

Bellantoni, M. F., & Blackman, M. R. (1988) Osteoporosis: Diagnostic screening and its place in current care. *Geriatrics, 43*(2), 63–70.

Carpenito, L. J. (1993). *Nursing diagnosis: Application to practice* (5th ed.). Philadelphia: Lippincott.

Cummings, S. R., Black, D. M., Devitt, M. C., et al. (1993). Bone density at various sites for prediction of hip fractures. *Lancet, 341*, 72–75.

Deahens, D. A. (1994). Teaching elderly patients about diabetes. *American Journal of Nursing, 94*(4), 39–44.

Gambert, S. R. (1985). Atypical presentation of thyroid disease in the elderly. *Geriatrics, 40*(2), 63–69.

Gambert, S. R. (1990). Atypical presentation of diabetes in the elderly. *Clinics in Geriatric Medicine, 6*(4), 721–729.

Kane, R. L., Ouslander, J. G., & Abrams, J. B. (1989). Decreased vitality. *Essentials of Clinical Geriatrics* (2nd ed.) (pp. 271–299).

Nathan, D. M. (1990). Insulin treatment in the elderly diabetic patient. *Clinics in Geriatric Medicine, 6*(4), 923–937.

Raisz, L. G. (1990). Osteoporosis. *Internal Medicine* (3rd ed.). Boston: Little, Brown.

Reed, A. T., & Birge, S. J. (1988). Screening for osteoporosis. *Journal of Gerontological Nursing, 14*(7), 37–38.

Storm, T., Thamsborg, G., Steiniche, T., Genant, H. K., & Sorensen, O. H. (1990). Effect of intermittent cyclical etidronate therapy on bone mass and fracture rate in women with postmenopausal osteoporosis. *New England Journal of Medicine, 322*(18), 1265–1271.

18

Problems With Continence

Objectives

1. Describe the physiologic changes associated with aging in bowel and bladder function.
2. Describe the psychosocial effect of urinary and fecal incontinence in the older adult.
3. List steps in the nursing assessment of an older adult with urinary and fecal incontinence.
4. Compare types of urinary and fetal incontinence.
5. Identify nursing diagnoses associated with urinary and fecal incontinence.
6. Design nursing interventions for the older adult with urinary and fecal incontinence.
7. Develop a nursing care plan for an older adult with urinary or fecal incontinence.

INTRODUCTION

INCONTINENCE, THE LOSS OF VOLUNTARY control over elimination, is never a normal consequence of aging, but rather a symptom of an underlying problem that should not be accepted as inevitable or irreversible. Yet millions of older people suffer from this physically, emotionally, and socially disruptive condition without seeking assistance from health care professionals. Without treatment, patients withdraw from social activities and often isolate themselves from family and friends.

Problems with incontinence can range from mild loss of bowel and/or bladder control to total incontinence. Most older adults do not report problems with maintaining continence, often accepting it as just another part of growing older. Other reasons cited include the embarrassing nature of the problem, frustration or fear that surgery may be indicated, lack of knowledge that treatment options exist, or, very often, a perceived lack of interest from health care professionals. Incontinence has been cited as the second leading cause of nursing home placement. The cost of incontinence care is astronomical and relates not only to supplies and laundry but also to nursing care time.

Recent conferences, including the 1988 National Institute of Health Consensus Conference on Urinary Incontinence and the Agency for Health Care Policy and Research 1992 Guidelines, drew much needed attention to urinary incontinence (National Institutes of Health, 1988; Agency for Health Care Policy and Research [AHCPR], 1992). Fecal incontinence, however, remains an area that is in need of increased attention by nurses. Incontinence problems consume a tremendous proportion of nursing resources at the bedside and are associated with a high degree of caregiver stress and frustration. Inadequate management of incontinence can lead to skin irritation, skin breakdown, and urinary tract infections.

No one is born continent. Continence, an acquired physiologic mechanism, is learned at varying ages during childhood through toilet training. Initially, infants rely on the sacral spinal reflex to control elimination. As the nervous system is more fully developed, the elimination reflexes come under voluntary control of the cortical control center. To remain continent, one must have an anatomically correct lower gastrointestinal and genitourinary tract, competent sphincteric mechanism (including adequate innervation and a coordinated reflex), adequate cognitive and physical functioning, motivation, and an appropriate environment for toileting. Remaining continent is taken for granted and toileting is done automatically and efficiently by most older adults.

NORMAL PHYSIOLOGIC CHANGES AFFECTING URINARY INCONTINENCE

Although aging alone does not cause incontinence, there are several age-related changes that my contribute to or make it more difficult to maintain bladder control.

Older adults often have a mild increase of residual urine, a slight decrease in bladder capacity, increased involuntary bladder contractions, and a decreased ability to postpone voiding. Although not well understood, there is also an increase in urine production and excretion at night. Decreased estrogen levels after menopause affect pelvic floor musculature and the sphincter support in women. This decrease in estrogen levels can cause atrophic vaginitis and urethritis, which affect continence. Childbearing may affect the pelvic supporting tissues secondary to perinatal trauma. Women are generally more susceptible to urinary tract infections due to the shortness of their urethra.

In aging men, the incidence of benign prostate enlargement increases the risk of incontinence. An enlarged prostate can press the urethra closed and result in decreased urine flow and/or obstruction. If patients have problems with chronic urinary retention or urinary tract infections, the detrusor muscle may become trabeculated or fibrotic, resulting in a less compliant bladder.

ABNORMAL PHYSIOLOGIC CHANGES AFFECTING URINARY INCONTINENCE

Urinary incontinence, simply defined as the involuntary loss of urine that is sufficient enough to be a problem (AHCPR, 1992), occurs more frequently than the loss of control over stool. Urinary incontinence affects more women than men, but is equally devastating to both. Commercial products allow urinary incontinence to be contained much easier than fecal incontinence and may contribute to lack of reporting.

Urinary incontinence is distinguished as either acute (transient) or persistent. Acute incontinence is of sudden onset, most often related to an acute illness, and subsides once the illness has been resolved. It is also associated with the use of medications, treatments, and other environmental factors. This type of incontinence is common in hospitalized older adults.

 ## Clinical Pearl

Intervention: Causes of acute incontinence can best be remembered by the acronym developed by Resnick (1990):

D	*Delirium, dehydration*
I	*Infection or symptomatic urinary tract infection*
A	*Atrophic vaginitis/urethritis*
P	*Pharmaceutical*
P	*Psychological, especially depression*
E	*Endocrine (hypercalcemia/hyperglycemia)*
R	*Restricted mobility, retention*
S	*Stool impaction*

The underlying causes for persistent incontinence may overlap several domains, including urologic, neurologic, functional/psychological, and iatrogenic/environmental factors. There are four basic types of persistent urinary incontinence that occur in the older adult: (1) urge incontinence, (2) stress incontinence, (3) overflow incontinence, and (4) functional incontinence.

Urge Incontinence. Urge incontinence is the sudden leakage of urine due to involuntary bladder contractions. Although the person senses a strong desire to void, he or she is still unable to hold urine long enough to reach the toilet.

Stress Incontinence. Stress incontinence is described as an involuntary leakage of urine associated with increased intra-abdominal pressure from activities such as lifting, coughing, sneezing, jumping, laughing, or bending. Stress incontinence occurs most frequently in women and is caused by inadequate urethral resistance. Often the anatomic support of the pelvic floor is weakened by perinatal trauma, generalized tissue weakening from aging and estrogen deficiency, pudendal nerve damage, or trauma from gynecologic or urologic surgery. Women who have had children often disregard this as normal urine leakage and an inevitable consequence of aging.

Overflow Incontinence. Overflow incontinence is the result of the bladder's inability to empty effectively, causing an overdistended bladder, which results in frequent, sometimes constant urine loss. The person is often unable to perceive a full bladder. Overflow incontinence is more common in men and may be caused by an atonic or underactive detrusor or an obstructive process. The detrusor may become underactive due to various neurologic conditions, diabetes, and medications that precipitate urinary retention. The urinary outflow can be obstructed by an anatomic obstruction, including prostatic hypertrophy, pelvic prolapse, strictures, tumors, or a neurogenic obstruction, such as with multiple sclerosis, suprasacral lesions, and detrusor–sphincter dyssynergia.

Functional Incontinence. Problems outside the urinary tract can affect continence. In functional incontinence, the lower urinary tract is intact, but continence is disrupted by immobility or cognitive impairment. Not all patients with cognitive impairment are incontinent, so it should not be expected or accepted. Potential causes and clinical clues for persistent incontinence are listed in Table 18-1.

PSYCHOSOCIAL ISSUES AFFECTING CONTINENCE

Both urinary and fecal incontinence carry tremendous psychosocial consequences. The fear of having an accident in a public setting is often strong enough to force older adults into social isolation. They frequently begin limiting fluid intake, urinating frequently, and avoiding activities that might cause urine loss. Unfortunately, this may lead to dehydration, constipation, irritable voiding patterns, and eventually interfere with social activities and relationships. Embarrassment, frustration, lowered self-esteem, and depression are very common among patients with incontinence. Many older adults view loss of bladder and bowel control as a sign of an impedance and therefore fear that their problem will be discovered. It is often identified as a key factor in the decision to seek nursing home placement. Family members and care providers feel helpless and inadvertently send the message that nothing can be done except conceal the leakage.

NURSING ASSESSMENT

The nursing assessment of urinary continence begins with the simple recognition that a problem exists. Unless the problem is of such severity that the person is requiring frequent clothing or linen changes, it is often unnoticed or easily concealed.

HISTORY AND INTERVIEW

A thorough history should begin with nonthreatening questions about normal bladder function and then proceed to targeted questions about incontinence. Asking the question in a nonthreatening, facilitative manner is essential for obtaining a good history. The question, "Do you have a problem with incontinence?" will get fewer responses than "Do you sometimes have to rush to the bathroom?" If you are asking specifically about incontinence, try rephrasing the question to, "Are there times when you can't make it to the bathroom without leaking urine?" Other questions include:

- Do you feel you go to the bathroom too often?
- Does this interfere with your lifestyle and things you enjoy doing?
- Are you using pads or protective devices?
- Do you wish you could hold your urine longer?

Voiding Symptoms. Once the patient has acknowledged having some degree of concern over bladder control, it is important to investigate specific

Table
18-1

TYPES OF PERSISTENT INCONTINENCE AND CLINICAL CLUES

Type	Causes	Clinical Clues

Urge (leakage of urine with a strong desire to void)	a. Detruser instability—Local irritating factors (not associated with neurologic impairment):
	    Infection
	    Stones
	    Tumor
	    Obstruction
	b. Detrusor hyperacitivity—CNS disorder (associated with neurologic impairment):
	    Cerebrovascular accident
	    Suprasacral spinal cord disease
	    Parkinson's disease
	    Dementia
	    Demyelinating disease
		Small bladder capacity
		Sense urge but unable to inhibit
		Moderate urine loss
		Urgency, frequency, nocturia
		Bladder irritants
		Positive urinalysis
		Increased blood glucose level

Stress (involuntary leakage of urine associated with increased intra-abdominal pressure)	a. Weakness/laxity of pelvic floor musculature b. Anatomic damage to urethral sphincter	Leakage associated with coughing, laughing, sneezing, jumping, or bending Usually daytime leakage only "Key in lock" syndrome Atrophic vaginitis Radical prostatectomy

Overflow (bladder's inability to empty effectively)	a. Bladder outlet obstruction:
	    Benign prostatic hypertrophy
	    Strictures
	    Tumors
	    Cystocele
	b. Underactive detrusor
	    Diabetes
	    Spinal cord disease
	c. Medication-induced retention
		Palpable bladder
		Enlarged prostate
		Poor/slow stream
		Hesitancy/straining
		Frequent/small voids
		Nocturia
		Periodic/continuous dribbling
		Difficult to catheterize
		Postvoiding residue > 100 mL

Functional (loss of control related to problems outside urinary tract)	a. Severe congnitive impairment
	b. Severe physical or mobility impairment
	c. Physical or chemical restraints
	d. Environmental barriers
	e. Psychosocial issues
	    Depression
	    Regression
	    Bipolar/Schizophrenia disorders
		Adequate urine volume and stream
		Functional frailty
		Toileting in inappropriate places
		Rule out obstruction, infection, etc.
		Voiding diary

Table 18-2	VOIDING SYMPTOMS	
	Symptom	Definition
	Urgency	Having to hurry to pass urine. Little warning before the need to toilet.
	Frequency	Numerous voids that may interfere with daily routine.
	Nocturia	Sensation to void awakens the person. Toilets frequently throughout the night. Try to distinguish between being awakened by the urge or simply toileting because he or she is awake.
	Hesitancy/straining	Delay in the ability to start the stream. Having to wait for the stream to start or expel urine.
	Slow stream	Force of stream is weakened or may be reported as divided/intermittent.
	Infrequent voids	Extended period of time between voids.
	Polyuria	Excessive volume of urine produced in a day.
	Dysuria	Pain with urination.
	Postvoid dribbling	Urine is expelled after voiding is complete. Generally a small amount of urine. May report incomplete emptying.

voiding symptoms. Specific voiding symptoms may help identify reversible factors contributing to incontinence and can lead to a thorough discussion of actual urine leakage. A very important question is, "Do you always sense the urge to go to the bathroom?" If patients fail to sense the urge, a more extensive neurologic evaluation is needed. Symptoms that should be investigated are listed in Table 18-2.

Normal urination can only be defined by the individual. In general, urinary frequency is often defined as toileting more than once every 2 hours. It is accepted that many older persons get up one to two times a night to void, presumably related to alterations in fluid elimination. If persons report getting up more than twice, sleep patterns will be interrupted, possibly interfering with daily functioning. Polyuria, generally accepted to be greater than 3 L per day, is often a sign of poorly controlled diabetes or is related to diuretic therapy.

Incontinence Symptoms. It is important to obtain an adequate description of the severity of the incontinence. Question the patient regarding the onset, duration, amount, and frequency of leakage. Attention should be paid to patterns of urine leakage, including nighttime and/or daytime accidents. In addition to determining the frequency or severity of voiding symptoms and actual accidents, it is important to look for circumstances around urine leakage. Persons may report urine leakage only when they laugh, cough, or sneeze. Others may report leakage associated with exercise or simply climbing stairs. Ask if the problem interferes with sexual relations. Lastly, many people report certain triggers that stimulate either the urge to urinate or actual urine leakage. Some commonly identified triggers are as follows:

- Unlocking the front door to their home
- Putting hands in cold water
- Hearing water run
- Noise from the shower
- Cold air from the refrigerator

Bowel Habits. Bowel functioning should always be questioned when evaluating patients with urinary incontinence. Does the patient have a long-standing history of constipation or chronic straining? Has he or she become laxative dependent? Does the individual have difficulty controlling defecation?

Voiding Diary. To thoroughly assess the nature of the incontinence, all patients should keep a voiding diary, which serves as an objective measure of the individual's bladder habits. If the patient is unable to keep a voiding diary, this record should be maintained by the care provider or the nursing staff. There are many different versions of voiding records that focus on frequency of voiding and/or accidents, amount or volume of urine expelled, and associated symptoms. Many include amount of fluid intake and documentation of bowel habits. Figure 18-1 shows an example of a voiding diary that is easy for patients to complete.

Fluid Intake. Patients frequently attempt to control accidents by decreasing daily fluid intake. Unfortunately, the risk of dehydration in older adults is great. Unless medical conditions prohibit, patients should strive for a minimum of 1500 mL a day. Inquire about the amounts and types of fluids consumed. It is helpful to have patients keep a record to identify actual intake. Note any relationship between intake of fluids in the late evening and nocturia. Determine the intake of potential bladder irritants. Caffeine, alcohol, citrus juices, and beverages with artificial sweeteners have been reported to cause irritable voiding symptoms.

Medical and Surgical Conditions Affecting Continence. Because acute and chronic medical conditions play a very important role in normal bladder function, all patients should be asked about any past genitourinary problems, including frequent urinary tract infections, pyelonephritis, kidney stones, hematuria, or any surgery or radiation to the pelvic cavity. Medical conditions to consider include diabetes, congestive heart failure, and numerous neurologic conditions. Bladder control is often affected in patients who have had a cerebrovascular accident, cognitive impairment, Parkinson's disease, or other neuromuscular disorders. Determine if the patient has had any surgical procedure or radiation therapy involving the spinal cord. In elderly women, inquire about gynecologic infections and problems, including those that may have been surgically corrected. Many women have undergone urethral dilatation procedures in an attempt to allow urine to flow more freely. Men should be asked about prostatic enlargement, prostatic surgery, urethral strictures, past urethral dilatations, and any history of sexually transmitted diseases.

Use of Containment Products. Question the individual about the type of containment products they have used to get an idea of the severity and frequency of incontinence. Products may include lightly absorbent pads, pant and pad systems, diapers, and external catheters (for men). Commercial containment products are costly. Be sensitive to other items that may be used to maintain dryness, such as washcloths or paper towels. Inquire about how of-

Voiding Record

Patient: _____

Day: _____

TIME:	Fluid intake # of glasses	Used urinal/ toilet If possible, indicate amount	Leaked urine "accident/wet" Indicate large or small amount	Reason or comments (see below)	Bowel movement Yes/No
6–8 AM					
8–10 AM					
10–12 N					
12–2 PM					
2–4 PM					
4–6 PM					
6–8 PM					
8–10 PM					
10–12 MN					
Nighttime voids					

*Reason: "accident on way to bathroom," occurred while coughing/laughing, opening the door, or describe "dribble vs. totally wet pants," or awakened wet.

Hickman, 1992

Figure 18-1. Sample voiding diary for patients.

ten the person changes pads during the day and night. Some patients may only change their pad when it becomes saturated versus mildly damp. Unless you ask specifics, you may overestimate or underestimate leakage.

Environmental Conditions. Environmental conditions may either hinder or assist an individual's ability to toilet. Are there adequate and accessible toilets and/or toilet substitutes? Can the person manipulate his or her walker to get in and out of the bathroom safely? Is the bathroom on a different level of the home, making access a problem? Does the height of the seat affect the individual's ability to get out of a chair or up from the toilet? In the hospital setting, are split side rails available to assist in getting out of bed? How far must the individual travel to get to the nearest bathroom? Will the wheelchair fit through the bathroom door? Is there adequate lighting and adaptive bathroom equipment, if needed? Can the person rise from the chair and/or toilet safely? If protective devices are used, are patients being provided access to a toilet?

Medical Conditions. Multiple disease states that occur more commonly in older adults, such as diabetes, heart failure, and stroke, can result in incontinence. In older adults who are normally continent, an exacerbation of an acute or chronic illness could cause incontinence. In addition, the use of an indwelling catheter during a prolonged hospitalization may interfere with bladder control after an illness has been treated.

MEDICATIONS

A number of medications affect normal urinary function, thus all patients should receive a thorough drug history. Table 18-3 lists medications and their potential effects on the bladder. If patients are on medications for a bladder control problem, have the medications helped? Many of the medications used to treat incontinence have difficult side effect profiles and should be closely monitored and reevaluated for efficacy.

PHYSICAL EXAMINATION

A performance-oriented functional assessment is important to evaluate for self-care deficits. Some patients will overestimate or underestimate their capabilities, making a performance-based assessment critical.

Cognitive and Psychological Status. When examining the older adult, determine if he or she desires to be continent. This can give you information about comprehension, motivation, and underlying depression or anger. Does he or she sense the urge to void? It often helps to ask the person to act out what he or she would do if he or she needed to use the bathroom. One could then identify how the individual would manage in an unfamiliar environment. This gives you insight into the cognitive level required to follow a multistage command.

Toileting Skills: Mobility, Transfer Ability, and Manual Dexterity. Always watch an older person ambulate. Determine if he or she is mobile, safe, and efficient. Can the person sit down and rise from a low seat, including the toilet seat? Watch the older adult undress and refasten clothing. How much time does it take? Are there modifications that could be made to clothing that would facilitate toileting?

Table 18-3

MEDICATIONS THAT CAN AFFECT CONTINENCE

Category	Potential Effects	Particular Medication
Diuretics	Increased urine volume (polyuria, frequency, nocturia)	Thiazides, furosemide
Sedatives/ hypnotics	Altered central nervous system— missed bladder cues dues to sedation	Lorazepam, furazepam, alprazolam, chloral hydrate
	Delirium	
	Bladder outlet relaxation	Triazolam, temazepam
Analgesics (narcotics)	Sedation	Codeine
	Bladder relaxation—urinary retention	Hydromorphone
		Meperidine
	Constipation/impaction	Morphine
Psychotropics: Antidepressants, neuroleptics	Altered central nervous system	Haloperidol
		Thioridazine
	Sedation	Thiothixene
	Rigidity/immobility	Amitriptyline
	Anticholinergic retention	Doxepin
		Imipramine
		Trazodone
Alpha-adrenergic blockers	Bladder outlet/urethral relaxation	Prazosin, terazosin
Alpha-adrenergic agonists	Increase urethral resistance	Ephedrine
	Retention	Phenylpropanolamine hydrochloride
		Pseudoephedrine
		Cold/flu remedies
Calcium channel blockers	Detrusor relaxation	Nifedipine
	Retention	Verapamil
Alcohol	Increase urine volume	Not applicable
	Altered central nervous system	
Anticholinergic agents	Detrusor relaxation	Propantheline bromide
	Retention	Diphenhydramine
	Constipation/impaction	Cold preparations

Physical Examination: Abdomen, Male and Female Genitourinary. Examine the abdomen for tenderness, masses, or bladder distension. Note any surgical scars. Check the perineal area for hygiene and intact sensation. If qualified, do a rectal exam to determine if constipation, impaction, or a rectal mass is affecting bladder control. When doing the rectal examination on men, palpate the prostate for any enlargement or pain that might indicate benign prostatic hypertrophy or infection. The absence of an enlarged prostate does not exclude an obstructive process. Any weakness or impairment noted with the anal sphincter should be reported.

For women, a vaginal examination by a qualified practitioner allows evaluation of the mucosa, urethral meatus, and rugal folds to ensure adequate estrogen stimulation. Extreme vaginal dryness or atrophic vaginitis is an important clinical finding. Have the patient bear down to check for pelvic floor laxity, which might include finding a cystocele, urethrocele, and/or rectocele. To evaluate the strength of pelvic muscles and teach pelvic muscle exercises, have the patient tighten her muscles around the examining finger. It may also be helpful to have the patient cough to determine urine leakage with increased intra-abdominal pressure.

DIAGNOSTIC STUDIES

To appropriately diagnose impaired bladder functioning, a number of tests may be ordered. When retention is suspected, a postvoid residual is performed to assess bladder emptying and determine the amount of urine left in the bladder after the patient has completed voluntary voiding. It is important to catheterize patients within 15 minutes of voiding. Always document the volume voided before the residual urine was obtained. Be certain that the patient is not severely constipated or impacted, because this may cause an elevated residual, not truly indicative of bladder functioning. A hand-held bladder scan is available for noninvasive determination of residual urine.

All patients with urinary incontinence, especially those with new onset incontinence, should have a urinalysis and a urine culture and sensitivity test. A urine dipstick test may be used to detect bacteriuria. Nitrite-positive urine indicates a high index of suspicion for bacteria in the urine. This quick test is less reliable if the patient is being actively diuresed or is dehydrated as evidenced by a high specific gravity. The presence of blood in the urine (hematuria) and glucose (glycosuria) are equally important to assess.

Depending on the clinical presentation and type of incontinence expected, various formal urodynamic tests may be ordered. If hematuria is present, patients may be sent for a cystoscopy to evaluate potential bladder disease (Table 18-4).

NURSING DIAGNOSES

After assessing for urinary incontinence and before planning for care, the nurse must determine the nursing diagnosis. The following is a listing of selected nursing diagnoses based on a patient with persistent urinary incontinence:

- Urinary Retention related to chronically overfilled bladder with loss of sensation of bladder distension, in neurogenic bladder
- Urge Incontinence related to disruption of inhibitory efferent impulses secondary to brain or spinal cord dysfunction
- Reflex Incontinence related to absence of sensation to void and loss of ability to inhibit bladder contraction
- Functional Incontinence related to inability or difficulty in reaching toilet secondary to decreased mobility or motivation

Table 18-4

URODYNAMIC TESTS FOR INCONTINENCE

Test	Explanation	Indication
Cystometrogram	Filling the bladder with air/water to determine bladder capacity, bladder compliance, presence of involuntary detrusor contractions, intravesical pressures, and intact sensation	Urge
Uroflow	Measurement of urine flow rate. Identifies abnormal voiding patterns	Overflow
Electromyography	Use of electrodes to determine the ability of the striated urethral sphincter to contract and relax.	Stress, urge
Urethral pressure profile	Measurement of resting and dynamic pressure along the urethra. Function of urethral sphincteric mechanism	Stress
Voiding cystourethrography	Evaluation of the bladder and urethra for proper position/angle, diverticulum, obstruction, and reflux	Stress, urge, overflow
Ultrasound	Identification of upper urinary tract dilatation and renal disease, such as hydronephrosis	Overflow
Intravenous pyelography	Invasive evaluation for upper urinary tract disease	Overflow

- Stress Incontinence related to pelvic floor muscle relaxation
- Total Incontinence related to motor and sensory losses
- Body Image Disturbance related to embarrassment and frustration with urine leakage
- Toileting Self-Care Deficit related to functional limitations

NURSING INTERVENTIONS

Interventions for acute urinary incontinence are aimed at the underlying problem that precipitated loss of bladder control. If patients have an active urinary tract infection, an attempt is made to eradicate the bacteria. When delirium or other major medical issues affect continence, it is appropriate to use containment measures (external/indwelling catheters or absorptive products) until the underlying medical problem has been resolved. If the patient has a low threshold for maintaining continence, it may take longer to regain bladder control. Do not accept that incontinence will be persistent. If for some reason difficulty does continue, initiate an aggressive evaluation and treatment plan.

PATIENT AND FAMILY EDUCATION

Before starting interventions for persistent incontinence, it is very important to set goals acceptable to the patient, because what is viewed as success by the patient may differ from that of the nurse. Interventions may be targeted to:

- Decrease the number of incontinent episodes
- Increase the ability to delay voiding
- Decrease nighttime voiding
- Decrease the volume of the accidents
- Resume social or physical activity
- Decrease size of absorptive product
- Feel more secure delaying the urge to void

Patient and family education are critical components of any continence promotion program. In general, the least invasive therapy is supported. Intervention options include behavioral approaches, medications, surgical intervention, and containment or management options.

Behavioral approaches to treating urinary incontinence are based on the principle that continence is a learned response to a physiologic mechanism. Behavioral approaches offer the advantage of being noninvasive and having no side effects. Treatment does require motivation and commitment of both the caregiver/staff and the patient. Hospitalization does not eliminate initiating behavioral therapies. If intervention is not possible, educate the individual that treatment is available and provide for follow-up. Because there are individuals in all settings with a range of functional capabilities and/or limitations, the treatment approach can either be patient driven or caregiver driven.

Pelvic Muscle Reeducation. Pelvic muscle exercises are a learned technique of paravaginal muscle contraction and a form of relaxation termed "pelvic muscle reeducation" (Wells, 1990). The muscles supporting urethral resistance can be improved through active exercise of the pubococcygeal muscle, thereby strengthening the outlet resistance and improving urine control. It is important to realize that Kegel exercises are not new to many individuals. They may state, "I've tried that before and it didn't work." Educate the patient that most individuals do not use the correct muscle and do not practice the exercises under a scheduled, well-monitored program. Pelvic floor muscle exercises do work if done correctly and routinely (Patient Teaching Box).

After patients are able to identify the appropriate muscle, it is very important to integrate the exercises into the daily routine. Lack of motivation and compliance with an exercise program are the primary reasons cited for failure. Instruct patients to consider doing the exercises while reading in bed, watching television, brushing their teeth, standing in the shower, or riding in the car. Remind them that no one can see them doing their exercises. Pelvic muscle exercises may be indicated for patients with urge, stress, and mixed incontinence.

Urge Suppression. Urge control involves teaching patients the best time to void. Rushing to the toilet can actually stimulate bladder contractions, increase intra-abdominal pressure, and increase the awareness of fullness. Individuals must be highly motivated to begin to accept that the brain does have control over the bladder.

The goal is to wait for a calm bladder state before toileting. Until individuals gain confidence with urge suppression, it is best to practice this at home. A voiding diary is critical to monitor progress. It may also be useful to begin by using this technique for certain urge triggers. As skill develops, it will become second nature to inhibit voiding. Urge suppression is primarily used for patients with urge incontinence. Provide patients with the specific individualized instructions on strategies to control the urge (Patient Teaching Box).

Patient Teaching Box
KEGAL EXERCISES

Use the following tips to help you to identify the appropriate muscle when performing the Kegal exercises.

Finding the right muscle:
• Stop the stream of urine.
• Tighten the muscle used to hold back gas/bowel movement.
• The sensation is one of "pulling in and up."
• Men: The penis should rise if doing this correctly.
• Do not use your stomach, legs, or buttock muscles.

Practicing the exercise:
• Tighten/squeeze this muscle and hold for a count of 10.
• Relax the muscle for a count of 10.
• Gradually you will be able to hold for a count of 10.
• Alternate doing the exercise lying, sitting, and standing.
• Avoid interruptions.
• Concentrate on the exercise.

Daily routine:
• Do exercises in three sessions each day
• Each session should consist of 15 exercises.
• Contract the muscle for 10 seconds and relax for 10.
• Repeat this 15 times to complete one session.

Initially, you will most likely be unable to sustain the contraction for 10 seconds, but with consistent practice it will happen. Be determined, as it may take 4 to 6 weeks for you to actually see any results.

Patient Teaching Box
METHODS FOR CONTROLLING URGENCY

Instructions for controlling urgency:

If the urge occurs and it has been less than _____ hours* from the last time you toileted, stop, stand still, and relax.
• Squeeze the pelvic floor muscle.
• Use relaxation, imagery, or diversional activities accompanied by slow deep breathing.
• Do not rush to the bathroom. This will increase the urgency and jiggle the bladder, making control more difficult.
• Tighten the pelvic floor muscle. This will help decrease the urge signal to void.
• Concentrate and you can make the urge go away. Tell yourself you can control your bladder.

After the urge subsides, wait _____ minutes.*

Take three slow, deep breaths, contract the pelvic floor muscle, and then walk slowly to the bathroom, whether or not you feel you need to go. The next urge will be much stronger and more difficult to control.

*Individualized based on voiding diary.

Biofeedback. Biofeedback, first introduced as an intervention modality for incontinence in 1948 by Kegel, uses highly sensitive probes, either vaginal or rectal, or surface electrodes, to measure the strength of the pelvic floor musculature. Visual and/or auditory feedback, regarding the periurethral muscle contraction, is provided to the individual as a form of reinforcement. This training technique is used to teach patients how to localize the pelvic muscles, increase the strength and duration of the contraction, and monitor ongoing progress. It has been shown to be an effective behavioral therapy for urge incontinence, female stress incontinence, postprostatectomy incontinence, and mixed incontinence.

Stimulation. Electrical stimulation is an intervention modality that can be used with pelvic muscle reeducation and biofeedback. A vaginal or rectal probe is used to deliver a faint electrical stimulus to assist in improving muscle tonus. The stimulus causes the muscle to contract, thereby improving the strength. This can be used to help persons identify the appropriate muscle group in addition to providing for passive exercise. The goal is to either increase the resistance of the pelvic floor or block uninhibited bladder contractions. Compact, in-home stimulators have been developed for private home use. Stimulation has been found helpful in patients with urge, stress, and mixed incontinence.

Toileting (Voiding) Schedules. Voiding schedules ranging from highly individualized treatment programs to basic staff-dependent toileting schedules are a very important intervention for treating persistent urinary incontinence. Bladder training, or bladder reeducation, can only be attempted in patients with adequate cognition and a fair degree of functional independence (Fantl et al., 1991; Hadley, 1986; Wyman & Fantu, 1991). The goal is to restore normal voiding patterns using urge-suppression techniques. Support and ongoing monitoring are essential to success. See Table 18-5 for an explanation of each voiding schedule. Voiding schedules are an essential part of treatment for patients with urge, stress, and functional incontinence.

MEDICATION THERAPY

The basic objective of introducing medications is to increase bladder capacity, increase urethral resistance and/or decrease uninhibited bladder contractions. Medications frequently used in urinary incontinence are listed in Table 18-6. Ensure that you avoid medications that can be making urine leakage worse, such as anticholinergic medications in patients with overflow incontinence.

DEVICES

Numerous new devices are available to assist women in managing stress incontinence. Weighted vaginal cones are available to provide assistance in pelvic muscle reeducation. These cones are thought to provide heightened proprioceptive feedback to the desired pelvic muscle contraction. Pessaries, a device similar to a diaphragm, may be fitted to help stabilize the bladder base and provide support to a relaxed pelvic floor. Pessaries and vaginal weights/ cones are useful in stress and mixed incontinence.

Men have used external penile clamps for many years to prevent leakage of urine. With new active treatments available, it is recommended that all other

Table 18-5

TOILETING SCHEDULES FOR URINARY INCONTINENCE

Toileting Program	Description	Goal	Indication
Bladder training	Scheduled voidings with progressive lengthening between voids Usually start with a prescribed interval that may be less than every 2 hours Controlling-the-urge strategies are used	Correct irregular voiding pattern Increase ability to inhibit contractions Urge suppression Increase intervals between voids Increase bladder capacity	Urge Stress Mixed
Habit training	Scheduled voidings based on voiding diary May increase/decrease interval based on voiding pattern	Void/toilet before accident occurs Void regardless of urge Does not work on urge suppression	Urge Mixed Functional
Timed/ scheduled voiding	Fixed voiding schedule Intervals between voids do not change	Increase opportunity for toileting Staff schedule	Urge Functional
Prompted voiding	Fixed toileting schedule that uses reinforcement techniques Able to monitor success with toileting and decide whether patients should be toileted or placed on a check-and-change protocol	Increase opportunity for toileting; staff schedule Reward when dry and for positive response/void when toileted Determine percentage of appropriate toileting	Functional
Patterned-urge response toileting	Scheduled voidings based on voiding pattern Use of a special electronic device to detect incontinent episodes and identify schedule	Increase opportunity for staff to toilet patient Staff schedule to keep patient dry	Urge Functional

options be exhausted before relying on a mechanical device. The commercially designed products usually provide more safety features than homemade devices used to constrict outflow of urine. However, any device that clamps off the urethra and surrounding tissues raises the risk of skin breakdown and actual penile necrosis. If the leakage of urine is so severe as to consider use of a penile clamp, the option of a surgically created artificial sphincter should be explored.

Table 18-6

MEDICATIONS USED TO TREAT INCONTINENCE

Category	Action	Specific Medications	Side Effects
Bladder relaxants	Decreases detrusor smooth muscle activity	Anticholinergic/antispasmodic • Oxybutynin (Ditropan) • Flavoxate (Urispas) • Propantheine (Pro-Banthine) Tricyclic antidepressant • Imipramine (Tofranil)	Retention Constipation Hypotension Delirium Increased intraocular pressure
Bladder stimulants	Stimulates smooth muscle in bladder	Cholinergic • Bethanechol (Urecholine)	Cardiac stimulation
Sphincter relaxants	Relaxes bladder outlet	Alpha-adrenergic blockers • Prazosin (Minipress) • Terazosin (Hytrin)	Hypotension Dizziness Drowsiness
Sphincter stimulants	Increases urethral resistance by acting on the smooth muscle of the internal sphincter	Alpha-adrenergic agonists • Pseudoephedrine (Sudafed) • Phenylpropanolamine (Ornade) Tricyclic antidepressant • Imipramine (Tofranil)	Cardiac stimulation Dizziness Headache Nausea Insomnia
Other	Improves periurethral tissues (strength and blood flow)	Conjugated estrogen • Premarin (oral/topical)	Endometrial Cancer Hypertension

SURGICAL INTERVENTIONS

There are several surgical options that should be considered if less invasive treatment strategies prove unsuccessful. For women with stress incontinence, surgical procedures aim to improve the angle or tighten the support at the bladder outlet. Frequently referred to as bladder neck suspension procedures, they are performed to raise the descended bladder and decrease hypermobility. Various artificial sphincters are available but are associated with a high rate of infection and erosion. For overflow incontinence, surgeries are prescribed for relieving the obstruction or widening the outlet. For men, a transurethral resection of the prostate is often indicated to allow free flow of urine out of the bladder. Chronic urine flow against an obstructed outlet results in trabeculation and scarring of the bladder wall, in essence, a less compliant bladder. Surgery may be indicated for repair of cystocele, rectocele, and urethrocele. A thorough evaluation is essential before any surgical approach is considered. Numerous risks are involved with any surgical approach, and many patients may still have problems with incontinence after the surgery.

ABSORPTIVE PRODUCTS

It is important that proper attention be paid to adequate diagnosis and treatment of the urinary incontinence before concluding that product management is necessary. Caution should be used when using various protective devices during a treatment program. Patients may become overdependent on the product and more reluctant to try behavioral interventions. Absorptive products should be viewed as a management strategy as opposed to a treatment strategy. The number of products available is rapidly increasing. These products should be tested for comfort, amount of liquid contained, and cost. Options range from reusable or disposable sanitary shields, to underpads, pant/pad systems, and diapers. A new drip-collector pouch is available for men who have a small amount of leakage. Nurses are key in helping patients select the most beneficial and cost-effective products.

CATHETERS

Indwelling catheters should be used with extreme caution in older adults and only rarely as an option for managing urinary incontinence. Most patients who have indwelling catheters have bacteriuria by the end of 30 days, with or without antibiotics (Warren, 1990). Often, male external catheters are used, however, these devices carry the risk of skin breakdown, penile necrosis, and bacteriuria. Little progress has been made in the development of external collection devices for women.

NORMAL PHYSIOLOGIC CHANGES AFFECTING FECAL INCONTINENCE

The relationship between the effect of aging on maintaining fecal continence is not well defined. It is generally accepted that older persons have slower peristalsis, decreased muscle tone, decreased resting anal sphincter tone, and less compliant rectums.

Smaller volumes of stool in the rectum inhibit the tone of the anal sphincter (Bannister, Abouzekry, & Read, 1987). Sphincter pressure decreases, presumably due to age-related changes in muscle mass and contractility. Elderly women may also have decreased maximal sphincter squeeze pressures. (McHugh & Diamant, 1987). Repeatedly ignoring the urge to defecate results in bulkier, harder, more difficult to pass stool. Excessive straining over time results in relaxation of the pelvic floor. Weakened anorectal muscles may actually protrude through the anus, resulting in a rectocele. Any of these variables that impair anorectal muscle function automatically decrease the support from the anorectal angle and decrease control of the external anal sphincter.

Although these mechanisms account for the physiologic aspects of continence, factors outside of the gastrointestinal tract affect bowel control. Functional impairments that contribute to fecal incontinence also affect bowel control, especially if abnormal bowel function is present. Decreased exercise or activity, even if just during an acute illness, affects normal bowel function. Environmental issues, such as lack of accessible toilets or toilet substitutes, will cause patients to postpone defecation. Bedpans do not allow for normal positioning and therefore may result in incomplete evacuation. Lack of privacy, especially relevant to hospitalized elderly, causes many patients to neglect normal bowel routines.

ABNORMAL PHYSIOLOGIC CHANGES AFFECTING FECAL CONTINENCE

Abnormal changes with aging result in fecal incontinence. Fecal incontinence may range from mild fecal seeping to total loss of control. Accidents may be formed stool or loose, watery stool.

Fecal incontinence—involuntary loss of stool from the rectum at inappropriate times—is extremely devastating to the patient and/or care providers. Fecal incontinence occurs in 10% to 25% of the hospitalized population and in up to 60% of persons in nursing homes (Abrams & Berkow, 1990; Wald, 1990). It is important to note that patients with fecal incontinence often report urinary incontinence as well. When working with patients who have both bowel and bladder control problems, it is best to address bowel problems first. Helping patients become continent of stool is much easier than helping them gain control over bladder function.

Gastrointestinal conditions affect bowel function and include diarrheal illnesses, chronic constipation, diverticular disease, rectal or colon cancer, inflammatory bowel disease, and bowel obstruction. Various medical problems, such as diabetes, stroke, and multiple neurologic disorders, may impair voluntary control over bowel elimination.

Fecal incontinence is very often multifactorial. Persons may report an acute episode of fecal incontinence versus a more persistent pattern of fecal soiling or actual bowel leakage. Fecal incontinence may be associated with impaired anorectal function, overflow, sphincter overload, neurologic diseases, or functional limitations in compromised individuals.

Impaired Anorectal Function. The supporting muscles of the pelvic floor, which support storage and emptying of fecal matter, are critical to maintenance of continence. The sphincteric support can be jeopardized by denervation, localized inflammation, or actual trauma. Denervation often results in an atrophied external sphincter or pelvic floor muscle, associated with chronic laxative abuse, straining to defecate, rectal prolapse, or pudendal nerve damage secondary to previous vaginal deliveries.

Overflow Incontinence. Overflow bowel incontinence is most often the result of fecal stasis or fecal impaction. If the stool at the entrance to the anal canal becomes excessively hardened, liquid stool may seep around the impacted stool. The resultant overflow leakage is often mistaken for diarrhea, and antidiarrheal agents are inappropriately prescribed. Stool may become hardened from inadequate dietary fiber, dehydration, medications, inactivity, repeatedly postponing defecation, and various bowel disorders. Rectal tumors or diverticula can serve as an anatomic obstruction to the passage of stool. Excessive laxative use results in a cathartic colon that fluctuates from constipation to diarrhea and makes treatment strategies more complex.

Clinical Pearl

Assessment: Fecal incontinence in institutionalized, impaired older adults is most commonly due to fecal impaction.

Sphincter Overload. Inflammatory bowel conditions may overload normally competent sphincteric support. Stool is propulsed rapidly through the gastrointestinal system, affecting fluid and electrolyte exchange and absorption. Stool is usually liquid or very loose from the inability of the bowel to absorb adequate water from the fecal content. The ability of the rectal canal to serve as a reservoir is impaired. Examples of these include an acute diarrheal illness.

Malabsorption disorders or diarrhea may be associated with diabetes. Numerous medications may cause diarrhea, particularly antibiotic therapy. This often occurs in patients who normally would be continent, but bowel inflammation decreases the ability to delay defecating and may impair the mechanism to signal the need to pass stool. Patients who have fecal incontinence from diarrhea should be monitored closely for dehydration or electrolyte disturbance. In compromised patients, this incontinence could result in delirium.

Neurologic Disorders. Disorders or injuries involving the spinal cord or central nervous system may impair normal bowel control. The location of the spinal cord lesion determines the extent of the damage. In general, the lower the lesion, the more impaired bowel control will be. Neurologic disorders impair the ability to interpret toileting needs, voluntarily control the external sphincter, or affect the sensation of rectal filling.

Functional Incontinence. Patients may have an intact gastrointestinal system but be unable to interpret the urge to defecate and/or find an appropriate place to toilet. Patients with functional incontinence generally pass formed stool at an inappropriate time or place. These patients require close nursing attention to bowel habits and a structured bowel management program to ensure they are toileted. Table 18-7 provides a classification of types of fecal incontinence, common causes, and clinical cues.

PSYCHOSOCIAL ISSUES

Social incontinence carries tremendous psychosocial consequences. Issues are similar to those for patients experiencing urinary incontinence (see page 278 for more information).

NURSING ASSESSMENT

Fecal incontinence should be aggressively evaluated in all patients, regardless of age or functional status. The nursing assessment of fecal incontinence involves a thorough evaluation of many conditions affecting the gastrointestinal system. In addition, because incontinence is often multifactorial, cognitive and functional status are essential components of the comprehensive assessment. Defecation is naturally a very personal bodily function, and therefore the assessment should be done in a setting that respects privacy.

Table 18-7	TYPES OF FECAL INCONTINENCE: COMMON CAUSES AND CLINICAL CLUES		
	Type	Common Causes	Clinical Clues
	Overflow	Fecal stasis or impaction Medications Rectal tumor, diverticula	Constipation Abdominal tenderness Impaction Diarrhea (leakage of stool) Fever Decreased appetite

	Impaired anorectal function	Trauma/denervation injury
		  Pelvic fracture
		  Anorectal surgery
		  Obstetric surgery
		  Excessive straining
		Anal sphincter disease
		Rectal prolapse
		Chronic straining to stool
			Loss of rectal tone
			Loss of anal reflex

	Sphincter overload:
	  Diarrhea
		Inflammatory process
		  Inflammatory bowel disease
		  Diarrheal states
		  Radiation enteritis
		Medication induced
			Frequent loose stools
			Urgency
			Normal rectal/sphincter tone and function

	Neurogenic	Central nervous system
		  Cerebrovascular accident (CVA)
		  Trauma
		  Tumor
		  Spinal
		  Multiple sclerosis
		  Tumor
		  Trauma
		  Peripheral nervous system
		  Diabetes
			Neurogenic bowel
			Reflex defecation
			Impaired perineal motor and sensory findings

	Functional	Central nervous system
		  CVA
		  Trauma
		  Tumor
		  Dementia
			Formed stool at inappropriate times/places
			Impaired cognitive or physical function

HISTORY AND INTERVIEW

A thorough assessment involves an extensive history of bowel functioning. Bowel habits are established early in life, and unfortunately, if these habits are poor, they often lead to problems with defecation later. Ask the following questions to discover the older person's usual routine for bowel elimination:

- How frequently do you move your bowels?
- Do you use the bathroom in the morning after breakfast or late in the evening?
- Do you use any natural bowel stimulants, such as warm coffee or foods?
- Do you always sense the urge to defecate, and if so, can you routinely make it go away?
- What do you consider a normal or desired frequency?
- Do you frequently postpone defecation, and if so, for how long?
- Do you feel pain with passing bowel movements?
- Are any of your medications affecting your bowel function?
- Have you noticed any recent changes in bowel habits, including blood or mucus in the stool?

It is very important to distinguish between real and perceived constipation. "Regularity" may indicate a bowel movement every day or less frequently. At what point would the patient feel constipated? How many days pass after the last bowel movement before the patient considers a laxative? Constipation may mean infrequent stools or very hard stools. Does the patient strain to move the bowels? Has the patient taken laxatives or ever required an enema? Is the patient currently using any laxatives, either over the counter or from the health care provider? Does the patient have any home remedies that work for constipation?

Stool Characteristics. Obtain information about the onset, frequency, volume, and the consistency of the stool as well as use of absorptive products. The following questions should be asked:

- Do you loose small amounts, sudden large volumes, or continuously ooze?
- Do you have the urge to defecate or does leakage occur without warning?
- How long after you get the urge are you able to delay toileting before stool will leak out?
- Are you able to hold back gas?
- Do certain situations make leakage more likely, such as exercise, coughing, stress, or medications?
- What type of foods trigger bowel accidents?
- What is the relationship of the accidents to meal time?
- Do the accidents occur during the day or night?

Medical and Surgical History Affecting Fecal Incontinence. Fecal incontinence may be a symptom of an underlying disease process. For example, 20% of people with diabetes have incontinence (Atchison, Fisher, Carter, McKee, MacCuish, & Finley, 1991). It is critical to obtain medical and surgical histories, which could indicate possible causes.

Bowel Record and Fluid/Dietary Habits. A bowel record provides objective data regarding the person's bowel function and will help identify defecation patterns. Pay particular attention to any patterns of stool loss. An example of a bowel record is included in Figure 18-2. It is important to obtain information about the amount and quality of fluid intake, because dehydration may lead to constipation. This can be added to the bowel record. Is the intake of fiber adequate? Cereal is thought to be a good source of fiber, however, many of the major brands contain very little bran. Poor dietary habits may have an insub-

Week: _____

Day and Time	Bowel Movement		Bowel Accident		Amount	
	H = Hard L = Loose S = Soft W = Watery		H = Hard L = Loose S = Soft W = Watery		1 = smear 3 = medium 2 = small 4 = large	

Weekly Information:
Check (   )
    Daily fluid intake: Daily fiber intake*:
        Less than 4 cups _____   Less than 2 servings _____
        More than 4 cups _____   More than 2 servings _____
    Exercise: Chairfast:
        Yes _____   Yes _____
        No _____   No _____
    Laxative Use:
        Yes _____   (Name: _____)
        No _____   When: _____

*Good sources of fiber: whole grain cereal and breads, bran, fresh fruits, vegetables, one teaspoon processed bran

Figure 18-2. Bowel record.

stantial effect on bowel function of very active older adults, but will play a major role if their activity level is decreased.

Medications. Many medications affect normal functioning of the gastrointestinal tract. In general, they either increase or slow transit time by altering the absorption of water. Because fecal incontinence can result in chronic constipation, it is important to evaluate medications that may cause constipation and possibly impaction. An acute diarrheal illness in patients who are normally continent can yield incontinence. Table 18-8 lists medications that often have adverse effects on the bowel.

PHYSICAL EXAMINATION

The physical exam must include a good neurologic exam to identify potential factors contributing to loss of bowel control. A basic neurologic examination should be performed, including a mental status examination. Examine the abdomen for tenderness, masses, surgical scars, and hyperactive or hypoactive bowel sounds. Does the person sense the urge to defecate? All patients should

Table 18-8	MEDICATIONS AFFECTING NORMAL BOWEL FUNCTION	
	Medications and Constipation	Medications and Diarrhea
	Analgesics (narcotics)	Alcohol
	Anesthetic agents	Antacids (magnesium)
	Antacids (calcium and aluminum compounds)	Antibiotics (broad-spectrum)
	Antiarrhythmics	Antidiarrheal agents
	Anticholinergics	Antineoplastics
	Anticonvulsants	Colchicine
	Antidepressants	Digoxin, quinidine
	Antihistamines	Nitrofurantoin
	Antiparkinson drugs	Nonsteroidal anti-inflammatory drugs
	Antipsychotics	(NSAIDS)
	Antispasmodics	Laxatives (stimulant)
	Barium	Lithium
	Diuretics	Hyperosmolar tube feedings
	Iron supplements	
	Laxative abuse	
	Opiates	

be checked for impaction, anal sphincter tone, and intact perianal sensation. Sensation can be tested by eliciting the bulbocavernosus reflex and the anal wink. Note any hemorrhoids, fissures, or anal gaping. A thorough functional and environmental assessment is performed to identify barriers to toileting. Refer to the information provided in the urinary incontinence section for key assessment strategies.

LABORATORY AND DIAGNOSTIC STUDIES

For patients with persistent diarrhea, a stool specimen may be obtained to look for various pathogens. If patients report irritable voiding symptoms or have urinary incontinence as well, a urine culture may be ordered to rule out a urinary tract infection. Bowel-incontinent patients are three times more likely to have urinary tract infections due to the contamination of the urethra (Lara, Troop, & Beadleson-Baird, 1990). If gastrointestinal causes are being evaluated, several serum values may be obtained to rule out infectious or malignant processes.

In addition to laboratory studies, numerous diagnostic tests are available to evaluate anorectal disorders or disease. In cases of persistent fecal incontinence, anoscope and flexible sigmoidoscopy may be ordered to rule out inflammatory or neoplastic processes. Abdominal x-rays or barium studies can be performed to evaluate for mechanical obstruction. Anal manometry, which measures pressures of the internal/external sphincters and rectum, can be used if anal sphincter competence is in question. Electromyography provides information regarding sphincteric strength, both at rest and during a contraction, to reveal neurologic involvement. Colonic motility studies may provide insight into chronic constipation.

To demonstrate fecal incontinence and provide valuable information about sphincter competence, physicians may elect to perform a saline infusion test to evaluate the ability of the rectum to retain an enema. Video defecography, a highly specialized test, evaluates the ability to hold rectal contrast and serves to document a poorly distensible rectum or check for the presence of internal prolapse. Defecating proctometrogram allows for a standard measurement of the anorectal angle and identifies any anatomic abnormalities. The last two tests are primarily done when surgical options are being considered.

NURSING DIAGNOSES

Fecal incontinence affects the lifestyle of the older adult, and the nurse needs to judge the patient's ability to cope. Selected nursing diagnoses for a patient with fecal incontinence include the following:

- Bowel Incontinence: Areflexic related to lack of voluntary sphincter control secondary to spinal cord injury involving sacral reflex arc
- Bowel Incontinence: Reflexic related to lack of voluntary sphincter control secondary to spinal cord injury above T-11.

NURSING INTERVENTIONS FOR FECAL INCONTINENCE

Nursing interventions for fecal incontinence depend on an accurate evaluation of the underlying problem that led to the bowel control problem. In the case of sphincter overload due to diarrhea, a thorough investigation is necessary to identify the potential causes. Fecal impaction should not be overlooked. More persistent forms of bowel incontinence will require a comprehensive treatment plan that uses numerous strategies. Treatment options include dietary and fluid management, exercise, toileting routines, medications, biofeedback, electrical stimulation, and, in some cases, surgery. The goal is for the individual to have a stool that is formed and easily passable without straining.

DIETARY AND FLUID MANAGEMENT

Patients with fecal incontinence or related bowel disorders will need information about dietary modifications. In general, patients who have fecal incontinence related to fecal stasis or impaction will need a diet high in fiber and at least six glasses of water per day. Foods high in fiber include peas, beans, green vegetables, prunes, blackberries, peaches, bran crackers, cereals, and breads. Patients should avoid foods that are constipating. Supplemental dietary fiber may be recommended if intake through food sources cannot be optimized. If patients are not drinking adequate fluids, it is best to avoid bulk-forming agents. Regularly scheduled meals will help with stimulation of the routine gastrocolic reflex.

EXERCISE AND ACTIVITY

Exercise and activity are essential components of any bowel program. Even patients with limited mobility can increase their activity and stimulate peristalsis by performing bed exercises. Bed mobility exercises can help improve abdominal muscle tone. Patients who are ambulatory should be encouraged to walk at least three times daily. Scheduling time to provide assistance in maintaining or improving a person's activity level is an extremely important nursing intervention, especially in frail older adults. Patients with impaired mobility are at high risk for impaction and subsequent fecal incontinence.

Clinical Pearl

Intervention: A home exercise program that becomes habit for the individual has greater potential for success.

TOILETING ROUTINES

To use the gastrocolic reflex to aid in defecation, recommend or assist patients in sitting on a toilet at regularly scheduled times after a meal. The best time for scheduling the toileting routine will be apparent after a good history of bowel habits is taken. For many patients, this can be accommodated by having them sit on a commode 20 to 30 minutes after breakfast. It may be beneficial to provide patients with any natural bowel stimulants routinely used, such as warm coffee or tea. Encourage patients to respond to the urge to defecate and avoid repeated delays. For patients who need better positioning, try placing their feet on a footstool and having them lean forward slightly. Applying pressure in a downward motion may help stimulate peristalsis. When possible, avoid the use of bedpans, because they are not compatible with normal positioning for defecation and may interfere with complete evacuation. Unless contraindicated, encourage use of Valsalva's maneuver by reminding patients to inhale against force while contracting their abdominal muscles.

Adaptive equipment may be helpful for patients with mobility impairments. Bedside commodes are often used for patients who have diarrheal illnesses in which warning time may be inadequate. It is important to remember that patients with dementia often rely on visual or tactile cues for performing routine daily activities. Having a bowel movement on a bedside commode in the center of a room will not be a familiar environment, and better results may be obtained by placing the patient in the bathroom setting. Elevated toilet seats are available to make getting on and of the toilet seat easier. It is always important to make every attempt to ensure privacy and allow adequate time for toileting.

Ideally, fecal impaction should be prevented by paying close attention to the bowel habits of older adults. Patients with fecal impaction often complain of abdominal pain or discomfort, nausea, and/or deceased appetite. Steps taken to clear the impaction are also generally uncomfortable for the patient and time consuming for staff. Appropriate nursing interventions should be taken to avoid actual impaction, because prevention is much simpler than working to resolve the impaction. Once the impaction has been cleared, a consistent bowel program can be initiated.

PATIENT AND FAMILY EDUCATION

Intervention is geared toward teaching appropriate techniques to eliminate continence stressors, maximize appropriate bowel performance, and maintain functional ability.

Pelvic Muscle Reeducation. When pelvic floor musculature and sphincter tone are weakened, pelvic muscle reeducation should be attempted. An exercise program targeted at improving the external anal sphincter tone of the pelvic floor has been shown to be effective in highly motivated patients. Success depends on consistent, daily exercise. The exercises are explained in the section on urinary incontinence. Individuals should be taught to focus on pulling in the muscles around the rectum. Teach the patient to perform three sets of 15 exercises per day. Contracting the muscle for 10 seconds and resting for 10 seconds will help strengthen the pelvic floor and subsequently increase anorectal control.

Biofeedback/Sphincter Electromyography. Biofeedback is a safe and effective intervention for fecal incontinence in patients who are cognitively intact and motivated. Two routes for conducting biofeedback to teach older adults how to produce a stronger external anal sphincter contraction include anal manometry and sphincter electromyography. Pelvic floor strengthening exercises should be accompanied by dietary and fluid modifications and increased activity. Weekly contact with the care provider is helpful to keep the patient motivated, especially early in the treatment plan.

Stimulation Therapy. Electrical stimulation, as used with urinary incontinence, is conducted to strengthen the pelvic floor musculature. The stimulus is not painful and is a good therapy to be used in addition to pelvic floor reeducation for patients with impaired support.

Medication Therapy. Medications, either laxatives or antidiarrheal agents, are frequently used to achieve formed, passable stool. There is probably an overreliance on medications in the case of constipation. If patients report a long-standing history of laxative use, some form of pharmaceutical intervention will probably be needed initially. With time, one can often decrease the use of highly irritative laxatives and suggest more natural methods for preventing constipation. One alternative that has been found to be successful is the use of a special recipe based on high-fiber foods (Behm, 1985). The special recipe can be used to help attain formed, passable bowel movements without the irritation often caused by laxatives. See the Patient Teaching Box for the special recipe.

In patients with fecal incontinence due to spinal cord involvement, the use

Patient Teaching Box
SPECIAL RECIPE*

Instruct the patient in use of the "Special Recipe."

Mix:
- 1 cup unprocessed bran
- 1 cup applesauce
- 1/2 cup to 1 cup prune juice

Use:
- 1 Tbsp (with a glass of water) to start
- May use in the evening for morning toileting
- Increase to 2 Tbsp each day until regular
- If more than 4 Tbsp are needed, give in divided portions
- Refrigerate between servings

*Bhem, RM (1985).

of glycerin suppositories and/or digital rectal stimulation has been found to be very helpful. This is also useful for patients with dementia who may lack the ability to voluntarily strain to pass stool. This stimulation of the rectal vault serves to heighten awareness of the defecation reflex.

SURGICAL INTERVENTIONS

Surgery may be indicated for persons who fail to respond to various nursing and medical interventions. Unfortunately, the surgical procedures available for fecal incontinence are very difficult and are associated with a high rate of complications. Surgical options include direct sphincter repair, postanal repair to restore the anorectal angle, anal encirclement, implantation of an artificial sphincter, and various muscle transfer procedures. While artificial sphincters would be useful in a number of patients with severe fecal incontinence, the procedure still carries a great risk of sepsis. In very severe cases, a diverting colostomy may be performed.

ABSORPTIVE PRODUCTS

Numerous absorptive products are available to assist in containing fecal matter. These products should be viewed as management, not treatment options. The type of product used will depend on the severity of the leakage and patient comfort. As with any absorptive product, meticulous skin care must be provided to maintain skin integrity. For watery diarrhea, external fecal incontinence pouches have been used with good success. The skin must be properly cleansed and dried before applying an external pouch.

Nursing Care Plan

FOR PATIENTS WITH URINARY INCONTINENCE

Nursing Diagnosis: Stress Incontinence, related to weakened pelvic floor musculature/decreased outlet resistance.

Definition: A condition in which the individual experiences urine leakage and increases in intra-abdominal pressure.

Assessment Findings:
1. Leakage with coughing, lifting, laughing, or exercise
2. Primarily daytime leakage
3. Amount of leakage is small
4. History of traumatic prostate surgery or bladder suspension surgery
5. History of urethral dilatation

Nursing Interventions with Selected Rationale:
1. Assess nature and frequency of leakage through use of a voiding diary.
   Rationale: Patients often overestimate or underestimate the severity of their leakage. Baseline information provided by the diary is essential for monitoring progress.
2. Assess amount and type of fluid intake.
   Rationale: Be aware that patients often dehydrate themselves to prevent urine leakage.

(continued)

Nursing Care Plan

FOR PATIENTS WITH URINARY INCONTINENCE *(Continued)*

3. Note any potential bladder irritants, such as caffeine and artificial sweeteners.
   Rationale: Irritants may contribute to the incontinence. If not contraindicated, advise a daily intake of six to eight glasses of water per day.
4. Conduct a medication review. Note medication that may increase the volume of urine, decrease the resistance of the bladder outlet, or result in urinary retention.
   Rationale: A medication history can provide clues about possible contributing factors to incontinence and allow for changes, if necessary.
5. Instruct the patient to perform meticulous skin care. In patients with atrophic vaginitis, conjugated estrogen may be indicated for friable tissues.
   Rationale: Incontinence predisposes the patient to skin irritation and possible skin breakdown.
6. Instruct the patient in measures to avoid constipation.
   Rationale: Constipation may further cause problems with bladder control.
7. Instruct the patient in pelvic floor muscle exercises. Remind the patient that success depends on consistent practice, progress is gradual, and lax muscles take time to strengthen.
   Rationale: Reassurance enhances patient motivation.
8. Encourage use of a voiding diary, exercise record, and audiotapes during the home program to monitor progress.
   Rationale: Record keeping promotes compliance and provides an objective means to evaluate progress.
9. Assist with incorporating the exercises into the patient's daily routine, for example, suggest doing the exercises while reading, watching TV, taking a shower, or standing in line. Reinforce that no one can see him or her doing the exercises.
   Rationale: Incorporation into daily routine promotes compliance and success of the exercise program.
10. Consider the use of sphincter electromyography/biofeedback to foster use of the correct muscle and monitor progress.
    Rationale: Electrical stimulation has also been shown to be helpful in muscle strengthening.
11. Instruct patient to contract the muscle before coughing, lifting, or performing other maneuvers that increase intra-abdominal pressure.
    Rationale: Conscious contraction prevents urine leakage.
12. Be aware that some patients may need additional support, such as pessaries, vaginal cones, and/or weights.
    Rationale: Additional measures may be necessary if other interventions do not succeed.

Desired Patient Outcomes/Discharge Criteria:
1. Patient will be able to contract the external sphincter and gradually hold contraction for 10 seconds.
2. Patient will experience fewer episodes of urine leakage after consistently performing the exercises for 6 to 8 weeks.
3. Patient will be able to contract the muscle during increases in intra-abdominal pressure and avoid urine leakage.
4. Patient will increasingly participate in social activities. Fear of accidents will decrease.
5. Patient will be able to prevent urine leakage associated with increases in intra-abdominal pressure through pelvic floor reeducation.

Nursing Care Plan

FOR PATIENTS WITH FECAL INCONTINENCE

Nursing Diagnosis: Bowel incontinence, related to fecal impaction.

Definition: A state in which the individual experiences leakage of stool from around the site of fecal impaction.

Assessment Findings:
1. Loose stool; often mistaken for diarrhea
2. Abdominal pain/tenderness
3. Possible fever
4. Impacted stool in rectum
5. Immobility

Interventions with Selected Rationale:
1. Assess bowel function, fluid and fiber intake, activity level, and history of laxatives. Be aware of the difference between real and perceived constipation. Investigate what is considered "normal" or "regular" for the patient.
   Rationale: Assessment of normal function provides a baseline for planning and intervention.
2. Review medications to identify potential effects on bowel function, such as constipation or diarrhea.
   Rationale: A medication history can provide clues to possible contributing factors and allow for changes if necessary.
3. Instruct the patient in critical components of an effective bowel program for fecal incontinence and impaction: fluids, fiber, activity/mobility, scheduled toileting, using gastrocolic reflex.
   Rationale: An effective bowel program attempts to reestablish the patient's control over bowel elimination.
4. Instruct the patient in the importance of responding to the urge to defecate.
   Rationale: Postponing the urge results in worsening constipation. The strongest defecation reflex is the initial urge, usually after the first meal of the day.
5. Offer the use of warm beverages such as water or coffee.
   Rationale: Warm beverages can act as a bowel stimulant.
6. Follow a prescribed bowel program, starting with an empty rectum, to prevent further episodes of impaction. Avoid alternating laxatives and antidiarrheal agents.
   Rationale: Adherence to a bowel program minimizes risking future impaction.

Desired Patient Outcomes/Discharge Criteria:
1. Patient will develop better bowel habits and avoid excessive or chronic use of laxatives.
2. Patient will develop soft, formed stool at scheduled times.
3. Patient will have no further episodes of fecal impaction.
4. Patient will have fewer or no episodes of fecal incontinence.

REFERENCES

Abrams, W., & Berkow, R. (Eds.). (1990). *The Merck manual of geriatrics.* Westpont, PA: Merck.

Agency for Health Care Policy and Research. (1992). *Clinical practice guidelines: Urinary incontinence in adults* (AHCPR Publication No. 92-0038). Rockville, MD: U.S. Department of Health and Human Services, Public Health Service.

Atichison, M., Fisher, B. M., Carter, K., McKee, R. MacCuish, A. C., & Finley, I. G. (1991). Impaired anal sensation and early diabetic fecal incontinence. *Diabetic Medicine, 8*(10), 960–963.

Bannister, J. J., Abouzrkry, L., & Read, N. W. (1987). Effect of aging on anorectal function. *Gut, 28*, 353.

Behm, R. M. (1985, July/August). A special recipe to banish constipation. *Geriatric Nursing,* 216–217.

Fantl, J. A., Wyman, J. F. McClish, D. K., Harkins, S. W., Elswick, R. K., Taylor, J. R., et al. (1991). Efficacy of bladder training in older women with urinary incontinence. *Journal of the American Medical Association, 265*(5), 609–613.

Hadley, E. (1986) Bladder training and related therapies for urinary incontinence in older people. *Journal of the American Medical Association, 256*(3), 372–379.

International Association for Intestomal Therapy. (1993). *Standards of Care for Urinary and Fecal Incontinence.*

Kegel, A. H. (1948). Progressive resistance exercise in the functional restoration of the perineal muscles. *American Journal of Obstetrics and Gynecology, 56*, 238–248.

Lara, L. L., Troop, P. R., & Beadleson-Baird, M. (1990). The risk of urinary tract infection in bowel incontinent men. *Journal of Gerontological Nursing, 16*(5), 24–26.

McHugh, S. M., & Diamant, N. E. (1987). Effect of age, gender and parity on anal canal pressures. *Digest of Disease Science, 32*, 726.

National Institutes of Health. (1988). *Urinary Continence Consensus Development Conference,* Bethesda, MD: Office of Medical Application of Research, NIH.

National Institutes of Health Consensus Development Conference Statement. (1989). Urinary incontinence in older adults. *Journal of the American Medical Association, 61*(18), 2685–2690.

Resnick, N. (1990). Initial evaluation of the incontinent patient. *Journal of the American Geriatrics Society, 38*, 311–316.

Wald, A. (1990). Constipation and fecal incontinence in the elderly. *Gastroenterology Clinics of North America, 19*(2), 405–418.

Warren, J. W. (1990). Urine-collection devices for use in adults with urinary incontinence. *Journal of the American Geriatrics Society, 38*, 364–367.

Wells, T. (1990). Pelvic (floor) muscle exercise. *Journal of the American Geriatrics Society, 38*, 333–337.

Wyman, J. F., & Fantu, J. A. (1991). Bladder training in ambulatory care management of urinary incontinence. *Urologic Nursing, 9*, 11–17.

BIBLIOGRAPHY

Colling, J. C. (1994). Urine volumes and voiding patterns among incontinent nursing home residents. *Geriatric Nursing,* 15(4), 188–192.

Diokno, A. C., Brock, B. M., Brown, M. B., & Herzog, A. R. (1986). Prevalence of urinary incontinence and other urological symptoms in the non-institutionalized elderly. *Journal of Urology, 136*, 1022–1025.

Engel, B. T., Nikoomanesh, P., & Schuster, M. M. (1974). Operant conditioning of rectosphincteric responses in the treatment of fecal incontinence. *New England Journal of Medicine, 290*(12), 646–649.

Fader, M. (1994). From wheelchair to toilet. *Nursing Times,* April 13, 90–115.

Gibb, H. (1994). How to choose: Nurses judgement of the effectiveness of a range of currently marketed incontinence aids. *Journal of Clinical Nursing,* 3(2), 77–86.

Herzog, A. R. (1990). Prevalence and incidence of incontinence in a community-dwelling population. *Journal of the American Geriatrics Society, 38*, 273–281.

Kane, R. L., Ouslander, J. G., & Abrass, I. B. (1989). *Essentials of Clinical Geriatrics* (2nd ed.). New York: McGraw-Hill.

Ouslander, J. G., Unman, G. C., & Urman, H. N. (1986). Development and testing of an incontinence monitoring record. *Journal of the American Geriatrics Society, 34*, 83–87.

Palmer, M. H. (1994). A health promotion perspective of urinary incontinence. *Nursing Outlook* 42(4), 163–169.

Resnick, N. M. (1992) Urinary incontinence in older adults. *Hospital Practice* 27(10), 139–142.

Schnelle, J. F. (1990). Treatment of urinary incontinence in nursing home patients by prompted voiding. *Journal of the American Geriatrics Society, 38*(3), 356–360.

Tobin, G. W., & Brocklehurst, J. C. (1986). Fecal incontinence in residential homes for the elderly: prevalence, aetiology and management. *Age and Aging, 15*, 41–46.

19

Problems With Elimination

Objectives

1. List the physiologic changes of aging that affect renal/urinary elimination and bowel elimination.
2. Describe psychosocial issues of elimination.
3. Identify the steps in the nursing assessment of renal and bowel elimination in the older adult.
4. List some major nursing interventions for older adults with renal/urinary elimination problems.
5. List some major nursing interventions for older adults with bowel elimination problems.

INTRODUCTION

PROBLEMS WITH BOWEL AND BLADDER functioning can have major physical and psychosocial implications for the older adult. Unfortunately, many treatable or preventable disorders associated with elimination have become an accepted part of growing older. The nurse can play an active role in early intervention. Although changes occur as a normal part of the aging process, the systems involved with elimination can generally maintain homeostasis unless placed under stress. The presence of disease, particularly involving the cardiovascular and neurologic systems, dramatically alters the functioning of the kidneys, bladder, and bowel.

NORMAL PHYSIOLOGIC CHANGES AFFECTING RENAL/URINARY ELIMINATION

The renal system undergoes dramatic changes, including a generalized loss of function and mass, as the adult grows older. The ability to store urine decreases and the frequency of urination increases with age.

Staab, AS and Hodges, LC: ESSENTIALS OF GERONTOLOGICAL NURSING,
© 1996 J. B. Lippincott Company

By age 90, the average weight of the kidney is 20% to 30% less than in the younger adult (Burkhart & Beck, 1990). The renal blood flow decreases partially due to sclerosis of the renal arteries. The direct result is a decrease in the glomerular filtration rate, or the filtering ability of the kidneys. The nephrons, the functioning units of the kidneys, decrease in size and number. The tubules, responsible for absorption and excretion, decrease in length and volume. The result is a loss of ability to concentrate or dilute urine.

Weakened bladder muscles result in incomplete emptying of the bladder and urinary retention. Chronic residual urine can predispose the older patient to infections. In women with a history of childbirth, surgery, urethral stenosis, or stricture, there may be difficulty in starting the urinary stream.

ABNORMAL CHANGES

Abnormal changes in the urinary tract and enlargement of the prostate can lead to urinary infections and obstructions in older men and women. Due to the loss of homeostatic mechanisms, the aging renal system tends to fail under stress, resulting in acute or chronic renal failure. The presence of other diseases, such as hypertension, diabetes, or cardiovascular disease, increases the incidence of these disorders.

Urinary Tract Infections. Urinary tract infections increase with age and are the most common cause of bacterial sepsis in the older adult. Although urinary tract infections are usually more frequent in women, the incidence increases in men after age 65. Early identification and intervention are essential to prevent serious complications.

Clinical Pearl

Assessment: The nurse should be alert for the following nonspecific symptoms of a urinary tract infection in the older adult, such as nausea, vomiting, anorexia, decreased alertness, and or low-grade fever.

Benign Prostatic Hypertrophy. The most common cause of bladder outlet problems in men is benign prostatic hypertrophy, an enlargement of the prostate gland (Brundage, 1988; Miller, 1990). Although rarely seen before the age of 50, 90% of men older than age 80 have enlarged prostates. Although the origin is unknown, the aging process and hormonal changes have been correlated with the condition (Brendler, 1990). As the prostate enlarges, urine outflow decreases and urinary retention increases. As a result, the older man is susceptible to urinary tract infections, calculi, and hydronephrosis.

Acute Renal Failure. Acute renal failure, a sudden, potentially reversible loss of kidney function, is caused by a decrease in the glomerular filtration rate resulting in ischemia. If the ischemia goes uncorrected, it will result in acute tubular necrosis or actual damage to the kidneys. The causes of acute renal failure can be grouped into three categories: prerenal, intrarenal, (intrinsic), and postrenal (see Display 19-1). The older adult may be unaware of the disease, because clinical manifestation can take up to a week to appear. Renal output may be relatively unchanged, so that the amount of urine output may be an unreliable indicator of renal function. Acute renal failure is potentially reversible if the causative factor is corrected. Irreversible damage and scarring of renal tissue can lead to chronic renal failure.

Chronic Renal Failure. Chronic renal failure, a permanent, irreversible loss of renal function, ranges from various stages of renal insufficiency to complete loss of function, which is known as end-stage renal disease. Most older adults can tolerate renal insufficiency with possible diet modifications and medications unless they are stressed by illness or surgery, which results in further loss of nephrons. Patients with end-stage renal disease must have dialysis or a kidney transplantation to survive.

Initially, treatment for chronic renal failure includes correction or control of the underlying cause to prevent further damage. Potentially fatal problems, such as fluid overload, acidosis, and hyperkalemia are corrected quickly. The mainstays of therapy for chronic renal failure involve dietary modification, drug therapy, and dialysis.

Display 19-1
CAUSES OF ACUTE FENAL FAILURE IN THE OLDER ADULT

1. *Prerenal* (any process that decreases blood flow to the kidneys, thereby decreasing glomerular filtration rate)
   • Hypotension
   • Cardiogenic shock (possibly due to myocardial infarction or congestive heart failure)
   • Surgery
   • Volume depletion
   • Septic shock
2. *Intrarenal* (any process involving severe inflammation or medication use that damages renal tissues)
   • Acute glomerulonephritis (inflammation of the glomerulus)
   • Nephrotoxic medications
      aminoglycosides
      chemotherapeutic agents
   • Radiologic contrast agents
3. *Postrenal* (any process causing blockage of urine outflow resulting in kidney damage from increased pressure)
   Renal calculi
   Obstructive uropathy
   Tumors

PSYCHOSOCIAL ISSUES

The signs and symptoms associated with changes in the urinary system, such as frequency and urgency, can cause embarrassment and social isolation. Older patients with urinary tract infections may present with nonspecific symptoms, such as altered sensorium. The pain associated with many disorders can cause depression and withdrawal from normal activities.

Uremic syndrome, or uremia, is caused by an excess of waste products in the blood. As the uremia worsens during renal failure, all of the body systems are affected, including the neurologic system, accounting for many of the psychological changes seen in end-stage renal disease before adequate treatment. Psychological changes that may be observed include depression, emotional lability, decreased libido, decreased concentration, irritability, and behavioral changes. These problems will generally improve or disappear after dialysis is initiated. Symptoms of uremia may reappear if dialysis is inadequate or if treatment is terminated. Every aspect of the older patient's life is changed in end-stage renal disease. Self-esteem and body image undergo drastic changes. Professional counseling is ideal if available and affordable.

NURSING ASSESSMENT

The nurse must be alert for subtle changes in the older patient that suggest an impairment in renal function (see Display 19-2). Many times the signs and symptoms of renal disease in the older adult are nonspecific and vary in severity depending on the degree of function lost.

HISTORY

General assessment of urinary elimination should include the chief complaint; past and current medical history; usual voiding patterns; amount of fluid intake and personal hygiene practices; volume, cloudiness, color, and odor of urine; current medications; unusual signs and symptoms, such as pain or frequency; and history of cancer (patient and family).

Because enlargement of the prostate is such a prevalent problem in the older man, the nurse should take a careful urinary history on all older men, focusing on the typical manifestations of the disorder. Many of the symptoms are very gradual at onset and may be ignored or considered a normal part of aging. Signs and symptoms of acute renal failure may be seen if hydronephrosis occurs (Smeltzer & Bare, 1992).

All medications should be assessed for potential nephrotoxic effects and degree of renal clearance. Unnecessary medications or improper dosing should be avoided. Geriatric dosages of drugs should be administered to ensure safe amounts. Because volume depletion is a major contributor to acute renal failure in the older adult, the nurse should be alert to those at risk for volume depletion, such as patients that are to receive nothing by mouth for tests or procedures, those on diuretic therapy, or those with gastrointestinal problems, such as nausea, vomiting, or diarrhea.

Display 19-2
CLINICAL FINDINGS ASSOCIATED WITH ACUTE OR CHRONIC RENAL FAILURE IN THE OLDER ADULT

Acute Renal Failure

Asymptomatic
Azotemia—increased nitrogenous wastes (urea) in the blood
Oliguria—decreased urine formation
Change in blood pressure
Fluid and electrolyte changes
Metabolic acidosis—a condition characterized by a low pH level and low
    bicarbonate level in the blood
Altered mental status

Chronic Renal Failure

Asymptomatic   Anemia
General malaise   Edema
Fatigue   Hyperkalemia
Muscle weakness/twitching   Hypertension
Elevated serum phosphorus level   Azotemia
Impaired cognitive ability   Oliguria
Psychological changes   Anorexia
   Depression   Weight loss
   Emotional lability   Nausea/vomiting
   Behavioral changes   Itchy, dry skin
Decreased libido

RISK FACTORS

Various factors place the older adult at risk for urinary problems. Patients with cardiovascular disease, hypertension, or diabetes are at far greater risk for renal failure than the average older adult. Factors that are associated with an increased incidence of infection include catheterization, decreased fluid intake, immobility, debilitating illness, sexual activity, anatomic abnormalities, and neurogenic bladder. Institutionalization in a hospital or long-term-care facility also places the older adult at high risk due to the number of antibiotic resistant organisms, decreased activity, and the number of indwelling urinary catheters (Smeltzer & Bare, 1992). Prostatitis is an inflammation of the prostate gland. In older men, it is a likely source of urinary tract infection if associated with a bacterial infection.

Older adults are at higher risk for acute renal failure because factors are more common in this population. Volume depletion, a major contributor to acute renal failure in the older adult, is often overlooked.

PHYSICAL EXAMINATION

Because urinary and renal problems can affect all body systems, a complete review of systems should be done. Additionally, the abdomen is inspected, percussed, and palpated for bladder fullness, pain, and any abnormalities. The costovertebral angle is palpated for tenderness, which may indicate a renal problem. Auscultation of the upper quadrants is done to assess for bruits (vascular sounds that might indicate renal artery stenosis). The external genitalia are inspected for any redness, irritation, inflammation, drainage, or lesions. The inguinal area is examined for enlarged lymph nodes. For men, a rectal examination is done to palpate the prostate gland.

Throughout the physical exam, the nurse should specifically assess the face and dependent body areas, such as the sacrum. Weight and intake and output should be evaluated (urine output is not a reliable indicator when used alone) as well as laboratory values of serum creatinine, blood urea nitrogen, electrolytes, and routine urinalysis. The lower extremities should be checked for edema. The nurse should observe the older patient for signs and symptoms of infection. If untreated, infection can lead to sepsis or, ultimately, septic shock, a prerenal cause of acute renal failure.

DIAGNOSTIC TESTS

Diagnostic tests commonly include the collection of urine specimens for routine urinalysis, culture and sensitivity, and a 24-hour urine collection. Dipstick urinalysis tests can be done to provide quick information about certain constituents, such as hemoglobin, protein, ketones, and leukocytes.

Clinical Pearl

Evaluation: The older adult at risk for dehydration should be carefully monitored when being prepared for diagnostic procedures using contrast dyes, particularly if he or she is not to receive anything by mouth or is receiving diuretic therapy.

Laboratory tests for serum creatinine, blood urea nitrogen, and electrolytes are commonly performed. Creatinine clearance and serum creatinine are laboratory tests typically used to assess renal function. Creatinine is a waste product from the breakdown of muscle mass, most of which is excreted in the kidneys by the tubules. Creatinine clearance, which involves a 24-hour urine test, measures how well the kidneys are excreting creatinine from the body. It measures glomerular filtration rate and indicates total renal status. Serum creatinine, a measure of creatinine in the blood, is less reliable due to the loss of muscle mass in the older patient. Creatinine clearance of less than 10 mL/minute indicates that the kidneys have lost the ability to filter waste products from the blood. Note that by age 80, the creatinine clearance has dropped by more than 50%. These values become especially important when administering medications that are primarily excreted by the renal system. See Display 19-3 for estimating creatinine clearance. Blood urea nitrogen can be used to assess renal function, but unlike creatinine, the values can be affected by hepatic function, hydration, and nutritional status.

Diagnostic studies involved in assessing an enlarged prostate include a rectal/digital prostate examination, ultrasound with fine-needle biopsy, cystoscopy, urinalysis with culture, and serum acid phosphatase (elevated with

Display 19-3

ESTIMATING CREATININE CLEARANCE

Using the following formula, the serum creatinine level can be used to *estimate* the creatinine clearance:

$$\text{Creatinine clearance} = \frac{(140 - \text{age}) \times \text{weight in kg}}{\text{serum creatinine} \times 72}$$

In women, multiply this value by 0.85. The result of this formula is the percentage of remaining renal function.

To demonstrate the marked change in renal function due to aging, the formula can be applied to a 60-kg woman at ages 20, 50, and 80 with a serum creatinine level of 1.0 mg/dL.

20 years old $\qquad \dfrac{(140 - 20) \times 60}{72} = 108 \times 0.85 = 92$

50 years old $\qquad \dfrac{(140 - 50) \times 60}{72} = 75 \times 0.85 = 64$

80 years old $\qquad \dfrac{(140 - 80) \times 60}{72} = 43 \times 0.85 = 43$

Note that by age 80, the creatinine clearance has dropped by more than 50%. These values become important, especially when administering medications that are primarily excreted by the renal system to the older patient.

bone metastasis). In addition, an intravenous pyelogram can be performed to identify obstructions or assess anatomy.

NURSING DIAGNOSES

Nursing diagnoses that can be used in the older adult with renal elimination problems may include the following:

- Fluid Volume Excess related to inability of kidney to maintain fluid balance
- Activity Intolerance related to fatigue and generalized weakness
- High Risk for Injury related to altered calcium and phosphorus metabolism (high risk for fractures)
- Altered Nutrition: Less Than Body Requirements related to increased catabolism and decreased intake
- Knowledge Deficit related to disease and plan of care
- Self-Esteem Disturbance related to changes in lifestyle.

NURSING INTERVENTIONS

Because many causes of urinary elimination problems are preventable or manageable, it is essential that the older adult comply with the plan of care. To help ensure compliance, the nurse should elicit input from the older adult and family when developing the plan of care.

PATIENT AND FAMILY EDUCATION

The nurse must discuss with the patient the signs and symptoms of urinary renal problems, and the patient must demonstrate an understanding of the potential complications of noncompliance of diet and medical therapy. Teach the patient to include foods in the diet that increase urine acidity (fish, poultry, and whole grains). Because problems with urinary elimination are so common among older adults, nurses need to provide education regarding the normal process of aging as compared with abnormal signs and symptoms. Older men need to be taught signs and symptoms of an enlarged prostate (see Patient Teaching Box). The nurse should carefully document teaching and evaluate the response of the patient and family. When using written materials for teaching the older adult, be certain they are written at the appropriate reading level and use an appropriate size print.

RESTORING AND MAINTAINING ELIMINATION

Interventions should be directed toward restoring and/or maintaining adequate urinary elimination and relieving pain. The use of indwelling urinary catheters should be avoided if possible due to the high incidence of urinary tract infections among older patients. Patients should be prompted to void regularly, especially in the presence of mental status changes. Adequate fluid intake and daily exercise will help prevent urinary stasis and improve output.

MEDICAL TREATMENT

To reduce the size of the prostate, some patients undergo long-term antiandrogen therapy. Prostatic balloons may be used to deflate the urethra to allow the outflow of urine. This is an alternative for the patient considered a poor surgical risk, but it is not considered a permanent treatment. The most common form of therapy is surgery for partial or complete removal of prostate tissue.

Patient Teaching Box
SYMPTOMS OF AN ENLARGED PROSTATE

As an older man, you should be aware of the following signs and syptoms of an enlarged prostate:
- Hesitancy in starting urinary stream
- Straining to void
- Decreased size and force of stream
- Interruptions of stream
- Sensation of incomplete emptying of the bladder
- Dribbling after urination
- Increased frequency of urination
- Excessive urination at night
- Sudden, compelling desire to urinate that is hard to control
- Pain or difficulty when urinating

If any of these symptoms occur, please call your doctor.

The type of surgery depends on the location and size of the prostate gland, the condition of the patient, and the possible need for bladder surgery.

Transurethral resection of the prostate is the most common prostate surgery performed. The Patient Teaching Box below provides discharge instructions for the patient with a transurethral resection.

DIALYSIS

It is imperative that the nurse not treat the patient with chronic renal failure as someone who is terminally ill. Although many changes in lifestyle may occur, most patients can maintain normal activities once they are stabilized on dialysis. The older adult and his or her support system must be motivated to follow the treatment plan. Self-care is essential, because renal failure affects so many aspects of the older patient's life. The nurse and other members of the health care team share the responsibility of education, health promotion, and referral to appropriate agencies.

The mainstays of therapy for chronic renal failure involve dietary modifications, drug therapy, and dialysis. The diet for the older patient with renal failure is restricted in protein, potassium, sodium, and phosphorous and high in carbohydrates and fat to maintain body weight. Fluids are restricted based on individual needs to prevent fluid overload. A dietary consultation is necessary so that the diet can be individualized according to the patient's needs and food preferences.

Patient Teaching Box
DISCHARGE INSTRUCTIONS AFTER TRANSURETHRAL RESECTION OF THE PROSTATE

- For the first 6 to 8 weeks after transurethral resection of the prostate (TURP), avoid the following because they increase pressure in the abdomen and may increase bleeding:
    Sitting for prolonged periods
    Taking long automobile rides
    Lifting heavy objects
    Straining at stool
- Resume sexual activities in 6 to 8 weeks unless otherwise ordered by the physician.
- Keep in mind that most surgeries do not result in impotence (it usually only occurs after total prostatectomy). Recommend sexual counseling or refer to specialists for treatment options.
- Remember that urine may become cloudy after intercourse due to retrograde ejaculation of semen into the bladder.
- Be aware that incontinence or dribbling are common after TURP and can last up to a year. To help with this,
    Perform Kegel exercises 10 to 20 times per hour
    Drink plenty of fluids (to increase bladder capacity), and void at least every 2 to 3 hours.
- Keep follow-up appointments, especially yearly exams, which are essential
    Benign prostatic hypertrophy can recur because only part of the tissue was removed.
    The remaining prostate gland needs to be assessed.

Human erythropoietin is now available as a medication to help replace the reduced production of erythropoietin in the kidneys and correct severe anemia. Phosphate binders, such as aluminum hydroxide gels and antacids, are administered with meals to help remove excessive phosphate from the body through the gastrointestinal tract. Patients on aluminum compounds need routine screening for aluminum levels, because toxic levels can accumulate in the body. Vitamin D and calcium supplements are given to help maintain serum calcium levels and prevent mobilization from the bone. Because most older adults have already lost bone mass due to osteoporosis, it is especially important to prevent further losses from the bone.

For the older adult with end-stage renal disease, dialysis is the key to survival. Dialysis treatments are necessary to clean the blood of waste products, remove excess fluid, and correct electrolyte imbalances. The two types of dialysis, hemodialysis and peritoneal dialysis, are available at most facilities, and the choice is based on the patient's condition, compliance, and preference.

For the older adult who progresses to end-stage renal disease, the financial costs can be devastating. Transportation, medications, laboratory and diagnostic testing, medical fees, and dialysis treatment and supplies can easily overwhelm the older patient, even with Medicare and other insurance benefits. Referral to a social worker experienced in dealing with patients receiving dialysis can assist the patient in exploring alternative funding.

TRANSPLANTATION

Transplantation, another option for patients with end-stage renal disease, has been successfully performed in the older adult. Unfortunately, there is a lack of available organs for transplant candidates in general, and the presence of chronic disease, such as cardiovascular disease and diabetes, usually prohibits most older adults from seeking transplantation. Based on the current physical status of selected older patients, transplantation should be explored as an alternative to dialysis (Brundage, 1988; Burkhart & Beck, 1990).

PHYSIOLOGIC CHANGES AFFECTING BOWEL ELIMINATION

Alterations in bowel function in the older adult can be attributed to a combination of factors, such as aging, lifestyle, diseases, and treatment practices. Although definite changes occur due to aging, the bowel can usually maintain homeostasis in the healthy older adult unless faced with a stressor.

Overall changes related to aging include mucosal and muscular atrophy, diminished innervation of the bowel, and decreased bowel transit time. Defecation is further affected by decreased muscle wall elasticity and possibly decreased innervation of the rectum and anus (Nelson & Castell, 1990).

ABNORMAL CHANGES

The three major abnormal bowel problems include diverticular disease, constipation, and colorectal cancer. The incidence of constipation, colorectal cancer, and diverticular disease (which includes diverticulosis and diverticulitis) increases dramatically with aging and is related to a low dietary intake of fiber and lifestyle behaviors.

Diverticular Disease. The aging colon responds to decreases in dietary fiber by developing muscle hypertrophy, which results in a narrowed lumen. Pressure increases within the colon push bowel contents, especially hard, formed stool, through a smaller opening. Herniation of the mucous membrane through the muscle wall of the intestines (diverticulum) results in the formation of a pouch or sac. The presence of diverticula without inflammation is called diverticulosis. When fecal contents collect in the sacs and begin to decompose, the inflammatory process is known as diverticulitis.

Diverticulosis is usually asymptomatic. Often referred to as "left-sided appendicitis," diverticulitis is characterized by low-grade fever, left lower quadrant pain, abdominal fullness, and discomfort, anorexia, nausea, and vomiting. A health history often reveals altered bowel function, such as constipation or alternating constipation and diarrhea. Blood may be found in the stool, especially with diverticular hemorrhage. Treatment may involve antibiotics or analgesics, or if obstruction or perforation occurs, a colon resection or temporary colostomy may be necessary.

Constipation. Although older adults often complain of constipation, it is not necessarily due to the normal aging process in the bowel. The causes of constipation are multifactorial and may involve a lifetime of poor health habits affecting the bowel. The immobile older adult is particularly susceptible to terminal reservoir syndrome, which involves the accumulation of feces in the left colon and rectum. The major contributing factors are poor dietary habits, medications that promote constipation, and a lack of routine or active exercise (Moll & Alford, 1989).

Contributing to the problem is the older adult's understanding of constipation. Constipation is described as a decrease in the frequency of bowel movements from the usual pattern. For many older adults, daily bowel movements are considered normal function, primarily a result of cultural influences and advertisements that encourage periodic purging for good health. Constipation is more objectively defined as the passage of hard, dry stool during which a defecation can be painful and difficult with a sensation of fullness or incomplete emptying of the bowel.

Colorectal Cancer. Colorectal cancer is very common in the older adult, with two thirds of the cases occurring in people older than age 65 (Cheskin & Schuster, 1990). Malignancies are usually adenocarcinomas developing from polyps in the epithelial lining of the intestines. Mortality rates in colorectal cancer are high, with a 5-year survival rate of less than 50%. Early detection and treatment are essential. Colorectal cancer is also associated with dull abdominal or rectal pain, anorexia, weight loss, or weakness. Routine occult blood testing of the stool is an inexpensive, simple method that can detect early, asymptomatic malignancies.

PSYCHOSOCIAL ISSUES

Bowel function is a major concern for many older adults. Time, energy, and finances are devoted to finding ways to maintain "normal" bowel patterns. Many grew up in an age that encouraged periodic purging to clear the body of excess waste. Advertisements encourage the use of over-the-counter remedies to maintain desired bowel function. Many older adults become dependent on laxatives or enemas to achieve regular, daily bowel movements. Unless they are weaned from these methods, the bowel will eventually lose tone and innervation, requiring long-term use of these interventions to maintain bowel function.

Psychological conditions may cause the older adult to fail to recognize or ignore the need to defecate. Dietary changes, as a result of depression, may decrease the amount of fluid and bulk in the diet, leading to changes in bowel function. Some older adults may refuse to have a bowel movement in situations in which they feel a loss of control.

NURSING ASSESSMENT

Nursing assessment should begin with a careful history of bowel habits and function. After obtaining the patient's history, a complete physical examination should be performed.

HISTORY

When obtaining the history, questions should focus on the following areas:

- Health history and the patient's chief complaint
- Past and current elimination patterns, especially any changes
- Use of elimination aids, such as laxatives and enemas
- Current medications
- Medical history, including any abdominal or gastrointestinal surgeries
- Family history of cancer
- Lifestyle patterns, including nutrition, exercise, stress, and emotional status
- Characteristics of the feces, including color, odor, consistency, and frequency
- Abdominal/rectal pain
- Presence of any of the following: straining, rectal pressure/fullness, diarrhea, constipation, bleeding, hemorrhoids, anorexia, fever, weight loss or flatulence
- Ability for self-care with toileting and preparation of meals
- Religious and cultural practices affecting diet or elimination

RISK FACTORS

Various risk factors have been associated with bowel elimination problems. Factors associated with constipation in the older adult include the following:

- Decreased activity, lack of exercise, immobility
- Dietary changes due to anorexia, poor dentition, financial problems, or inability to prepare meals
- Medications that reduce peristalsis or cause dehydration
- Inattention to the urge to defecate
- Abuse of laxatives or enemas
- Change in daily routine
- Decreased abdominal muscle strength

- Organic disease (diabetes, hypothyroidism)
- Depression or mental illness
- Decreased fluid intake or excessive fluid loss

Colorectal cancer also has been associated with certain risk factors. These include a family history of colon cancer, history of rectal polyps or inflammatory bowel disease, and/or a diet low in fiber and high in fat.

PHYSICAL EXAMINATION

Before beginning the physical examination, ask the patient to empty the bladder or assist him or her in doing so. Begin by inspecting the abdomen for contour and symmetry. Note any scars or visible masses. Occasionally, peristalsis or pulsations will be visible. Listen for bowel sounds and document frequency and character. Percuss the abdomen in all four quadrants. Areas of tympany (bell-like or resonant) usually occur over gas in the gastrointestinal tract. The presence of masses, feces, or fluid produces a duller sound. Palpate the abdomen to identify distention, masses, or tenderness.

Inspect the perianal area for hemorrhoids, fissures, and irritation. Digital rectal examination should be performed to further assess the hemorrhoids and the amount and consistency of stool in the rectum. Rectal masses should be reported to the physician, because the digital exam can detect many of the large bowel and rectal malignancies.

DIAGNOSTIC TESTS

Diagnostic tests include stool analysis, sigmoidoscopy, colonoscopy, barium enema, and computed tomography scan. Fiberoptic sigmoidoscopy or colonoscopy with biopsy or barium studies can assist with diagnosis. Laboratory studies include an anemia profile. Surgical treatment of colorectal cancer may involve colon resection or colostomy. The older adult may undergo radiation therapy and/or chemotherapy as a substitute or addition to surgery.

NURSING DIAGNOSES

A partial listing of nursing diagnoses to consider when planning care for the older adult with problems with bowel elimination might include:

- Constipation related to effects of medication on bowel function
- Constipation related to health habits
- Pain related to constipation

NURSING INTERVENTIONS

The major goal of nursing care is to restore or maintain normal, healthy bowel elimination in the older adult. This goal is achieved primarily through patient education.

PATIENT AND FAMILY EDUCATION

Older adults and their families may need education about bowel elimination. The older adult needs to learn to separate signs and symptoms of abnormal changes from the normal age-related changes. Misconceptions about bowel elimination, such as the necessary daily bowel movement, must be corrected with realistic explanations. Patients should be instructed in the safe use of laxatives to prevent laxative abuse.

Education about allowing sufficient time for toileting and a regular schedule for bowel elimination is important. The nurse should work with the patient to establish a time that is most helpful. Rocking the trunk from side to side and back and forth while sitting on the toilet can help stimulate a bowel movement.

Instructions about diet and activity are key to promoting bowel elimination. A diet high in bulk and fluids can promote bowel elimination. The nurse should review with the patient foods that might be effective, such as prunes, coffee, and bran, and these should be incorporated into the diet. The Patient Teaching Box outlines dietary and bowel habits that can help prevent serious complications if adopted into the older adult's lifestyle.

Additionally, all older adults should be taught warning signals and have routine physical examinations. They may notice a change in bowel habits and characteristics of stool.

Patient Teaching Box
HEALTH PROMOTION FOR BOWEL ELIMINATION

Use the following as guidelines to promote bowel elimination:

- Increase dietary fiber and bulk in the diet. Add small amounts of unprocessed bran slowly to the diet by sprinkling in orange juice or mixing with muffins or other recipes. Add high-fiber cereal to breakfast menu, but be careful when increasing the amount of bran in the diet, because it can cause abdominal distension, loose bowel movements, and loss of electrolytes.
- Drink at least six to eight glasses of water per day (unless contraindicated).
- Avoid use of laxatives or enemas. Changes in dietary habits will usually decrease the need for these remedies. Use of laxatives and enemas over a long time may interfere with normal bowel function.
- Remember that daily bowel movements are not essential for good health. The average bowel movement is about every 2 to 3 days.
- Avoid using mineral oil, because it can interfere with the vitamins being absorbed in the bowel.
- Stay as active as possible.
- Respond as soon as possible when you feel the urge to move your bowels.
- Report any change in bowel habits, such as constipation, diarrhea, blood in the feces, dull abdominal or rectal pain, loss of appetite, weight loss, or weakness.

Nursing Care Plan

FOR THE OLDER ADULT WITH A URINARY TRACT INFECTION

Nursing Diagnosis: Altered Urinary Elimination, related to inflammation and irritation of the urinary tract.

Definition: The state in which the individual experiences or is at risk of experiencing urinary elimination dysfunction.

Assessment Findings:
1. Urgency/frequency
2. Dysuria/pain
3. Fever/chills
4. Flank pain
5. Nausea/vomiting
6. Anorexia
7. Altered sensorium

Nursing Interventions with Selected Rationale:
1. Encourage frequent, routine voiding (every 2 to 3 hours) and prompt response to the urge to void.
   Rationale: Stasis or pooling or urine contributes to bacterial growth.
2. Teach patient the rationale for completing all prescribed antibiotics. Discuss dosage, schedule, and major side effects with the patient.
   Rationale: Adherence to the medication regimen promotes resolution of infection.
3. Assess the patient's ability to obtain and self-administer prescribed medications.
   Rationale: Ability to self-medicate properly ensures compliance and promotes effective therapy.
4. Review proper perineal hygiene with older women.
   • Encourage wiping from front to back after elimination.
   • Discourage the use of bubble baths and feminine hygiene products.
   • Recommend showers rather than tub baths.
   Rationale: Proper perineal hygiene measures are helpful in preventing urinary tract infections.
5. Encourage use of sitz baths or mild analgesics for burning or pain.
   Rationale: Sitz baths and analgesics promote comfort.
6. Discuss the need for adequate fluid intake of at least 6 to 8 glasses of water per day (unless contraindicated).
   Rationale: Adequate fluid intake maintains dilute urine and helps prevent infection.

Patient Outcomes/Discharge Criteria:
1. Patient consumes adequate fluids.
2. Patient has established a regular, frequent pattern of voiding without urgency or frequency.
3. Patient (and family) can identify the signs and symptoms of urinary tract infections.
4. Patient can describe measures that will relieve discomfort.
5. Patient describes/demonstrates health promotion activities to help prevent recurrence.

Nursing Care Plan

FOR THE OLDER ADULT WITH CONSTIPATION

Nursing Diagnosis: Constipation, related to inadequate health habits.

Definition: The state in which the individual experiences or is at high risk of experiencing stasis of the large intestine resulting in a decrease in the frequency of bowel movements and/or the passage of dry, formed, hard stool.

Assessment Findings:
1. Changes in normal bowel habits; decrease in bowel movements
2. Decreased appetite
3. Hard, dry stools, less than three times per week
4. Straining, painful defecation
5. Feelings of rectal fullness or incomplete defecation/abdominal distension

Nursing Interventions with Selected Rationale:
1. Unless contraindicated, encourage the older patient to drink at least 6 to 8 glasses of water or fluid daily.
   Rationale: Sufficient fluid intake is necessary to maintain bowel patterns and promote proper stool consistency.
2. Provide the older patient with a cup of hot liquid (lemonade, tea, prune juice) 30 minutes before breakfast.
   Rationale: Hot liquids taken before meals act as a peristaltic stimulant.
3. Establish a toileting schedule for the patient according to his or her usual bowel pattern. The best time to attempt defecation is after breakfast or dinner. If tolerated, the patient should stay on the toilet for 20 minutes to encourage defecation.
   Rationale: Establishing a routine for defecation aids in defecation.
4. Encourage foods that increase the amount of fiber and bulk in the diet, such as bran, whole-grain cereals, bread, nuts, and fresh fruits and vegetables.
   Rationale: A diet high in fiber-rich foods promotes normal bowel movements.
5. Teach the patient to avoid foods high in refined sugar and flour, such as pastries, pasta, and bread (unless made from whole grain).
   Rationale: Refined foods produce small hard stools increasing the colon's suceptibility to disease.
6. Assist the older patient in assuming as normal a position for defecation as possible. Leaning forward in an upright position on a toilet/bedside commode with the feet on the floor or small stool is best. Provide privacy for defecation. Massaging the colon may also stimulate the urge to move the bowels.
   Rationale: Normal positioning allows for voluntary contraction of abdominal muscles, aiding in feces expulsion.
7. Encourage daily exercise, including active/passive range-of-motion exercises if immobile. Teach abdominal strengthening exercises.
   Rationale: Exercise stimulates peristalsis.
8. Instruct patient and family members to modify home environment (nightlight, handrails, removal of scatter rugs) for nighttime safety.
   Rationale: Environmental modifications promote self-care with bowel elimination while maintaining safety.

(continued)

Nursing Care Plan

FOR THE OLDER ADULT WITH CONSTIPATION *(Continued)*

Desired Patient Outcomes/Discharge Criteria:
1. Patient has established a routine bowel pattern.
2. Patient consumes adequate fluids and fiber.
3. Patient uses appropriate positions to assist with defecation.
4. Patient demonstrates an increased activity level.
5. Patient and family have prepared the home environment to provide safety with toileting activities.

REFERENCES

Brendler, C. B. (1990). Disorders of the prostate. In W. R. Hazzard, R. Andreas, E. L. Bierman, & J. P. Blass (Eds.), *Principles of geriatric medicine and gerontology* (2nd ed.) (pp. 582–591). New York: McGraw-Hill.

Brundage, D. J. (1988). Age-related changes in the genitourinary system. In M. A. Matteson & E. S. McConnell (Eds.), *Gerontologic nursing: Concepts and practice* (pp. 279–289). Philadelphia: W. B. Saunders.

Burkhart, J. M., & Beck, L. H. (1990). Renal diseases in the elderly. In W. R. Hazzard, R. Andes, E. L. Bierman, & J. P. Blass (Eds.), *Principles of geriatric medicine and gerontology* (2nd ed.) (pp. 565–581). New York: McGraw-Hill.

Cheskin, L. J., & Schuster, M. M. (1990). Colonic disorders. In W. R. Hazzard, R. Andes, E. L. Bierman, & J. P. Blass (Eds.), *Principles of geriatric medicine and gerontology* (2nd ed.) (pp. 645–653). New York: McGraw-Hill.

Miller, C. A. (1990). *Nursing care of older adults: Theory and practice*. Glenview, IL: Scott, Foresman/Little, Brown.

Moll, J. A., & Alford, D. M. (1989). Gastrointestinal changes. In K. K. Esberger & S. T. Hughes, Jr. (Eds.), *Nursing care of the aged* (pp. 91–107). Norwalk, CT: Appleton & Lange.

Nelson, J. B., & Castell, D. O. (1990). Aging of the gastrointestinal system. In W. R. Hazzard, R. Andes, E. L. Bierman, & J. P. Blass (Eds.), *Principles of geriatric medicine and gerontology* (2nd ed.) (pp. 593–608). New York: McGraw-Hill.

Smeltzer, S. C., & Bare, B. G. (1992). *Brunner and Suddarth's textbook of medical surgical nursing* (7th ed.). Philadelphia: Lippincott.

BIBLIOGRAPHY

Anderson, S. (1990). Nephrology/fluid and electrolyte disorders. In C. K. Cassel, D. E. Riesenberg, L. B. Sorensen, & J. R. Walsh (Eds.), *Geriatric medicine* (2nd ed.) (pp. 301–311). New York: Springer-Verlag.

Moore, P. G. (1993). *Health assessment in nursing* (2nd ed.). Springhouse, PA: Springhouse.

Robbins, A. (1989). Genitourinary changes. In K. K. Esberger & S. T. Hughes, Jr. (Eds.), *Nursing care of the aged* (pp. 109–151). Norwalk, CT: Appleton & Lange.

Staab, A. S., & Lyles, M. F. (1990). *Manual of geriatric nursing*. Glenview, IL: Scott, Foresman/Little, Brown.

Problems With Psychosocial Functioning

20

Promoting Healthy Psychosocial Functioning in the Older Adult

Objectives

1. Discuss the role of psychosocial functioning in promoting health in the older adult.
2. Discuss the concept of "connectedness."
3. Discuss the role of music, dance, creative arts, pet therapy, reminiscence, and life review in promoting psychosocial functioning.
4. Describe the way self-transcendence is related to healthy aging.
5. Identify several nursing interventions used to promote psychosocial functioning in the older adult.

INTRODUCTION

THE AGING PROCESS BRINGS ABOUT MANY changes in psychosocial functioning. Grief, depression, anxiety, behavioral changes, loss of mobility, loss of intimacy, and even suicide are frequently outcomes of these changes. Yet, a growing number of older adults are able to use the losses they experience throughout life as lessons that help them grow toward wisdom and fullness of life. Nursing interventions aimed at the whole person help to lessen the negative outcomes of nursing diagnoses like loneliness, fatigue, hopelessness, grief, powerlessness, social isolation, and spiritual distress.

Music, art therapy, reminiscence and life review, pet therapy, dance, and movement are measures that promote a sense of connectedness. This sense of connectedness plus transcendence or spirituality help a person toward a fuller, more meaningful old age.

Theories about aging differ, but psychosocial and biophysical components affect each other (Ryan, 1991). For example, it has been shown that a relationship exists between stress and lowered immunity, and between lowered immunity and depression (Gueldner & Bramlett, 1994; Houldin, Lev, Prystowsky, Redei & Lowery, 1991). Therefore, interventions designed to promote wellness in the older adult include both physical and psychological components.

A pleasurable emotional state decreases stress, thereby helping avoid depression and physical illness. For many older people, memories of past pleasant experiences are comforting and satisfying and can reduce stress. Music may help a person recall wonderful moments in the past. Remembering those moments recalls the pleasant feeling one had when hearing the music for the first time—a feeling in the body as well as in the mind. Memories that evoke certain emotions can be explained by a phenomenon called "state-dependent memory." When a memory is encoded, or stored in the brain, not only the word or picture is stored, but also the emotion one felt as one experienced the event (Dossey, 1988). When the memory is recalled, so is the emotion.

Although theories about aging differ, most agree that the older person has a number of tasks in later life which, if done well, promote health. One of those tasks is "body transcendence versus. body preoccupation," a way of saying that one is less preoccupied with the body, which seems to be declining, and more preoccupied with finding ways to maintain feelings of well-being despite the body's decline (Miller, 1991). Other tasks include maintaining high activity levels and remaining in contact with the rest of society and with family.

Holistic nursing interventions designed to address those tasks include the use of music and other techniques that help the person recognize the environment outside of self and how he or she fits into it, yielding predictable outcomes for the growth and well-being of the older adult. Each intervention can be used individually or in groups and requires that the nurse become competent in the use of the technique. Some of the interventions, such as visualization or the creative arts, require further study to become proficient. Often, other health care providers can be consulted for help.

Promoting psychosocial function improves physiologic function. For example, improving coping skills may make is possible for the patient to develop the exercise program needed for improving pulmonary function. Conversely, a planned exercise program decreases social isolation.

MUSIC

The music that stays in one's long-term memory is usually acquired between the ages of 15 and 25 (Randall, 1991). It is therefore available to the older person if access to it can be found. The planned use of music may have many positive effects. Music promotes exercise, socialization, and a sense of continuity of relationships and of life.

Music provides mobility through tapping toes, patting thighs, clapping hands, playing an instrument, dancing, and heel-to-toe stepping. Communication is enhanced through singing with others and setting new words to music. Music can promote connectedness through stimulation of sharing past events or musical highlights of the past and talking or dancing with others at musical events. Music can evoke pleasant memories, lessen anxiety, and lift depression (if the music is meaningful).

Playing the kazoo, for example, may sound childish for a mature adult, but if that person played the kazoo in the past, as many older persons did, it evokes a sense of connectedness that those not of the generation that used kazoos find hard to imagine. Also, there is the benefit of deep respirations when blowing into the tiny instrument. It is necessary to be sensitive to the person who does not want to use a kazoo but who may respond to a harmonica or other music maker. Some musical instruments promote fine muscle movement and improve function of hands and coordination.

INDIVIDUAL MUSIC THERAPY

When planning music therapy used for an individual, headphones should be used so conversation around the patient is not interrupted. In planning music therapy for an individual, the nurse should consider the following:

- The type of music must be meaningful to the patient
- The volume of the music must be adjusted for the patient's hearing level
- Headphones shared between patients must be properly cleaned between use
- Headphones left on for long periods of time lose their effectiveness
- A good rule for length of a music session through headphones is 20 minutes at a time, unless the patient asks for a longer session

Music can be helpful to patients who have had a stroke as well. A person who is aphasic because of a stroke in the speech center may be able to sing words set to music. Neurologists have found that for some people, music is processed on the opposite side of the brain from the speech center. Thus, a creative nurse or music therapist who teaches the patient to sing "I am hungry, I am hungry, I am hungry Clementine" to the tune of the familiar old song, may be teaching the patient a method of communication (Randall, 1991). In addition, some people do not need to have new words set to old tunes, but find that they can sing even though they cannot talk. These people can be encouraged to use the songs they know to communicate or to sing along with others and feel a part of a group. This decreases the sense of loneliness.

GROUP MUSIC THERAPY

Music can be used as therapy for groups. Knowledge of the musical culture of the group is helpful. Other people of the same age in the group can be of great assistance in planning group music. Individual preference must still be acknowledged, depending on the cultural or ethnic background of the group, but most often the people in the group are willing to provide a list of favorite songs. Sometimes there is a person who can play the piano or other instrument, lead the singing, or create a list of musical selections for playing compact discs or tapes. Some songs may evoke sadness, reminding patients of the death of loved ones. Crying is an excellent way to release intense emotion and cope with sad feelings, but the group members must be willing to support this means of coping.

Music therapists, often available for consultation to nurses in large hospital settings, may be able to give good advice about the type of music and setting to accomplish a specific goal for groups. For example, music used for a group of old people to guide exercise is likely to be faster and perhaps louder than music used to stimulate reminiscence. Music used to calm an agitated patient is likely to be slower. People of similar ethnic groups may enjoy ethnic music. For example, a German Lutheran home for the elderly might find many residents able to sing the old German hymns. However, if music therapists are not available, the following commonsense rules will help the choice of music and setting:

- Music must be meaningful to the patient.
- Faster music stimulates; slower music calms.
- Calming music is usually slower than an average patient's pulse (72 beats/minute).
- If patients are expected to sing along, words will need to be provided, either by repetition or in written form.
- If patients are expected to exercise, demonstration must be provided with the music.

Be sensitive to the needs of the group about quality. A group of retired professional musicians may not welcome a kazoo player, even if they understand the goal is socialization. A separate group for kazoo players may be a better option. Groups of people with a special interest in music can be used to convey appropriate messages and attitudes. For example, a senior citizens' group in South Carolina formed a group of older people and teenagers who go to various meetings and homes of older adults. They sing songs like "bubble gum and bifocals" to support intergenerational connections.

DANCE

Dance is a major movement therapy, along with range-of-motion exercises, walking, and other forms of exercise. Dancing, or movement to music, can benefit the older patient both physically and emotionally. It is particularly appropriate for older persons because they belong to a generation of people for whom dancing was a significant part of their lives. Dancing can promote flexibility, muscle strengthening, improve cardiovascular function, and improve respiratory fitness as well as touch, socialization, a sense of connectedness, and good memories. Like music therapy, dancing can be done alone or with partners, depending on the goal of the therapy. Many dances for groups are ethnic in origin, promote a sense of community among the participants, and evoke pleasant memories.

Some dance therapists describe dance as the ability to use one's body as a tool of "release and joy" (Helm, 1985). There is some risk for the older person who is beginning to increase physical activity. Therefore, one of the first steps in promoting exercise or dance is a risk assessment. Table 20-1 lists things to be considered before starting dance/movement sessions for an older person. The presence or absence of any of the risk factors does not prohibit dance. Risk factors may influence the choices of kinds of dance and length of sessions and require a careful assessment before beginning a dance routine.

INDIVIDUAL DANCE THERAPY

Dance for the individual may be no more than range of motion set to music and done in one's room. Many older people stretch and go through a regular routine before getting out of bed in the morning to avoid early morning stiff-

Table 20-1	RISK ASSESSMENT FACTORS
	1. Medical history • Poor cardiovascular status • Chronic obstructive lung disease • Reports of vertigo • Degenerative musculoskeletal problems • Muscle atrophy 2. Past exercise patterns • History of exercise patterns • Dyspnea on mild exertion 3. Obesity 4. Personal habits • Smoking • Alcohol consumption 5. Other assessment parameters as suggested by nursing history

ness and aches. These highly motivated individuals often do not use music and do not ask for help. Sometimes they can be persuaded to perform their exercises to music. It may be necessary to provide time for them to complete their routines when they are hospitalized.

A more formal dance that is increasingly popular is the t'ai chi. Used for centuries in Asia, t'ai chi has rapidly gained popularity in the United States as a form of gentle exercise (Fig. 20-1). This dance is a series of formal motions involving concentration, relaxation, strength, and symbolic movements to create a sense of connectedness with nature and the universe. In t'ai chi, the dance movements are unhurried; precise; involve the whole body in graceful, pleasing, slow movement and posture; and promote both exercise and a sense

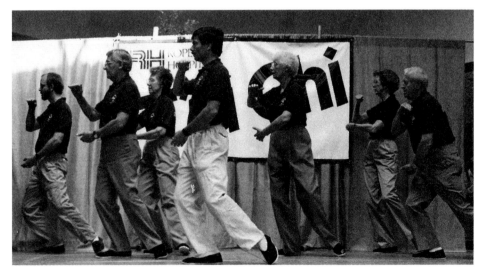

Figure 20-1. T'ai chi is a gentle form of dance therapy popular among older adults.

of peace and calm. It is often done outdoors, adding the dimension of the outside environment to the movement. Inside, it is performed in a pleasing, quiet environment that enhances feelings of relaxation and calm. Many of the graceful, pleasing, movements can be adapted to sitting in a chair for those unable to stand. Once learned, it can be done individually, without a class or group.

GROUP DANCE THERAPY

Dance for groups is more common in America. People at any level of physical ability can participate, achieving a sense of unity with others by tapping their toes, patting their thighs in time to the music, and increasing proficiency to include the intricate steps of the waltz, fox trot, or polka. Dances are often organized by volunteers, recreational therapists, or physical therapists. Provision of space, appropriate music, and help getting people to the dance room may be all that is required of the nurse, although more participation is usually appreciated. For dance movements with specific goals, dance/movement therapists may be involved.

▷ *Clinical Pearl*

Intervention: For senior citizens, the benefits of touch, reminiscence, and a sense of well-being are often the results of dancing.

CREATIVE ARTS

There are a variety of creative arts, such as art therapy, bibliotherapy, drama, and writing workshops, which can be used with older adults to improve their sense of well-being. They create connections between people, give a sense of self-esteem and productivity, often improve mobility, and help the older adult focus on things outside self (transcendence). Creative arts can be used by experts as therapy or in conjunction with other forms of therapy. The nurse can use the common form of the art as a tool to create a healthy environment.

BIBLIOTHERAPY

Bibliotherapy uses literature, such as short stories, poetry, or remembering stories everyone in the group once read, for example, Swift's (1985) "Gulliver's Travels," to communicate and share messages within the group. Goals might include increasing self-awareness, increasing awareness of others, improving reality orientation, and giving people a new way of communicating (Hynes & Hynes-Berry, 1986). The group may read literature ahead of time and discuss it at the meeting, choose to read poetry and other short selections at the meeting itself and then discuss it, or choose to write their own selections, like poetry or short prose, and share it at the meeting.

ART THERAPY

Art therapy, in many forms, achieves tactile stimulation as well as a product, often supporting one's sense of self. Art therapy commonly is used as an adjunct to psychotherapy because of its use of symbolism. Often, people can say in art what they cannot say in words. Pictures people draw sometimes are used to assess or identify patterns of behavior or thought that has meaning in the therapeutic process. Simply allowing people to draw, make pottery, or paint ceramic objects, however, is a good way to involve them in a group activity, and it can be done without getting involved beyond the skill level of the nurse in interpretation of symbols.

PET THERAPY

Pets have been used successfully in therapy for older patients both in hospital settings and for those who live at home alone. It has been shown that for older adults, pets can provide companionship, a source of love and affection, and a sense of security and belonging that is often missed when the older adult loses a spouse and/or loved ones (Fig 20-2). The comfort of having a familiar pet can counteract feelings of loneliness and isolation. Pets also can promote more physical activity and social interaction for the older person living at home, because of the responsibilities of caring for a pet. Animals in nursing homes or residential settings can be used as the focus for beginning reminiscence groups or other activities to help residents interact and participate. The pets

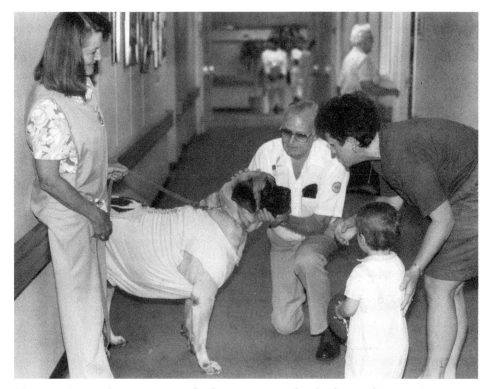

Figure 20-2. In long-term-care facilities, pets can be the focus of interaction among small groups or can provide one-on-one companionship. (Photo courtesy of Roper Hospital, Charleston, SC)

often remind the older person of pets they had in the past, thus eliciting pleasant memories and comfort.

Long-term care facilities are using resident pets to allow residents to care for and interact with them, giving the resident a sense of responsibility and promoting self-esteem in individuals who believe that no one needs them. Dogs and cats as well as fish, birds, guinea pigs, turtles, and even rabbits (wearing rubber pants) make good resident pets.

Pets living in the home of an older adult can sometimes present some health risks. For example, for a person with failing sight, there is the danger of tripping over a cat or dog and falling. A solution might be to place a bell on the pet to signal its whereabouts to warn the elderly person.

The nurse can help in selecting the appropriate pet for the needs and abilities of the individual or group. The needs of both the individual and the pet should be considered. The following are some helpful guidelines to assess for pet therapy:

- For frail older adults, make sure the animal is calm, good-natured, gentle, and nonthreatening.
- If the person has had a pet in the past, choose the same sort of pet to which he or she can relate and recall pleasant memories.
- If the person is frail, have cats declawed.
- Assess for any possible safety considerations, for example, tripping, over the pet.
- Assess the individual's ability to adequately care for a pet, such as financial resources to support the pet, ability to transport the animal to the veterinarian when sick or needing shots, ability to feed and groom the animal, and ability to keep the pet area clean.
- Plan for who will care for the animal in case of a patient's future illness or inability to care for the pet. Many older pet owners fear what will happen to their pets if they go to the hospital or die—a source of stress and worry to them. Appropriate pet care plans can relieve this fear and allow them to benefit fully from pet therapy.

If well planned, pet therapy can be quite beneficial to those older adults living alone at home or those in acute care or long-term care settings. Dogs have been trained to assist the sight-impaired and the hearing-impaired. Training animals to assist older adults with certain functions they are unable to perform, such as by fetching things for the chairbound individual and opening doors or carrying heavy packages, is currently under study. Pets may be able to be trained to help improve the quality of life for older persons.

Clinical Pearl

Intervention—Pet Therapy: Using volunteer pets at acute care centers and long-term-care centers is extremely valuable and beneficial in drawing patients out and helping them interact. Dressing a large, gentle dog in a bright-colored T-shirt helps patients recognize him as a volunteer pet and also helps control dander and shedding.

REMINISCENCE AND LIFE REVIEW

Remembering the past is a natural thing to do. Butler (1963) suggested the idea of structuring that natural reminiscence into steps and using it as therapy. He reasoned that reminiscence did not signal the onset of senility, as some people believed, but that it helped a person to see how all of life fit together. Reminiscence seems to help integrate one's sense of self and make life more meaningful.

LIFE REVIEW

Life review provides structure for the reminiscence process. Developed to a large extent by nurses (Haight, 1991), life review divides one's remembering into the stages of life from earliest memories to the present (Table 20-2). Life review differs from spontaneous remembering because each stage of life must be remembered, remembering painful episodes as well as pleasant. The outcome of that work is thought to be less depression, less suicide, greater integration of self, and greater satisfaction with life in general.

Life review can be done in groups or with individuals and is effective in both contexts. The choice of whether to do it with groups or individuals can be made based on individual preference or setting. In groups, people laugh together and cry together, gaining comfort from knowing others have experienced the same things. One person's memories often trigger another's, opening the door for further discussions.

 Clinical Pearl

Planning: Reminiscence is unstructured and fun. It distracts, promotes connectedness, and requires little planning. Be spontaneous and get into the spirit of the moment.

In group life review, the role of the leader is to be sure the group stays focused on the stage of life being discussed. If the task for one session is to discuss adolescence (or middle age, or any other stage), then the group should focus only on that time period. Each stage should be complete before moving to another. The leader also makes sure that each person in the group participates and is able to share thoughts and feelings, whatever they are. The leader should ensure that support is given by the group when sad or unpleasant memories cause discomfort for any members. The leader should not attempt to direct the group beyond these simple rules. Questions should be open-ended, and answers should not be judged as right or wrong. Two people may share the memory of a similar event but remember it differently. Each person's perception, thoughts, and feelings should be accepted and respected as having value and meaning for that individual.

When doing the review with an individual, the same rules apply. Memories should be allowed to direct the conversation within time periods, and the older person should finish the time period before going on to the next stage. All per-

Table 20-2

HAIGHT'S LIFE REVIEW AND EXPERIENCING FORM

Childhood

1. What is the very first thing you can remember in your life? Go as far back as you can.
2. What other things can you remember about when you were very young?
3. What was life like for you as a child?
4. What were your parents like? What were their weaknesses, strengths?
5. Did you have any brothers or sisters? Tell me what each was like.
6. Did someone close to you die when you were growing up?
7. Did someone important to you go away?
8. Do you ever remember being very sick?
9. Do you remember having an accident?
10. Do you remember being in a very dangerous situation?
11. Was there anything that was important to you that was lost or destroyed?
12. Was church a large part of your life?
13. Did you enjoy being a boy/girl?

Adolescence

1. When you think about yourself and your life as a teenager, what is the first thing you can remember about that time?
2. What other things stand out in your memory about being a teenager?
3. Who were the important people for you? Tell me about them. Parents, brothers, sisters, friends, teachers, those you were especially close to, those you admired, those you wanted to be like.
4. Did you attend church and youth groups?
5. Did you go to school? What was the meaning for you?
6. Did you work during these years?
7. Tell me of any hardships you experienced at this time.
8. Do you remember feeling that there wasn't enough food or necessities of life as a child or adolescent?
9. Do you remember feeling left alone, abandoned, not having enough love or care as a child or adolescent?
10. What were the pleasant things about your adolescence?
11. What was the most unpleasant thing about your adolescence?
12. All things considered, would you say you were happy or unhappy as a teenager?
13. Do you remember your first attraction to another person?
14. How did you feel about sexual activities and your own sexual identity?

Family and Home

1. How did your parents get along?
2. How did other people in your home get along?
3. What was the atmosphere in your home?
4. Where you punished as a child? For what? Who did the punishing? Who was "boss"?
5. When you wanted something from your parents, how did you go about getting it?
6. What kind of person did your parents like the most? The least?

(continued)

Table 20-2

HAIGHT'S LIFE REVIEW AND EXPERIENCING FORM (Continued)

7. Who were you closest to in your family?
8. Who in your family were you most like? In what way?

Adulthood

1. What place did religion play in your life?
2. Now I'd like to talk to you about your life as an adult, starting when you were in your 20s up to today. Tell me about the most important events that happened in your adulthood.
3. What was life like for you in your 20s and 30s?
4. What kind of person were you? What did you enjoy?
5. Tell me about your work. Did you enjoy your work? Did you earn an adequate living? Did you work hard during those years? Were you appreciated?
6. Did you form significant relationships with other people?
7. Did you marry?
   (yes) What kind of person was your spouse?
   (no)   Why not?
8. Do you think marriages get better or worse over time? Were you married more than once?
9. On the whole, would you say you had a happy or unhappy marriage?
10. Was sexual intimacy important to you?
11. What were some of the main difficulties you encountered during your adult years?
    a. Did someone close to you die? Go away?
    b. Were you ever sick? Have an accident?
    c. Did you move often? Change jobs?
    d. Did you ever feel alone? Abandoned?
    e. Did you ever feel need?

Summary

1. On the whole, what kind of life do you think you've had?
2. If everything were to be the same, would you like to live your life over again?
3. If you were going to live your life over again, what would you change? Leave unchanged?
4. We've been talking about your life for quite some time now. Let's discuss your overall feelings and ideas about your life. What would you say the main satisfactions in your life have been? Try for three. Why were they satisfying?
5. Everyone has had disappointments. What have been the main disappointments in your life?
6. What was the hardest thing you had to face in your life? Please describe it.
7. What was the happiest period of your life? What about it made it the happiest period? Why is your life less happy now?
8. What was the unhappiest period of your life? Why is your life more happy now?
9. What was the proudest moment in your life?
10. If you could stay the same age all your life, what age would you choose? Why?
11. How do you think you've made out in life? Better or worse than what you hoped for?

(continued)

Table 20-2	**HAIGHT'S LIFE REVIEW AND EXPERIENCING FORM** *(Continued)*

12. Let's talk a little about you as you are now. What are the best things about the age you are now?
13. What are the worst things about being the age you are now?
14. What are the most important things to you in your life today?
15. What do you hope will happen to you as you grow older?
16. What do you fear will happen to you as you grow older?
17. Have you enjoyed participating in this review of your life?

NOTE: Derived from new questions and two unpublished dissertations:

Gorney, J. (1968). *Experiencing and Age: Patterns of Reminiscence Among the Elderly.* (Unpublished Doctoral Dissertation, University of Chicago).

Falk, J. (1969). *The Organization of Remembered Life Experience of Older People: Its Relation to Anticipated Stress, to Subsequent Adaptation and to Age.* (Unpublished Doctoral Dissertation, University of Chicago).

(© 1982 Barbara K. Haight, RNC, Dr.PH., Professor of Nursing College of Nursing, Medical University of South Carolina, Charleston, SC 29425–2404)

ceptions and feelings should be accepted and respected by the leader. Specific steps to be used in conducting a life review are listed in the Patient Teaching Box.

SELF-TRANSCENDENCE

Self-transcendence is one of the most important components of spiritual care for the older person. Self-transcendence is characterized by "an expansion of self-boundaries and an orientation toward broadened life perspectives and purposes" (Reed, 1991). Coward (1991) expanded on this idea, showing that all people facing personal tragedy, like diagnosis of a fatal illness, were often able to move beyond self-concern, without devaluing the self, and find a new and important meaning in life. This meaning included greater connection with

Patient Teaching Box
LIFE REVIEW

Instruct the patient in the following principles of life review:

1. Life review involves work for at least eight sessions, meeting at a regular place and time each session.
2. All memories can be shared and may not be the same as another person's; all memories and feelings are meaningful and important.
3. Each stage of life is important and will be discussed separately, including childhood; adolescence; family and home; adulthood; and a summary of life to date.*
4. Some memories will be sad, but it is appropriate to cry, grieve, get angry or thoughtful during some life review sessions.

*See Haight's Life Review and Experiencing Form (Table 20-2) others and with the universe. Reed (1991) identified self-transcendence as a characteristic of healthy aging. Reed believed that the older person expands the sense of self inwardly by introspective experiences; outwardly by reaching out to others; and temporally by integrating the present with the past and with one's perception of the future.

The nurse can help the patient grow through introspective experiences in a number of ways. Ensuring access to the patient's preferred religious services and practices is one way. Meditation, self-reflection, journal keeping, and life review all help the patient to know himself or herself better. Some of these techniques, like successful life review, also help a person reach out temporally, realizing a place in history and a having a hand on the future.

Meditation and/or prayer are examples of introspective experiences, a transcendence from self to something larger than self, toward God or the universe. People meditate to touch something within themselves that they are only dimly aware of at other times. Meditation is a discipline which, according to LeShan (1974), helps us discover our fullest "humanhood." Prayer is a meditation, or discipline, which unites one's humanhood with the divine.

Nurses are seldom asked to teach an older adult or any other patient how to meditate or pray, but nurses should always respect the individual's need for time and privacy to do so. The nurse who is asked by a patient to join in on a prayer and feels comfortable doing so may not only give emotional support to that person in his or her own transcendent experience, but also may strengthen the nurse–patient relationship and a sense of trust.

Visualization or imagery is used throughout life for relaxation, pain management, stress management, and for improving coping skills. Visualization can be used to move from self toward other people. It is also a technique that can be taught to older adults individually or in groups. General guidelines for using imagery as well as a variety of relaxation formats include the following:

- Create a quiet, pleasant environment.
- Use some form of relaxation exercises before starting the specific imagery.
- Use images that are familiar to the older adult.
- Use images that incorporate all of the senses.

When using imagery as an intervention to help older adults achieve a sense of transcendence, two specific goals can be considered. One goal of imagery is to support the positive effects of reminiscence; another is to provide comfort near the time of death.

Using visualization with reminiscence, a group of older adults can be led to remember positive experiences with other people, to reconnect with a sense of being with a part of a group, to feel less alone, and to develop a stronger sense of identity. The group decides on an experience that is common to all members. All five senses should be incorporated into the image created. The leader (usually the nurse) reads a script prepared ahead of time. The session starts with a relaxation exercise that the group has practiced. The nurse uses knowledge of the needs of the aged and the culture as well as intuition and creativity to write a script that is relevant and promotes a sense of reaching beyond self to touch those in the past and present.

Similar principles involve the use of imagery to comfort the dying. A nurse who is experienced in the care of the dying and is sensitive to their needs may help a patient to imagine what death is like and what must be done to prepare appropriately for it (Zahourek, 1988). Patients may use imagery to rehearse talking to their families about their feelings of death. Helping the dying to communicate with families is one of the most important and rewarding responsibilities of the nurse.

The older adult is not the only person who experiences or works toward transcendence. Anyone who is experiencing end-of-life issues may find himself or herself working on the task of broadening life perspectives and purposes. Such perspectives include developing a sense of connectedness with the past and the future as well as with people in the immediate surroundings.

REFERENCES

Butler, R. N. (1963). The life review: An interpretation of reminiscence in the aged. *Psychiatry, 26,* 65–76.

Coward, D. D. (1991). Self-transcendence and emotional well-being in women with breast cancer. *Oncology Nursing Forum, 19*(5), 857–863.

Dossey, B. M. (1988). The psychophysiology of body/mind healing. *Holistic nursing: A handbook for practice.* Rockville, MD: Aspen.

Gueldner, S. H., & Bramlett, M. H. (1994). Influences of behavior and age on the immune system. Lecture at Seminar on Aging, sponsored by the Georgia Consortium on Psychology of Aging, University of Georgia, Athens, GA, Nov. 4, 1994.

Haight, B. K. (1991). Reminiscing: The state of the art as a basis for practice. *International Journal of Aging and Human Development, 33*(1), 1–32.

Helm, J. (1985), Can you grab a star? In N. Weisberg & R. Wilder (Eds.), *Creative arts with older adults: A sourcebook.* New York: Human Sciences Press.

Houldin, A. D., Lev, E., Prystowsky, M. B., Redei, E., & Lowery, B. (1991). Psychoneuroimmunology: A review of the literature. *Holistic Nursing Practice, 5*(4), 16.

Hynes, A. M., & Hynes-Berry, M. (1986). *Bibliotherapy—The interactive process: A handbook.* Boulder, CO: Westview.

LeShan, L. (1974). *How to meditate.* Toronto: Bantam.

Miller, M. (1991), Factors promoting wellness in the aged person: An ethnographic study. *Advances in Nursing Science, 13*(4), 38–51.

Randall, T. (1991). Music not only has charms to soothe. *Journal of the American Medical Association, 266*(10), 1323–134l.

Reed, P. (1991). Toward a nursing theory of self-transcendence: Deductive reformulation using developmental theories. *Advances in Nursing Science, 3*(4), 64–77.

Ryan, J. E. (1991). Building theory for gerontological nursing. In E. M. Baines (Ed.), *Perspectives on gerontological nursing,* Newbury Park: Sage, 29–40.

Swift, J. (1985). Gulliver's travels. New York: Modern Library.

Zahourek, R. P. (1988). *Relaxation and imagery: Tools for therapeutic communication and intervention.* Philadelphia: W. B. Saunders.

BIBLIOGRAPHY

Burnside, I., & Haight, B. (1994). Reminiscence and the life review: Therapeutic interventions for older people. *Nurse Practitioner, 19*(4), 55–61.

Dennis, P. (1991). Components of spiritual nursing care from the nurse's perspective. *Journal of Holistic Nursing, 9*(1), 33.

Olson, M. (1991). Expanded dimensions of nursing care for the older adult. *Nursing update: The older adult.* Raleigh, NC: North Carolina Nurses Association.

21

Problems Associated With Behaviors

Objectives

1. Identify normal aging behaviors.
2. Identify abnormal behaviors.
3. Develop assessment strategies to deal with older adults with behavioral problems.
4. Design nursing interventions to meet the emotional needs of older adults with behavioral problems.

INTRODUCTION

PROBLEM BEHAVIOR IS ONE OF THE MOST important and perhaps one of the most poorly understood areas encountered in the care of the older adult. Behavior is any observable, recordable, and measurable act, movement, or response of an individual. In short, behavior is everything a person does. A nonspecific symptom can develop into a primary physical illness or a behavior disorder. Abnormal behaviors may be a source of anxiety and stress for the caregivers as well as for the older adult, directly affecting the quality of the older adult's life, frustrating the efforts of caregivers, and affecting discussions about institutional placement.

PHYSIOLOGIC CHANGES AFFECTING BEHAVIOR

Normal changes that can interfere with behavior and functioning include receiving messages from the sensory organs, altered by losses in hearing and vision; changes in integrating messages, altered by decreased cerebral blood flow and decreased rate of conduction between neurons; and changes in the sending of messages to the sensory effector neurons, altered by nerve cell loss.

Staab, AS and Hodges, LC: ESSENTIALS OF GERONTOLOGICAL NURSING,
© 1996 J. B. Lippincott Company

Physical decline and the need to conserve energy may cause the older adult to express emotion more subtly.

ABNORMAL CHANGES

All behavior reflects human need states and is present to some degree in every individual. The behaviors are not a problem unless they occur in the extreme. A behavior becomes extreme as the need that generates it becomes more pressing (Billings, 1991). Some of the abnormal behaviors found in older adults include anxiety, sounding or repetitive babble, aggressive behavior, and wandering.

Sounding. Sounding is incoherent or repetitive speech that is an expressive process that occasionally accompanies aging. It is frequently seen as meaningless babble and often occurs when meaningful communication has been interrupted.

Sounding can serve several purposes for older adults:

• Reaffirming their presence
• Testing how people respond to their needs
• Discharging pent-up tension
• Providing self-stimulation
• Establishing their personal space or territorial boundaries

Aggressive Behavior. Agitation, diminished sleep, increased energy, increased irritability, angry outbursts, and paranoid ideation may predominate the older adult's clinical picture. As the level of anxiety increases, mental capacities become overworked, are paralyzed, and decompensate. Anxious, aggressive behavior is manifested as agitated behavior, such as constant moaning, wringing of the hands, continuous pacing, acting uncooperative, and being demanding. Verbal and physical aggression are symptomatic ways of attempting to handle stress or a potentially maladaptive effort to overcome feelings of helplessness and powerlessness. Restoration of a sense of autonomy and personal control is essential.

Wandering. Wandering is a tendency to move about either in a seemingly disoriented fashion or in pursuit of an unobtainable goal. This becomes a problem for families and institutions who have a moral and legal obligation for the older adult's safety. Wandering is often an avoidance behavior in response to stress. Wanderers move about more than other older adults, spend more time screaming or calling out, spend less time in social behaviors, and are generally disoriented. The wandering may be goal directed, such that the person searches for someone or something or calls out repeatedly. Goal-directed, industrious behavior is such that the wandering represents the individual's need to recapture a sense of security and belonging by searching for situations that bring comfort.

PSYCHOSOCIAL ISSUES AFFECTING BEHAVIOR

The losses of aging can result in self-destructive behavior, such as refusing to eat, refusing medication, and not taking care of one's physical needs. These behaviors may be interpreted as being stubborn, cantankerous, or confused.

Neglect of physical needs could be viewed as forgetfulness or carelessness. Sensory deprivation from living alone or social isolation can lead to loss of mental function and personality disintegration. Cognitive appraisal of the older adult's self and life situation is important, because negativism can result in depression and anxiety. The losses inherent in aging can result in a decreased perception of control over life and an inability to improve the situation.

NURSING ASSESSMENT

It is often difficult to assess behaviors in older adults who are anxious, defensive, or confused. There may be no reliable source of information. If a supporter or caregiver is available, he or she should be included in the interview. The assessment information should be comprehensive, multidisciplined, and aimed at conclusions about what is causing the problem and what interventions would be helpful. It is important to remember that older adults are sensitive to fatigue, boredom, medications, and environmental influences, which can affect their mental status.

HISTORY AND INTERVIEW

All data should be gathered in a milieu that is free of distraction. The nurse needs to establish a supportive and trusting relationship. Patience and attentive listening promote a sense of security. Placing the older adult in a situation that interferes with an already compromised sensory apparatus only heightens his or her anxiety and compromises the nurse's ability to accurately assess the behavior. The nurse should ask questions regarding all past and present medical conditions and any changes in health status.

Some areas to question include:

- Sensory impairments to judge presence of deprivation and distortion
- Diet history, with particular attention to hydration, because dehydration can cause confused behavior
- Falls that may have resulted in head trauma
- Medication use, especially sedative and hypnotics, with an awareness of toxicities and adverse reactions
- Alcohol consumption, because alcohol is a central nervous system depressant, and intoxication may mimic behaviors similar to dementia

The history should include an assessment of cognitive functions, including memory, reasoning, abstractions, calculations, and judgment. Psychological history and family history may reveal coping styles, level of intimacy, family expectations, and family's perceptions of the older adult. Give examples of the patient's behavior and, when appropriate, use direct quotations to substantiate inferences and to present a vivid picture. The history should include:

- Overall mood, affect, and response to the interview
- Impressions of interactions with family and others
- Coping skills and defenses used by the patient
- Educational level and cultural factors
- Speech, thought continuity, impulse control, and frustration tolerance

If wandering behavior is suspected, the following questions should be considered:

- Does the person have a pattern or route of wandering?
- Is it searching behavior combined with calling out or looking for an unobtainable person or goal? For example, is the person searching for a pet or dead spouse?
- Is it searching behavior directed toward an obtainable but lost object? For example, is the person looking for dentures or clothing?
- Is it apparently non–goal directed, characterized by multiple goals and aimlessness or a poor attention span?
- Is it the result of a lifelong pattern of coping with stress, as in walking or running away from stress?
- Is it related to previous work roles, such as mail carrier or security guard?
- Is the person fearful or anxious and searching for security?
- What is the timing of the wandering? Is it seasonal or at a particular time of the day?
- What is the person's affect and behavior during the wandering?

Objective data regarding the person's psychological and emotional status include the nurse's impressions from the content and process aspects of the interview. These include descriptions of the person's overall mood, affect, and responses; impressions of interactions with family; evaluation of coping skills and defenses used by the patient; insight into illness; and observance of speech and frustration tolerance.

PHYSICAL EXAMINATION

The physical examination should be aimed at level of self-care or a functional assessment. Besides weight and vital signs, the examination should include a description of the physical appearance of the person. The loss of mobility and independence are real fears that may be underlying factors for abnormal behaviors. Special attention to a complete neurologic exam and thorough medical workup will help to rule out disease processes and may yield answers to some behavioral problems. Abnormal behavior may precipitate the need for nutritional evaluation, because some problems may involve need for assistance in eating or monitoring of nutritional intake. A psychiatric consultation may be helpful to evaluate for possible functional illness.

DIAGNOSTIC TESTS

Diagnostic tests to discern the possibility of disease underlying the behavior should include a standard diagnostic laboratory screen, including blood chemistries, thyroid studies, urinalysis, and a chest x-ray. The dexamethasone suppression test may be useful in identifying major depression in persons with early and/or mild to moderate dementia (Albert, 1994). An electrocardiogram reviewed for arrhythmias or heart disease and serum drug levels may be helpful in determining the underlying cause, especially if the patient is receiving digoxin, theophylline, or benzodiazepine. A computed tomography scan and electroencephalogram may demonstrate cerebral atrophy or other brain disease. A serologic test for syphilis, B_{12}, and folate levels should be included.

NURSING DIAGNOSES

The nursing diagnosis is the culmination of data collected about the older adult's behaviors. Behavioral interpretations help the nurse intervene in dysfunctional or disruptive processes. Some possible nursing diagnoses of behavioral problems include:

- Self-concept Disturbance related to the aging process
- Altered Thought Processes related to medication
- Powerlessness related to feelings of loss of control
- High Risk for Violence related to anger and frustration
- Impaired Social Interaction related to behavioral problem

NURSING INTERVENTIONS

Nursing interventions should build on the older adult's strengths and not encourage disability. Effectiveness of the interventions is related to the extent to which needed changes are incorporated into the older adult's long-established life patterns. Older adults often have the self-awareness to assess changes in their sense of well-being. Nursing interventions should be geared toward minimizing the loss of self-care capacity and supporting cognition, returning the older adult to the previous or the highest possible level of functioning.

 Clinical Pearl

Intervention: Encourage older adults to be involved in their own care, because the more independent a person is, the more his or her self-esteem will be enhanced.

In treating behavioral illnesses, such as dementia, no treatment is available for the underlying disease, so treatment is aimed at the symptoms. The nurse must identify specific behaviors and target them for intervention, which is best accomplished by assessing the older adult, attempting to find the solution to the situation, and using a trial-and-error approach. Change may be accomplished through behavioral interventions, such as weekly activity schedules, graded task assignments, and logs of mastery or pleasures. Behavior modification is possible by manipulating environmental cues prompting the behavior or environmental consequences and reinforcing its occurrence. The nurse must forget the behavior and analyze the antecedents and consequences that normally occur in an attempt to increase the occurrence of the desired behavior. If increased social interaction is desired, the interventions can include living environment modifications, such as rearrangement of furniture; reminders of social activities; and refreshments for reinforcement of social interaction in the past. The frequency of inappropriate behavior, such as wandering, can be decreased by using colored symbols that have been paired with noxious noises to mark areas in the institution the patients should not enter. New behaviors can be shaped, including coping strategies for sleep disturbances, increasing social interactions of those institutionalized patients who feed themselves, or teaching staff to acknowledge appropriate verbalization and to ignore inappropriate statements or shouting behaviors.

Pharmacotherapy generally is indicated only when symptoms are at least moderately severe. Some behaviors are not amenable to medication therapy and should be treated by environmental manipulation. For example, wandering, shouting, and touching are best addressed by identifying precipitating factors, reducing stress, and distracting the patient. Attempts to suppress such behaviors with medication may result in oversedation, immobility, falls, and decreased cognition. Reality orientation, validation therapy, relaxation therapy, resocialization, reminiscent therapy, and pet therapy are some of the methods used for older adults.

REALITY ORIENTATION

Reality orientation is a behavioral approach that attempts to increase awareness of time, place, and person in severely impaired patients who have short attention spans and who need verbal and visual stimulation. It may be very effective in some conditions but can be frustrating and ineffective in cases of dementia. The two basic approaches used are 24-hour reality orientation and classroom reality orientation. In 24-hour reality orientation, everyone who comes in contact with the confused older adult acts as a team in trying to help orient the patient by providing truthful, timely information. Many times it is used in conjunction with activities and physical or occupational therapy. The person may attend structured reality orientation classes alone or in conjunction with reality orientation. Classroom structured reality orientation involves small group sessions with the goal of reducing the person's confusion. The environment reinforces contact with reality and with the present and is kept simple and focused. Effectiveness of treatment is evaluated by the person's ability to state time, place, and date.

VALIDATION THERAPY

Proponents of validation therapy believe that disoriented behavior is not meaningless and that continually correcting it systematically neglects the true meaning of the confused behavior (Feil, 1982). The neglect is perceived by the patient and increases anxiety and isolation. For example, if an institutionalized person still thinks he or she is at home, then he or she may become upset when a reality orientation program is aimed at removing that belief. Validation therapy involves searching for the meaning of and emotion behind the patient's words and validating these verbally with the patient. A series of verbal cues or steps are involved that allow the patient to simply focus on key words or phrases in the confused interaction, and the nurse validates the patient by asking for description, more detail, or clarification.

RESOCIALIZATION

Resocialization incorporates techniques for facilitating socialization and group interaction. The group creates unity and a sense of belonging through touching and joining hands. Friends are kept together, and activities are designed to meet the needs of group members, not the abstract or complicated ideas of an oriented leader.

MILIEU THERAPY

Milieu therapy is the scientific structuring of the environment to promote health, foster individual strengths, and effect personal growth. Behavioral principles and group process theory form the major theoretical foundations for constructing a therapeutic milieu. Milieu therapy focuses on interactions and contact with the world. Music, touch, warmth, and sensory stimulation all focus on positive aspects of behavior and downplay the negative aspects.

MEDICATION THERAPY

Medications often can be helpful in the treatment of older adults with such behavioral problems as anxiety, wandering, aggressiveness, and restlessness. Older adults tend to be more sensitive to the side effects of psychotropic drugs, so the potential benefits need to be clear to justify their use. The nurse needs to be aware of any oversedative and anticholinergic effects. Careful administration of these medications could reduce the unwanted consequences of oversedation, orthostatic hypotension, mental deterioration, bowel and bladder dysfunction, and falls leading to hip fractures. The nurse needs to observe the older adult for problems with dressing, personal hygiene, mobility, toileting, and urinary continence.

PATIENT AND FAMILY EDUCATION

Older adults and their families often question the physiologic and cognitive (memory) changes that occur naturally in aging. Some changes that may be interpreted as pathologic include slowed response time, benign memory loss, alterations in gait, and interrupted sleep pattern. Dispelling myths and stereotypes related to the aging process is a primary goal for patient education. Families should be advised to purchase one of the numerous books available commercially that address problems such as agitation, wandering, withdrawal, resistance, insomnia, anorexia, and restlessness. Mealtimes can be especially trying for the older adult with a behavior problem as well as for the caregivers. See the Patient Teaching Box for some helpful hints for mealtime.

Information on the extent of impairment and on community resources helpful for managing these patients can be critically important to families and caregivers. Support groups are available in many cities. Family members should be encouraged to periodically seek respite care so that they can have time for themselves.

Caregivers can be instructed to use activities for older adult patients to decrease isolation and sensory deprivation:

- Use arts and crafts to enhance sight, smell, and texture sensation by using colorful materials and different textures, such as working with colored yarns, hooking rugs, and working with colored clay.
- Use nature walks, hikes, or demonstrations to note different colors and examine differences in animals and plants. Stimulate hearing by having the older adult listen to the sounds of birds, frogs, and insects; stimulate touch by having the older adult feel the textures of plants; stimulate smell by having the older adult smell leaves or flowers; and stimulate taste by having the older adult taste berries.
- Restore social communication by relocating the person or planning visits by members of the team.

Patient Teaching Box
HELPFUL HINTS FOR MAKING MEALTIMES MANAGEABLE

These hints may help create a more pleasant mealtime with the older adult with a behavior problem:

• Provide a calm environment at mealtime.
• Use simple one-step instructions, such as "Pick up your fork," "Raise it to your mouth."
• Repeat instructions when necessary.
• Limit the number of choices the person has to make.
• Put only one utensil and only one food in front of the person at a time.
• Use finger foods.
• Avoid placing condiments on the table until requested, because they may be used inappropriately.
• Use a plate with no design to reduce confusion.
• Try not to keep anything around that may look like food, such as flower bulbs, artificial flowers, or artificial fruit.

• Allow the older adult to have control and to participate in decision making.
• Help increase memory by having the older adult reorganize his or her possessions.
• Assist spiritually and socially by encouraging the older adult to be a foster grandparent, engage in late-life learning, and reminisce or act as a mentor for a younger person.

REDUCING WANDERING

Wandering behavior may be especially hazardous because of its association with falls in the older adult (Gurwitz, Sanchez-Cross, Eckler, & Matulis, 1994). One of the predominant concerns with the problem of wandering is the risk of falls. Falls can be a result of fatigue, as many occur in the early evening hours, or may be related to the adverse effects of tranquilizers, sedatives, diuretics, or hypotensive agents (Blixen, 1989). One remedy has been to restrain the patient, either chemically or mechanically, to maintain safety. Although this approach may reassure the caregiver, it is believed to increase the risk for cognitive impairment and further psychological, if not physical, deterioration. Common treatment for wandering is to institutionalize the older adult or to manage wandering with the use of medications, door locks, geri-chairs, and other restraints. However, these actions may produce or even exacerbate wandering behavior. Restraints may increase hostility as well as decrease security, orientation, and stimulation. Rehabilitation approaches should include efforts to orient the person and to provide a schedule of physical and social activities that is carried out consistently.

Nurses need to observe the patient carefully to identify the situations that contribute to wandering behavior. Actual mapping of the behavior might be helpful. Interventions should be tailored to the mood of the wanderer. If wandering meets the needs for attention, efforts to control the behavior may actually reinforce it. Placid wanderers may be bored or may be repeating a real or imagined activity and need to be approached casually and perhaps channeled into a less disturbing behavior.

Some people are extremely sensitive to stress and tension in the environment. Agitated wanderers may be releasing frustration and tension through motor activity. They need to be listened to, kept at a distance from the caregiver to keep the patient from hitting, and given outlets for their aggression. Happy wanderers may be exploring and need to be left alone but watched or taken on "guided tours." In general, wandering decreases if a regimen of exercise, walking, or getting outside is established. Persons with potential wandering behavior should be given a special identification bracelet listing their name and a phone number to call if they become lost. Concrete, simple, exact instructions done in a calm tone of voice should be taught to all caregivers to be used in patient care.

ENVIRONMENTAL STRUCTURING

Environmental structuring helps promote cognitive functioning. The use of familiar objects from home, such as a rocking chair, photos, or favorite slippers help to orient the patient and decrease untoward behaviors. Easily read clocks, orientation boards, and a consistent daily routine help orient the patient. To allay anxiety, arguing with the patient about verbal discrepancies should be avoided. Rather, the patient should be directed toward areas of interest that are familiar and pleasurable. If the patient uses confabulation to fill in a memory gap, it should be noted, and reality-based conversation should continue. The nurse should give the patient direction without giving choices, since the patient is unable to choose. For example, it is more appropriate to say "Brush your teeth" than to say "Do you want to brush your teeth?" The nurse should always call the patient by name, approach the patient so that he or she can see the nurse clearly, give simple directions, and refrain from touching the patient.

Restlessness and wandering can be dealt with by allowing the patient with dementia to wander in a closed milieu. Crowds or large open spaces without boundaries should be avoided. If the patient is disorganized at night, the room should be well lit (a night-light works well) and without shadows. Environmental design can be used to camouflage doorways or to incorporate distractions.

REDUCING AGITATION

Agitation can occur if the older adult is rushed to do something unfamiliar or unclear. Explanations of expectations should be clear, complete, and concise. Choices should be offered only if the patient can make them. An individual daily schedule of activities that the patient has helped to plan can be used. If a patient refuses to participate in an activity, continued insistence usually increases agitation, and sometimes the loss of behavioral control can cause a catastrophic response. The best approach is to wait a few minutes and then return to see if the patient will agree to the request. If the person becomes agitated and cannot be calmed, a change of subject or a sign of friendship, such as a smile or a handshake, is often effective.

REDUCING AGGRESSION

The caregivers should make a conscious effort not to react negatively to the patient's hostility. Helping the older adult to express anger in a socially acceptable way prevents anger from building. It is important to anticipate the patient's demands, support a sense of autonomy, and give the person an opportunity to participate in the planning of care. Because anxiety is felt empathetically and communicated interpersonally, the caregiver will need to address his or her own level of anxiety to reduce the spiraling effect of tension.

Anger displayed toward the nurse may not be meant for the nurse. It can reflect a misunderstanding of a situation or simply the patient's justifiable frustration with his or her disabilities or memory losses. Irritability and belligerence may be a sign of physical pain. Ask the person if he or she is experiencing pain; be aware of the nonverbal signs of pain. Keep in mind that inappropriate or annoying behavior is usually unintentional. Often patients simply do not remember what is expected of them or may be frustrated with their own disabilities. Try not to let your anger show and avoid explanations or arguments, because the memory-impaired person may be frustrated by his or her misunderstanding of the situation. A belligerent attitude may be a patient's defense against negative feelings about himself or herself. A warm, positive, accepting approach indicates that you accept the person for who they are. A doll or stuffed animal may be effective in calming or soothing the older adult with dementia.

Different approaches for handling hostile or demanding behavior may work at different times:

- Sometimes, ignoring demands is the best approach.
- If you simplify the task rather than demand that the patient perform it as is, the patient may be able to do it.
- Saying "no" calmly and firmly and then redirecting the resident's attention may diffuse a tense situation.
- Take the person to a quiet room, have a drink of tea or coffee, or go for a walk.

If the person becomes violent, call for assistance and protect yourself. Remove anything that may be used as a weapon, and call emergency numbers if needed.

Some shouting and acting out may be a result of paranoia or hallucinations, which require antipsychotic medications. Isolation keeps older adults from a stimulating environment that connects them to reality, so caregivers need to demonstrate understanding, encouragement, and social support to help the older adult build trust.

Nursing Care Plan

FOR A PATIENT WITH ABNORMAL BEHAVIOR

Nursing Diagnosis: Impaired Social Interaction, related to unmet security and personal contact needs.

Definition: Diminished social functioning or unacceptable social functioning due to unmet security and social needs causing noisy or wandering behavior.

Assessment Findings:
1. Calling out
2. Crying and wailing

(continued)

Nursing Care Plan

FOR A PATIENT WITH ABNORMAL BEHAVIOR *(Continued)*

  3. Screaming for long periods of time
  4. Repetitive rambling
  5. Lack of interest in surroundings
  6. Wandering

Nursing Interventions with Selected Rationales:

  1. Schedule time with the older adult in short, frequent blocks.
     Rationale: Scheduled, short time periods to offer reality orientation and to assure the older adult that he or she will have human contact.
  2. Have family and/or staff on a planned schedule of interaction time.
     Rationale: This planned time ensures patient contact but spreads it so that one person does not get overloaded and increases the quantity and variety of interaction opportunities.
  3. If patient is institutionalized, encourage family contact and visitors, such as friends, chaplain, and staff.
     Rationale: These visits and contacts increase interactive situations for the patient and may reduce the restlessness and agitation secondary to dementia.
  4. Include the patient on trips and take outdoors whenever possible.
     Rationale: These are attempts at distraction. Increased social interaction will provide distraction therapy, thereby limiting time spent alone.
  5. Keep patient physically active.
     Rationale: Wanderers tend to be people who handle stress by being physically active.
  6. Attempt to find reasons for the abnormal behavior.
     Rationale: Wandering or shouting may be a purposeful behavior, such as calling for a real or imagined person or looking for a toilet.
  7. Keep the patient in view of the staff or in a safe, confined area to protect him or her from harm or hazards, such as swimming pools, stairways, balconies, or highway traffic. Place locks on gates and electronic buzzers or chimes on doors, or place a pressure-sensitive mat at the door or person's bedside.
     Rationale: Wanderers may be regressing to a more childlike state and need a more protective, observant environment.
  8. Educate local police and neighbors as to what process to follow if they find the person wandering. Have a current photograph and physical description of the person available. Offer suggestions about where the police might find the older adult, such as in old neighborhoods, former workplaces, or favorite places.
     Rationale: These actions will facilitate assistance if others find the person wandering away from home.

Patient Outcomes/Discharge Criteria:

  1. The older adult will respond to social contacts, and noisy behavior will stop or decrease within an acceptable range.
  2. The patient and/or family will have increased and more socially acceptable interactions with each other.
  3. The family and/or staff will be more willing to care for the older adult.

REFERENCES

Albert, M. S. (1994). Cognition and aging. In W. R. Hazzard, E. L. Bierman, J. P. Blass, W. H. Ettinger, & J. B. Halter (Eds.), *Principles of geriatric medicine and gerontology* (3rd ed.). New York: McGraw-Hill.

Billings, C. (1991). Nursing strategies: Managing extreme behaviors. In *Nursing update: The older adult*. Raleigh, NC: North Carolina Nurses Association.

Blixen, C. E. (1989). Aging and mental health care. *Journal of Gerontological Nursing, 14*(11), 11–15.

Feil, N. (1982) *Validation: The Feil method*. Cleveland: Edward Fell Productions.

Gurwitz, J. H., Sanchez-Cross, M. T., Eckler, M. A., & Matulis, J. (1994). The epidemiology of adverse and unexpected events in the long-term care setting. *Journal of the American Geriatrics Society, 42*(1), 33–38.

BIBLIOGRAPHY

Barry, P. P. (1993). Differentiating confusion delirium or dementia? *Emergency Medicine, April 30*, 96–103.

Beck, C., & Heacock, P. (1988). Nursing intervention for patients with Alzheimer's disease. *Nursing Clinics of North America, 23*(1), 92–124.

Birren, J. E., Sloane, R. B., & Cohen, G. D. (1992). *Handbook of mental health and aging* (2nd ed.). New York: Academic Press.

Blair, D., & New, S. (1991). Assaultive behavior: Know the risks. *Journal of Psychosocial Nursing, 29*(11), 25–30.

Dawson, G. (1987). Wandering. *Gerontologist, 27*(1), 104–110.

Kermis, M. D. (1986). *Mental health in later life*. Boston: Jones and Bartlett.

Kikuta, S. (1991). Clinically managing disruptive behavior on the ward. *Journal of Gerontological Nursing, 17*(82), 4–8.

Negley, E., & Manley, J. (1990). Environmental interventions in assaultive behavior. *Journal of Gerontological Nursing, 16*(37), 29–33.

Rawlins, R. P., Williams, S. R., & Beck, C. K. (1993). *Mental health–psychiatric nursing* (3rd ed.). St. Louis: Mosby–Year Book.

Stolley, J. M. (1994). When your patient has Alzheimer's disease. *American Journal of Nursing, 94*(980), 34–41.

Stuart, G. W., & Sundeen, S. J. (1995). *Principles and practice of psychiatric nursing* (5th ed.). St. Louis: Mosby–Year Book.

Valente, S. M. (1994). Recognizing depression in elderly patients. *American Journal of Nursing, 94*(12), 19–24.

Weick, M. D. (1992). Physical restraints: An FDA update. *American Journal of Nursing, 92*(11), 74–80.

Wilson, H. S., & Kneil, C. R. (1992). *Psychiatric nursing* (4th ed.). Redwood City, CA: Addison-Wesley.

22

Problems With Cognition

Objectives

1. Describe physiologic and psychological changes of aging that may affect cognition.
2. Differentiate abnormal changes in cognition from normal age-related changes.
3. Describe the components of a comprehensive assessment of cognitive function in the older adult.
4. List common causes of cognitive impairment in the older adult.
5. Compare and contrast etiology, behaviors, and treatment of dementia, depression, and delirium.
6. List potential nursing diagnoses for the older adult experiencing dementia, depression, or delirium.
7. Discuss desirable nursing interventions for older adults experiencing problems with cognition.

INTRODUCTION

COGNITIVE FUNCTION IS ESSENTIAL FOR the older adult to be able to make some sense of the surrounding environment and to respond in appropriate ways to meet daily needs. Cognition refers to the complex mental processes taking place between one's experience of the environment (the stimulus) and one's outwardly observable behavior (the response). These processes include perception of the environment; the ability to remember what is perceived; the ability to reason or think about what has been perceived; the ability to make decisions and to solve problems; and the ability to form complex patterns of information that can be stored as knowledge. Stored knowledge is formed with symbols that represent information and that serve as the basis for language and outward communication. For the older adult to be truly functional, these cognitive processes must all operate at an effective level.

Effective cognitive function requires health of both the perceptual organs and the brain itself. Critical to perception are the senses of hearing and vision and, to a lesser extent, the senses of touch, taste, and smell. Adequate vision and hearing are essential to taking in clues about the environment. Normal brain structures, including neurons, nerve endings, and the cerebral cortex, are required for cognitively processing these clues.

An older adult whose perceptual organs are impaired or whose brain and neurons are damaged, for whatever reason, is likely to experience difficulties with cognition. Impaired cognition can interfere greatly with activities of daily living and put the individual at risk for other health, safety, and interpersonal problems. Recognizing cognitive limitations is essential to helping the patient and family minimize their effects and cope with the related problems for maintenance of optimal function.

PHYSIOLOGIC CHANGES WITH AGING

Overall, cognitive function is not necessarily affected to any great extent by the normal physiologic changes that occur with aging. The normal human brain has far more capacity than is effectively used. Normal aging does lead to a decrease in brain weight and a decrease in the number of neurons, beginning at age 20 and accelerating after age 60 (Brody, 1987). However, in most individuals, this loss is not noticeable in terms of function. There is evidence that some neurons in the cerebral cortex will show dendrite deterioration with aging, thereby decreasing their ability to send and receive messages. There appears to be an increase in the number and thickening of dendrites in other cortical neurons, which may compensate for decreased transmitting ability of those that have deteriorated (Brody, 1987). Unless the deterioration is great or damage occurs in critical areas of the cortex, reasonable cognitive function can continue into advanced years.

It is common for aging persons to experience several cognitive changes, including some difficulty with recent memory, some degree of psychomotor slowing, a decrease in simple reaction time, alteration in mode of problem-solving, production deficiency, and increased cautiousness. These changes may interfere with daily living.

Although everyone forgets things occasionally, as persons age, forgetfulness becomes more noticeable when it occurs more frequently. The forgetfulness associated with normal aging relates to recent memory (the processing and storing of new memories). In contrast, for most older adults, their older, long-held memories generally remain intact.

Psychomotor slowing and a decrease in simple reaction time are normal changes with aging often requiring physical responses, such as driving or avoiding falls when losing balance. In an alert person, awareness of these changes usually allows compensation so that accidents are avoided and the slowness does not significantly interfere with function.

There is evidence that the manner in which older adults solve problems is different from the way younger people solve problems, although the causes for this difference are not always agreed on (Salthouse, 1989). Differences may be related to use of a different problem-solving mode based on developmental aging (such as Piaget's developmental theory extended to older ages) or may reflect an actual decrease in performance.

Increased cautiousness or hesitancy about risk taking has been observed as a common cognitive change with increased age. It may be attributed to slowing of the nervous system and a slower behavioral response when quick responses are normally required or expected, such as driving. This change may put the older adult at risk for safety problems in situations when quick thinking or judgment is needed.

Normal physiologic changes in perceptual organs can greatly affect cognition. When the primary sensory modes of vision or hearing are diminished for whatever reason, the older adult may not obtain sufficient stimulation or information from the environment to maintain effective cognitive function. Misperceptions or understimulation can lead to difficulties with interpersonal relationships, withdrawal, and overall cognitive decline that otherwise could be prevented.

ABNORMAL CHANGES

Although some cognitive change may be considered normal with advancing age and temporary changes in memory, concentration, and thinking considered normal during times of stress, loss, or bereavement, more serious, sudden, or prolonged changes must be considered pathologic. Memory loss (amnesia) progressing in extent or severity is not a normal expectation with aging. If it occurs it should be carefully investigated to determine the possible cause.

Similarly, the noticeable onset of difficulties with learning or problem-solving or a decrease in attention span is a sign that pathologic changes may be occurring. Such symptoms should be monitored and thoroughly investigated.

Agnosia, the inability to recognize objects or nonverbal symbols, is a sign that visual–spatial recall or perception is not operating correctly in the brain. For example, a patient does not recognize a common object, such as a hairbrush, and does not know what to do with it. The development of agnosia indicates pathologic changes in the brain.

Language or communication problems in an older person usually indicate an underlying problem that may also have a pathologic basis in the brain. Anomia is the inability to name common objects correctly. Aphasia has several forms. One form is the inability to express oneself or use intended words. Either anomia or aphasia can interfere with verbal communication. Both are indicative of brain disease and require careful assessment.

Cognitive impairment can be a sign or a result of many, varied disturbances. Some of them are treatable, in which case most symptoms are reversible, whereas others are not and require special care to assist the patient to function as well and as long as possible. Determining the cause of the impairment can be of critical importance to the patient's long-term well-being. Some primary disorders that result in cognitive impairment include anxiety, delirium, depression, and dementia. These disorders can occur independently or together, greatly compounding a patient's inability to function.

Anxiety. Anxiety is a feeling of dread, uneasiness, or distress with no recognizable cause. Anxiety is found in at least two forms: trait anxiety (anxiety in an individual as a relatively stable characteristic that persists over time regardless of the situation) and state anxiety (transitory anxiety that arises in regard to a specific situation). Older people have generally been found to display anxiety in similar ways as do younger people. Therefore, older adults are no more prone to developing anxiety than are younger people; however, they will demonstrate anxiety if they have lived with it throughout their lives. They will also respond with anxiety in given situations.

Anxiety states may be difficult to identify in older adults, because society's expectations have tended to normalize problems with aging. Thus, the older person may actually assume that uncomfortable feelings have to do with growing older and may not complain or may not look for other reasons. Detection of changes in levels of anxiety is therefore vital.

Anxiety interferes with cognitive function because it narrows perception. An individual experiencing anxiety is less able to focus on environmental stimuli and therefore may not take in important information needed for appropriate functioning. It also shortens the attention span and interferes with thinking, logic, and problem-solving. Although a moderate level of anxiety is believed to heighten awareness and the ability to perform, as anxiety persists or increases, it narrows the individual's focus, drains energy, and erodes mental functioning. This is increasingly evident as anxiety escalates.

Delirium. By definition, delirium is an acute state of organic brain dysfunction that is potentially reversible but that can progress into chronic mental dysfunction if not treated. It can be caused by a wide variety of disorders. An individual who displays acute anxiety, is often unable to focus, maintain attention, or think logically, and may develop altered consciousness is described as being in a state of delirium. The key is to determine the presence of symptoms before they progress, identify the cause, and treat the patient according to the cause. Early medical referral is crucial so that thorough medical evaluation, diagnosis, and treatment can be performed in a timely manner.

Depression. Depression in persons older than age 60 is most frequently related to experiencing a major loss, such as retirement, assumption of a major caregiver role (with loss of usual role or normal partner), or the death of a spouse or other loved one. Loss-related depression is often resolved normally without the necessity of treatment, yet it can interfere with cognitive function while it is present, as can depression that arises for other reasons.

An important component of depression among older adults may be a perceived lack of control over their lives or their current situation. Older adults who believe they do not have control to any real extent will usually demonstrate decreased motivation to respond to stimuli or to act for themselves, decreased cognitive function, and signs of depression. This pattern of behavior has sometimes been described as learned helplessness. Perceiving that one has little or no control can lead to giving up or to feeling and then behaving in an increasingly helpless manner. This is more likely to occur when the individual believes his or her own behavior has little or no effect on outcomes.

Dementia. Dementia is a progressive loss of cognitive function characterized by decreased memory, thinking, judgment, and problem-solving. The ability to communicate becomes impaired, and the individual becomes increasingly dependent on others to perform even the simplest tasks of daily living. Although there are a number of causes of dementia, the process is generally considered irreversible once it has progressed to any degree.

The incidence of dementia increases with aging. Therefore, as increasing numbers of people live to older ages, the scope of the problem of caring for persons with dementia is also greatly increasing. It is believed that more than half the population of nursing home residents in the United States has some form of dementia. An even greater number of persons living with dementia are cared for by the family members in the home. Of those persons who have dementia, at least half are believed to have Alzheimer's disease. This dementia is sometimes referred to as dementia of the Alzheimer's type or primary degenerative dementia, the causes of which are still unknown. Approximately 15% of other dementia patients have multiinfarct dementia resulting from repeated cerebrovascular accidents, which leave significant brain damage. The remainder are dementias of mixed type (dementia of the Alzheimer's type and multiinfarct dementia combined), rare types of dementia, and chronic problems that were not successfully treated (postdelirium). For information comparing dementia, depression, and delirium, see Table 22-1.

Table 22-1

COMPARISON OF DEMENTIA, DEPRESSION, AND DELIRIUM

Factor	Dementia	Depression	Delirium
Etiology	Varied: Strokes (multi-infarct dementia [MID]) Unknown (dementia Alzheimers type [DAT]) Genetic or viral factors possible	Varied: Loss Bereavement Hormonal or metabolic disorder Drug reaction Genetic factors	Varied: Tumor Metabolic disorder High fever Drug reaction Acute anxiety Alcohol intoxication Alcohol withdrawal
Onset	Gradual	Gradual or sudden in response to loss or other factors	Acute
Course	Progressive Irreversible	Variable May be chronic and progressive or temporary and reversible	Reversible with treatment or removal of cause
Memory	Recent loss first progressing to remote; eventually lost completely	Intact	Intact
Orientation	Diminished to time, then place, and eventually person, including self	May be dimished with time	Variable but temporary
Attention	Short span Easily distractible	May not be affected	Very short span
Psychomotor speed	Normal or slowed as disease progresses	Slowed	Rapid hyperactive
Energy level	Normal or agitated until late in disease	Minimal energy	Hyperactive May need assistance to avoid fatigue

(continued)

Table 22-1

COMPARISON OF DEMENTIA, DEPRESSION, AND DELIRIUM (Continued)

Factor	Dementia	Depression	Delirium
Language	Aphasia Anomia "Nonsense" talk meaningless to others	No difficulties May not volunteer unless prompted	No difficulties Rapid speech
Hallucinations	Possible or may misinterpret visual cues in environment	None unless psychotically depressed	Common, tend to be visual and tactile, "crawling" sensation
Affect	Emotional lability Apathy or blunting of affect later in disease	Depressed Low self-esteem Guilt-ridden	Anxious May be dulled
Special tests for diagnosis	Mini-Mental State Exam No history of other factors Computerized tomography (CT) scan to rule out other causes	Beck depression inventory (BDI) Geriatric depression scale (GDS) History of loss or depressive episodes	Neurologic exam CT scan History of causative factors
Medical treatment	None known (Experimental drugs to improve memory being tested)	Antidepressants Psychotherapy Electroconvulsive therapy Combination therapy	Antianxiety agents Antipyretics or removal of toxic or other agent based on cause
Desired or possible outcome	Maintain function as long as possible	Return to normal function	Complete recovery, with return to normal function

Abstract problem-solving is strongly diminished (compounded by memory loss), as are learning, concentration, and attention span. The clinical course of dementia is marked by symptoms that compound memory impairment (such as agnosia and anomia), so that the person's performance is even poorer overall. Lacking the ability to make sense of environmental cues or to understand what is going on because the brain itself is deteriorating leaves the person with dementia mystified and even more dependent.

Clinical Pearl

Assessment: Asking a patient to name a common object is useful in assessing the extent and nature of cognitive impairment. An older adult who cannot name a rubberband, but who picks it up and tries to "pop" the nurse with it is able to recognize the object and its use. This patient has anomia, but not agnosia.

PSYCHOSOCIAL ISSUES

As people age, losses tend to occur with increasing frequency. Such losses include spouses, other family members, and peers. Changes in roles, such as retirement from lifelong work, also can be perceived as a loss. Too often, the circumstances of aging can result in perceived lack of control over one's life and one's choices. These changes may affect cognitive function in several ways. Preoccupation with multiple losses or a dissatisfaction with life can cloud perception of the external environment. Either may be a factor in actual depression, which, in turn, is evidenced by slowing of the mental processes that include thinking, decision making, and problem-solving. A vicious cycle involving inadequate stimulation from the environment, slowing of mental processes, decreased receptivity to new stimuli, and further slowing and withdrawal is set in motion. Once begun, this cycle can severely hamper overall cognitive function and limit the effectiveness and quality of daily living.

NURSING ASSESSMENT

Overall cognitive function is best assessed through observation of outward behavior over time. A thorough assessment must include a careful history of the older adult's behavior and observation of current function in relation to activities of daily living. Because the assessment must focus on the patient's perception, thinking processes, and communication, the approach to the patient and manner in which assessment occurs is critical to obtaining accurate and meaningful results. A warm, nonthreatening approach is essential. Providing an environment with minimal distractions will help the patient to focus and perform at an optimal level.

To conduct an assessment of cognitive function, the nurse should follow these steps:

- Arrange a quiet location for the interaction to minimize stimuli and distractions.
- Approach the patient in a calm, direct, unhurried way.
- Tell the patient you will be asking him or her to answer some questions and perform some simple tasks to better understand how he or she is functioning, but that there are no right or wrong answers. The information will be used to better help you plan his or her care.
- Allow a family member to remain with the patient if this seems to be reassuring.
- Ask questions or give directions in a clear, simple manner, using only one question or direction at a time. Allow the patient time to respond. Proceed at a pace comfortable for the patient.
- Repeat questions or directions at least once if necessary. If the patient is still unable to respond or perform the task, proceed to the next item.
- Allow interruption if the patient's anxiety level or lack of concentration requires this. Proceed as the patient is able to tolerate. Discontinue if the patient is unable to concentrate or perform or becomes frustrated.
- When the assessment is completed, reassure the patient that information obtained will help in planning his or her care. Be sure to acknowledge frustration if it has occurred, and provide positive feedback about areas in

which effective functioning was observed. For example, state, "You were able to name all three objects you were shown and were able to write a sentence when asked. This will help me know how to take care of you."

A patient whose attention span is shortened may have some difficulty concentrating, may become easily distracted, or may get up and walk away. Allowing the patient to expend some energy may actually improve the likelihood of completing the assessment and of achieving accurate results. Such interruptions should be handled calmly and matter-of-factly by the nurse. If a patient cannot tolerate the length of time needed for a complete assessment, the most important focus should be on how the patient is functioning at the moment. Family members then can be questioned separately and in more detail about the patient's history and usual patterns of behavior.

HISTORY AND INTERVIEW

A careful history should include a report on normal patterns of behavior and changes in behavior, including information about the times when they occurred. The history needs to include past and current abilities in maintaining activities of daily living, particularly self-care behaviors, such as feeding, toileting, bathing, dressing, grooming, getting in and out of bed, activity levels, and interest and daily pastimes. It is important to ask questions about medication use, alcohol intake, and dietary intake patterns. Analysis of these factors can give important clues about brain function and possible causes of any interference.

Assessment of depression among older adults can be difficult. Depression affects cognitive function, but the precise effects may be difficult to assess, because the same symptoms often occur with other age-related problems, such as dementia. During the history, the nurse should question and be alert to symptoms, including a decreased energy level, psychomotor slowing, disturbance with sleep and/or appetite, and an increase in somatic concerns. Noticeable difficulty in these areas, particularly if they are accompanied by persistent sadness, withdrawal, or a pervasive negative outlook, should be investigated carefully. Symptoms of depression among older adults differ from those of younger adults in that older adults who are depressed tend to report a mood disturbance with less intensity (so that it may be overlooked) and tend to put more emphasis on somatic symptoms.

Assessment of dementia is dependent on observation of a pattern of behavior that develops over time and reveals progressive cognitive decline. Disruption of thought processes becomes pervasive and appears as widespread mental deterioration. Memory impairment is so severe that it alone can impair the older adult's ability to perform any cognitive task. An example commonly observed is the person with dementia who tries to fix a meal. The individual cannot complete such a task because he or she cannot remember the steps to follow from one moment to the next, cannot remember what equipment is needed or where to find it, and cannot recall the intended task in even a very short space of time.

PHYSICAL EXAMINATION

In addition to performing a review of systems, current cognitive function is assessed by observation or measurement of orientation of time, place, and person; of recent and remote memory; of the use of language; and of the ability to solve problems. Comparison of a patient's current function with earlier function can be important to understanding patterns and potential progression of disease.

Mood and affective or emotional state are also important to assess, particularly when attempting to differentiate causative factors for cognitive change. Abnormalities in cognitive function or affective state in the older adult patient should be reported to the physician so that a thorough physical examination that includes a neurologic examination can be performed.

DIAGNOSTIC TESTS

Routine laboratory testing, including serum lab tests, radiography, and nuclear imaging scans, should be performed to rule out a pathophysiologic basis for cognitive problems. Although a physician should perform thorough neurologic testing when any abnormalities are found to persist, the nurse can readily perform an assessment of overall cognitive function to serve as the basis for planning care and initiating referral. A straightforward and simple test that can alert the nurse to abnormalities and/or changes in a patient's cognitive function is the Mini-Mental State Exam (Folstein, Folstein, & McHugh, 1975) (see Display 22-1). This test combines simple questions and simple commands that allow a maximum score of 30 points if all responses are correct. In addition to a score that indicates relative health of cognitive function, responses reveal functional ability or disability in a full range of mental functions, including orientation, registration of information, attention and calculation, recall of information, and use of language. The Mini-Mental State Exam can be administered quickly (in as little as 10 minutes) yet reveals a great deal of important information, making it ideal for use with patients who are potentially cognitively impaired. Comparing a patient's responses over time can assist in identifying whether the patient is improving, maintaining function, or deteriorating progressively. A feeling of success is important to maintain optimal performance. Tests of mental functioning are a threat to persons whose cognitive abilities are already impaired. When assessing cognition, always leave patients with a request they can perform, so that they will be left with a feeling of success rather than frustration or defeat.

Depression may be evaluated in older adults by two commonly used depression rating scales. The Beck Depression Inventory and the Geriatric Depression Scale are self-report symptom checklists that screen for the presence of depression and provide a measure of the severity of depressive symptoms (Spreen & Strauss, 1991). If clinical depression exists in older adults, medical treatment with antidepressant medication or psychotherapy or a combination of the two can be effective in reversing it.

NURSING DIAGNOSES

Nursing diagnosis is the culmination of problems identified from the data collected about the older adult's cognitive function. Some possible nursing diagnoses for older patients with problems with cognitive functioning include:

- Altered Thought Processes related to cognitive impairment secondary to delirium, depression, or dementia

---

Display 22-1

MINI-MENTAL STATE EXAMINATION

Patient _____

Date _____

Maximum Score	Patient Score	
		Orientation
5	_____	What is the (year) (season) (date) (day) (month)?
5	_____	Where are we: (state) (county) (town) (hospital) (unit)?
		Registration
3	_____	Name three objects—1 second to say each. Then ask patient to name all three after you have said them.
		Give 1 point for each correct answer. Then repeat until patient learns all three. Count trials and record. Trials:
		Attention and Calculation
5	_____	Serial 7's. One point for each correctly given. Stop after 5 answers. (Alternative: spell "world" backwards.)
		Recall
3	_____	Ask for three objects repeated above. Give 1 point for each correct answer.
		Language
9	_____	Name a pencil and a watch. (2 points)
		Repeat the following: "No ifs, ands, or buts." (1 point)
		Follow a three-stage command: "Take a paper in your right hand, fold it in half, and put it on the floor. (3 points)
		Read and obey the following: "Close your eyes." (1 point)
		Write a sentence. (1 point)
		Copy design. (1 point)
Total	_____	

The test scores a maximum of 30 items; patients scoring 24 or below are to be considered cognitively abnormal. (From Rabins & Folstein, [1983]. "The dementia patient: Evaluation and care." *Geriatrics*, 38:8.)

- Self-Care Deficit related to cognitive impairment
- Ineffective Individual Coping related to cognitive impairment secondary to delirium, depression, or dementia
- Impaired Verbal Communication related to cognitive impairment secondary to delirium, depression, or dementia
- Sleep Pattern Disturbance related to hyperactivity secondary to delirium (agitation secondary to dementia)
- High Risk for Injury related to cognitive impairment secondary to delirium, depression, or dementia

- Altered Nutrition, Less than Body Requirements related to agitation, withdrawal, and short attention span secondary to delirium, depression, or dementia
- Altered Family Processes related to effects of condition on relationships, role responsibility, and finances secondary to delirium, depression, or dementia
- Impaired Social Interaction related to withdrawal secondary to depression or dementia

NURSING INTERVENTIONS

The older adult experiencing problems with cognition will need empathetic, supportive care. Care should be planned to ensure that basic needs and activities of daily living are fulfilled and safety needs are met without depriving the patient of autonomy and self-esteem. Meeting these criteria presents one of the greatest challenges a nurse can face. It is difficult to empathize with a patient whose mental deterioration makes the surrounding environment virtually incomprehensible. It is difficult to feel or understand what that experience must be like and to avoid the temptation of doing for the patient what the patient seems reluctant, slow, or unable to do for himself or herself. The patient who is cognitively impaired must be allowed and encouraged to perform self-care activities as long as he or she is able.

Clinical Pearl

*Intervention: Perceived control is crucial to mental health. The nurse can foster a sense of control by providing choices for the older adult, even in small areas, such as food or clothing preferences, and by being sure that the patient knows the choice is there and **makes** the choice freely. These are the most critical principles applicable to the care of older adults with cognitive deficits.*

PROTECTIVE MEASURES

Protective measures to maintain both the patient's safety and sense of security must be initiated as soon as possible. The cognitively impaired person may not recognize surroundings or people, may not correctly interpret the use of equipment or objects, and may not be able to reason clearly or use proper judgment. Such persons are therefore at risk in a number of ways. They may wander, become lost, and have difficulty finding the way back. Communication problems compound this risk because of the inability to explain their predicament or ask for help. They are likely to be easily frightened if they are unable to recognize others, especially in unfamiliar surroundings. The use of everyday equipment, including cars, stoves, and even scissors or knives, presents serious safety risks related to failure to recognize their use (in dementia), short attention span, and poor judgment. A car might be left running or a stove left burning because the cognitively impaired person has completely forgotten about it.

Because changes in function can occur very rapidly or slowly (depending on the cause), it is important that an ongoing assessment of the patient's current abilities be made frequently. Doing things *for* the patient can foster unnecessary dependency and remove autonomy too soon. However, holding unrealistic expectations of the patient's performance creates serious safety risks. A balance between expectations of the patient's function that are either too high or too low can be found only with careful, regular assessment of the patient's current abilities.

ORIENTATION MEASURES

Many older adults with recent memory loss can be helped to maintain orientation by means using specific cues and purposeful orientation. For example, the nurse should not assume that a cognitively impaired patient will recognize the nurse or other caregiver regardless of how frequently they interact. On approaching the patient, nurses should reintroduce themselves each time in such a way as to avoid assumptions or insult, for example, "I'm Janice and I'll be caring for you today." Printed schedules can help the patient who is able to read. Visual cues about daily events, holidays, and seasons can serve as reinforcement to discussions about what is or will be taking place.

Clinical Pearl

Planning: A patient with dementia may be able to maintain continence and toilet himself or herself if able to find the bathroom. A picture of a toilet placed on the bathroom door provides a visual cue and can prevent confusion in a hall with many doors, thus helping the patient find the bathroom autonomously.

Some patients with memory loss can be helped to learn or retain important information, such as self-care measures or a prescribed health regimen, if their specific needs are incorporated into the teaching plan. Use of both oral and visual presentation of information to be learned has been found to be effective in increasing recall among older adults (Ressler, 1991). In addition to explaining instructions to the older patient in words, the nurse can reinforce learning through demonstration, use of pictures or diagrams, and written instructions (Fig. 22-1).

COMMUNICATION TECHNIQUES

Communication with the cognitively impaired person is enhanced if the nurse empathetically recognizes the loss of self-esteem or loss of one's real self that the patient is experiencing. A caring approach involves at least some degree of understanding of the patient's experience, as difficult as this might be.

A calm, simple statement or request should be given while allowing sufficient time for a response. Choices should be offered but kept simple so that they are not overwhelming. The patient should always be treated with respect. Regardless of the severity of impairment, the patient is still a person of worth and value and still deserves to be treated with dignity and respect.

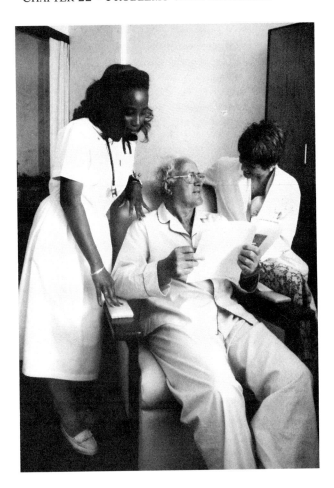

Figure 22-1. Combining visual with oral presentations helps reinforce messages, increasing recall among older adults. (Photo courtesy of Ron Ferrell, Duke Photo Department, Durham, NC)

With patients who display extreme cautiousness, feelings of fear and anxiety can be minimized by the nurse who conveys that the patient is valued as a person regardless of the lack of ability or quality of performance. The patient who is valued in such a way is more likely to attempt a task rather than avoid it (thereby increasing helplessness and dependence), particularly when the nurse conveys that the consequences of trying and taking risks are likely to be positive. The nurse who demonstrates positive acceptance of the cognitively impaired patient regardless of the patient's performance on a task, such as bathing, is more likely to earn the patient's cooperation in self-care. The patient, in turn, is more likely to maintain feelings of accomplishment and self-esteem.

HEALTH PROMOTION

All cognitively impaired patients are at risk for not meeting their basic physiologic needs for varied reasons that relate to the nature of their impairment or its causes. Short attention span, short-term memory loss, inability to reason, and perceptual problems with recognizing objects and surroundings can result in interference with self-feeding, toileting, bathing, grooming, dressing, mobility, and sleep. The specific problems may vary depending on whether the patient is extremely anxious or depressed or is experiencing delirium or dementia. For all of these patients it becomes the nurse's responsibility to monitor activities of daily living and self-care tasks and to ensure that basic needs are met when the patients are unable to do so for themselves.

Regarding depression and early stages of dementia, monitoring of activities and verbal reminders may be all that are required. Regarding delirium, when the patient cannot function (or loses consciousness), and advanced dementia, the nurse must be prepared to provide complete care to meet basic physiologic needs. During the middle stages of dementia and during more severe depression, the nurse must be able to take cues from the patient's behavior and modify approaches to match the level of need. Approaches may need to progress from verbal reminders to the patient, to assisting the patient to initiate a self-care task, to providing more active assistance or complete care.

 Clinical Pearl

Intervention: An individual with a short attention span and recent memory deficit due to dementia may be unable to complete normal activities of daily living (ADLs), such as dressing or feeding self without assistance. Providing complete assistance is not only strenuous on the caregiver but also deprives the patient of autonomy, control, and self-esteem. Both ADLs and autonomy can be maintained by giving the patient simple, single-step verbal reminders that allow the patient to complete a task one step at a time without being physically assisted.

Many approaches have been used to assist older adults to maintain or improve declining cognitive function. Research has suggested that exercise can improve cognitive function. However, results are not conclusive.

Regardless of whether cognitive abilities are actually improved with exercise programs, regular exercise can help older adults maintain normal physiologic function, including circulation, mobility, elimination, and sleep. Maintaining these functions is especially important for patients with psychomotor slowing and withdrawal (patients with depression) and for patients who are forgetful, apathetic, or inattentive (patients with dementia). Regardless of whether cognitive abilities can be improved, functional abilities can be maximized, even for patients with dementia, depending on the care they receive.

PATIENT AND FAMILY EDUCATION

The nature of cognitive deficits means that the patient will be dependent on others either temporarily or progressively for daily care. This dependency creates challenges not only for the nurse but also for the family. Many families will develop unique and creative ways to care for the older adult with cognitive deficits. Other families will require a considerable amount of support, assistance, and instruction to learn to cope with the multitude of daily problems that challenge them as caregivers. A great deal of support and teaching may be necessary. Families should be reassured that as unique problems arise, there is usually no absolute right or wrong answer. They can be offered ideas, alternatives, suggestions, and encouragement to try to adapt these approaches to the patient's needs, problems, and abilities (see the Patient Teaching Box, "Maintaining Self-Care in Patients With Dementia").

COMMUNITY RESOURCES

An excellent source for referral of families whose family member is suffering from dementia is the Alzheimer's Disease and Related Disorders Association. The Alzheimer's association has affiliated chapters located throughout the country that sponsor family caregiver support groups. Attendance at support group meetings can provide families with information, emotional release, and much-needed encouragement to cope with the daily burdens of caring for a loved one with dementia.

The challenges presented by the older person with cognitive impairment are among the greatest the nurse will ever face. The older adult with cognitive impairment and the family will benefit from the nurse's thorough attention to their problems in order to preserve the older adult's function and satisfaction with life as long as possible.

Patient Teaching Box
MAINTAINING SELF-CARE IN PATIENTS WITH DEMENTIA

To assist the patient with dementia to maintain self-care in specific daily tasks, do the following:

- Identify the task or activity to be performed by the patient.
- Break the task down into its smallest component parts (ie, each single step required to complete the task).
- Give the patient directions to perform only one step at a time, using simple, clear, slowly stated directions.
- Allow time for the patient to complete each step before giving the direction for the next step.
- Repeat for each step of the task.
- Provide verbal reinforcement for each step completed adequately, such as, "You have put your arm into your shirt sleeve." This allows the pateint to recognize a successful action and to feel a sense of accomplishment.
- If a task or step seems to frustrate or overwhelm the patient, gently offer assistance with that step. Then provide verbal direction for the next step. Avoid "taking over," even if the task is not done as well as you would like to see it done. Accomplishment and a degree of autonomy are more important at this point than perfection.
- If the patient is completely unable to perform the task or becomes agitated, distract the patient with a neutral topic or divert attention to something else going on in the environment. Patients with dementia are easily distracted and will usually forget momentary frustration as soon as their attention is focused elsewhere.

Nursing Care Plan

FOR PATIENTS WITH COGNITIVE IMPAIRMENT

Nursing Diagnosis: Self-Care Deficit: feeding, bathing/hygiene, dressing/grooming, toileting, related to cognitive impairment.

Definition: A state in which the individual experiences an impaired ability to perform or complete activities of daily living.

Assessment Findings:
1. Inability to bring food from receptacle to mouth
2. Inability to wash body parts, to obtain or get to water source, and to regulate water flow or temperature
3. Impaired ability to put on or take off necessary items of clothing, to obtain or replace articles of clothing, to fasten clothing, and to maintain appearance at satisfactory level
4. Inability to locate or get to toilet or commode, to manipulate/remove clothing for toileting, to sit on/rise from toilet or commode, to carry out proper toilet hygiene, and to flush toilet or empty commode
5. Inability to remember; short attention span

Nursing Interventions with Selected Rationales:

Self-Feeding Deficits
1. Assess the patient's physical capability; note range of motion, swallowing ability.
   Rationale: Mechanical and physical requisites to feeding are essential to self-feeding.
2. Provide food in a quiet environment away from others.
   Rationale: Minimizing distracting stimuli increases likelihood that patient will focus on eating and avoids distraction before consuming sufficient nourishment.
3. Present patient with one food at a time; provide the next food item after the first one is eaten; include foods the patient likes.
   Rationale: Complex choices and excess stimulation easily overwhelm the patient, thus preventing him from eating. Simplifying choices fosters appropriate responses. Using food the patient likes enhances the possibility of compliance.
4. Provide nutritional finger foods.
   Rationale: Foods that do not require recognition of objects (utensils) and their use will increase likelihood of patient feeding self.
5. Allow the patient to continue self-feeding even if messy in appearance.
   Rationale: Self-feeding preserves a sense of autonomy and accomplishment, which reinforces behavior.
6. Feed the patient or assist with feeding only when necessary.
   Rationale: Minimum nutrition will be maintained.
7. Instruct the family in measures to enhance self-feeding.
   Rationale: Family education promotes continuity of care and enchances compliance.

Patient Outcomes/Discharge Criteria:
1. Patient will feed self using appropriate methods (hands or single utensil).
2. Patient will tolerate eating for a sufficient length of time to consume reasonable portions or will consume smaller amounts more frequently.
3. Patient will continue self-feeding when prompted.
4. Patient will maintain desired weight.

(continued)

Nursing Care Plan

FOR PATIENTS WITH COGNITIVE IMPAIRMENT *(Continued)*

5. Family will describe ways to handle feeding by providing simple directions, adapting the environment, and offering limited choices based on the patient's behavior.

Self-Bathing/Hygiene Deficits
1. Assess patient's personal preferences and usual bathing habits (time of day, tub or shower), and respect if possible.
   Rationale: Preserving long-standing habits increases the likelihood of cooperation in bathing.
2. Recongize terrors attached to nonrecognition of objects and surroundings (fear of tub, running water). Explain what you are going to do.
   Rationale: Explanations and reassurance may decrease fears and resistance.
3. Remind patient of the steps to follow for bathing, washing hands, brushing teeth, and using deodorant; provide directions one step at a time.
   Rationale: Breaking down tasks into individual steps allows the patient to comprehend and follow more easily.
4. Assist with bath if necessary.
   Rationale: Maintaining cleanliness, skin integrity, and freedom from infection is important to well-being.

Patient Outcomes/Discharge Criteria:
1. Patient will cooperate in bath and hygiene measures without resistance or undue fear.
2. Patient will be free of unpleasant body odor.
3. Patient's skin will be clean and free of skin breakdown or infection.

Dressing/Grooming Deficit
1. Ascertain personal preferences/habits regarding clothing, comfort, and order of putting on clothing.
   Rationale: Respecting habits and preferences increases the likelihood of maintaining self-care and cooperation in dressing.
2. Arrange clothing in the order it is to be put on. Provide verbal directions one item at a time when the patient is dressing.
   Rationale: This simplifies information the patient must process so that the patient is able to respond.
3. Offer simple choices, such as only two colors of sweater.
   Rationale: Exercising choice preserves autonomy and meaning.
4. Adjust clothing to temperature.
   Rationale: The patient may lack judgment; patient safety and comfort must be preseved by the nurse.
5. Provide grooming items, such as hairbrush, one item at a time, or demonstrate each item's use.
   Rationale: Demonstrating use compensates for presence of agnosia and fosters the patient's autonomy in using items correctly.

Patient Outcomes/Discharge Criteria:
1. Patient will be dressed appropriately for situation and weather.
2. Patient will accomplish dressing/grooming with minimum assistance.
3. Patient will be acceptable to others in appearance.

(continued)

Nursing Care Plan

FOR PATIENTS WITH COGNITIVE IMPAIRMENT *(Continued)*

Toileting Deficit

1. Note need for elimination on a regular basis and provide reminders.
   Rationale: This promotes regular elimination based on habits.
2. Provide privacy to extent possible.
   Rationale: Privacy generally fosters successful elimination.
3. Attend to the patient while toileting to ensure proper usage, and provide assistance as needed.
   Rationale: Attendance allows adjustment to patient needs as they arise.
4. Demonstrate or assist with clothing removal and sitting on the toilet.
   Rationale: Assisting the patient in initiating an activity increases the likelihood of success.
5. Instruct patient in use of toilet paper and hand washing.
   Rationale: This ensures good hygiene and preserves habit.

Patient Outcomes/Discharge Criteria:

1. Patient will use the toilet successfully on a regular basis for both urinary and bowel elimination.
2. Patient will maintain hygiene during toileting process.

REFERENCES

Brody, H. (1987). Central nervous system. In G. L. Maddox (Ed.), *Encyclopedia of aging* (pp. 108–112). New York: Springer-Verlag.

Folstein, M. F., Folstein, S. E., & McHugh, P. R. (1975). Mini-Mental State: A practical method of grading the cognitive state of patients for clinician. *Journal of Psychiatric Research, 12,* 189–198.

Ressler, L. E. (1991). Improving elderly recall with bimodal presentation: A natural experiment of discharge planning. *Gerontologist, 31*(3), 364–370.

Salthouse, T. A. (1989). Age-related changes in basic cognitive processes. In M. Storandt & G. R. VandenBos (Eds.), *The adult years: Continuity and change* (pp. 7–40). Washington, DC: American Psychological Association.

Spreen, O., & Strauss, E. (1991). *A compendium of neuropsychological tests: Administration, norms, and commentary.* New York: Oxford University Press.

BIBLIOGRAPHY

Abraham, I. L., Neundorfer, M. M., & Currie, L. J. (1992). Effects of group interventions on cognition and depression in nursing home residents. *Nursing Research, 41*(4), 196–202.

Abraham, I. L., & Reel, S. J. (1992). Cognitive nursing interventions with long-term care residents: Effects on neurocognitive dimensions. *Archives of Psychiatric Nursing, 6*(6), 356–365.

Bashore, T. R. (1989). Age, physical fitness, and mental processing speed. *Annual Review of Gerontology and Geriatrics, 9,* 120—144.

Bromely, D. B. (1990). *Behavioral gerontology: Central issues in the psychology of aging.* Chichester, IL: Wiley and Sons.

Fiedler, I. G., & Klingbell, G. (1990). Cognitive-screening instruments for the elderly. *Topics in Geriatric Rehabilitation, 5*(3), 10–19.

Fromholt, P., & Larsen, S. F. (1991). Autobiographical memory in normal aging and primary degenerative dementia (dementia of Alzheimer's type). *Journal of Gerontology, 46*(3), 85–91.

Kausler, D. H. (1991). *Experimental psychology, cognition, and human aging.* New York: Springer-Verlag.

Keane, S. M., & Sells, S. (1990). Recognizing depression in the elderly. *Journal of Gerontological Nursing, 16*(1), 21–25.

Lindenmuth, G. F., & Moose, B. (1990). Improving cognitive abilities of elderly Alzheimer's pa-tients with intense exercise therapy. *American Journal of Alzheimer's Care and Related Disorders Research*, 5(1), 31–33.

Mace, N. L. (1990). The management of problem behaviors. In N. L. Mace (Ed.), *Dementia care: Patient, family, and community* (pp. 74–112). Baltimore: Johns Hopkins University.

Mace, N. L., & Rabins, P. V. (1991). *The 36-hour day: A family guide to caring for persons with Alzheimer's disease, related dementing illnesses, and memory loss in later life* (rev. ed.). Baltimore: Johns Hopkins University.

McElvoy, C. L. (1990). Behavioral treatment. In J. L. Cummings & B. L. Miller (Eds.), Alzheimer's disease: Treatment and long-term management. *Neurological Disease and Therapy, 4*, 207–224. New York: Marcel Dekker.

Moore, L. W., & Proffitt, C. (1993). Communicating effectively with elderly surgical patients. *AORN–Journal 58*(2), 345, 347, 349–350.

Puckett, J. M., & Reese, H. W. (Eds.). (1993). *Mechanisms of everyday cognition*. Hillsdale, NJ: Erl-baum Associates.

Ressler, L. E. (1991). Improving elderly recall with bimodal presentation: A natural experiment of discharge planning. *Gerontologist, 31*(3), 364–370.

Rosswurm, M. A. (1990). Attention-focusing program for persons with dementia. *Clinical Gerontol-ogist, 10*(2), 3–16.

Scharnhorst, S. (1992). AIDS dementia complex in the elderly. *Nurse Practitioner, 17*(8), 37–43.

Valentine, J. L., & Valentine, C. R. (1989). Overview of Alzheimer's disease. In G.D. Miner et al. (Eds.), *Caring for Alzheimer's patients: A guide for family and healthcare providers* (pp. 9–21). New York: Insight Books.

Wands, K. et al. (1990). A questionnaire investigation of anxiety and depression in early dementia. *Journal of the American Geriatrics Society, 38*(5), 535–538.

Yesavage, J. (1987). The use of self-rating depression scales in the elderly. In L. W. Poon (Ed.), *Handbook for clinical memory assessment of older adults* (pp. 213–217). Washington, DC: Amer-ican Psychological Association.

Problems With Sexuality

Objectives

1. Describe changes in sexuality that occur with aging and chronic illness.
2. Identify types of alterations in sexual health and related nursing interventions.
3. Outline strategies to assess sexuality in older adults as well as a plan of care to prevent and overcome sexual problems.

INTRODUCTION

SEXUALITY IS A COMPLEX PHENOMENA for older adults. Many jokes about the elderly either stereotype them as asexual or imply that continued sexual interest and sexual activity are abnormal. Health care providers and older adults themselves may believe that a decreased interest in sex is natural and expected. Most studies show that nurses ignore the sexual concerns of patients of all ages and especially those of older adults due to these stereotypes (Matocha & Waterhouse, 1993). It is true that physiologic changes occur with aging that affect sexuality. Chronic illnesses can have a profound effect on sexual health as well. However, many older adults retain the ability and the interest to maintain a sexually active, intimate lifestyle. Others may need assistance from nurses to overcome the effects of aging and the health problems that often accompany old age. By addressing sexuality, the nurse may uncover other problems that the patient may have originally been reluctant to discuss.

Sexuality is far more than just intercourse. Sexual function (the way individuals express themselves sexually or the ability to give and receive pleasure), sexual self-concept (body image, sexual identity, and feelings of adequacy as a man or woman), and sexual role/relationships (patterns of intimacy, values about sexual expression, and sex-role behaviors) are three important dimensions of sexuality in older adults (Woods, 1987). Sexual development continues throughout the life span, with each component of sexuality being influenced by biologic development as well as sociocultural forces. Some of the significant developmental experiences related to sexual function, sexual self-concept, and sexual role/relationships are outlined in Table 23-1.

PHYSIOLOGIC CHANGES WITH AGING

The effects of aging on sexual function can be detected as early as age 40 or late as age 70. These changes make the older adult more prone to sexual dysfunction; however, once experienced, the difficulties may be overcome.

Kaplan (1990) described human sexual response as consisting of three phases: desire, excitement, and orgasm. These phases are related components of sexual response governed by separate neurophysiologic systems. The concept of sexual response is useful for understanding the physiology of sexual response, the consequences of aging and pathophysiology, and the etiology of sexual dysfunctions.

DESIRE PHASE

The desire phase of sexual response refers to the experience of sexual appetite or drive that motivates the older adult to seek out sexual activity. Bonding to another person and love are powerful stimuli to sexual desire. Other stimuli that may be conditioned by culture include sight, smells, and other sensory cues. Fear and pain are the most potent inhibitors of sexual desire.

Desire may change with aging. One of the misconceptions of desire is that desire increases with abstinence. Older adults who continue to engage in sexual activities as they age report that desire decreases somewhat. Those who have ceased to express themselves sexually report that as time without sex increases, desire continues to decrease.

EXCITEMENT PHASE

In the excitement phase of sexual response, the level of sexual tension intensifies with swelling of the genitalia and vaginal lubrication. Erections in men and vaginal swelling and lubrication in women are considered corollary excitement phase responses controlled by two centers in the spinal cord (S-2 to S-4 and T-11 to L-2, associated with arteriole dilation). Because vasocongestion is primarily a parasympathetically mediated response, an intense sympathetic response such as fear or anxiety can lead to loss of vasocongestive changes, including erection.

Men often notice that with age, achieving and maintaining an erection requires more direct penile stimulation and more time. When erect, the penis may be softer. Ejaculation is not as forceful, and ejaculation may not occur with each sexual encounter. These changes are thought to occur from changes in genital blood circulation interfering with penile engorgement, a diminished sensitivity of the penis to vibration and touch, and prostate changes (Kaiser, 1991). Women also tend to notice sexual changes, particularly decreased vaginal secretions and lubrication.

Table 23-1	SIGNIFICANT DEVELOPMENTS RELATED TO SEXUAL FUNCTION, SEXUAL SELF-CONCEPT, AND SEXUAL RELATIONSHIPS			
	Developmental Stage	Sexual Function	Sexual Self-Concept	Sexual Role/Relationship
	Infancy	Orgasmic potential present Erectile function present	Gender identity reinforced Association of sexuality and good/bad Distinction between self and others	
	Toddler	Genital pleasuring and exploration Sensual activity (eg, hugging)	Core gender identity solidified (by age 3)	Sex role differences learned Discrimination between male and female role models Sexual vocabulary learned
	Preschool	Sex play—exploration of own body and those of playmates Self-pleasuring (masturbation)	—	Sex roles learned Parental attachment and identification
	School age	—	Curiosity about sex Sexual fears and fantasies Interest in aspects of sexual development Self-awareness as sexual being	Same-sex friends
	Prepubertal adolescence	Menarche Seminal emissions	Concerns about body image	Sexual experiences as part of friendship, same-sex friends

Early adolescence	Awkwardness in first sexual encounter (50% not sexually active)	Sexual thoughts, fantasies Anxiety over inadequacy, lack of partner, virginity	Appropriate-sex friendships Dating
Late adolescence	Masturbation, petting May or may not be sexually active	Responsibility for sexual activity	Intimacy in relationships learned Sex role behaviors, life styles explored
Young adult	Experimentation with sexual positions, expression Exploration of techniques	Responsibility for sexual health (eg, contraception, sexually transmitted disease prevention Development of adult sexual value system, tolerance for others	Giving and receiving pleasure learned Long-term commitment to relationship developed
Middle adult	Adaption to altered sexual function (eg, vaginal dryness of menopause, slower erections)	Accepts body image changes related to aging	Adjustment of relationship as roles change
Late adult	More gradual sexual function	Accepts slowed sexual response cycle without ending sexual aspects of relationship	New ways of sharing sexual pleasure and intimacy developed Adaptation to loss or illness of partner

Source: Mims, F., & Swenson, L. (1980). Sexuality: A nursing perspective (pp. 62–65). New York: McGraw Hill Book Co. From: Woods, N.F. (1987). p. 4. Used with permission.

ORGASM PHASE

Orgasm, the peak and release of sexual tension, is a phase of sexual response characterized by a genital reflex governed by spinal neural centers. Orgasm consists of reflex contractions of certain genital muscles. Some older women report that uterine contractions experienced during orgasm are even painful. These changes are most often attributed to a decrease in estrogen with menopause. However, it is likely that the neuronal and circulatory changes that occur in men also occur in women.

Some couples adapt well to these changes by paying attention to each others' needs, taking more time during intercourse, and increasing the amount of genital fondling and caressing during lovemaking. For these couples, sexual satisfaction may even be greater in old age than when younger. Other couples do not adapt as well. Some couples may have never found sex to be that important or pleasurable, and the changes with aging may be a welcome end to a part of the relationship that was never very satisfying. A woman's fear of pain during intercourse or a man's fear of erectile failure may lead a couple to discontinue the sexual portion of the relationship. However, dyspareunia and erectile dysfunction are not a normal part of aging.

ABNORMAL PHYSIOLOGIC CHANGES

With menopause, women experience decreased estrogen levels, and some may have vaginal thinning as well as decreased vaginal lubrication. These changes may produce symptoms of vaginal dryness, burning, and itching. The lack of lubrication may make vaginal intercourse painful (dyspareunia). Vaginal dryness and dyspareunia may lead women to feel less desire for sexual activity, and they may abstain from masturbation and sexual intercourse. Abstinence may make decreased vaginal lubrication even worse. In addition, chronic illnesses, such as diabetes and hypertension, and many medications, such as antihypertensives, contribute to vaginal dryness. Although the effect of antihypertensives on a man's ability to achieve an erection has been known for some time, the corollary effect of these medications on women has been ignored by health care professionals until recently.

The inability to experience an erection occurs in most men at some time. The more commonly used term for erectile dysfunction is impotence. However, "impotence" has a negative connotation and implies permanent dysfunction, thus "erectile dysfunction" is a more acceptable term. Older men have a greater likelihood of experiencing erectile dysfunction because of the changes that occur in sexual function with age and the effects of chronic illnesses and medications. Feldman, Goldstein, Hatzichristou, Krane, and McKinlay (1994) estimated that erectile dysfunction affects 18 million American men 40 to 70 years old.

Until recently, most erectile dysfunction was thought to be psychological rather than physiologic in origin. Current estimates are that 90% of impotence is due to chronic illnesses. The most common cause of erectile dysfunction is due to atherosclerosis of the vessels in the penis. Other major causes include hormonal alterations due to decreased testosterone and chronic illnesses such as diabetes. Medications, including antihypertensives and antidepressants, and alcohol abuse also are major contributors. Chronic illnesses that cause pain and/or decreased mobility, such as arthritis, chronic obstructive pulmonary disease, and Parkinson's disease, are also a factor. Finally, psychogenic causes, such as bereavement, anxiety, and depression can play a role. Often, erectile dysfunction is caused by a multitude of factors. Erectile dysfunction should never be ignored, because it may be the presenting symptom of heart or vessel disease, diabetes, or hypertension (Kaiser, 1991).

PSYCHOSOCIAL ISSUES

Changes in sexual self-concept with aging have not been studied as thoroughly as the physiologic changes, however, many of the physical, psychological, and socioeconomic changes that occur with aging are thought to influence an older adult's sexual self-concept. Physical changes, such as loss of hair, loss of body tone, and the wrinkling of the skin, can affect how sexy and vibrant a person feels. The changes in sexual response in both men and women may contribute to thoughts that sex is no longer desirable. Other psychological changes and the sexual effects of these changes are more difficult to identify. Although depression and alcoholism are known to be prevalent in the elderly and affect sexual self-concept, the relationship between these problems and sexuality has not been studied.

Cultural expectations also have an effect on sexuality. Stereotypes still abound in which youth is associated with being sexy. Older people who remain sexually active may be labeled "lecherous old men" and "dirty old women." Older adults are still often seen as being sexually conservative, especially by health care providers. Older adults who have been sexually active since their 20s have 40 to 50 years of sexual experience. No doubt most older adults have experienced many sexual changes throughout their lives; if they have overcome these changes, they may have much more experience and expertise than many younger adults.

Changes also occur with sexual role and sexual relationships throughout the life span. For example, a couple who are in their 70s and have been married since they were both in their 20s may have experienced several role and relationship changes due to careers and child rearing. Maintaining a lifelong intimate relationship through these experiences is difficult. Another stereotype in American society is that a person who has had many sexual partners is a great lover. However, keeping one person sexually satisfied for a lifetime is also the sign of a great lover. Chronic illness and the death of a partner also have a profound effect on sexual relationships.

Many older women no longer are sexually active because their partner has a sexual dysfunction. Access to a partner for women may be the primary problem in remaining sexually active. Women outlive men at all ages, thus women may lose a partner and not have the opportunity to establish a new sexual relationship.

Retirement for either a man or a woman may have either a positive or negative effect on sexuality. For those who considered work a burden, the relief of not having to work and the increase in free time may give a boost both to an older person's sexual self-concept and to a sexual relationship. Others find the loss of a career devastating to their self-esteem, with resultant sexual dysfunction. After retirement, leisure activities become the focus of one's life. Couples who share leisure activities often find that intimacy increases.

Widowhood, divorce, and remarriage are all common among married adults as people age. Gay and lesbian older adults may experience the same losses. Little is known about the sexual adjustment after the loss of a partner, but for many, these events may mean the end of sex with another person forever. Nurses can do much by acknowledging this sexual loss as well. However, not all older adults who experience this feel remorse.

▷ Clinical Pearl

Assessment: The loss of a partner may seem like a new lease on life, especially for a spouse who has endured a bad marriage with a person who was cruel or abusive. It is best first to ask how a person feels about the end of a relationship before offering sympathy.

Developmental changes in employment and relationships may mean a change of residence for some older adults. Many move to new environments as diverse as age-segregated communities, assisted-living centers, nursing homes, or with adult children. Nursing homes are often seen as being the most restrictive of these options in permitting sexual activities among patients. Rules about cohabiting with members of the same or opposite sex may exist in all of these environments, which can profoundly affect the ability of an older adult to explore sexual options.

Older adults are a sexually diverse group of people. Some older adults engage in sexual activity with partners of the same sex, although few of these people had been exclusively gay or lesbian. Because of negative stereotypes associated with homosexuality, sexual orientation may be hidden, with some older adults "coming out," or revealing their homosexuality, in their 50s and 60s. Heterosexual relationships, including marriage, may occur before this coming-out period. Studies reveal that among older lesbian women, greater than 40% had formally been married and that from 16% to 35% have children (Deevey, 1990).

Approximately 10% of the general population is believed to be gay or lesbian. It is difficult to estimate if this percentage persists across all ages. However, nurses are likely to encounter gay or lesbian elders at some time during their practice. Because older adults who are gay and lesbian have most likely spent a lifetime hiding their sexual orientation, they may not indicate their true sexual preference even if asked (Deevey, 1990). Stevens (1994) found that lesbians may feel vulnerable to mistreatment by health care professionals and may limit information about themselves to meet their own needs for safety. Therefore, it is likely that a gay or lesbian elder may not seek sexual advice from nurses. Because the nurse may not know the sexual orientation of the patient, it is recommended that language appropriate for older adults of any sexual orientation be used. For example, during assessment, the nurse should ask, "Who is most important to you?" rather than asking about marital status and should use the term "significant other," although somewhat out of vogue in nursing, instead of the term "family" or "friends" to inquire about social support.

> *Clinical Pearl*
>
> *Assessment: A nurse should not automatically assume an older adult is heterosexual because he or she either has been married or has children.*

Although rare, nurses may encounter an older adult who is seeking a sex-change operation. There are many commonly held, often false, stereotypes about aging and transsexuals.

Marital fidelity is practiced by most married older adults. However, some married and single older adults have sex with multiple partners. There is a need for safe-sex education aimed at older adults to curtail the spread of sexually transmitted diseases (STDs) and acquired immunodeficiency syndrome (AIDS). These diseases are not prevalent in this population, and prevention efforts can be very effective if geared toward the over-50 age group.

A few older men report engaging in sex with a prostitute after age 50. Information on women is not available in the literature. Prostitution is legal in Las Vegas. Many retirement areas are developing in the South, and no doubt some older adults go to Las Vegas to shop, gamble, see entertainment, and possibly engage in sex with a prostitute. Older adults also need to be aware of safe-sex practices necessary to avoid the transmission of AIDS or other STDs.

Sexually explicit materials (eg, books and magazine articles, films, photographs) may be used by older adults to generate fantasies before engaging in sexual activity, during sexual activity with partners, or alone while masturbating. Viewing sexually explicit films and masturbating may become more common in all age groups as a safe-sex activity. Older adults may confide in the nursing staff about using sexually explicit materials to verify that this is a "normal" activity. Sex therapists have routinely advocated the use of sexually explicit materials as one method of treating sexual dysfunction. Nurses may also recommend this to older adults who voice an approval of sexually explicit films and books but who have not tried them.

NURSING ASSESSMENT

Nurses should include a 5- to 10-minute assessment of sexuality as a routine part of their care of older adult patients. By doing so, the nurse can help the patient to prevent or overcome sexual problems resulting from or coexisting with illness and the aging process.

HISTORY AND INTERVIEW

The sexual assessment should be completed near the end of the nursing assessment to allow time to establish rapport as well as identify problems with other areas, such as mobility and elimination, which many contribute to sexual dysfunction. Chronic illnesses can also have a profound effect on sexuality and should be noted in the history (Billhorn, 1994). Table 23-2 lists several chronic illnesses that can affect sexuality. If the patient acknowledges any of these chronic illnesses during the nursing assessment, then the nurse should assess

Table 23-2

EFFECT OF CHRONIC ILLNESSES ON SEXUALITY AND POTENTIAL NURSING INTERVENTIONS

Chronic Illness	Potential Effect of Sexuality	Interventions
Heart disease Hypertension Peripheral vascular disease	Decreased circulation to the genitals and antihypertensive medications may cause erectile dysfunction in men and vaginal dryness in women. May have fear of chest pain during sex.	Stopping smoking combined with an exercise program may increase genital circulation. Encourage couple to walk together to increase endurance and intimacy. Patient can ask physician if medications can be changed.
Diabetes	Peripheral and autonomic neuropathy cause decreased genital sensation and erectile dysfunction in men and vaginal dryness in women.	Explain that symptoms vary over time. Encourage close blood sugar monitoring and weight control to decrease neuropathy.
Chronic lung disease	Loss of stamina, fatigue, and chronic cough all may contribute to loss of sexual desire. Fatigue may preclude sexual activity. Changes in sex roles due to dependence may affect the sexual relationship.	Enhance breathing and reduce fatigue with low-level exercises and breathing techniques that will also increase desire. Adopt sexual positions that prevent shortness of breath. Wear oxygen canula during sexual activity. Encourage exploring a rehabilitation program to increase independence in ADLs.
Alcohol abuse	High intake of alcohol will cause erectile dysfunction and vaginal dryness. Sexual function problems, relationship problems, and sexual self-concept problems may contribute to alcohol abuse.	Explain the relationship between alcohol intake and lack of sexual excitement. Encourage treatment of alcohol problems to resolve sexual dysfunction.

Parkinson's disease Arthritis	Impaired mobility may limit sexual acitivity. Pain, depression, and dependence can lead to decreased feelings of self-worth and sexual desire.	Plan for sex at time of day when pain and spasticity are less. Adopt positions that don't cause pain or spasticity. Encourage planning time for intimacy and sexual expression to combat depression.
Urinary incontinence	Underlying cause may also coincide with erectile dysfunction, vaginal dryness, and dyspareunia. Incontinence leads to embarrassment and loss of self-esteem. Sexual partner may find incontinence distasteful.	Learning Kegel exercises may not only treat the incontinence but also increase vaginal tone. Recommend medical evaluation to ensure that any vaginal infections are treated. Encourage showering and bathing as a part of sexual activity.
Prostate surgery	After prostate surgery, may have retrograde, or "dry" ejaculation. Will have concerns of when to resume sex after surgery and fear of erectile dysfunction.	Inform patient to resume sex after a few weeks when healing has occurred. Inform patient that ejaculation may be dry and that few men experience erectile dysfunction.
Dementia Alzheimer's disease	Memory loss means loss of the lover and confidant the partner has known. Some lose inhibitions and become more sexually aroused. Others may lose sexual desire completely. Are concerns whether demented partner can consent to sex.	Encourage partner to discuss feelings. Provide anticipatory guidance that these sexual changes may occur. Encourage redirecting the uninhibited person to a more appropriate activity.

whether the patient has any of the potential sexual concerns. During the history, the nurse should identify prior surgeries that can effect sexuality, for example, older women who have undergone mastectomies for treatment of breast cancer, which has a major effect on body image and sexuality (Johnson, 1994), and older men who have undergone surgery for cancer of the prostate, which may affect erection. The following introduction and four questions will identify sexual problems. The questions can be tailored to the individual, based on the reason for admission to the health care setting, or to other problems identified during the assessment. Start with the less sensitive question about roles and relationship and then move to sexual function.

The nurse may start with the following statement:

"Now I am going to ask a few questions about sexuality. Many patients with (back pain, incontinence, heart disease, etc.) have sexual concerns, and I may have some information that will help you.

> Has your (illness, hospitalization) interfered with your being a (husband, wife)? If so, how? (If the patient has acknowledged a sexual partner) Has your (pain, incontinence, etc.) interfered with the relationship with your (spouse, sexual partner)? If so, how?
> Has your (heart attack, Parkinson's disease, mastectomy, etc.) changed the way you see yourself as a (woman, man)? If so, how?
> Has your (colostomy, hysterectomy, etc.) changed your ability to function sexually (or your sex life)? If so, how?
> Have you noticed any open sores on your genitals (privates, penis, vagina) or discharge from your (penis, vagina)?"

When conducting a nursing assessment, screening for STDs can be done by asking the older adult if he or she has either a penile or vaginal discharge or open lesions or sores on the genitals. These two questions will identify most of the older adults with STDs. Although an older adult may indicate the presence of lesions or discharge when asked, he or she probably will not offer this information unless asked. Elders grew up when many STDs were either untreatable or poorly treated. A person may not have sought treatment because of embarrassment or a misperception that the disease is untreatable.

 Clinical Pearl

Assessment: Asking about sexual concerns may reveal additional (nonsexual) problems that would remain uncovered if sexuality was not assessed.

Initially, a nurse may become anxious asking these questions. With practice, the comfort level will increase. Most nurses experience a great deal of anxiety when giving their first intramuscular injection, yet no one argues that this is an acceptable reason for not learning to administer them. Unfortunately, anxiety over asking about sexual concerns on the part of the nurse often means that the sexuality of many older patients is ignored.

PHYSICAL EXAMINATION

Sexuality is best assessed by means of a sexual history. However, a nurse should complete a review of body systems and be alert for genital discharge when providing perineal hygiene, particularly with older adults who cannot communicate this on their own. Discharge and other genital abnormalities, such as uterine prolapse, should also be noted and reported for treatment. Older adults should routinely undergo genital exams as a part of routine physical exams by their usual health care provider.

DIAGNOSTIC TESTS

Few diagnostic tests are used in evaluating sexuality problems in older adults. If STDs or AIDS is suspected, the appropriate blood test or genital discharge culture may be obtained. Blood tests to evaluate thyroid function or hormone levels may also be conducted. When evaluating erectile dysfunction in men, Doppler pressures, penile duplex ultrasonography, or cavernosometry may be performed to evaluate genital blood flow. Studies that measure a man's erectile ability during sleep (nocturnal penile tumescence) are not helpful in older men (Kaiser, 1991).

NURSING DIAGNOSES

Based on the assessment, the following potential nursing diagnoses can be generated to plan interventions.

- Sexual dysfunction related to impaired sexual self-concept, sexual function, and sexual role/relationships resulting from self-care deficit
- Low self-esteem related to loss of sexual partner
- Altered sexuality patterns related to mobility restrictions
- Sexual dysfunction related to vaginal dryness and painful intercourse
- Knowledge deficit related to lack of information about potential treatments for erectile dysfunction
- Sexual dysfunction related to premature ejaculation
- Altered sexuality patterns related to pain and fatigue
- High risk for infection related to lack of safe-sex practices
- Body image disturbance related to mastectomy
- Altered sexuality patterns related to stress incontinence

NURSING INTERVENTIONS

Five strategies are used when addressing sexual problems: (1) providing patient education, (2) providing anticipatory guidance throughout the life cycle, (3) promoting a milieu conducive to sexual health, (4) validating normalcy about sexual concerns, and (5) performing sexual self-care. Education, anticipatory guidance, validation, and health promotion are commonly used among nurses. Nurses are not expected to be sex counselors or sex therapists, because this is beyond most nurses' preparation. However, many of the sexual prob-lems nurses encounter with patients can be addressed through these ᶠ strategies.

PATIENT AND FAMILY EDUCATION

Many medications affect sexual abilities. The major groups of medications known to affect either sexual excitement or desire are hypoglycemics, cardiac drugs, vasodilators, and antihypertensives (Feldman et al., 1994). These medications are commonly used with the older adult. Patients need to be informed of these side effects when the medications are prescribed. Although nurses, physicians, and pharmacists are usually aware of these problems, they may not think this information is important or know how to approach the issue. Nurses should inform patients of the potential side effects and encourage the patient to discuss other options for medications if problems are experienced. Often, changing from one drug to another in the same class will relieve the untoward effect (Steele, 1989).

Nurses may have several opportunities to provide sexual education to older adults. For older men experiencing difficulty with erections, a common sexual problem among this group, nurses can begin treatment by focusing on the underlying causes. For example, diabetic men may find that better control of their blood sugar lessens erectile dysfunction. Furthermore, patients with vascular disease may benefit from stopping smoking, reducing their cholesterol and fat intake, and adopting an exercise program. These strategies have been shown to actually reduce the amount of coronary artery disease and probably have a long-term effect on penile circulation.

If treating the underlying factors does not relieve sexual dysfunction, penile implants, pharmacologic erection programs (injecting medication into the penis), and vacuum tumescent devices (plastic cylinder pump) may be used to correct the problem of erectile dysfunction (see Table 23-3).

When dealing with older women, nurses can intervene by asking if they are experiencing vaginal dryness, dyspareunia, purulent vaginal discharge, or uri-

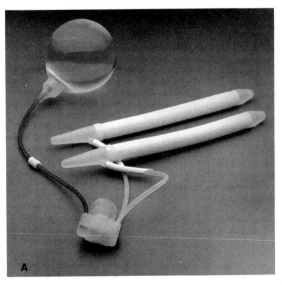 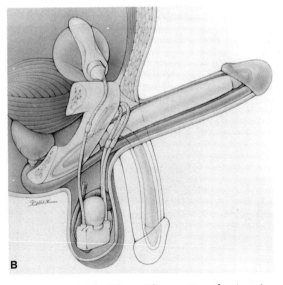

Figure 23-1. Inflatable penile prosthesis—the AMS 700 Ultrex Plus. *A.* Prosthesis prior to insertion. *B.* Prosthesis in erect and flaccid position.

Table *23-3*	MEDICAL AND SURGICAL TREATMENTS FOR PENILE ERECTILE DYSFUNCTION	
	Penile implants	Implants are surgically placed into the penis by a urologist. The two most common types are semirigid rods or inflatable devices. The penile implant only affects the ability to get an erection; the ability to reach orgasm and penile sensation are not affected. A photograph of one type of inflatable penile prosthesis is included in Figure 23-1.
	Pharmacologic erection programs (PEP)	Pharmacologic erection programs are offered by urologists who specialize in the treatment of erectile dysfunction. As part of an extensive educational program, men are taught to self-inject the penis with doses of vasoactive drugs to achieve an erection that lasts from 30 to 40 minutes and is sufficiently hard to permit intercourse. A small syringe and needle are used. Papaverine hydrochloride, used alone or in combination with phentolamine mesylate has a reported success rate of between 65% and 100%, with a very low rate of side effects. These agents only affect the ability to get an erection; they do not affect orgasm or ejaculation. PEPs are widely used by men with erectile dysfunction due to diabetes, hypertension, pelvic trauma, and arteriosclerosis who want to continue intercourse and do not wish to have a penile implant.
	Vacuum tumescent device	A vacuum tumescent device with constriction/retention bands is another option that does not require surgery or injections for men. The vacuum device consists of a plastic cylinder that is placed over the penis. Pumping the device creates negative pressure, and blood is drawn into the penis, leading to an erection. The erection is maintained by applying a constriction/retention band to restrict the venous flow of blood out of the penis. Erections may last from 15 to 30 minutes. A photograph of one brand of vacuum tumescent device is shown in Figure 23-2.

nary incontinence. Those with such symptoms should be instructed to seek medical treatment. Nurses should educate older women about treatment for common sexual dysfunctions, the most common being vaginal dryness (see the Patient Teaching Box, "Treating Vaginal Dryness").

Older women also need to be taught vulvar self-examination, because they are more prone to vulvar cancers. Many older women were taught *not* to look at their "privates," and nurses can do much to reassure them that this practice is essential to their health. They should report any vulvar discoloration, bleeding, or abnormal growth on the vulva to their physician (Bachmann, 1990).

Several resources are available to assist nurses in providing sex education. These books are specifically written to address the sexual concerns of older adults (Boston Women's Health Book Collective, 1992; Butler & Lewis, 1993; Cutler & Garcia, 1992; Doress–Worters & Siegal, 1994; Edelman, 1992; Gershenfeld & Newman, 1991; Kroll & Klein, 1992). Information can also be gained through newsletters that focus on topics specific to the older adult, including the effect of health problems on sexuality, such as *Sex Over Forty* (DKT International, P.O. Box 1600, Chapel Hill, NC 27515).

Students and nursing staff can also develop their own educational materials for patients, or nurses can obtain professionally written patient education ma-

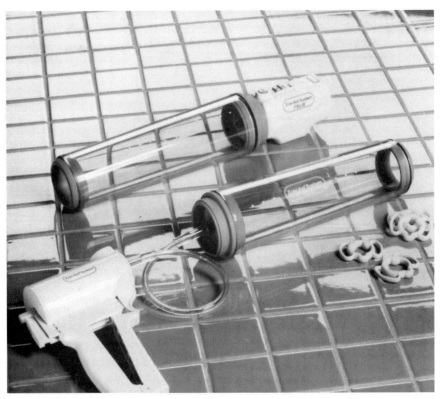

Figure 23-2. Vacuum tumescence device—the Erec Aid. (Courtesy of Osbon Medical systems)

Patient Teaching Box
TREATING VAGINAL DRYNESS

If you are experiencing vaginal dryness, you should know the following:
• Vaginal dryness predisposes you to vaginal infections and urinary incontinence.
• With vaginal dryness, even though you may have no desire to be sexually active, you should seek treatment.

Treatment for vaginal dryness can include the following:
• Estrogen replacement therapy (ERT), which can be administered orally, through a skin patch, or by vaginal cream. Discuss with your physician or nurse practitioner if ERT may be helpful.
• Vaginal lubricating agents, which can be obtained over the counter at a local drug-store and applied once or twice a week to maintain lubrication. These include the following brand-name products: Replens, Lubrin, Gyne-Moistrin, and Slippery Stuff.
• Wear loose-fitting cotton underwear to reduce the incidence of vaginal infections.
(Bachmann, 1990)

terials from such sources as the American Cancer Society and the American Arthritis Association. The use of a written handout for patients that addresses a specific sexual concern may help to break the ice in discussing sexuality with older adults. The handouts can be given to all patients, telling them to throw it away if they do not want it. Patients often will be grateful, not offended. With or without written or film resources, nurses can provide older adults with information about sexuality. For example, a patient with an indwelling catheter can be taught how to care for the catheter during intercourse. Men can fold the catheter back over the penis and then apply a latex condom, which will prevent irritation of the urinary meatus during lovemaking. Women should be instructed to tape the catheter up to the abdomen during intercourse. Some women prefer to wear crotchless underwear to cover the catheter during intercourse.

ANTICIPATORY GUIDANCE

Nurses are often in strategic positions to provide anticipatory guidance about sexuality to older adults. By informing individuals about the usual changes expected with aging, nurses can assist older adults to adapt their lovemaking to accommodate these changes in their bodies. For example, the nurse can inform the patient and partner that men tend to take longer to get erections and that women may notice less vaginal lubrication. However, additional genital stimulation during intercourse often compensates for these changes and is pleasurable to both partners.

Loss of sexual desire may occur with stressful life events and with a change in health. Nurses can intervene by reassuring the patient and partner(s) that a decrease in sexual desire commonly occurs. The couple should be encouraged to talk about it and seek help to correct any underlying causes, such as medications or symptoms of chronic illness.

Nurses can also assist older adults to anticipate and prevent problems that might interfere with sexual activity. A woman who is afraid of leaking urine during intercourse can be told to empty her bladder before sexual activity and to use positions, such as side-lying or the woman on top, that minimize the potential for leakage. As an added preventative, the mattress can be covered with a waterproof overlay, so that if an accident occurs, the mattress will not be soiled. Dyspareunia often accompanies incontinence, so a water-soluble lubricant should also be used to prevent pain and further irritation (Wheeler, 1990). K-Y jelly is the most commonly recommended lubricant in the literature, but it unfortunately gums up quickly. Better water-soluble lubricants such as Slippery Stuff (Wallace–O'Farrell, Tacoma, WA), PrePair (Trimensa Pharma, Newbury Park, CA), and Astroglide (Biofilm, Inc., Vista, CA), may be sold in the condoms or women's hygiene products section of stores or may be available through mail order.

Anticipatory guidance can also be given to patients who have undergone disfiguring surgery to assist them with sexual concerns that are likely to arise when they return home. For example, a woman who has had a mastectomy can be advised that she probably will not feel like having sex until her incision heals. Both she and her partner may have concerns about how her body will look. She will need information about specially designed bras and breast prostheses. Finally, she may benefit from being advised that friends and family will be curious about how she looks, and she may find them staring at her breasts.

Although nurses cannot prevent this reaction from occurring, they can help patients think through how they will handle this situation if and when they experience it.

PROMOTING A MILIEU CONDUCIVE TO SEXUAL HEALTH

The first step in promoting a milieu conducive to sexual health is to give a patient permission to ask about intimacy and sexual concerns. By including sexuality as a routine part of a comprehensive nursing assessment, the nurse is saying that it's okay to talk about sensitive issues. Another approach is providing time for privacy and intimacy for patients and their partners while in the hospital or other health institution. Patients and families experience tremendous crises during admissions and often need time alone to help each other cope effectively. Family members often ask if it is okay to kiss or hug a patient. One woman, whose husband had a head injury, found that lying down on the bed with him when he became agitated helped him to relax. Some patients and partners may want to have intercourse in the hospital or institution. Hospital staff often object to this, but the objections are justified only if the sex act will jeopardize the patient's physical condition (Schmidt, 1993). Guidelines have also been written for providing opportunities for intimacy (Wright, 1993) and for managing sexual relationships (Wallace, 1992) among elderly residents in long-term-care facilities.

VALIDATING NORMALCY ABOUT SEXUAL CONCERNS

Validating normalcy is a strategy that nurses can perform. Older adults may seek information stating that physical changes in genitalia or sexual function are a normal part of the aging process. They may seek out the nurse for validation of sexual normalcy. Older adults may be concerned about sexual thoughts, fantasies, dreams, and feelings as well as perceptions of sexual behaviors regarded as "dirty" or "perverted." It is up to each individual to decide what is okay and what is unacceptable. An older woman may have been told while growing up that to fondle or stroke a man's penis is wanton and may seek reassurance that this is okay. However, the opposite may be true as well. A woman in her 70s who had recently remarried stated that her husband was having difficulties getting an erection. She wanted reassurance that it was okay to refuse to "put his penis in my mouth" because this was unacceptable to her.

Clinical Pearl

Intervention: Nurses often ask, "When should I bring up the topic of sexuality?" Three natural times to address sexuality are (1) during the admission assessment, (2) as part of routine teaching, and (3) during discharge planning. Think about the sexual implications of the content being taught and then include sexuality in the teaching plan.

SEXUAL SELF-CARE PROMOTION

A final strategy nurses can use is promoting sexual self-care. Promoting self-examination of the genitals and breasts to detect early warning signs of cancer and other diseases is one example that is often recommended by nurses. Using safe-sex techniques to prevent STDs is another example.

Older adults who are sexually active need to be aware of safe-sex practices to prevent STDs and AIDS. The variety of nursing practice settings allows for unique opportunities for nurses to assess human immunodeficiency virus (HIV) risk and to provide protective sex education for older adults (American Nurses Association, 1994). The risk of transmission of HIV during various sexual practices is shown in Display 23-1. Protective sex includes sexual activities in which no semen, vaginal secretions, or blood is exchanged between sexual partners. Such activities include hugging, kissing, caressing, genital handling in the absence of an open lesion, and vaginal or anal intercourse provided a condom and spermicide are used correctly (Flaskerud & Ungvarski, 1992). Older adults have not been the target of AIDS prevention education because the current incidence of STDs and AIDS in older adults is low. Most older adults are aware of AIDS and the national push to use condoms from the me-

---

Display 23-1

RISK OF SEXUAL TRANSMISSION OF HUMAN IMMUNODEFICIENCY VIRUS

Absolutely Safe
  Abstinence
  Mutually monogamous sex with noninfected partner—any sexual activity
    between noninfected partners is safe
  Telephone sex, erotic videos or magazines, fantasy
  Solo or mutual masturbation
Very Safe (Assuming intact skin and no lesions)
  Noninsertive sexual practices
  Manual stimulation of partner
  Massage
  Unshared sex toys
  Dry kissing
Probably Safe
  Insertive sexual practices with the use of condoms and spermicide.*
    Penile–vaginal and penile–anal intercourse with a barrier, as well as
      cunnilingus
    Fellatio
    Anilingus with a barrier
Risky
  Everything else

---

*Condoms, either the male condom, which fits over the penis, or the female condom, which is inserted into the vagina, must be used correctly in conjunction with a spermicide (Nonoxynol-9) See Hatcher et al., 1994, or Anastasi, 1993, for complete information on condom usage.

Adapted from Flaskaerud and Ungvarski (1992).

dia but may need more explicit information. However, because the focus is on the young, older adults may not think they are at risk of contracting STDs and AIDS, even if sexually active with more than one partner. An often overlooked issue is that problems in one area of self-care, such as mobility, may have a concurrent effect on sexuality. Addressing sexual concerns may promote the adoption of other healthy habits by patients. For example, nurses are taught to teach patients with chronic obstructive pulmonary disease to maintain optimal levels of endurance with low levels of exercise, stop smoking, use pursed-lip and abdominal breathing techniques, and comply with medications and breathing treatments. All of these activities not only serve to stabilize the disease and increase the ability to perform activities of daily living, but also can increase sexual performance. The nurse also can suggest that these patients wear their nasal oxygen cannula and use proper breathing techniques during lovemaking.

Sexual concerns may be a motivator to promote self-care. An older woman with multiple sclerosis sought out home health care services to assist her in learning to perform her own intermittent catheterization for bladder management. Even though her multiple sclerosis had caused visual problems, poor hand and wrist strength, and paraplegia, the home health nurse and occupational therapist were able to teach her to catheterize herself with the use of a "cock up" wrist splint, "labia spreader," lighted magnifying mirror, hard rubber catheters, and a urinal. The patient expressed her gratitude that her husband no longer needed to perform this activity for her.

Documentation of nursing interventions related to the older adult's sexual concerns is important. To maintain confidentiality and also accurately document nursing care when addressing sexual concerns, the nurse can simply write, "Patient (and partner) expressed sexual concerns related to (underlying health problem). Discussed options to overcome these concerns. Will follow up as needed." More specific information is not necessary. The patient should be told about what is written. For more information about appropriate nursing care, see the Nursing Care Plan for older adults with sexual dysfunction.

Nursing Care Plan

FOR OLDER ADULTS WITH SEXUAL DYSFUNCTION

Nursing Diagnosis: Sexual Dysfunction, related to impaired sexual self-concept, sexual function, and sexual role/relationships resulting from self-care deficit.

Definition: The state in which an individual experiences or is at risk of experiencing a change in sexual functioning that is viewed as unrewarding or inadequate. Inability to participate in sexual activities or relationships.

Assessment Findings:
1. Verbalization of problems of:
   • decreased sexual arousal
   • erectile dysfunction or vaginal dryness/dyspareunia
   • orgasmic dysfunction

(continued)

Nursing Care Plan

FOR OLDER ADULTS WITH SEXUAL DYSFUNCTION *(Continued)*

2. Mobility limitations in selected areas of self-care deficit (dressing, ambulation, toileting)
3. Poor sexual self-concept, poor self-esteem
4. Role confusion, difficulty communicating with partner

Nursing Interventions with Selected Rationales:

1. Assess level of impairment and the impairment's effect on the patient's ability to communicate, participate in sexual activities, and maintain a sexual relationship.
   Rationale: Obtaining baseline information about the patient's problems provides a foundation on which to design and plan appropriate interventions.
2. Assess effect on body image and sexual self-concept.
   Rationale: Changes in sexual function can have a negative effect on body image and sexual self-concept.
3. Encourage communication between partners about fears, desires, and effect of disability on the relationship.
   Rationale: Open communication fosters trust and promotes closeness between partners.
4. Provide information on adapting lovemaking activities to overcome sensation loss and limitations on mobility (eg, side lying, the partner superior, or in a wheelchair instead of a bed).
   Rationale: Adaptations help to minimize the change in sexual functioning, thereby promoting participation between partners.
5. Encourage nonsexual intimate time together, such as hugging, touching, and kissing, and then resuming sex slowly.
   Rationale: Nonsexual intimacy promotes closeness and sharing between partners, enchancing self-esteem.
6. Encourage lifestyle changes that can increase both self-care ability and sexual ability.
   Rationale: Incorporation of lifestyle changes enhances the patient's ability to adapt to the changes, promoting optional level of functioning.

Patient Outcomes/Discharge Criteria:

1. Patient and sexual partner will identify potential barriers to sexual function and options to overcome these barriers concurrently or independently of changes in self-care ability.
2. Patient and partner will verbalize understanding of all instructions.
3. Patient and sexual partner will verbalize an increase in positive self statements, reduced anxiety about sexual activities, and improved sexual arousal.

REFERENCES

American Nurses Association. (1994). *Nursing and HIV/AIDS*. Washington, DC: Author.

Bachmann, G. A. (1990). Sexual changes and dysfunction in older women. *Medical Aspects of Human Sexuality, 24*(8), 49–54.

Billhorn, D. R. (1994). Sexuality and the chronically ill older adult. *Geriatric Nursing, 15,* 106–108.

Boston Women's Health Book Collective. (1992). *The new our bodies, ourselves: A book by and for women. Updated and expanded for the 1990's.* New York: Simon & Schuster.

Butler, R. N., & Lewis, M. I. (1990). *Love and sex after sixty* (rev. ed.). New York: Ballantine.

Cutler, W. B., & Garcia, C. R. (1992). *Menopause: A guide for women and those who love them* (rev. ed.). New York: W. W. Norton.

Deevey, S. (1990). Older lesbian women, an invisible minority. *Journal of Gerontological Nursing, 16*(5), 35–39.

Doress–Worters, P. B., & Siegal, D. L. (1994). *The new ourselves, growing older: Women aging with knowledge and power.* New York: Simon & Schuster.

Edelman, D. S. (1992). *Sex in the golden years: What's ahead may be worth aging for.* New York: Donald Fine.

Feldman, H. A., Goldstein, I., Hatzichristou, D. G., Krane, R. J., & McKinlay, J. B. (1994). Impotence and its medical and psychosocial correlates: Results of the Massachusetts male aging study. *Journal of Urology, 151,* 54–61.

Flaskerud, J. H., & Ungvarski, P. (1992). *HIV/AIDS: A guide to nursing care* (2nd ed), Philadelphia: W. B. Saunders.

Gershenfeld M., & Newman, J. (1991). *How to find love, sex, and intimacy after 50: A woman's guide.* New York: Fawcett Columbine.

Johnson, J. R. (1994). Caring for the woman who's had a mastectomy. *American Journal of Nursing, 94*(5), 25–32.

Kaiser, F. E. (1991). Sexuality and impotence in the aging man. *Clinics in Geriatric Medicine, 7,* 63–72.

Kaplan, H. S. (1990). Sex, intimacy, and the aging process. *Journal of the American Academy of Psychoanalysis, 18,* 85–205.

Kroll, K., & Klein, E. L. (1992). *Enabling romance: A guide to love, sex, and relationships for the disabled (and the people who care about them).* New York: Harmony.

Matocha, L. K., & Waterhouse, J. K. (1993). Current nursing practice related to sexuality. *Research in Nursing & Health, 16,* 371–378.

Schmidt, J. (1993). John had AIDS—and one romantic wish. *Nursing, 23*(1), 55–56.

Steele, D. (1989). Drugs causing sexual dysfunction and their alternatives: A reference tool. *Urologic Nursing, 9*(6), 10–12.

Stevens, P. E. (1994). Protective strategies of lesbian clients in health care environments. *Research in Nursing & Health, 17,* 217–229.

Wallace, M. (1992). Management of sexual relationships among elderly residents of long-term care facilities. *Geriatric Nursing, 13,* 308–311.

Wheeler, V. (1990). A new kind of loving? The effect of continence problems on sexuality. *Professional Nurse, 5,* 492–496.

Woods, N. F. (1987). Toward a holistic perspective of human sexuality: Alterations in sexual health and nursing diagnoses. *Holistic Nursing Practice, 1*(4), 1–11.

Wright, B. A. (1993). Behavior diagnoses by a multidisciplinary team. *Geriatric Nursing, 14,* 30–35.

BIBLIOGRAPHY

Anatasi, J. K. (1993). What to tell patients about the female condom. *Nursing, 23,* 71–73.

Burgener, S., & Logan, G. (1989). Sexuality concerns of the post-stroke patient. *Rehabilitation Nursing, 14,* 178–181, 195.

Chatauvert, M., Duffie, A., & Gilmore, N. (1991). Human immunodeficiency virus antibody testing: Counseling guidelines from the Canadian Medical Association. *Patient Education and Counseling, 18,* 35–49.

Docter, R. F. (1985). Transsexual surgery at 74: A case report. *Archives of Sexual Behavior, 14,* 271–277.

Hatcher, R. A., Trussel J., Stewart, F., Stewart, G. K., Kowal, D., Guest, F., Cates, W. Jr., & Policar, M. F. (1994). *Contraceptive technology* (16th rev. ed.). New York: Irvington.

Mulligan, T., & Katz, P. G. (1991). Urologic considerations in geriatric erectile failure. *Clinics in Geriatric Medicine, 7,* 73–84.

Tichy, A. M., & Talashek, M. L. (1992). Older women: Sexually transmitted diseases and acquired immunodeficiency syndrome. *Nursing Clinics of North America, 27,* 937–949.

24

Problems With Substance Abuse

Objectives

1. Identify the physiologic changes associated with alcohol, drug, and tobacco abuse in the older adult.
2. Identify methods of assessing substance abuse in the older adult.
3. Describe how the nurse can organize and plan nursing care to promote a successful health protection program for older adults with substance abuse problems.

INTRODUCTION

MANY OLDER ADULTS FIND LITTLE RELIEF from the stresses of aging except through the use of alcohol, psychoactive drugs, over-the-counter (OTC) drugs, tobacco, or a combination of all four. The use of such agents in the older population presents a significant problem, which has only recently been identified. Society's historic inability to recognize substance abuse among older adults is symptomatic of its general failure to identify and treat those with significant substance abuse problems. That aging can further complicate matters is rarely considered. Therefore, substance abuse among older adults needs to be viewed from the context of the physiologic, sociologic, psychological, and economic processes of aging.

ALCOHOL ABUSE IN THE OLDER ADULT

Excessive alcohol consumption is a multifaceted public health problem of medical, social, legal, and economic importance. One group receiving limited attention in this area is the older adult population (Fig. 24-1) (Molgaard, Nakamura, Stanford, Peddecord, & Morton, 1990). Constituting 12.2% of the

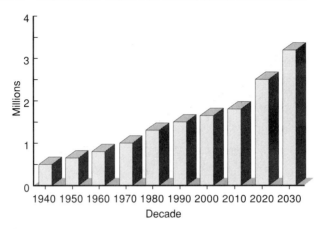

Figure 24-1. Estimated numbers of elderly alcoholics by decade.

population, people older than age 65 represent the fastest growing segment of society and include many more people of increasingly advanced age. Because the quality of life for these people is greatly enhanced by the maintenance of health, it is appropriate to investigate how age and alcohol can interact to compromise the health and even the lives of older adults.

PHYSIOLOGIC CHANGES OF AGING

General physiologic changes associated with aging are important to consider in determining the extent to which alcohol and other chemical substances affect the older adult. With age there is a decrease in lean body mass and an increase in fat-storing (adipose) tissue, which result in higher concentrations of drugs accumulating within organs. Because of the diminution in hepatic detoxification that occurs with age, blood alcohol is cleared more slowly. Given a loading dose of alcohol controlled for body surface area, the average 60-year-old will exhibit a peak blood alcohol concentration about 20% higher than the average 45-year-old. At age 90, this peak is 50% higher than it was at age 20. In real terms, this means that relatively small amounts of alcohol can cause noticeable intoxication in the aging adult. In the elderly, all heavy drinking is problem drinking, but drinking need not be heavy to be problematic.

Age tends to slow down the processes of metabolism and elimination. As a result, the elimination process may be particularly affected by the pressure of medications. The liver may be operating at suboptimal efficiency and may be required to process multiple substances at one time. All of these factors affect the alcohol tolerance level, which decreases with age (Table 24-1).

PSYCHOSOCIAL ISSUES

Several researchers have observed that older problem drinkers are a hidden population. Even though the use and abuse of alcohol among the elderly requires treatment, statistics indicate that older adult alcoholics are underrepresented in alcohol treatment environments. Instead, they tend to show up in acute care and psychiatric institutions, which is testimony to both the seriousness of alcohol use in the elderly and the difficulty in detecting it. Several reasons could account for this, including:

Table 24-1

DRUGS THAT INTERACT WITH ALCOHOL THAT ARE COMMONLY PRESCRIBED FOR ELDERLY PATIENTS

Generic	Trade	Category	Effect With Alcohol
Amphetamines Caffeine	Coffee, tea cola, Vanquish Benzedrine Dexedrine	CNS stimulants	Can reverse effects of alcohol, giving false sense of security.
Phenytoin	Dilantin	Anticonvulsants	Reduces effect. May enhance CNS depression
Cyclobenzaprine	Flexeril	Skeletal/muscle relaxant	Increased CNS depression
Hydrochlorathiazide Furosemide	HydroDIURIL, Lasix Diuril	Diuretics	Increase BP. Lowers effect of diuretic. May cause postural hypotension
Salicylates	Bayer ASA, Bufferin Alka Seltzer	Analgesics	Increase potential for GI bleeding
Codeine Morphine Opium Oxycodone Propoxyphene Pentazocine Meperedine	Paregoric Percodan Darvon Talwin Demerol	Narcotic Analgesics	Reduce functioning of CNS
Nitroglycerin Isosorbide	Nitrostat Isordil Sorbitrate	Antianginals	Decreases BP (to potentially dangerous level)
Brompheniramine maleate Chlorpheniramine malecte	Dimetane Chlor-Trimeton (many others, OTC and Rx)	Antihistamines	Enhances CNS depression
Reserpine Methylodopa	Serpasil, Aldomet	Antihypertensive	In moderate amts. alcohol will increase BP, which lowers effects of these drugs. This can cause postural hypotension. Increased CNS depression with Aldomet
Fenoprofen Ibuprofen	Nalfon Motrin, Mediprin Rufen, Advil, Nuprin	NSAIDS	May increase chance of GI bleeding. Some increase pro-thrombin time, and alcoholics may have clotting problems. May cause CNS depression

(continued)

Table 24-1

DRUGS THAT INTERACT WITH ALCOHOL THAT ARE COMMONLY PRESCRIBED FOR ELDERLY PATIENTS (Continued)

Generic	Trade	Category	Effect With Alcohol
Indomethacin	Indocin		
Naproxen	Naprosyn		
Piroxicam	Feldene		
Furszolidone	Furoxone	Antibiotic	May have disulfiram-like reaction
Metronidazole	Flagyl	Anti-infective	
Nitrofurantoin	Cyantin or Macrodantin		
Pargyline	Eutonyl	MAOI	Beer, wine contain tyramine, which interacts with MAOI to produce a hypertensive, hyperpyrexive crisis
Isocarboxazid	Marplan		
Phanelzine	Nardil		
Tranylcypromine	Parnate		
Nortiptyline	Aventyl	Antidepressant	Increased CNS depressant effect
Amitriptyline	Elavil		
Doxepin	Sinequan		
Imipramine	Tofranil		
Warfarin	Coumadin	Anticoagulants	Chronic alcoholism inhibits effect. With acute alcohol use the effect is enhanced and can lead to hemorrhaging
Coumarin	Dicumarol		
Chlorpropamide	Diabinase	Antidiabetics Hypoglycemics	May have severe and unpredictable interactions. Hypoglycemia or hyperglycemia. May have disulfiram-like reaction
Tolbutamide	Orinase		
Tolazamide	Tolinase		
Glyburide	Diabeta		
insulins	Regular NPH		

CNS: central nervous system; BP: blood pressure; GI: gastrointestinal; NSAID: nonsteroidal anti-inflammatory drug; MAOI: monoamine oxidase inhibitor.

This is not meant to be a complete list of drugs that may interact with alcohol. It is intended to make the home care nurse aware of the multitude of drugs the elderly patient may be taking that can have adverse effects when that person also uses alcohol.

Compiled and modified from: (1) *Understanding Alcohol,* 1982 (used by permission of J. Kinney.)
(2) *Physician's Desk Reference for Prescription Drugs,* 1989
(3) *Nursing 89 Drug Handbook,* 1989
(4) *Micromedex,* 1974–1990

- Subtle presentation of symptoms
- Inaccurate diagnosis of symptoms related to other medical or psychological problems
- Reluctance of care providers to identify problems or intervene
- Lack of awareness of the amount of alcohol being consumed on part of the elderly
- Reluctance to self-disclose
- Existence of denial and enabling within family units

Enablers or rescuers are those in the alcoholic's social environment who make continued drinking possible by direct encouragement or by failure to acknowledge the existence of the problem.

NURSING ASSESSMENT

Recognizing alcohol and other substance abuse in the older adult population is complex. Rarely do older adults who abuse psychoactive substances engage in criminal activity, drive under the influence, or cause community disturbances (Marcus, 1993). Persons older than 65 years are not likely to be in the mainstream of the job market, thus making it difficult to assess, assist, and recognize the often subtle warning signs of a potential problem.

History and Interview

History-taking is perhaps the most important step in assessing the use and abuse of alcohol in the older adult. Questioning patients about the following aspects of their drinking behavior can be particularly useful for identifying abuse (Gupta, 1993):

- Early drinking behavior
- Current drinking patterns
- Reasons for drinking
- Feelings about drinking
- Alcohol-related problems

Because alcoholism threatens personal relationships, it can create many social problems for the drinker. The mood swings, denial, and/or hostility that can accompany alcohol intake often lead to depression or belligerence. These behaviors, in turn, create conflict between drinkers and their families, friends, and employers and may lead to loss of self-esteem, feelings of uselessness, and isolation. Questioning family members as well as friends in an effort to detect such conflicts is another way of obtaining additional information that may confirm a problem.

Notable symptoms associated with loss-of-control drinking behavior include hangovers, blackouts, memory loss, and confusion. Other indicators may include anxiety and nervousness, insomnia, hand tremors, loss of appetite, and prolonged periods of isolation.

Risk Factors

Although alcohol abuse begins for many in earlier years, numerous older adults turn to alcohol for relief from the stresses of aging. These stressors include retirement, loss of loved ones, poor health, loneliness, and depression. Whether the abuse is one of lifelong alcoholism or late-onset excessiveness, the older adult faces a range of unique complications. Overall, the older adult is more sensitive to the negative effects of alcohol because of normal and patho-physiologic changes. Specifically, older adults are often prescribed a number of medications and therefore are at a heightened risk of complications when these drugs are used in combination with alcohol. Alcohol has a stronger effect on the older adult's brain, which may result in dementia. Furthermore, the abuse of alcohol provokes physical risks, such as falls and injuries, malnutrition, and self-neglect. Finally, the older adult may not receive necessary treatment if the family denies or ignores the problem. Often, this is so because the family believes it is too late to help the older adult or that the patient deserves to enjoy a few drinks in his or her last years. Display 24-1 provides an alcoholism fact sheet that offers more insight into the risk factors an older adult may encounter.

Physical Examination

Tolerance to alcohol deceases with age as a result of slowed metabolism and elimination. The decreased efficiency of these processes may result in intoxication, as evidenced by the blood level of alcohol being held for a longer period of time. Symptoms commonly associated with alcoholic intoxication in the older adult include:

- Confusion
- History of falls
- Anorexia
- Insomnia
- Anxiety
- Nausea
- Weight loss/gain
- Difficulty controlling blood pressure

Withdrawal symptoms should be noted during an initial physical exam. Early signs of alcohol withdrawal include tremors, dehydration, vomiting, diarrhea, and hallucinations. As the condition worsens, convulsions (acute alcohol withdrawal) and ongoing violent activities occur. Furthermore, tremors and hallucinations intensify (Scherer, 1995). Cumulative toxic effect of excess alcohol and nutritional deficiency may also be present in patients experiencing withdrawal.

Diagnostic Studies

Laboratory abnormalities are insensitive and tend to be of little use in the diagnosis of alcoholism in older adults. Hospitalized older alcoholics are somewhat more likely than younger alcoholics to have abnormalities in aspartate transaminase (AST), gamma glutamyl transferase, and mean corpuscular volume. However, even the test results of the most sensitive test, AST, is only abnormal in 55% of those hospitalized for alcoholism. Presumably, older persons with less severe alcoholism would be even less likely to have abnormalities in laboratory examination (Egbert, 1993).

NURSING DIAGNOSES

On the basis of a complete assessment of the older adult, common nursing diagnoses associated with the use of alcohol can be determined. The following is a list of selected nursing diagnoses:

Display 24-1

ALCOHOLISM FACT SHEET FOR OLDER ADULTS

1. Among the 25 million Americans age 65 or older, an estimated 2.5 to 3.7 million are addicted to alcohol.
2. Diagnostic problems constitute perhaps the greatest barrier to treatment of alcoholism among senior citizens. What is perceived as frailty, senility, or simply the unsteadiness of old age may, in fact, be alcoholism.
3. One in five older adults receiving treatment for medical, surgical, or psychiatric difficulties is an alcoholic or problem drinker.
4. Health care providers not sensitized to the problems of older alcoholics frequently see physical and mental disorders as syptoms of aging rather than conditions aggravated or caused by alcoholism.
5. Medical problems prominent in the older alcoholic include amnesia, delirium, convulsions, gastritis, anemia, cardiomyopathy, ulcers, pneumonia, and fractures from falls.
6. Alcoholism exaggerates psychological problems, such as anxiety, depression, and suicidal contemplation and can mimic senility.
7. Indications of alcoholism in the older adult include self-neglect, injuries, depressive moods, anorexia, confusion, paranoia, and having more than two drinks a day.
8. Alcohol combined with sleeping pills may cause severe depression of the central nervous system, even to the point of death. The interaction of alcohol and insulin may cause blood sugar levels to plummet rapidly.
9. Elderly widowers appear to be the most vulnerable to alcoholism.
10. The two groups of older adults who have drinking problems are those who have adopted drinking as a reaction to one or more of the stresses of aging and those who have a long history of alcohol abuse and continue to drink excessively in their later years.
11. Older problem drinkers, who include long-term alcoholics who have survived into old age, are among the least visible of the nations's problem drinkers as a whole because many of them are retired and have retired from the mainstream of society. Unless they are public inebriates, and a few of them are, their drinking goes largely unnoticed.
12. A family may actually encourage or tolerate the older person's excessive drinking, believing that it makes him or her easier to deal with. As a result, many older adults are able to drink themselves into difficulty with little interference and few offers of help.
13. In nationally randomly selected communities, 305 of all alcoholism information and referral calls come from persons older than 65 years of age.
14. Studies indicate that excessive use of alcohol, when it is either the primary psychiatric problem or a symptom of a depressive illness, is an important factor in suicide among older adults.

(Adopted from Care Unit Program, Monticello Medical Center, Monticello, CA.)

- Knowledge Deficit, related to alcohol effects
- Powerlessness
- Altered Nutrition: Less than body requirements related to alcoholic intake
- Alteration in Self-concept, related to drinking behaviors
- Self-care Deficit, related to intoxication
- Risk for injury

NURSING INTERVENTIONS

A supportive and trusting nurse–patient relationship is the ideal situation in which to approach the older adult problem drinker. The nurse should avoid the label "alcoholic" as well as judgmental, blaming, or punitive statements. Also, it has been shown that characterizing alcoholism as an addictive disease rather than a problem of morality or willpower increases the likelihood that the person will accept the diagnosis (Haldeman and Gafner, 1990).

The nurse can face the problem with the patient by offering a choice of treatment modalities, a supportive environment, and practical help. It is important to show a positive attitude when working with the elderly, because it enhances their ability and willingness to meet goals and overcome disappointments. Everyone needs an occasional pat on the back. Friends and relatives can help older adults build self-esteem by taking an interest in their activities and offering encouragement and praise.

Learning more about the disease of alcoholism and its implications for the older adult is the responsibility of every nurse. Working with older adult alcoholics gives the nurse an opportunity to offer prevention, education, and treatment as a part of the team approach to better health. Nursing has proven that the older adult is never too old to change, learn, and recover from a life driven by alcohol consumption. See the nursing care plan for a patient with alcohol abuse problems.

DRUG ABUSE AND MISUSE IN THE OLDER ADULT

Older persons are more likely to use drugs. This can lead to a number of problems, including polypharmacy, misuse of medications (both overmedication and undermedication of symptoms), drug abuse, and related issues of dependency. These problems, like those that accompany alcoholism, are often underdiagnosed. Below is a review of the terminology used in talking about drug-taking behavior.

Drug use is defined as the introduction into the body of any chemical for the purpose of affecting the body in a specific manner. According to this definition, taking an aspirin would qualify as drug use. *Drug abuse*, on the other hand, is a value-laden term used to suggest that drug use causing legal, social, and medical problems can be traced directly to some moral deficiency in the drug abuser. For a diagnosis of drug (or substance) abuse to be made, the older adult must be taking the substance for other than its intended purpose and be experiencing some negative effects as a result of drug use; also, continued drug use in the face of its negative effect on life is usually observed.

Drug addiction is defined as a state of chronic intoxication that is detrimental to the individual, which is produced by repeated consumption of a drug. It is characterized by:

• Overpowering need or desire to take the drug
• Willingness to obtain the drug by any means, including illegal means
• Tendency to increase dose
• Physical dependency on effects of drug

Although nurses have been trained to recognize and treat any person with a drug dependency, their attention is often focused on detecting the problem among those younger than 65. This is perhaps due to the perception that be-

Nursing Care Plan

FOR A PATIENT WITH ALCOHOL ABUSE PROBLEMS

Nursing Diagnosis: Powerlessness, related to disease process, low self-esteem, loss of control

Definition: A condition in which an individual experiences, or could experience, a feeling of insuffient control, influence, and/or authority over the immediate environment.

Assessment Findings:
1. Malnutrition
2. Tachycardia
3. Tachypnea
4. Mild hypertension
5. Tremor
6. Anxiety
7. Delerium tremors, which may result in alteration of consciousness
8. Hallucinations
9. Heightened withdrawal symptoms

Nursing Interventions with Selected Rationales:
1. Train the patient to tolerate increased stress and to learn improved methods of coping with stress.
   Rationale: Improvements in stress management make it less likely that the patient will resort to alcohol to relieve tension.
2. Prepare the patient for difficult or painful events.
   Rationale: Warning of potential difficulties allows the patient to plan ahead and thus reduces stress.
3. Reduce irritating or frustrating environmental stress.
   Rationale: A neutral or comfortable environment is less likely to provoke an unpleasant reaction from the patient and increases compliance with treatment regimen.
4. Reduce patient's social isolation.
   Rationale: Ensuring that the patient has a network of social contacts promotes interpersonal interaction and self-reliance.
5. Attempt to alter alcoholic beverage chemically to lessen addictive qualities.
   Rationale: Removing the addicitive component of alcohol lessens its allure.
6. Help patient to identify factors that may contribute to feelings of powerlessness.
   Rationale: Overcoming feelings of powerlessness will alleviate the need to seek artificial strength in alcohol.
7. Document the plan of care as agreed on by the nurse and the patient in the nursing care plan.
   Rationale: In addition to providing legally verifiable proof of nursing care, the nursing care plan helps to promote consistency of care among all health care providers involved with the patient.

Desired Patient Outcomes/Discharge Criteria:
1. Patient identifies factors that contribute to a sense of powerlessness.
2. Patient verbalizes feeling control over environment.
3. Patient verbalizes feeling control over the plan of care.
4. Patient participates in decision making regarding the plan of care.

cause late-onset addiction to illicit drugs is virtually nonexistent among the elderly, their difficulties with the use of prescription and OTC drugs must be similarly rare. However, this is not the case.

Even though older adults make up only 12.2% of the total population, it is estimated that they use 25% to 30% of all drugs prescribed in the United States. Noninstitutionalized Medicare beneficiaries purchased or otherwise obtained 486.6 million prescriptions in 1987. The expenditure associated with these prescriptions totaled $8 billion. In practical terms, the high rate of prescription drug use among the elderly means that many adults are taking up to or more than five prescribed drugs at a time (polypharmacy). These drugs are sometimes dispensed by different physicians who give conflicting directions for appropriate use of the medications. This pattern of polypharmacy can lead to many problems. Some of the most common problems include:

- Failure to take the prescribed dose of medication at the correct time
- Taking the wrong medicine to treat a specific symptom
- Not taking into account the interaction of multiple drugs

Potential consequences from drug abuse and misuse can be discussed in a thorough nursing assessment.

PHYSIOLOGIC CHANGES

Older adults are at particular risk for the negative consequences of drug misuse and abuse for several reasons. They have slowed metabolic turnover of drugs, altered body fat:water ratio, and age-related organ changes that affect metabolism and increase or decrease sensitivity to drugs (Chenitz, Salisbury, & Stone, 1990).

The body's ability to metabolize and excrete drugs declines with age. Drug binding is reduced, which in turn increases the availability of unbound drug for distribution among body tissues. This can result in a buildup to harmful levels even when a drug is taken at recommended doses. For example, in the case of digoxin, the higher frequency of toxicity in older adults may be partially explained by higher blood levels of the drug, which are, in turn, attributed to slower clearance. Measurements of serum drug levels coupled with adjusted nomograms may be especially useful for calculating drug dosage in older patients.

 Clinical Pearl

Intervention: Always ask the patient or the patient's family to bring in all medications, regardless of whether they were prescribed by a physician or bought over the counter.

PSYCHOSOCIAL ISSUES

The most commonly overused drugs are psychoactive medications. The average older adult in America receives 3.6 prescriptions per year for psychotropic medications. This means that 15% to 20% of all older noninstitutionalized individuals receive such medications. The most commonly used psychoactive drugs are benzodiazepines (Valium, Dalmane) and other sedatives or analgesics.

In addition to coping with clinical changes, such as decreased mobility, poor eyesight, and loss of hearing, taste, and smell, the older adult must often adjust to loss of income, social isolation, chronic pain, and worry. These concerns are often what bring the older person to the physician. For such problems, a "quick fix" is expected, often in the form of a prescription. Feeling pressured to respond immediately to consumer demands, many physicians offer medicines instead of counseling or education. This approach to treatment is used because patients have been conditioned to get something tangible on presenting themselves to the physician. With the appropriately prescribed medications in hand, the patient may fall into the habit of unintentional misuse. A single sedative or narcotic may cause mild confusion, ataxia (unsteady gait), or incontinence. Patients who are already compromised may forget they took their medication and take another, which produces further instability and increases the potential for complications.

Older adults are predisposed to polypharmacy, which can take many forms. The problem can involve misuse of nonprescription or prescription medications or both and be associated with:

- Medication without apparent cause
- Duplication of medicines (for example, digoxin and lanoxin) for the same problem
- Use of OTC drugs that interfere with prescription medications (eg, taking antacids and tetracycline concomitantly)
- Use of aspirin for patients with a history of peptic ulcer disease
- Use of aspirin for patients on anticoagulants, such as Coumadin

Multiple medication side effects often provide the evidence of misuse. The concurrent ingestion of several medications contributes to more serious adverse drug reactions and often leads to unnecessary hospitalization or injury. The opposite problem of undermedication among older adults is also of concern. A percentage of older adults seek no medical care. Instead, they may use outdated drugs, purchase OTC medications, or borrow medication from friends or relatives to treat their conditions. The result is that many chronic illnesses afflicting the older adult—depression, arthritis, diabetes mellitus, and osteoporosis among them—may be undertreated by physicians and unacknowledged or misunderstood by families.

The most common clinical presentation of prescription drug abuse includes confusion, lethargy, or depression. Because the older adult may unwittingly consume extra doses of the medication, family members must often be consulted for reliable information about the patient's pattern of drug use.

In most cases of drug abuse, older persons have no history of drug abuse and do not consider themselves drug abusers. They are likely to have inadvertently become addicted to prescription drugs (Chenitz et al., 1990).

As mentioned previously, late-onset addiction to illicit drugs is virtually nonexistent. In fact, heroin and opiate abuse is much less prevalent than alcoholism in people older than 65 by a factor of 1:5. Most older addicts began using drugs in their younger to middle years. If they survive to old age, most have either given up the habit, restricted their addiction to alcohol, or substituted methadone for the previously abused drug. It is also possible that they have switched to prescription drugs, such as codeine, barbiturates, or benzodiazepine. Morbidity among this age group also exceeds that of their nonaddicted peers by 2.5:1. Overdosing is rare, and deaths tend to be only indirectly related to the drugs. This population dies from accidents, assaults, and complications of their addiction (Bienenfeld, 1990).

NURSING ASSESSMENT

The nurse is often the first person to recognize an older adult's potential abuse or misuse of medications. However, because drug abuse among the elderly is often masked by a variety of other symptoms, nurses must make a special effort to see the signs in older adults. Anxiety and depression are common observable consequences of drug dependence in general and are complicated if there is also a history of alcoholism.

A thorough nursing assessment of drug usage is essential for prescribing safe, effective drug therapy in older adults. This assessment includes obtaining an accurate drug history, with particular emphasis on:

- Polypharmacy, which includes drug interactions (new and old medications)
- Deliberate overmedication
- Use of OTC drugs

History and Interview

An accurate nursing assessment should always include information on what drugs the patient is taking and why. Some typical questions the nurse might ask include the following:

- What drugs are you currently taking? Please list all prescription, illicit, and over-the-counter drugs and why you are taking them.
- How many physicians are prescribing medications for you? Do they coordinate their drug-dispensing behaviors?
- Do you always follow all directions for appropriate drug use? If not, why not?
- Have you ever noticed unusual symptoms, such as rashes, dizziness, or lethargy, after taking a drug or a combination of drugs?

The nurse should determine whether several people are responsible for the care of the older adult. If this is the case, physicians need to be informed so that they can give all caregivers consistent information. Finally, every attempt should be made to find out if the older adult is and has been competent to self-medicate. Families may have let the cognitively impaired older adult assume primary responsibility for dispensing the medication, even though he or she clearly did not understand the potential consequences of inappropriate self-medication.

Risk Factors

Normal aging can change the absorption, distribution, metabolism, and excretion of drugs in the body, as described in Chapter 10 on drug administration. Physiologic changes affect medication-taking patterns and drug effects, as listed below:

- Decreased drug efficiency
- General slowing down of activity

  • Different rates of decreasing function in systems is expressed in different persons of the same age
  • Decreased homeostatic reserve to compensate for the effect of drugs

Vision and memory changes may lead to erratic or dangerous drug-taking behavior. The older adult may misread bottles or fail to recall side effects and to report them. Some adverse effects of drugs may mimic aging. In the older adult, the inadequacy of homeostatic mechanisms to provide control systems, such as the hypotension that frequently occurs when antihypertensive drugs are combined, are much less efficient and have a narrower margin to compensate. Age-related changes in receptor sensitivity may be the basis for an increased or decreased response to some drugs and could lead to increased adverse effects.

Other risk factors include polypharmacy, which contributes directly to increased risk of drug reactions, environmental factors, and nutritional deficits. Errors in self-administration of drugs, such as dose omissions, combining of doses, and noncompliance, increase the risk of interactions. Display 24-2 outlines additional major and contributing risk factors for older adults.

Physical Examination
The physical examination of the older adult with a suspected drug abuse problem should include the assessment of weight (with and without clothes) and blood pressures in two positions to observe for orthostatic hypotension. Vision and hearing tests and tests of normal dexterity, including the ability to open bottles, will assist in the assessment of the older adult. Display 24-3 identifies some physical signs of adverse drug reactions.

Diagnostic Studies
With decreased gastric emptying time combined with a rise in the pH of gastric juices, the risk of drug irritation to the delicate mucous membranes may cause stomach irritation. Older adults receiving long-term therapy, such as aspirin or nonsteroidal anti-inflammatory agents, should be assessed for gastrointestinal bleeding with the use of stool sample tests for blood and total blood count evaluations.

Normal aging does not lower serum albumin significantly, but chronic illness and poor nutrition can cause a decrease. When the level of serum albumin decreases, the number of protein-binding sites also decreases, which

---

Display 24-2
RISKS FACTORS DEMONSTRATED BY OLDER ADULTS

Major Risk Factors	**Contributing Risk Factors**
Chronic diseases	Lack of disease knowledge
Long-term therapy	Lack of drug knowledge
Multiple medications	Experiencing side effects
Multiple pharmacies	
History of depression	
Isolation/lives alone	

Display 24-3

IDENTIFYING POTENTIAL ADVERSE DRUG REACTIONS

- Never assume a change in behavior is the result of aging.
- In the elderly, toxic reactions can occur even at low drug dosages.
- The more medication the client takes, the greater likelihood of a drug–drug effect.
- The longer an individual is on a drug, the greater the likelihood of an adverse reaction.
- Do not ignore everyday drugs such as antacids, laxatives, or cold medicines as possible culprits if a drug reaction is suspected.
- The effects of an adverse drug reaction can appear as an isolated symptom (drowsiness) or in symptom clusters (depression and confusion).
- If your client suffers a major depressive or confusional episode, investigate the use of or sudden withdrawal of any drugs acting on the central nervous system.
- Stay alert to any signs of involuntary movements. Drug-induced parkinsonism is a commonly encountered clinical problem following the administration of antipsychotic medications. These medications may also cause tardive dyskinesia and/or akathisia.
- Look for abnormal movements of the tongue, lips, and jaws (tardive dyskinesia) and/or pacing, inability to sit or stand still, continuous agitation (akathisia).
- Drugs are a major cause of dizziness in persons over age 60. Every client complaining of dizziness should be evaluated for orthostatic (sudden) drops in blood pressure.
- Inappropriate timing of diuretic administration is a common and easily remedied cause of incontinence.
- Fatigue and weakness can be caused by beta-blocking drugs, diuretics, tricyclic antidepressants, antipsychotics, barbiturates, benozodiazepines, antihistamines, and certain antihypertensives.
- Fatigue and weakness may be an early sign of a depressive reaction to medication. Look for early-morning awakening, appetite disturbances, and multiple physical complaints.
- Difficulty standing or walking (ataxia) can be a side effect of anticonvulsants and hypnosedatives. Drugs such as Sinemet, Indocin, Dilantin, and Valium are typical of the drugs that cause ataxia.

Focus on Geriatric Care & Rehabilitation, Volume 2, Number 8, February 1989. Permission to photocopy this page is granted by Aspen Publishers, Inc., 1600 Research Blvd., Rockville, MD 20850. Direct inquiries regarding the newsletter to the Newsletter Editor at the above address.

raises the concentration for the free or unbound portion of certain drugs and increases the risk of toxicity.

Other lab values that may be necessary are dependent on the medication regimen being followed:

- Antibiotics: Monitor renal function by examining urine-specific gravity, intake/output, blood urea nitrogen, and creatinine levels
- Narcotics: Check blood pressure to assess for hypotension and monitor electrolytes
- Oral anticoagulants: Schedule prothrombin times
- Cardiovascular agents: Monitor side effects of drugs (eg, dizziness, depression, confusion) as well as serum potassium, digoxin, and quinidine levels

NURSING DIAGNOSES

Because substance abuse often mimics depression or dementia, it is difficult to recognize in the older adult. Related nursing diagnoses that suggest depression, dementia, and, by implication, substance abuse are listed below:

- Ineffective Individual Coping, related to defensive coping
- Impaired Self-concept, related to drug effects
- Altered Nutrition: Less than body requirements, related to drug side effect
- Knowledge Deficit, related to drug use

Once substance abuse has been diagnosed, treatment that focuses on enhancing the patient's ability to self-medicate without harmful consequences can be implemented. See the Patient Teaching Box for safe and effective medication use.

Patient Teaching Box
COMMONSENSE STRATEGIES FOR SAFE AND EFFECTIVE MEDICATION USE

- If childproof containers are hard for you to handle, ask your pharmacist for easy-to-open containers. Always be sure, however, to keep them out of the reach of children.
- Make sure you understand the directions printed on the drug container and that the name of the medicine is clearly printed on the label. Ask your pharmacist to use large type on the label if you find the regular labels hard to read.
- Discard old medicines; many drugs lose their effectiveness over time.
- When you start taking a new drug, ask your doctor or pharmacist about side effects that may occur, about special storage, and about special foods or beverages, if any, to avoid. Pharmacists are drug specialists and are able to answer most questions about drug use. Ask for the drug insert if possible.
- Always call your doctor promptly if you notice unusual reactions, such as rash, nausea, vomiting, dizziness, and confusion.
- New information about drugs and about how they affect the older adult is available. You and your doctor should always review your need for medicines at least twice a year, or more often if you think it is necessary.
- Take exactly the amount of drug prescribed by your doctor and follow the dosage as closely as possible. If you have trouble or questions, call your doctor or pharmacist.
- Medicines do not produce the same effect in all people. Never take drugs prescribed for a friend or relative, even though your symptoms may be the same.
- Always tell your doctor about past problems you have had with drugs (eg, rash, indigestion, dizziness, or loss of appetite). When your doctor prescribes a new drug, be sure to mention all other medicines you are currently taking, including those prescribed by another doctor and those you buy without a prescription.
- Keep a daily record of the drugs you are taking, especially if your treatment schedule is complicated or if you are taking more than one drug at a time. The record should show the name of the drug, the doctor who prescribed it, the amount you take, and the time of day for taking it. Include a space to check off each dose as you take it. Keep a copy in your medicine cabinet and one in your wallet or pocketbook.

NURSING INTERVENTIONS

There appears to be a major problem of drug noncompliance among older adults. Noncompliance can be defined as the failure of the patient to use the specified drug in the specified manner. Noncompliance, or rejection of schedule, can lead to several negative consequences, such as undertreatment, relapse, toxicity, increased incidence of side effects, unnecessary hospitalization, and increased medical expenses.

Nurses understand how risk factors (see Display 24-2) can inhibit patient compliance and impair their understanding and ability to follow a simple medication format. Even normal aging changes can affect the most compliant patient. Loss of hearing, poor vision, or impaired memory may prevent a willing patient from adhering to his or her medication schedule.

Cognitive decline and its effect on the ability to use medications correctly is also a concern in the older adult. Older adults who cannot manage independent activities of daily living (IADL) or activities of daily living (ADL) often have similar problems with their medications. Clear, simple instructions repeated over time will produce greater adherence to the treatment plan. Nurses, with their holistic view of the older adult patient, should provide quality information in a clear, concise, and nonthreatening manner and use this knowledge to enhance the well-being of their patients (Fig. 24-2).

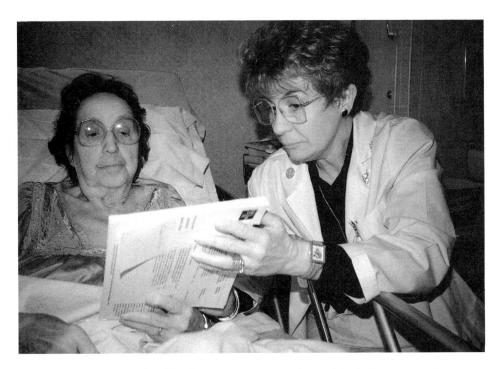

Figure 24-2. Nurses should take extra care to review with their patients the proper methods and schedules for medications as well as the side effects and risk factors associated with each prescription. Clearly illustrated charts and tables help enhance the patient's understanding of this vital information.

Older adults may have functional reasons for noncompliance, such as environments that are not user-friendly. For example, bathrooms may be too far away or inaccessible. In addition, physical difficulties such as joint disease or the neuromotor consequences of stroke could greatly affect the patient's ability to comply. Some tips for detecting noncompliance in the older adult are:

- Frequent refill requests
- Long periods between refill requests and acquisition of required prescription drugs
- Use of multiple health care providers/facilities
- Acute changes in health or behavior
- Acute mental changes
- Excessive/inappropriate OTC drug use
- Saving of old drugs
- Frequent falls
- Complaints of physical weakness and fatigue
- Requests for new or additional drugs

Medications can enhance the older adult's ability to function and maintain homeostasis. Health care providers who understand this as well as how compliance and noncompliance can alter the effects of drug therapy can better ensure that the elderly reap the maximum benefit from proper drug use. The following strategies may be used by the nurse for assessing and optimizing medication compliance in the older adult:

- Encourage patients to bring all their medications to each visit.
- Determine if there are risk factors that can influence compliance, such as chronic disease, impaired vision, hearing loss, or impaired cognition.
- Assess medication compliance through open, nonthreatening conversation, reviewing refill patterns, pill counts, and drug levels.
- Recruit active patient and family involvement, stressing the importance of compliance.
- Provide written and verbal drug information to the patient and family.
- Consider the use of compliance-enhancing aids, such as drug record, medication record, and medication boxes. (See also the Patient Teaching Box on commonsense strategies for safe and effective medication use.)

SMOKING AMONG OLDER ADULTS

Smoking is a modifiable behavior with serious health consequences, no matter what the age of the smoker. Unfortunately, the body of knowledge directly applicable to helping older smokers quit is limited, because, as a group, they have been lower on the priority list for research than the younger population. Although the prevalence of smoking is somewhat lower in the older population than in younger groups, older adults are at least equally interested in personal health promotion. The consequences of continued smoking are especially serious for them, and the benefits of their quitting are substantial.

Recent evidence indicates that by quitting, older smokers with existing coronary heart disease can reduce their risk of myocardial infarction and death, even after years of accumulated exposure to smoke (Hermanson,

Omenn, Dronmal, & Gersh, 1988). Clearly, older adults should quit smoking, but the how and why of smoking cessation are rarely addressed in the literature.

PHYSIOLOGIC ISSUES

In the United States and other developed countries, more than 80% of all deaths due to coronary heart disease occur among people who are 65 or older, as do two thirds of the deaths due to cancer (LaCroix et al., 1991). Cigarette smoking is known to cause coronary heart disease and cancer in middle age. However, it remains undetermined whether long-term smokers who survive to old age remain at higher risk of death resulting from cigarette smoking than nonsmokers.

As people live longer and escape the threat of death from infectious or acute illness, chronic health conditions, such as heart disease, cancer, and lung disease, are accounting for increased morbidity and mortality. In recent annual surgeon general's reports, it was estimated that smoking causes 30% of cancer deaths (Smith, Shultz, & Morse, 1990), 30% of deaths from coronary heart disease, and 80% to 90% of deaths from chronic obstructive disease each year. The estimated annual number of deaths attributable to smoking from these three causes of death is more than all the American lives lost in World War I, Korea, and Vietnam combined.

Smoking-related cancer deaths account for 41% of cancer deaths in men age 65 years and older and 15% of cancer deaths in women age 65 years and older (Keintz, 1988). Among adults age 55 to 64 years, there are 996 deaths from coronary heart disease per 100,000 men for smokers, compared with 542 for nonsmokers. For adults age 65 to 74 years, the rates are 1400 for nonsmokers compared with 2025 for smokers (Keintz, 1988). Determinations such as these have prompted the surgeon general to conclude that smoking is a preventable cause of premature death and disability in the United States. However, despite widespread publicity about the dangers of smoking, nearly one of three adults continues to smoke (Smith et al., 1990).

ECONOMIC EFFECT OF SMOKING

Older adults represent approximately 12% of the population, but they account for 36% of health care expenditures. These expenditures totaled more than $150 billion and averaged $5,000 per year for each older person, more than four times that spent for younger persons. About one fourth of the average expenditure, came from direct (out-of-pocket) payments by or for older people. The costs associated with smoking exacerbate the rising health care costs incurred by older adults.

Older people accounted for 31% of all hospital stays and 42% of all days of care in hospitals in 1987. The average length of a hospital stay was 8.6 days for older people, compared with 5.4 days for people younger than age 65. Current and former older smokers spent more days in the hospital than did their nonsmoking counterparts. They also lost more days from work and have higher mortality rates than nonsmokers.

The most important costs of smoking are those of diseases and the attendant morbidity, mortality, medical care costs, indirect losses, and intangible losses from pain, suffering, and other quality-of-life changes. Almost $5.67 billion in direct costs were attributable to smoking for adults age 65 years and older. As persons age, their health care costs are borne not only by themselves but also by the government and employers. At an average cost of $1.69 per pack of cigarettes, it could literally pay to stop smoking.

HEALTH BENEFITS OF SMOKING CESSATION

The older adult smoker should be counseled concerning the risks of smoking and the overall benefits of smoking cessation. These benefits include the following:

- Smoking cessation has major and immediate health benefits for men and women of all ages; benefits apply to persons with and without smoking-related diseases.
- Former smokers live longer than continuing smokers.
- Smoking cessation decreases the risk of lung cancer, other cancers, heart attack, stroke, and chronic lung disease.
- The health benefits of smoking cessation far exceed any risks from the average 5-lb (2.3 kg) weight gain or any adverse psychological effects that may follow quitting.

In the 1990 surgeon general's report, life-table projections of mortality by smoking status were performed using data from follow-up of more than 1 million subjects for 4 years. These calculations showed substantially lower mortality with sustained abstinence from cigarettes over all age groups through 70 to 74 years. For example, for women who had smoked less than one pack of cigarettes daily and quit at 65 to 69 years of age, the projected 15-year mortality was 39%, compared with 46% for those who continued to smoke (Samet, 1990).

NURSING ASSESSMENT

Cigarettes and other forms of tobacco are addicting. Nurses have a responsibility to treat and advise patients who are addicted to illicit drugs or alcohol.

History and Interview
Although the prevalence of smoking is somewhat lower in the older population than in younger groups, older adults are at least equally interested in personal health promotion. The consequences of continued smoking are especially serious for them, and the benefits of their quitting are substantial. Therefore, the nurse must assess the following:

- Smoking history
- Daily habits that support the use/abuse of tobacco products
- Interest in smoking-cessation programs
- Alternatives to decrease nicotine withdrawal

The interview should include a discussion of health beliefs with the older adult and family, and the nurse should encourage discussion of preventive health measures specific to the needs of the person, cessation of smoking, dietary needs, stress reduction, and implementation of an exercise program. Informational resources (community) specific to health maintenance needs of the person/family as well as multidisciplinary patient care conferences that discuss health maintenance needs can add much to the older adult's ability to limit tobacco use.

Risk Factors

Smoking is considered a major risk factor in 8 of the top 16 causes of death for people age 65 and older (Hermanson et al., 1988). Smoking continues to affect lung function into old age, with 55% of the respiratory system disease deaths among men 65 years and older attributed to smoking and 38% of women's deaths. Deaths from chronic obstructive pulmonary disease rise linearly to about 425 per 100,000 adults among smokers age 75 to 84 years compared with about 50 per 100,000 for nonsmokers (LaCroix et al., 1991). Exposure to passive smoking is a problem for older adults, especially those with compromised health status. Passive smoking exacerbates both the onset of angina and the symptoms of bronchial asthma. Smoking complicates existing illnesses, which are likely to be more prominent in older adults than in younger ones. Smoking affects every aspect of life and health, from increased morbidity and mortality to effects of acute and chronic illness on quality of life.

Clinical Pearl

Assessment: Pack Years: Multipy each pack per day by the number of years smoked. For example, 2 packs per day times 40 years equals 80 pack years.

Cost: Multiply the initial 80 pack-year old person by

$$\$1.69 \times 2 \times 365 = \$ \ 1,233.70$$
$$\textit{Total cost} \qquad = \$49,348.00$$

Other problems associated with smoking in the older adult include reduced bone demineralization, as in osteoporosis; decline in body weight; decline in muscle strength; a higher incidence of oral cancer; and a higher incidence of smoking-related accidents, such as home fires and body burns.

Physical Examination

The physical examination should include inspection of posture, shape of the chest, symmetry of chest expansion, respirations, capillary refill of nail beds, skin color, and sputum (color, odor, amount, consistency). Palpation of the ribs for tenderness should be included, along with skin temperature, turgor, and moisture. Examination of the chest should include percussion for dullness or flatness, with bilateral comparisons and ausculation of breath sounds for crackles or wheezes.

DIAGNOSTIC STUDIES

Diagnostic studies for the older adult smoker should include a chest x-ray for baseline assessment. If deficits are suspected, arterial blood gases when breathing room air and/or oxygen saturation may be ordered.

NURSING DIAGNOSES

Selected nursing diagnoses based on a specific patient with a history of to-bacco abuse are as follows:

- Activity Intolerance, related to smoking
- Altered Tissue Perfusion (cardiovascular), related to smoke inhalation
- Altered Tissue Perfusion (respiratory), related to smoke inhalation
- Ineffective Airway Clearance, related to bronchial disease
- Ineffective Breathing Pattern, related to airway congestion
- Impaired Gas Exchange, related to smoking
- Altered Health Maintenance, related to smoking behavior

NURSING INTERVENTIONS

Older adults may need special help to quit smoking, because they tend to be long-term heavy smokers. There is substantial evidence that several factors improve success in quitting, including the use of multiple cessation methods, presence of illness or risk factors that enhance motivation to quit, and good maintenance procedures for long-term support.

A variety of smoking cessation methods have been used over the years. The most recent method is the use of transdermal nicotine patches. All trans-dermal nicotine doses significantly decrease the severity of nicotine withdrawal and significantly reduce cigarette use by patients who do not stop smoking (Christen, Hatsukami, Rennard, & Lichtenstein, 1991). Although studies based on the use of patches have not included older adults, the potential for smoking cessation with a transdermal patch should be considered based on smoking habit, health factors, and willingness of the patient to quit smoking. Nicotine patches may have adverse side effects. Nurses and health care providers should caution their older adult patients to look for the following:

- Erythema
- Itching
- Burning under the patch (approximately 25% to 50% of patients)
- Other side effects reported less often, including a generalized rash, headache, nausea, vertigo, dyspepsia, myalgias, increased cough, insomnia, and nightmares

Although overdose, dependency, and abuse have not been reported with the patches, experience is still limited.

Nicotine poisoning can cause signs and symptoms ranging from pallor, dizziness, and nausea to hypotension, convulsions, and respiratory failure. There are a variety of approaches to treatment that appeal to different patient preferences and budgets. Smoking cessation can include behavior modification, group support, hypnosis, and specialized clinics and agencies, such as the American Lung Association, American Cancer Society, and American Heart Association. See also the nursing care plan for a patient with tobacco abuse problems.

Nursing Care Plan

FOR A PATIENT WITH TOBACCO ABUSE PROBLEMS

Nursing Diagnosis: Altered Health Maintenance, related to health benefits and disease process.

Definition: A condition in which an individual is or could be unable or unwilling to learn or to maintain optimal wellness.

Assessment Findings:

1. Hypertension
2. Body lesions
3. Obesity
4. Smoking
5. Unclean physical appearance
6. Elevated serum glucose level

Nursing Interventions with Selected Rationales:

1. Provide a nonjudgmental environment in which patient and patient's family can share health beliefs.
   Rationale: The patient is more likely to share important health information if the nurse meets all patients with nonjudgmental acceptance.
2. Encourage discussion of preventive health measures specific to patient needs, such as dietary changes, cessation of smoking, stress reduction, implementation of exercise program.
   Rationale: If the patient understands how and why such changes need to be made, compliance is more likely.
3. Evaluate patient's and family's ability to perform learned skills after discharge by requesting a return demonstration.
   Rationale: Deficits in the patient's (and the family's) understanding of care techniques can be remedied before the patient is discharged.
4. Offer information on community resources specific to health maintenance needs of the patient and the patient's family
   Rationale: Community resources may provide the peer support the patient needs to adhere to smoking-cessation programs.
5. Initiate a multidisciplinary patient care conference to discuss health maintenance needs with patient and family.
   Rationale: Understanding how smoking affects the body as a whole may impress upon the patient the need to adhere to health maintenance regimens.

Desired Patient Outcomes/Discharge Criteria:

1. Patient verbalizes knowledge of adverse effects of previous health beliefs.
2. Patient acknowledges necessity for assistance.
3. Patient verbalizes willingness to follow nursing/medical regimen.
4. Patient demonstrates knowledge of preventive health measures.

REFERENCES

American Association of Retired Persons. (1989). A profile of older Americans. *AARP Fulfillment.* Available from AARP, 1909 K St., NW, Washington, DC 20049, PF3049 (1289) D996.

Bienenfeld, D. (1990). Substance abuse. In *Verwoerdt's clinical geropsychiatry* (3rd ed.), Bienenfeld, E. & Verwoerdt, A. 164–176). Baltimore: Williams & Wilkins.

Chenitz, W. C., Salisbury, S., & Stone, J. T. (1990). Drug misuse and abuse in the elderly. *Issues in Mental Health Nursing, 11,* 1–16.

Christen, A., Hatsukami, D., Rennard, S., & Lichtenstein, E. (1991). Transdermal nicotine for smoking cessation. *Journal of the American Medical Association, 266*(22), 3133–3138.

Egbert, A. M. (1993). The older alcoholic: Recognizing the subtle clues. *Geriatrics, 48*(7), 63–69.

Gupta, K. L. (1993). Alcoholism in the elderly. *Alcoholism, 93*(2), 203–306.

Haldeman, K., & Gafner, G. (1990). Are elderly alcoholics discriminated against? *Journal of Psychosocial Nursing, 28*(5), 7–11.

Hermanson, B., Omenn G. S., Dronmal, R. A., & Gersh, B. J. (1988). Participants in the coronary artery surgery group. Beneficial six-year outcome of smoking in older men and women with coronary artery disease; results from the CASS registry. *New England Journal of Medicine, 88*(319), 1365–1369.

Keintz, M. K., Rimer, B., Fleisher, L., & Engstrom, R. (1988). Health promotion and problems: Aging, smoking among older adults: Cosequences and possible solutions. *The Gerontologist, 28*(4), 481–490.

LaCroix, A. Z., Lang, J., Scherr, P., Wallace, R. B. Cornoni-Huntley, J., Berkman, L., Curb, J. D., Evans, D., & Hennekens, C. H. (1991). Smoking and mortality among older men and women in three communities. *New England Journal of Medicine, 324*(23).

Marcus, M. T. (1993). Alcohol and other drug abuse in elders. *Journal of E. T. Nursing, 20,* 106–110.

Molgaard, C. A., Nakamura, C. M., Stanford, E. P., Peddecord, K. M. & Morton, D. J. (1990). Prevalence of alcohol consumption among older persons. *Journal of Community Health, 15*(4), 239–251.

Samet, J. M. (1990). The report of the surgeon general: The health benefits of smoking cessation. *American Review of Respiratory Disease, 142,* 993–994.

Scherer, J. (1995). *Introductory medical surgical nursing* (6th ed.). Philadelphia: J. B. Lippincott.

Smith, P. E., Shultz, J. M., & Morse, D. L. (1990). Assessing the damage from cigarette smoking in New York State. *New York State Journal of Medicine, 90,* 56–60.

BIBLIOGRAPHY

Beresford, T. P., Blow, F.C., & Brower, K. J. (1990). Alcoholism in the elderly. *Comprehensive Therapy, 16*(9), 38–43.

Busby, W. J., Campbell, A. J., Borrie, M. J., & Spears, G. R. S. (1988). Alcohol use in a community-based sample of subjects ages 70 and older. *Journal of the American Geriatrics Society, 36,* 301–305.

Huntington, D. D. (1990). Home care of the elderly alcoholic. *Home Health Care Nurse, 8*(5) 26–32.

Laforge, R. G., & Mignon, S. I. (1993). Alcohol use and alcohol problems among the elderly. *Rhode Island Medicine, 76,* 21–25.

Ticehurst, S. (1990). Alcohol and the elderly. *Australia and New Zealand Journal of Psychiatry, 24,* 252–260.

Miller, N. S., Belkin, B. M., & Gold, M. S. (1991). Alcohol and drug dependence among the elderly: Epidemiology, diagnosis, and treatment. *Comprehensive Psychiatry, 32*(2) 153–165.

Nicotine patches. (1992). *Medicine Letter, 34*(86), 37–38.

U.S. Bureau of the Census. (1990). *Census of the population: subject reports, American Indians.* Washington, DC: U.S. Government Printing Office.

Problems Associated With Abnormal Cell Growth

Objectives

1. Compare normal physiologic changes in the older adult with changes related to abnormal cell growth.
2. Describe nursing assessment of older adults with abnormal cell growth.
3. Identify potential nursing diagnoses appropriate for the needs of the older adult with abnormal cell growth.
4. Identify the nurse's role as health promoter in carrying out interventions related to education, prevention, and early detection of abnormal cell growth in the older adult.
5. Describe the nurse's role when cancer is diagnosed in the older adult.
6. Describe the nurse's role during the period of cancer therapy.
7. Describe the nurse's role in the care of the older adult cancer survivor.
8. Describe the role of hospice in the care of the older adult patient with cancer.

INTRODUCTION

CANCER IS A LARGE GROUP OF DISEASES characterized by the uncontrolled growth and spread of abnormal cells. This abnormality may result in death. There is a steady increase in the incidence of cancer in aging adults, suggesting that at least some aspect of the aging process increases one's susceptibility to cancer. One theory is that as the body ages the immune system deteriorates, losing its ability to serve as a buffer against the abnormal cancer cells that form in the body throughout life. As the body ages, impaired integrity of the immune system allows new cancers to develop by failing to detect and eliminate abnormal cells. This theory is supported by the incidence of cancer in pa-

Staab, AS and Hodges, LC: ESSENTIALS OF GERONTOLOGICAL NURSING,
© 1996 J. B. Lippincott Company

tients with acquired immunodeficiency syndrome. The immune system breaks down, giving rise to the emergence of multiple rare forms of cancers. In addition to a breakdown in the immune system, the older patient has generally experienced a longer duration of exposure to carcinogens and the long duration periods required for the development of clinical cancers.

Cancer is the second leading cause of death in adults older than 65 years of age in the United States. The leading cause of cancer deaths among men and women is lung cancer (American Cancer Society, 1993). The highest incidence of cancer in the older adult male are those of the prostate, lung, colon, and rectum. Breast, colon, rectum, and lung cancers rank high in incidence among older females.

Many of the older population still believe that a cancer diagnosis is synonymous with impending death. The number of older adults who survive cancer has increased so significantly that cancer is now considered a chronic life-threatening illness rather than a terminal disease. This rising number of cancer survivors will require continuing care throughout periods of recurrence, subsequent treatment, and remission. Although aggressive medical treatment remains the initial primary focus of patients with cancer, the nurse and other health professionals must begin to focus on the changing needs of the patient at various points along the continuum of recurrence and remission.

With early detection and a wide choice of aggressive therapies, cancer is almost always treatable and often curable. There is always hope and, usually, there is reason for optimism, because an older adult cancer patient's life can be extended and its quality improved. The nurse should view the older adult with cancer as a patient with a chronic illness who should be cared for and managed accordingly.

NORMAL PHYSIOLOGIC CHANGES WITH AGING

The Oncology Nursing Society Position Paper on Cancer and Aging (McCaffrey Boyle et al., 1992) reports that many barriers hinder the provision of quality care to older adults with cancer. A major barrier cited in this report is the limited knowledge base about the relationship between cancer and aging. The older adult may delay reporting an early cancer warning signal because of the tendency to credit body changes to the aging process. To differentiate between what is normal and what might be cancer, the older adult should know the changes in body systems associated with aging.

BOWEL AND BLADDER CHANGES

Colon motility slows but bowel habits are not altered by aging if diet and activity remain the same, if no constipating medications are given, and if response is prompt to the urge to defecate. Structural alterations in the urinary system, such as atrophy and muscle weakening, occur with aging. The overall bladder capacity decreases. Nocturia, urgency, frequency, dysuria, and retention may occur.

MALE AND FEMALE REPRODUCTIVE CHANGES

Men may experience benign enlargement of the prostate and the resultant inability to urinate or to start urination only with difficulty. The urinary stream may be weak with slight hematuria. In women, relaxation of perineal muscles may lead to incontinence. There should be no vaginal discharge of blood post-menopause. There should be no discharge from the urethra after an ileal conduit. Breasts may become pendulous, elongated, and flaccid as the result of muscle atrophy, and nipples may retract due to nipple atrophy and fibrotic changes.

UPPER GASTROINTESTINAL CHANGES

Weight loss may occur due to changes in the upper gastrointestinal tract, including thinning of the oral mucosa. The mouth becomes drier and taste buds are less sensitive. Gum disease, root cavities, and cracked teeth may develop. Poorly fitting dentures and improper mastication related to joint changes may also contribute to this weight loss. Lowered esophageal sphincter pressure is considered a normal finding in people older than 60 years of age. Heartburn and possible esophageal erosion may result from acid reflux. Reduced gastrointestinal motility may lead to constipation, flatulence, and abdominal discomfort.

SKIN CHANGES

General dryness, laxity, uneven pigmentation, variety of proliferative lesions, and loss of dermal thickness (thin skin) are considered normal aging changes of the skin. Such factors as genetic tendencies and sun exposure affect the rate of the skin's aging process.

LUNG CHANGES

In the aging lung, there is a decline in tissue elasticity. There is a general loss of strength in respiratory muscles and the diaphragm and a reduction in compliance of the bony thorax as the rib cage becomes more rigid. As a result, breathing requires more work, and tolerance of exercise and stress decreases. There is a normal diminished ability to cough.

ABNORMAL PHYSIOLOGIC CHANGES AFFECTING CELL GROWTH

The older adult needs to be alert to body changes. The American Cancer Society has identified seven warning signals of cancer. The initial letters of the seven signals form the acronym "CAUTION." It is important that the older adult exhibiting any of these signals sees a physician immediately. Even if the signal turns out to be a false alarm rather than an indication of cancer, the potential lifesaving benefits of early detection and reporting should outweigh any embarrassment about going to the doctor.

PSYCHOSOCIAL ISSUES

The older adult with cancer will range from one who is performing all activities of daily living to one who is already coping with a chronic, disabling illness. During the diagnostic phase, activities will be interrupted. There may be a knowledge deficit about physicians' exams, fear and anxiety related to the

Display 25-1
CANCER'S SEVEN WARNING SIGNALS (CAUTION)

1. Change in bowel or bladder habits
2. A sore throat that does not heal
3. Unusual bleeding or discharge
4. Thickening or lump in breast or elsewhere
5. Indigestion or difficulty in swallowing
6. Obvious change in wart or mole
7. Nagging cough or hoarseness

The warning signals can save your life . . . if you see your doctor (American Cancer Society).

uncertainty of test results, and discomfort from symptoms and loss of control related to schedules.

When there is confirmation of the cancer diagnosis, the response of the patient and family will reflect the meaning of cancer to them. The nurse may observe signs of shock, anger, fear, crisis, and spiritual distress. During the period in which the treatment choice is being decided by the professional team, sensory overload, depression, and despair may be evident after physician, patient, and family conferences.

The patient must regain control when it is time to give informed consent to treatment. Dialogue with the health care team about details of treatment will enable the older adult to enter the program as a partner. All involved must consider that the patient may elect not to receive treatment.

Potential stressors related to the treatment period include factors associated with recovery from surgery, discomforts of adjunct treatment, depression over the length of the treatment, financial burden, and lengthy family stress. There is continued need for a support system.

The last stage on the health–illness continuum is the return of the individual to optimum activities of daily living and the recognition that the period of survivorship is being entered. Health promotion should continue, as should emphasis on the seven warning signals.

NURSING ASSESSMENT

Much of the assessment of an older adult with cancer can be collected through a history and interview. The nurse should use an unhurried approach and conduct the interview in a comfortable, private location. The goal of the interview is to obtain all of the facts that will ultimately influence both the nursing diagnoses and the plan of care.

HISTORY AND INTERVIEW

The history of the current complaint is very important. For example, the chief complaint of change in bowel habits in the older adult would generate the following questions:

- What are your normal bowel habits?
- What is the difference in your current bowel habits?

- How long ago did the change occur?
- What is the shape of your bowel movements?
- Have you noticed any blood in your stool?
- Have you had any stomach discomfort, such as bloating, fullness, cramps, or gas pains?
- After your bowels move, do you feel that they have emptied completely?
- Have you had an unexplained weight loss?
- Have you noticed an increase in fatigue?

The nurse will learn how much the patient knows about his or her body. This will also demonstrate his or her alertness to variations from the normal.

The older adult should be given ample time to answer the questions thoroughly and time to ask for clarification of any questions not understood. The older adult with a history of colon cancer will probably show evidence of higher anxiety but will be more familiar with the questions. For patients presenting with a chief complaint suspicious of cancer, the combination of questions, both open-ended and direct, relating to normal aging and early warning cancer signals should be the format.

RISK FACTORS

Of particular concern to the nurse are risk factors in the older patient's history that might lead to abnormal cell development. Risk factors include those outside a person's control, such as age and family history, and those under personal control, such as dietary habits and habits related to lifestyle (see Table 25-1 for risk factors and warning signals of cancer for the older adult). The nurse can help the patient differentiate between the risk factors that are uncontrollable and those that may be personally controllable. Heightening awareness of risk factors for cancer and warning signals could create the perception of personal vulnerability and thus stimulate preventive self-care actions. These self-care actions to decrease cancer risk include the following:

- Changing from a diet high in fat to foods in the cabbage family, more fiber in the diet, and an increase in foods high in vitamins A and C
- Stopping cigarette smoking
- Wearing a mask when spraying chemicals (avoids skin and lung irritation)
- Smoothing rough edges on dentures (avoids oral mucosal irritation)
- Limiting alcohol intake

PHYSICAL EXAMINATION

Cancer screening includes procedures that should be done during physical examination by the nurse. The sequence below follows that of cancer's seven warning signals, as presented in Table 25-1. Screening tests for older adults are used for the detection of:

- Bladder cancer—urinalysis every year
- Prostate—digital-rectal examination every year when older than age 50
- Oral cavity cancer—general physical examination should include yearly examination of the oral cavity for cancers (should be included in a twice-yearly dental checkup using the techniques of inspection and palpation)
- Cervical and endometrial cancer—should include Pap smear and pelvic exam every year: after three or more consecutive satisfactory normal an-

Table 25-1

RISK FACTORS AND WARNING SIGNALS FOR TYPES OF CANCER

Warning Signals	Risk Factors
Colon Cancer	
• Diarrhea or constipation	• Increasing age (after 60)
• Bloody stools	• Colorectal polyp(s)
• Stools narrower than usual	• Family history of colorectal cancer
• General stomach discomfort (bloating, fullness, cramps)	• Inflammatory bowel disease
• Frequent gas pains	• Diet low in fruits and vegetables containing vitamins A and C
• Feeling that the bowel doesn't empty completely	• High-fat, low-fiber diet
• Weight loss with no known reason	• History of genital or bladder cancer
• Constant fatigue	
Bladder Cancer	
• Hematuria ranging from microscopic to gross, present through entire stream, rarely profuse, usually intermittent and painless	• Male, white, older than age 50 years
	• Smoking
	• Exposure to chemical carcinogens
• Prostate cancer (asymptomatic in early stages)	• Personal history of bladder cancer
	• Increasing age
• Back and/or hip pain	• Black males
Oral Cavity Cancer	
• Painless sore in the mouth that bleeds easily and does not heal in 2–3 weeks	• Occurs twice as often in males as in females older than 60 years of age
• Painless lump in the cheek that can be felt with the tongue	• Smoking and tobacco use
• White or red patch on gums, tongue, or lining of mouth	• Use of smokeless tobacco
• Soreness or a feeling that something is caught in the throat	• Poor oral hygiene
• Difficulty chewing or swallowing	• Ill-fitting dentures
• Difficulty moving jaw or tongue	
• Numbness of tongue or areas of mouth	
• Swelling of the jaw that causes dentures to fit poorly	
Cervical and Endometrial Cancer	
• Increased or abnormal vaginal discharge	• Early age at first intercourse
• Any bleeding after menopause	• Multiple sex partners
• Pap smear Class III, IV, V	• Smoking, condylomata, or warts
• Bleeding from bladder/colon	• Postmenopausal, late menopause, infertility
	• Diabetes, hypertension
	• Irregular menses
	• Personal history of breast/ovarian cancer
	• Prolonged estrogen therapy

(continued)

Table 25-1

RISK FACTORS AND WARNING SIGNALS FOR TYPES OF CANCER
(Continued)

Warning Signals	Risk Factors
Breast Cancer • Lump or thickening in the breast with less distinct borders • Painless, immobile lump (pain with more advanced disease) • Usually solitary, unilateral lesion • Nipple drainage (bloody) or eversion • Skin dimpling or retraction • Skin edema or peau d'orange	• Majority of cases in women older than 50 years of age • Familial history (mother or sister), precancerous lump • First-born after age 30 • Obesity, never had children • History of benign breast lump • Being single or Jewish • Alcohol consumption • High socioeconomic status • Diet high in fat • Early menarche, late menopause

Skin Cancer
• Obvious change in wart or mole:
  Asymmetry
  Border irregular
  Color not the same all over
  Diameter wider than 1/4" or growing larger
• Most common sites are face, ears, neck, lip, hand, head, shoulders, shin, ankles, lower leg, palms, skin, under nails, soles of feet
	• Increasing age (incidence rises between 30–60 years of age)
	• Light-skinned, fair-haired, freckles; albinism
	• Burns easily; history of severe sunburn when younger than 30 or excessive sunbathing
	• History of congenital moles or dysplastic nevi or cutaneous melanoma
	• Outdoor occupation

Lung Cancer • Nagging cough or hoarseness • Cancer of the lung or larynx • Silent disease in the early stages • Cough that changes from dry and hacking to productive, with thick, purulent sputum • Blood-tinged sputum, particularly in the morning • Recurring fever • Unresolved pneumonia	• Older than age 50 years • Voluntary smoking and involuntary passive smoking • Occupational exposure, such as asbestos • Excessive alcohol intake
Esophageal Cancer • Vague sense of pressure, fullness, indigestion, difficulty swallowing • Occasional substernal distress, may be advanced even though symptoms have been noticeable for only weeks/months	• Increasing age (older than age 50) • History of chronic irritation from heavy intake of alcohol and tobacco use • Hiatal hernia/gastric reflux • Esophagitis, diverticula • Eating extremely hot foods • Postingestion of caustic agent • Poor oral hygiene

(continued)

Table 25-1	RISK FACTORS AND WARNING SIGNALS FOR TYPES OF CANCER (Continued)	
	Warning Signals	Risk Factors
	Stomach Cancer • Stomach upset or chronic stomach problems • Vague, poorly defined symptoms of variable duration • Fullness, heaviness, moderate distension after meals • Overt symptoms usually mean advanced disease	• Age above 70 years • Low socioeconomic status • Poor nutritional habits • Vitamin A deficiency • Use of food additives, smoking • Pernicious anemia, benign peptic disease, gastric polyps, hypochlorhydria, alcohol consumption

nual exams, the Pap test may be performed less frequently at the discretion of the physician; endometrial biopsy at menopause if high risk
• Breast cancer—monthly breast self-examination
• Skin cancer—yearly examination of all skin surfaces to evaluate changes of moles, blemishes, freckles, and other lesions
• Lung cancer—chest x-ray is not included in routine cancer exam but might be indicated if patient has history of long-term smoking habit; sputum cytology when history indicates

There is no screening for esophageal cancer, but data gathered in the history and interview would indicate high-risk factors that need to be eliminated. There is no screening for stomach cancer. At-risk patients should consult their physicians for chronic stomach problems.

DIAGNOSTIC STUDIES

There are two major diagnostic studies for early detection of cancer: the proctologic examination (proctoscopy, sigmoidoscopy, total colonoscopy) for colon and rectal cancer and mammography for breast cancer. Indication of an early warning signal during this history and interview of a patient or a stool sample with occult blood would justify a visual colon examination. The test most frequently used as a diagnostic tool for occult blood in the stool is the Hemoccult slide test. This is a test completed by the patient at home. A paper is dropped into the commode after each stool, or a stool sample is applied to a card. The paper turns purple if there is blood present. The extent of the colon examination would be decided by the physician based on Hemoccult slide reactivity. The older adult who is at high risk for colon and rectum cancer should have a proctologic examination annually for 2 years. In the absence of detectable cancer, proctologic examination may then be reduced to once every 3 to 5 years, as the physician advises.

The older adult woman should have an annual mammogram unless the presence of high-risk factors dictates more frequent assessment. The patient who has scheduled diagnostic tests may lack knowledge related to the examination, experience fear and anxiety related to the uncertainty of test results or discomfort related to symptoms, and have a feeling of loss of control related to schedules imposed. It is the role of the nurse and other health care workers who have contact with the patient during the diagnostic process to provide knowledge by giving written and verbal instructions. The patient's questions should be answered and the instructions reinforced. The patient's concerns should be heard and privacy, comfort, and safety provided. When appropriate, the patient should participate in the scheduling of the examinations.

NURSING DIAGNOSES

Once the assessment of the older adult with abnormal cell growth has been completed, the patient's needs can be identified and stated as nursing diagnoses on which the nurse can base an individualized plan of care for the patient. The following are nursing diagnoses related to normal aging changes and the patient's having received treatment for cancer:

- Risk for Impaired Skin Integrity, related to aging changes in the immune system and skin
- Altered Oral Mucous Membrane, related to disease process or radiation/chemotherapy
- Potential Knowledge Deficit, related to behavior during the period of frequent examinations and while undergoing treatments
- Body Image Disturbance: Alopecia, related to cancer therapy
- Altered Nutrition: Less than body requirements, related to diminished appetite
- Activity Intolerance: Fatigue, related to disease process or treatment side effects
- Pain: Alteration in Comfort, related to disease process
- Anticipatory Grieving, related to loss of control/normal lifestyle
- Potential Knowledge Deficit, related to the need to continue health behavior

NURSING INTERVENTIONS

Efforts to maintain good health in the older adult are widespread. Older adults show a remarkable willingness to accept responsibility for health promotion, education, and support as cancer survivors. Older adults may require nursing assistance as they evaluate life's meaning and reassess priorities as a result of recognizing the limits of their own mortality. Cancer survivors who respond favorably to treatment may feel guilty when comparing their progress with that of cancer survivors whose course has been less successful. The nurse needs to be aware that these reactions are normal. The nursing care plan should incorporate normal changes of aging and early symptoms of cancer when teaching the older adult.

PATIENT AND FAMILY EDUCATION

More than 80% of the causes of cancer are theoretically avoidable, which demonstrates that cancer is not inevitable and that cancer prevention is feasible and practical. The nurse needs to promote prevention as effectively as care (Cohen & Frank Stromberg, 1990). For cancer survivors, mortality is disproportionately higher in older adults than among their younger counterparts,

Nursing Care Plan

FOR A PATIENT MAKING COMPARISON OF NORMAL AGING CHANGES AND EARLY CANCER SIGNALS

Nursing Diagnoses: Knowledge Deficit, related to the difference between normal aging changes and early symptoms of cancer

Definition: State in which patient does not know if physical symptoms require medical attention

Assessment Findings:
1. Unaware that body changes may be caused by disease
2. Body change in functioning of lungs, colon, breast, prostate, mouth, or skin

Nursing Interventions With Selected Rationales:
1. During the history, collect data on current body functions and habits.
   Rationale: This initial assessment provides baseline measures of physical function.
2. If a change is identified, ask how long the change has been present.
   Rationale: Identifying symptoms and determining their duration allows the nurse to set priorities for the treatment of symptoms in their order of potential severity.
3. Collect specific data on symptoms related to change using knowledge of seven warning signals as basis for questions.
   Rationale: Targeting assessment of potentially vulnerable areas allows health care provider to rule out or treat common cancers in a timely fashion.
4. Document all data on the nursing history form, including the chief complaint(s) on the nurse's notes.
   Rationale: Accurate documentation ensures consistency of care for the patient by providing a historical and dynamic record of interventions
5. If the nursing history does not correlate with the medical history, discuss the differences with the physician.
   Rationale: Reconciling differences between medical and nursing records ensures that all health care personnel have the same accurate picture of the patient's health status. This prevents them from providing contradicting care.

Desired Patient Outcomes/Discharge Criteria:
1. Patient is aware of own body structures, functions, and habits and how they change with aging.
2. Patient recognizes what is normal for self.
3. Patient recognizes changes from what has been normal.
4. Patient knows seven warning signals.
5. Patient exhibits sense of responsibility for own health.
6. Patient consults physician when a signal appears.

---

which may indicate a reluctance of older adults to change lifelong high-risk practices. Nurses must advocate both primary and secondary cancer prevention and early detection activities for older adults. Patients' willingness can be a strong motivating factor, yet the problem of changing lifelong habits can be very stressful for older adults (Staab & Lyles, 1990). The nurse should encourage the older adult to lead a healthier life and to reduce cancer risks by following the 10 steps listed in Table 25-2.

Table *25-2*	**TEN STEPS TO A HEALTHIER LIFE AND REDUCED CANCER RISK** (Primary Factors)

Protective Factors
(Add to your life)

1. Eat more cabbage-family vegetables.
2. Add more high-fiber foods.
3. Choose foods with vitamin A.
4. Do the same for vitamin C.
5. Add weight control.

Risk Factors
(Subtract from your life)

6. Trim fat from your diet.
7. Subtract salt-cured, smoked, and nitrite-cured foods.
8. Stop cigarette smoking.
9. Go easy on alcohol.
10. Respect the sun's rays.

Taking Control: 10 Steps to a Healthier Life and Reduced Cancer Risk. American Cancer Society, MM No. 2019.05

MAMMOGRAPHY

The National Cancer Institute's cancer control objectives for the year 2000 are to increase the percentage of women 50 to 70 years of age who have an annual breast examination from 45% to 80% (Cohen & Frank Stromberg, 1990). Reasons that the older adult woman may not adhere to the recommended yearly mammogram include fear of radiation dosage and the discovery of cancer, embarrassment of exposure, and discomfort during the procedure. As a health educator, the nurse can help dispel the patient's fear of the test and explain the early detection benefits (see the Patient Teaching Box on mammography).

Patient Teaching Box
MAMMOGRAPHY PROCEDURE

- The screenfilm mammography or the xeromammography process used to film the breast produces minimal and safe radiation.
- The mammography procedure may detect a cancerous tumor too small to be felt at a very early stage of development.
- Although the breasts are exposed one at a time during the procedure, the rest of the body is covered with a hospital gown, exposing only the area being filmed. Usually the mammogram is done in a small, private room used specifically for that purpose.
- The breast is compressed between two plates, causing a feeling of tightness. Tissue compression improves the quality of the image and reduces the amount of primary and scatter radiation.

BREAST SELF-EXAMINATION

Seventy percent of breast cancers occur in women older than 50 years of age. Because 80% of breast tumors are detected by patients themselves, breast self-examination (BSE) should be included in the teaching plan of all older adult women. Breast examination is included in routine physical examinations, and the importance of a monthly self-exam is stressed. An opportune time for the nurse to evaluate the patient's knowledge of BSE is while giving hygienic care. The nurse may find that the older adult is uncomfortable feeling her own body or considers the procedure too complex to master. The nurse's teaching intervention should include:

- Providing information on the increased incidence of breast cancer with aging
- Demonstrating the technique of BSE on the patient
- Requesting that the patient return the demonstration
- Letting the mention of BSE serve as a reminder to the patient who does BSE regularly
- Asking the patient for a demonstration to ensure the patient that her technique is correct
- Answering any questions the patient may have about the procedure

The American Cancer Society has published several brochures that include diagrams to help the patient remember the technique (see accompanying display).

DETECTION OF COLORECTAL CANCER

Ninety-three percent of colorectal cancer occurs in persons age 50 or older. Failure of the older adult to know his or her own body may result in a missed symptom of colorectal cancer. The nurse who questions the patient about frequency, color, consistency, shape, and composition of the stool when taking a history of the pattern of elimination is establishing basic guidelines for evaluation. This enables the patient to know what changes to look for in the bowel pattern. The patient will come to know what is normal, when this pattern changes, and how to describe the change. Blood in the stool, constipation, narrowing of the stool to a pencil-like shape, mucous diarrhea, and a feeling of incomplete evacuation may be early indications of colorectal cancer. Pain is a late symptom.

The Hemoccult slide test is the leading test for fecal occult blood, yet of every 100 persons given the kits, only 52 complete and return them. In socioeconomically disadvantaged groups, the results are even more discouraging. Only 5 to 20 of any 100 tests are returned (Zanca, 1992). Failure of the older adult to return the Hemoccult slide test kit may result in a missed early warning sign of colorectal cancer.

Research reveals that noncompliance may be related to the fact that the person does not understand what is expected or how to use the test properly. One study demonstrated a way to improve participation in colorectal cancer screening for a group of older adults at a center where they came together daily for a hot meal. Older adult educators originated the idea of using peanut butter to demonstrate the procedure for collecting the stool specimens required for the Hemoccult slide test. After the peanut butter demonstration, the test yielded a 96% return at one site and 100% at another. Three cases of col-

Display 25-2

BREAST SELF-EXAMINATION TECHNIQUE

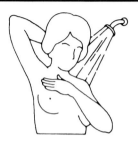

1. In the shower.

Examine your breasts during bath or shower; hands glide easily over wet skin. With fingers flat, move then gently over every part of each breast. Check for any lump, hard knot, or thickening.

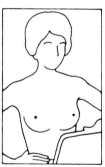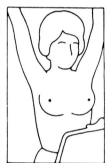

2. Before a mirror.

Inspect your breasts with arms at your sides. Next, raise your arms high overhead. Look for any changes in contour of each breast—a swelling, dimpling of skin, or changes in the nipple. Then rest palms on hips and press down firmly to flex your chest muscles. Left and right breast will not match exactly—few women's breasts do. Regular inspection shows what is normal for you and will give you confidence in your evaluation.

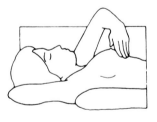

3. Lying down.

To examine your right breast put a pillow or folded towel under your right shoulder. Place your right hand behind your head—this distributes breast tissue more evenly on the chest. With left hand, press gently in small circular motions around an imaginary clock face. Begin at outermost top of your right breast for 12 o'clock, then move to 1 o'clock, and so on around the circle back to 12. A ridge of firm tissue in the lower curve of each breast is normal. Then move in an inch, toward the nipple, keep circling to examine every part of your breast, including the nipple. This requires at least three more circles. Now slowly repeat the procedure on your left breast with a pillow under your left shoulder and your left hand behind your head. Notice how your breast structure feels. Finally, squeeze the nipple of each breast gently between your thumb and index finger. Any discharge, clear or bloody, should be reported to your physician immediately.

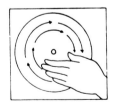

orectal cancer (9% of those tested) were found, which was significantly higher than the expected rate of 5% (Zanca, 1992). Nurses should ensure that when giving a Hemoccult kit to a patient, the procedure is described in detail and the patient is questioned to verify understanding.

> ### Clinical Pearl
>
> *Assessment: The nurse should identify where the older adult is in the cancer experience.*

NURSE AS SUPPORTER

When the confirmation of a cancer diagnosis has been made following diagnostic studies, biopsy, or surgery, the first role of the nurse as supporter is to interpret and validate information given to the patient and family. There will be consultations among the health care team followed by meetings between physicians, patient, and family. A visit from the chaplain may be helpful during this period, when there may be decisions to be made regarding treatment choices such as chemotherapy or surgery and consent forms to be signed. The nurse can help patients to deal with personal feelings of despair, helplessness, and loss of control while helping them to become actively involved in decision making and treatment.

Coping with the stress of having lost control of one's life may be the most difficult and discomforting emotional experience accompanying the overall ordeal of cancer. Much of this sense of lost control comes from the patient's perception that he or she lacks the information and knowledge needed to participate in self-care and the decisions about treatment. Therefore, by giving patients information and empowering them with knowledge, the nurse can restore the sense of self-control that is so critical to perceived quality of life. Nursing research has shown that most patients want maximum information about their illness. Moreover, the enhanced sense of self-control associated with having increased information can improve both functional status and perceived sense of well-being in patients with cancer (Camp-Sorrell, 1992). If the patient elects not to have the recommended treatment, the health care team members may need support in dealing with their personal feelings in relation to the patient's decision not to pursue treatment.

SUPPORT GROUPS

In the role of supporter, the nurse can refer the patient to a variety of support groups that are available for the older patient with cancer. Table 25-3 contains a list and descriptions of support groups usually offered by an active unit of the American Cancer Society. The groups consist of fellow patients, caregivers, family members, and members of the health care team who serve as facilitators. A nurse, psychologist, family counselor, or clergyman may serve as facilitator.

Support groups are designed to help patients and caregivers adapt to cancer and its treatment. The network of support comes from sharing and serves as

Table 25-3

SUPPORT GROUPS FOR CANCER PATIENTS AND CAREGIVERS

Support Group	Type of Patient	Services Offered
Reach to recovery	Mastectomy survivors	• Visit from former mastectomy patient • Must have physician referral for visit • Visitor must be 1 year postsurgery • Visitor must be recommended for American Cancer Society training course by surgeon
Look Good—Feel Better	Survivors taking chemotherapy or radiation	• Skin care and wig care • Cosponsored by American Cancer Society, Cosmetic Toiletry and Fragrance Association, and National Cosmetology Association • Cosmetics are free but wigs are not
Ostomy Support	All types of ostomy survivors	• Meet regularly as a group • American Cancer Society provides guidelines
Nu Voice	Laryngectomy survivors	• Group support • American Cancer Society provides guidelines
I Can Cope	Survivors with multiple diagnoses	• American Cancer Society has a scheduled agenda for a series of programs for survivors and families
Road to Recovery	All types of survivors who are receiving radiation or chemotherapy	• Volunteer drivers transport patients to treatments • Drivers take a brief course sponsored by the American Cancer Society

an outlet for the expression of fears, feelings, and frustrations. Attendance needs to be monitored. Patients with breast cancer may discontinue attending sessions that include patients with other types of cancer, because their problems relating to self-image and sexuality are too personal to share with those not experiencing the same concerns. This may be an indication of the need for a specialized group for breast cancer patients only, patterned after the ostomy and laryngectomy support groups, in which all patients have similar physical and psychological problems.

ONE-TO-ONE CANCER SURVIVOR SUPPORT

When the newly diagnosed patient is trying to make a decision about treatment choices, someone who has survived the same type of cancer can often offer support and comfort, help with difficult treatment decisions, and answer many questions based on his or her own personal cancer experience. Seeing a cancer survivor who has returned to an active lifestyle can give the newly diagnosed person hope and encouragement. What may begin as a telephone relationship may develop into personal visits. The cancer survivor as a support person expresses interest in the patient by making a commitment of time, energy, and knowledge to that patient. The patient may then come to the decision that resources enable them to cope with treatment or the results of surgery and altered lifestyles. An example of a one-to-one survivor support relationship can be found in the nursing care plan for an older adult with an ostomy.

Nursing Care Plan

FOR THE OLDER ADULT WITH AN OSTOMY

Nursing Diagnosis: Potential Body Image Disturbance, related to an ostomy

Definition: Response to physical changes created by ostomy

Assessment Findings:
1. Has had no previous exposure to person with ostomate
2. Does not want to discuss ostomy
3. Does not participate in ostomy care
4. Verbalizes depression

Nursing Interventions With Selected Rationales:
1. Include a cancer survivor with an ostomate as a support person on the health team.
   Rationale: An ostomate who has had the same type of cancer and returned to an active lifestyle can give the new ostomate hope and encouragement.
2. Schedule the support person's visits with regularity.
   Rationale: The visitor, though encouraging verbalization, will understand the patient's reluctance to talk and that it may take some time to draw out the patient's feelings.
3. Encourage the visitor, nurse, and enterostomal therapist to share information on the types of available appliances, products for skin care, and characteristics of the aging skin. Also have them demonstrate products and ask for return demonstration by the patient.
   Rationale: This information about the variety of resources of care may provide the patient with concrete facts indicating choices in care and techniques that can be mastered.
4. Encourage the patient to look and touch the stoma in the nurse's presence.
   Rationale: This indicates the nurse's acceptance of the stoma and understanding that the patient needs help in accepting the stoma as a new part of the body.
5. Ask the visitor to share his or her initial reluctance to participate in care.
   Rationale: This will indicate to the patient that such a reaction is normal. The older adult with a new stoma would face the same adjustments as any other person but, because of maturity tempered by life experiences, might not experience the intense emotional reaction that a younger ostomate would (Phillips, 1986).

Desired Patient Outcomes/Discharge Criteria:
1. Patient will establish an ongoing relationship with the visiting ostomate as a support person.
2. Patient will discuss the ostomy.
3. Patient participates in ostomy care.
4. Patient will adjust to the diagnosis of cancer in addition to that of the ostomy.

NURSE AS SUPPORTER DURING CANCER TREATMENTS

The nurse's responsibility when the older adult is receiving chemotherapy is to teach the patient what side effects to expect and which of those to report. Aging suppresses the immune system, especially in the presence of chronic disease, and many chemotherapy drugs cause bone marrow depression. The nurse needs to teach the patient to report common symptoms of these problems, such as elevated temperature, bleeding, shortness of breath, fatigue, and palpitation.

Adequate nutrition while receiving chemotherapy is important to replace normal tissues destroyed by the medication. Therefore, monitoring of gastrointestinal side effects, such as vomiting and diarrhea, is crucial to ensuring maintenance of body weight. Because the thin oral mucosa and drier mouth of the older adult places the chemotherapy patient at a higher risk for mouth sores, oral hygiene will be of particular concern. When stomatitis (inflammation of the mucosa of the mouth) is an expected side effect of the prescribed chemotherapy, the physician may start an older adult on a medicated mouthwash at the beginning of therapy before he or she is symptomatic. An older adult with a history of constipation taking chemotherapy will receive a stool softener to ease evacuation.

Teaching should include measures to help the patient deal with the physical and psychological aspects of alopecia (hair loss), a side effect of some medications. Physical assessment and accurate height and weight are essential data needed to determine dosage of the drug and expected tolerance. Dosage of the drug, which is determined by body surface, may be lowered if there is a decrease in function of the liver (which degrades the drugs given in chemotherapy) or kidneys (which excrete the drugs). The nurse needs to monitor liver enzymes and maintain an accurate intake and output on the patient. Numbness and tingling in the extremities may signal nerve damage, another potential side effect of chemotherapy. Chemotherapy may be given frequently for a period of 12 to 18 months. Leukemia, a second malignancy, and neurologic or cardiac symptoms may develop as a result of treatment months or even years after chemotherapy is discontinued.

The nurse has the added responsibility of monitoring the patient's skin when the older adult is receiving radiation therapy. There is the potential for tearing of the skin anywhere on the body during transportation of the patient or during positioning on the treatment table. Generally, the older adult tolerates the 5 days a week of radiation over a 5- to 6-week period. However, if the patient is debilitated from chronic disease, medication problems, or effects of cancer at the time of radiation, the radiation team assesses the tolerance of the patient, monitors the patient's skin, prescribes the type of preparation should the skin become damaged, and decides whether the treatments will continue or be terminated. The nurse reinforces these instructions with the older adult.

During therapy treatments, the older adult often establishes a bond with the treatment team. This relationship may make the patient feel comfortable about continuing with treatment. Patients telephone the staff to ask about symptoms while receiving treatments. A particular challenge to the team lies in not fostering patient dependency as they follow the older adult over an extended period of time. The team members should, therefore, not give out their home phone numbers. They should encourage care of the patient by more than one nurse and encourage the patient to reach out for support.

ROLE OF THE NURSE IN PROVIDING CARE TO CANCER SURVIVORS

The National Coalition of Cancer Survivors charter defines a survivor as a person diagnosed with cancer who has survived an episode of the disease (National Coalition for Cancer Survivorship, 1992). The survivor concept is a positive philosophy thought to affect the patient's outlook and, by association, enhance the immune system. The nurse encourages the patient to assume the survivorship philosophy, encourages attendance in a support group, resumes health promotion, and continues to watch for warning signals of cancer. Regular checkups are initially scheduled for every 3 to 4 months and then once or twice a year thereafter.

 Clinical Pearl

> *Intervention: After the nurse has given health promotion information to the older adult, that individual must make the ultimate decision about changing lifelong habits in an effort to prolong life.*

A major characteristic of cancer is its ability to metastasize and recur at different body sites. One common fear of all survivors is that after what appears to be successful treatment and remission of symptoms, cancer cells will appear at another body site. A consequence of the lengthened period of survivorship may be the appearance of another cancer in a different location. This new cancer, which appears at what is termed a "secondary primary site," is not a metastasis but rather cancer of a different cell type.

The occurrence of a second cancer experience may result in depression and despair for the patient and family. It is important that the nurse and members of the health care team continue to support and encourage the patient during this period. Patients and their families may need to confront more complicated issues, such as severe changes in body image and possible persistent physical debility, which make it difficult to fulfill their roles within their families and communities. They may need to look at alternative lifestyle changes and the necessity of preparing families and self for the issues of death and dying.

THE ROLE OF HOSPICE CARE

There is, however, the possibility that palliation will become the goal of nursing care. When the remission of symptoms is not possible, treatment measures have been exhausted, and life expectancy is limited, the older adult patient may seek the services of hospice. Hospice is an organization that creates a special environment in the home, not in the hospital, where staff is limited and family members are encouraged to care for the patient. The provision of hospice care will help to bridge the gap between what the patient may view as abandonment when treatment stops and the order needed to deal with the chaos of the rest of life (West, 1989). The multidisciplinary hospice team functions as follows:

- The nurse's role is symptom control, monitoring physical care, and patient/family teaching.

- The chaplain supports and encourages the coping abilities of the older adult as beliefs are tested and struggles with questions of fear and faith occur.
- The social worker supports the family in their efforts to attain available resources, handle circumstances that arise, and fill out forms. The social worker educates them about options to pursue legal issues, if necessary.
- Trained volunteers relieve family members who need time away from the patient.
- The patient's physician remains in contact with the team.

All members of the team continually assess the family situation and communicate with each other about the need for a change in the plan of care. When death is near, the team gives the family confidence and physical support to maintain care at home as long as the situation remains under control. The Medicare hospice benefit helps relieve the family of the financial burden of terminal care. An additional service offered by hospice is bereavement follow-up after the patient's death.

REFERENCES

American Cancer Society. (1993). *Cancer facts and figures*, 93-400M, No. 5008.93, 10–14.

American Cancer Society. *Seven warning signals that can save your life*, 777.

American Cancer Society. *Taking control: 10 steps to a healthier life and reduced cancer risk*. MM No. 2019.05.

Camp-Sorrell, D. (1992). Patient involvement in therapeutic decision making. *Oncology Patient Care, 3*(1), 1–12.

Cohen, R., Frank Stromberg, M. (1990). Cancer risk and assessment. In Groenwald S. L., Frogge, M. H., Goodman, M. & Yarbo, C. H. (Eds.), *Cancer nursing principles and practice*, (2nd ed., p. 115). Boston: Jones & Bartlett.

McCaffrey Boyle, D., Engelking, C., Blesch, K., Dodge, J., Sarna, L., & Weinrich, S. (1992). Oncology nursing society position paper on cancer and aging: The mandate for oncology nursing. *Oncology Nursing Forum, 19*(6), 913–931.

National Coalition for Cancer Survivorship. (1992). *Networker*. Silver Spring, MD: Author.

Phillips, R. (1986). The "Senior" with an ostomy, In R. Phillips, *Coping with an ostomy*. Wayne, NJ: Avery.

Staab, A., & Lyles M. (1990). *Manual of geriatric nursing*. Glenview, IL: Scott, Foresman/Little Brown.

Zanca, J.A. (1992). If people understand what to do, they'll do it. *Cancer Nursing News, 10*(2), 1,5.

BIBLIOGRAPHY

American Cancer Society. (1993). *Cancer facts and figures*. 93–400M. No. 5008.93, 10–14.

Bloch, R. (1994). Weighing your words: Instilling hope that doesn't have to mean holding out. *Cope, 10*(3), 48.

Eakes, G. (1993). Chronic sorrow: A response to living with cancer. *Oncology Nursing Forum, 20*(9), 1327–1333.

Johnson, J. (1994). Caring for the woman who's had a mastectomy. *American Journal of Nursing, 94*(5), 24–31.

National Cancer Institute. (1991). *Facing forward: A guide for cancer survivors*. NIH publications, 90-2424. p. 17.

Taylor, E. (1993). Factors associated with meaning in life among people with recurrent cancer. *Oncology Nursing Forum, 20*(9),1399–1405.

Welch-McCaffrey, D., Leigh, S., Loescber, L., & Hoffman, B. (1990). Psychosocial dimensions: Issues in survivorship. In Groenwald, S. L., Frogge, M. H., Goodman, M. & Yarbo, C. H. (Eds.), *Cancer nursing principles and practices* (2nd ed., pp. 375–377). Boston: Jones & Bartlett.

Zerwekh, J. (1994). The truth-tellers: How hospice nurses help patients confront death. *American Journal of Nursing, 94*(2), 30–34.

Problems in the Home and Community

26

Problems Associated With Issues of Death and Dying

Objectives

1. Describe the role of the courts in establishing legal precedents regarding the right to die.
2. Discuss the ethical principles that guide the nurse in supporting the older adult's right to die.
3. Discuss the factors that influence determinations of competency in the older adult.
4. Define the methods available to ensure the rights of older adults to govern end-of-life decisions.
5. Describe the role of the nurse in assisting the older adult in end-of-life decision making.

INTRODUCTION

IN THE LAST 20 YEARS, TECHNOLOGICAL advances in medicine have radically changed health care. Health care providers, relying on technological advances, can now sustain a person's life even in the presence of severe physical disability and dysfunction. Before medicine had attained its current level of life-sustaining technology, the right to die was rarely a conscious decision that had to be made. Death and the right to die were simply a fact of life. However, technological advances have widened the gap between life and imminent death and in so doing have prompted patients, families, health care providers, and the general public to contend with a wide variety of issues that revolve around death and dying.

Staab, AS and Hodges, LC: ESSENTIALS OF GERONTOLOGICAL NURSING,
© 1996 J. B. Lippincott Company

Patients can no longer assume that they have the right to die a natural death unmediated by medical intervention. In fact, the patient's right to die is often superseded by a presumed right to treatment. To resolve any potential decision-making complications, individuals should now indicate before an illness or any potential adverse aspects of the aging process whether they would wish to have medical and technological interventions to forestall death.

The ethical and legal guidelines concerning the right to die are designed to promote patient well-being and self-determination (the ability to make one's own decision). The court's role is to set legal precedents related to the right to die and establish the procedures for enacting the wishes or presumed wishes of the older adult in that regard. The nurse is ethically responsible for assisting the older adult in making end-of-life decisions.

THE ROLE OF THE COURTS

The courts have played a major role in establishing legal guidelines regarding the right to die. There are two landmark Supreme Court decisions in this area. Each case revolves around a comatose patient and the efforts of concerned family members to remove life-sustaining technology and allow the patient to die.

In 1975, Karen Ann Quinlan became comatose. After a year in a persistent vegetative state, there was no evidence that she would ever regain consciousness. The patient's father petitioned the courts to become his daughter's guardian. It was his wish to remove the patient's mechanical ventilator so that she might die. When the court refused to grant Quinlan's request, he appealed to the Supreme Court. The Supreme Court responded by reversing the decision of the lower court and awarding Quinlan legal guardianship of his daughter. As the patient's legal guardian, Quinlan's request to remove Karen Ann from life support was granted. Much to everyone's surprise, the patient continued to breathe on her own for almost 10 years. In 1985, Karen Ann Quinlan died in a nursing home.

The ruling in Quinlan was a landmark decision that was based in part on the constitutional right to privacy. New Jersey Supreme Court Chief Justice Hughes held that the notion of privacy guarantees individuals the right to control their lives. The court noted that the right to privacy, as recognized by the Supreme Court, was "broad enough to encompass a patient's decision to decline medical treatment under certain circumstances" (*In re* Quinlan, 1976, p. 40), even if such a decision led to the patient's death.

In addition to the constitutional right to privacy, there is also the acknowledged common-law right of individuals to decide what should be done with their bodies. The courts have determined that any competent older adult has a common-law right to be "free from nonconsensual bodily invasions" (Annas & Glantz, 1986, p. 98). By according this right, the courts recognize the individual's right to privacy in making personal health-related decisions. This right is to be upheld over any medical indications for treatment. Judge Cardozo wrote in 1914, "Every human being of adult years and sound mind has a right to determine what shall be done with his own body. . . ." (*Schloendorff v. Society of New York Hospital*, 1914, pp. 129–130). Hence, when a competent individual who is terminally ill wishes to have life support withdrawn or withheld, the courts have ruled that the right of the individual should be respected.

Although there is little dispute within the legal system that a competent patient has the right to make treatment decisions, the situation is different for the person who has been deemed incompetent. Since the Quinlan case, numerous states have reviewed cases regarding treatment decisions for incompetent patients. In most states, the courts have sought to honor the rights of these individuals by stating that surrogates, or individuals designated to make decisions on their behalf, may make treatment decisions for incompetent persons. An exception to this, however, is the state of Missouri, which was the setting for the second landmark case concerning the rights of incompetent patients.

Nancy Cruzan was injured in an automobile accident in 1983 and as a result of the accident was in a persistent vegetative state. She required artificial feedings to remain alive. Her parents and her sister believed that she would not want to live in this condition. Their belief was based in part on their knowledge of Nancy and on previous statements she had made stating that she would not want to live if she were not "at least halfway normal" (Annas, 1990, p. 670). Although the trial judge gave her parents permission to have Cruzan's tube feeding stopped, the Missouri Supreme Court reversed the decision. This court ruled that the feedings could be stopped only if "clear and convincing evidence" could be shown that Cruzan would want the feeding discontinued. At this point, Cruzan's parents appealed to the Supreme Court. The Supreme Court essentially upheld the Missouri court's decision by stating that life support could be withdrawn only if "clear and convincing evidence" is in place that the patient would desire discontinuation of treatment. In this ruling, the Supreme Court strengthened the individual's right to refuse or discontinue treatment so long as the person makes those wishes known in a clear and convincing manner while competent. One of the benefits of this ruling has been to highlight the responsibility of individual patients to make clear their wishes regarding end-of-life treatment decisions.

Although these court rulings have helped to open up for public discussion the importance of clarifying one's wishes regarding treatment decisions while one is competent, it is the opinion of many that the role of the courts is being abused and overused (Capron, 1986). The courts are invaluable in situations involving a dispute between family members, yet some have argued that an over-reliance on the courts for right-to-die decisions strains not only the court system but also the patient's relationship to the physician or the nurse. In a 1988 ruling, the judge observed that judicial intervention in right-to-die cases should be minimal. "Courts are not the proper place to resolve the agonizing personal problems that underline these cases. Our legal system cannot replace the more intimate struggle that must be borne by the patient, those caring for the patient, and those who care about the patient" (*In re* Conservatorship of Morrison, 1988, p.534).

The shift of decision making from patients, families, and health care providers to the courts has had harmful consequences in many areas. These consequences could include:

• Introducing an adversarial component into health care decisions
• Diminishing trust between the health care provider and the patient
• Depriving some patients of rights to make decisions that directly affect their well-being
• Undermining efforts of family members who seek what they perceive as

best for an incapacitated family member. Regardless of one's opinion about the benefits of court involvement, it remains indisputably clear that the courts have had a major influence on right-to-die decisions in health care since the Quinlan decision.

▷ *Clinical Pearl*

Assessment: A competent adult who can consent to treatment is likewise qualified to refuse treatment.

THE NURSE'S RESPONSIBILITY

The following nurse's story illustrates a caring, ethically responsible intervention by a nurse in the care of a patient who refused treatment. This nurse's decision to respect the patient's wishes was supported by the moral concerns of care and the ethical principle of patient autonomy, or self-determination.

A nurse in the surgical intensive care unit was caring for an older adult who had been injured in an accident. He had had one arm amputated in the accident and the other amputated in surgery. He was a very devout Jehovah's Witness. He had specifically stated in the emergency room that he did not want to receive any blood. In the middle of the night, the nurse received an order from the physician to administer two units of blood. The nurse was in a moral bind. The physician, a colleague whom she respected and liked, was telling her to give the blood; the patient, who was alert and competent, had stated in the emergency room that he did not want the blood. Further, the nurse knew the patient might die without the blood. She was not a Jehovah's Witness and had difficulty understanding the patient's refusal of the transfusion.

In an effort to resolve the dilemma, she went to the patient once again and asked him if he wanted the blood. He was intubated so he could not speak, but he shook his head indicating a negative response. Despite her conflicting feelings, the nurse believed she must respect the wishes of this clearly competent patient. She called the head nurse, who supported her decision to refuse to give the blood. She then called the hospital's clinical ethicist, who also strengthened her resolve to respect the patient's refusal of treatment. The blood was not given. After the crisis had passed, the nurse went to the physician to discuss their different perspectives regarding the treatment decisions made. After much dialogue, both physician and nurse were able to see and appreciate the viewpoint of the other.

In situations in which the patient's competence is *not* in question, the ethical responsibility of the nurse lies in determining the patient's wishes and upholding them while ensuring that unnecessary treatment, pain, and suffering are avoided. It is the professional, legal, and ethical duty of the physician to discuss treatment and termination of treatment options with the patient. The patient should be informed of any and all treatment options and of the risks involved. In general, it is the responsibility of the physician to provide the medical facts to allow the patient to make an informed decision. Ideally, the physician discusses these options with the patient at the time of the patient's entry into the health care system and before the initiation of treatment. In these discussions, decisions must be guided by a concern for the patient's well-being and allow the patient room to exercise self-determination. The outcome of the discussions should be communicated to the nurse and other members of the treatment team so that the patient's wishes can be supported or adapted as the situation unfolds.

However, it is not always the case that these discussions occur, that the patient fully understands the nature of the discussion, or that the conclusions of the conversation between physician and patient are communicated to the nurse. In these cases, the nurse has an independent ethical duty to make sure that end-of-life options are addressed and that the patient's resultant decisions are fully informed. If the nurse does not believe that the patient has participated in these discussions or that the patient has understood the nature of the exchange, the nurse should relay these concerns to the physician. Together, they must ensure that the competent patient participates in an informed decision-making process. Once patient preferences have been determined, the nurse then makes every effort to see that the patient's wishes are recorded on the chart, the proper documents are completed, and the wishes of the patient are respected. In instances when an older adult is transferred from one facility to another, the nurse should determine whether previously stated preferences regarding treatment or termination of treatment still apply. If so, it is the nurse's responsibility to see to it that these preferences are recorded in the patient's new chart.

The patient's decision regarding treatment, including its termination, may change as the situation unfolds. Patients have the right to change their minds about treatment at any point. It is often the nurse who is in the best position to note whether the patient or family members are comfortable about their treatment decisions. The nurse's role is to assist in clarifying patient preferences and values regarding treatment decisions, particularly those involving life-sustaining measures. The nurse may need to initiate conversations with other health care professionals about the patient's preferences, particularly if they change during the course of treatment. The nurse might choose to encourage the physician to talk with the patient or simply inform the physician about what the patient has already revealed concerning these matters.

The nurse is supported in these efforts on behalf of the patient by the ethical principle of patient autonomy, or self-determination. This principle ensures respect for individual freedom and human dignity in decisions that have a direct effect on an individual and do not harm others. The American Nurses Association Ethical Code for Nurses states, "The fundamental principle of nursing practice is respect for the inherent dignity and worth of every client" (American Nurses Association, 1985, p. 2), regardless of the nature of the health problem. This respect should be accorded to the dying patient as well. Another ethical principle guiding the nurse in these matters is the principle of fidelity, which implies a promise to faithfully respect and support all patients.

Both of these ethical principles are practiced within a framework of a caring concern for the patient. Within this caring relationship, the nurse's primary concern is to be responsive to the patient's needs as they arise, whatever may be the nature of these needs. It is essential that nurses respect the dignity of their patients even as they respond to the patients' needs for care. A caring response by the nurse involves affirming the patient's decision regardless of whether the nurse agrees with the patient's choices. It is in this way that the nurse ensures that the dehumanizing effects of technological interventions are confronted and softened by the humanizing concerns of care.

PATIENT SELF-DETERMINATION ACT

The Patient Self-Determination Act, which became effective in 1991, was instituted to ensure that the patient plays a vital role in end-of-life decisions. This national law applies to all health care institutions that receive Medicare or Medicaid. It stipulates that every individual who receives medical care through these institutions must be informed in writing of his or her rights to make decisions about medical care. The patient is given the opportunity to define personal choices in advanced directives (which function as a living will) or a durable power of attorney. Patients are not required to complete any document related to their choices about medical care, but if they choose to do so, they are assisted in the completion of the document. Once the documents are completed, they are placed in the patient's chart. Patients are not to be discriminated against based on whether they have executed an advanced directive. The Patient Self-Determination Act is implemented by giving the patient written information at the time of admission to a hospital, skilled nursing facility, health maintenance organization, or hospice. The nurse's role in implementing this law is determined by the specific institution. However, all nurses need to be aware of this legislation, because the patient may choose to complete advanced directive forms at any point during participation in the health care system.

DETERMINATION OF COMPETENCY

The determination of an individual's competency is a complex issue, partly because competency is itself a difficult capacity to define. When advanced medical technology has complicated the fundamental nature of death and dying, determining competency and its correlate, capacity, has become a matter of great importance for both the health care and legal professions. Older adults often must give informed consent to initiate or withhold treatment. When their decisions conflict with accepted medical opinions, these older patients may find themselves in the position of having their competency to render these decisions challenged.

The courts have sought to eliminate some of the guesswork involved in determining competency by defining a competent person as one who is "duly qualified; answering all requirements; having sufficient ability or authority; possessing the requisite natural or legal qualifications" (*Black's Law Dictionary*, 1979, p. 257). According to this definition, a competent patient must be able to demonstrate three capacities: 1) awareness of the situation, 2) understanding of the issues, and 3) the ability to make a decision based on awareness and understanding. Legally, competency is generally understood to be founded on sound mental capacity. But how is the nurse or any other health care provider to judge competency in a patient given its inexact and sometimes changeable nature?

Competency may be imagined to exist on a continuum, along which there exist no set points for complete competence and total incompetence. To further complicate matters, an individual may be competent in one area and incompetent in another. For example, an older adult may not be able to manage business affairs, although that same individual may be competent to make fine moral distinctions between suicide, assisted suicide, and refusal of medical treatment. Or, consider those adults who may function competently outside of the health care setting but, when faced with the intimidation of hospitalization and health care personnel, may be so threatened that they lose the ability to exercise their autonomy. In these situations, the older adult may be more or less competent depending on familiarity with the environment or experience with the health care system (Beauchamp & Childress, 1989).

The nurse, by virtue of the amount and quality of time spent with the patient, may be able to assess a patient's competency to make specific treatment decisions. However, the nurse must be careful to make the distinction between a patient's capacity to make decisions and the patient's status as legally competent. Patient capacity, as opposed to competency, is specific to a particular decision and situation, can change with the circumstances, and is determined apart from legal rulings on competency. In other words, a patient who has been deemed by the courts incompetent to manage the daily affairs of life may be capable of making a decision regarding treatment or termination of treatment in health care. In contrast, legally competent persons may be found incapable of making an informed health care decision.

It is the nurse's responsibility to be aware of the patient's capacity to make particular health care decisions. In 1987, the Hastings Center, a center for the study of ethical and legal issues related to health care, set out guidelines regarding determinations of patient capacity to make informed decisions (Smith & Veatch, 1987). According to these guidelines, the patient should exhibit the capacity to:

- Comprehend information relevant to the decision
- Think about choices as they relate to the patient's values
- Communicate either verbally or nonverbally with health care providers (Smith & Veatch, 1987, p. 131).

Recall the case of the Jehovah's Witness patient and how he met these three requirements of capacity: he understood that he needed to receive a blood transfusion; he was able to justify his choice to refuse treatment based on his own religious values; and he communicated these values and his decision to the health care providers (see Table 26-1 for nursing responses to competent older adults who request either the initiation or termination of treatment).

PRECAUTIONS IN DETERMINATIONS OF COMPETENCY

In considerations of competency, special care should be taken not to discriminate against the older adult based on advanced age alone. This is particularly important to remember in determinations of competency related to right-to-die issues, in which the decision to initiate or, more often, withhold treatment may be based primarily on the patient's age. Although age can be a decisive factor, it should always be secondary to considerations of the patient's functional ability and whether such ability can be enhanced by the proposed treatment.

	NURSING RESPONSES TO THE COMPETENT OLDER ADULT WHO REQUESTS INITIATION OR TERMINATION OF TREATMENT
Table *26-1*	• Ensure that the patient has adequate information to make an informed decision. • Discuss with the patient values related to treatment decisions and life-sustaining measures. • Determine what the patient perceives to be good quality of life. • With the patient's permission, discuss the patient's expressed values and course of treatment with family members. • Facilitate conversations between the patient, family members, and other health team members as needed. • Familiarize the patient with the Patient Self-Determination Act. • Provide appropriate forms for the patient to sign, if the patient so desires. • Ensure that the patient's wishes are recorded in the patient's chart. • Rely on the ethical principles of respect for persons in any efforts to ensure the rights of the older patient.

If the nurse is convinced that unfair or prejudiced standards of competency have been imposed on the older patient, the nurse should speak up for the patient and, if necessary, seek assistance from a hospital ethics committee on the patient's behalf. Once again, recall the case of the Jehovah's Witness. In that situation, the nurse believed that medical values were obscuring the religious values of the patient. When her attempts to promote the patient's wishes were frustrated, she turned to appropriate resources for help.

INCOMPETENT OLDER ADULTS AND THE RIGHT TO DIE

The patient's right to exercise self-determination in right-to-die situations becomes more complicated when the patient has been declared incompetent, because although the incompetent patient's right to self-determination has been effectively overruled by the courts, the patient still retains the right to die or refuse treatment. The rationale for this was explained in a ruling from a Massachusetts case as follows:

In a Massachusetts case, the court stated, "The recognition of that right [to refuse treatment] must extend to the case of an incompetent, as well as a competent patient, because the value of human dignity extends to both" (*In re* Brophy v. New England Sinai Hospital, Inc., 1986, p. 634). The rights of the incompetent older adult can be exercised by a surrogate decision maker who makes decisions on behalf of the patient while keeping the patient's own best interests in mind.

There are two categories of incompetent individuals: those who were once competent and those who have never been competent. If the incompetent individual was once competent, as in the previously cited case of Nancy Cruzan, and had expressed a preference concerning continued life support, then that preference should be honored. If the patient has never expressly stated a preference, then the court will determine the patient's competency in one of two ways: it may allow testimony of friends and family about previous value-related choices of the patient, or the court may make a determination based on its own evaluation of the patient's circumstances. In the case of patients who have never been competent, surrogate decision makers must act on behalf of the patient. These surrogates might ask, "What would the patient want if the patient had ever been competent?"

Clinical Pearl

Assessment: In the absence of evidence to the contrary, the nurse should assume that the patient has the capacity to make personal health care decisions.

There are several procedures concerning the incompetent patient's rights, including the right to die. These procedures fall into two categories:

- Advanced directives, which are documents devised by previously competent individuals in which directions about future medical decisions are clearly laid out
- Surrogate decision making, which is used in the absence of advanced directives for once-competent and never-competent individuals

ADVANCED DIRECTIVES: LIVING WILLS

One of the most widely used advanced directives is the living will. In this document, an individual simply declares that he or she desires to die a natural death without the use of extraordinary medical treatment.

The living will is a legal document, with certain statutory requirements, that enables a competent patient to oversee the future course of medical treatment in the event that the patient becomes incompetent. This instrument may authorize and direct the withholding or withdrawal of life support in certain situations. In most states, revocation of the living will may be accomplished by informing the physician of one's wish to revoke the document. It is often the nurse who is the first member of the treatment team to learn that the patient wishes to implement or revoke a living will. Any changes in the patient's self-determination choices should be communicated by the nurse to the physician.

There are serious limitations to any documents, such as living wills, that set out advanced directives (Areen, 1987):

- In most states, the living will becomes operative only when more than one physician determines the patient to be terminally ill.
- There is much disagreement regarding the meaning of "terminally ill," which may not include many sick older adults.
- In some states, the living will is legally binding only if the patient, after becoming terminally ill, reaffirms a desire for the living will to be effective.
- There is no requirement that health care providers follow the patient's wishes, and failure to do so does not result in any punishment.
- Although living will statutes do not prohibit the administration of care, they do not require health care providers to offer palliative care to a patient who has refused medical treatment.

Despite these limitations, the use of the living will has risen dramatically since the Cruzan decision by the Supreme Court and the passage of the Patient Self-Determination Act.

ADVANCED DIRECTIVES: POWER OF ATTORNEY

State laws define the rights and privileges associated with drafting a power of attorney. Power of attorney is defined as "an instrument authorizing another to act as one's agent. . . ." (*Black's Law Dictionary*, 1979, p. 1055). The appointed agent acts for and under the direction or control of the principal.

The powers assigned to the agent may be either general or specific. When warranted, the nurse should note whether the patient who has appointed a general agent has also given that agent health care power of attorney. The health care power of attorney is designed to allow, in advance, for the appointment of an individual to make health care decisions for the patient once the patient becomes incapable of decision making. The power of the agent to act for the principal is terminated at the death of the principal.

Because statutory requirements may vary from state to state, the adult who desires to appoint an agent should consult an attorney for assistance in drafting a document to provide for the older adult's specific needs. The previously described Patient Self-Determination Act also provides a means for patients to create a health care power of attorney (Fig. 26-1).

SURROGATE DECISION MAKING

In the absence of advanced directives, health care providers must rely on surrogate decision makers. There are numerous types of surrogate decision makers. Ideally, designated family members serve in this capacity. This was the situation in both the Quinlan and Cruzan cases. When family members serve as surrogate decision makers, the nurse may need to remind the family that decisions should be based on the patient's previously expressed wishes or on what the family thinks the patient would want. This is a difficult role to fulfill for family members who are faced with the potential loss of a loved one, possible financial pressure, or the ongoing stress of coping with the patient's extended illness. Family decision makers need to be properly counseled regarding the relevant factors in each situation in order to make informed decisions. They need to be given time to decide these issues and supported in their efforts on behalf of the patient. In those situations where the nurse thinks the family is not acting in the best interest of the patient, the nurse should discuss these concerns with the nurse supervisor and the physician.

When there is no family member who can serve as a surrogate decision maker for the patient, there are other means of surrogacy for the incompetent older adult. Legal guardianships allow for the appointment of a legal guardian by the courts; in most cases, this person can make medical decisions for the patient. The requirements for guardianship and the extent of the guardian's power vary from state to state. Guardianship decisions are made on the basis of "substituted judgment," that is, the guardian makes the decision based on the best estimate of what the patient would have wanted. These decisions frequently entail selecting treatments that provide the **patient** with the **greatest** quality of life while ensuring the least possible suffering.

Another means of surrogate decision making is through adult protective ser-

Durable Power of Attorney   SAMPLE*

FOR HEALTH CARE

I; _____

hereby appoint: _____

name _____

home address _____

home telephone number _____

work telephone number _____

as my agent to make health care decisions for me if and when I am unable to make my own health care decisions. This gives my agent the power to consent to giving, withholding or stopping any health care, treatment, service, or diagnostic procedure. My agent also has the authority to talk with health care personnel, get information, and sign forms necessary to carry out those decisions.

If the person named as my agent is not available or is unable to act as my agent, then I appoint the following person(s) to serve in the order listed below:

1. name _____

home address _____

home telephone number _____

work telephone number _____

2. name _____

home address _____

home telephone number _____

work telephone number _____

By this document I intend to create a power of attorney for health care that shall take effect upon my incapacity to make my own health care decisions and shall continue during that incapacity.

My agent shall make health care decisions as I direct below or as I make known to him or her in some other way.

(a) Statement of desires concerning life-prolonging care, treatment, services, and procedures:

_____
_____
_____
_____

(b) Special provisions and limitations:

_____
_____
_____
_____
_____
_____

(Continued)

BY SIGNING HERE I INDICATE THAT I UNDERSTAND THE PURPOSE AND EFFECT OF THIS DOCUMENT.

I sign my name to this form on _____
                                    (date)

My current home address:

_____
_____

_____
(You sign here)

WITNESSES

I declare that the person who signed or acknowledged this document is personally known to me, that he/she signed or acknowledged this durable power of attorney in my presence, and that he/she appears to be of sound mind and under no duress, fraud, or undue influence. I am not the person appointed as agent by this document, nor am I the patient's health care provider, or an employee of the patient's health care provider.

First Witness
Signature: _____
Home Address: _____
Print Name: _____
Date: _____

Second Witness
Signature: _____
Home Address: _____
Print Name: _____
Date: _____

(At least one of the above witnesses must also sign the following declaration.)

I further declare that I am not related to the patient by blood, marriage, or adoption, and, to the best of my knowledge, I am not entitled to any part of his/her estate under a will now existing or by operation of law.

Signature: _____
Signature: _____

I further declare that I am not related to the patient by blood, marriage, or adoption, and, to the best of my knowledge, I am not entitled to any part of his/her estate under a will now existing or by operation of law.

Signature: _____
Signature: _____

Check requirements of individual state statute.

Figure 26-1. Sample durable power of attorney for health care.

vices and public guardianships. In all states, there is some form of adult protective services. The activities of this service vary from state to state and range from the prevention of abuse and neglect of the elderly to investigating and ruling on treatment decisions.

SUICIDE AND EUTHANASIA

Some individuals argue that if a competent older adult has the right to terminate treatment, a decision that may result in death, then the competent older adult also has the right to request assisted suicide or voluntary euthanasia. Ethical and health care traditions in this culture do not support this action on the part of nurses or physicians, despite the numerous cases in which the unbearable suffering of patients might have been humanely ended had the patients been granted assistance in ending their lives. In our society, there is a clear distinction made between withdrawing treatment at the patient's request (even though doing so may lead to death) or either assisting a patient to commit suicide or participating in voluntary euthanasia. In most situations, when a patient refuses treatment, it is usually because further treatment will cause needless suffering and may be burdensome. It is not because a patient primarily desires to bring about death. Hence, for the nurse to support a patient's informed choice to forgo treatment demonstrates above all else an effort to honor the patient's choice, not to assist in the patient's death (Smith & Veatch, 1987) In contrast, if the nurse supports a patient's informed choice to end his or her life, this action honors the patient's choice but also supports the primary intent of the patient to bring about death. This is not generally morally acceptable within the health care community.

It is important that the nurse make the ethical distinction between assisted suicide or voluntary euthanasia and the patient's decision to forgo treatment. This distinction is complex and not always clear to the health care team. However, at this stage in the debate over these issues, the policy and traditions in health care are useful guides for the nurse. Policy is based on the effort to protect the rights of individuals. Policy makes the clear distinction between withdrawing or withholding treatment at the patient's request, which falls within the domain of the health care provider, and assisting in voluntary euthanasia or suicide, which falls outside of the ethical and legal guidelines established in health care. The power of health care professionals in these areas is extreme. There are concerns that this power might be misused or abused, even when intentions are good. Hence, policy and traditions in health care are designed to limit this power and to ensure that it is carefully and wisely used (Smith & Veatch, 1987).

Because the nurse is on hand to fully witness the full extent of the patient's suffering, the nurse might empathize with the patient's request for assisted suicide from the health care team. This sympathy, although understandable, may create a conflict for the nurse, whose nursing role demands that the nurse fulfill what have become essentially incompatible goals: the alleviation of suffering and the protection of the patient's wishes. In these situations, it is the nurse's responsibility to ensure that the patient has access to every available medical means of pain relief. Although the administration of these palliative medications may hasten the patient's death, this consequence is not the primary intent of the nurse.

ETHICAL CONCERNS OF THE NURSE

There are two ethical principles at stake in all issues surrounding either patient competency and capacity to make health care decisions or the patient's right to die: autonomy and beneficence. Autonomy has been previously described as the patient's enactment of self-determination. Beneficence means to do good, or *benefit* the patient. The principle of beneficence is often used to support decisions to treat the patient because it is usually assumed that treatment will benefit the patient. In decisions supported by the ethical principle of beneficence, it is critical that the patient and the health care provider share the same understanding of what is of benefit to the patient. It is not always the case that the patient's perception of benefit is similar to that of the health care provider. When there is a disagreement between the patient and health care provider or when disagreement exists among several health care providers about the benefits of treatment or termination of treatment, the ethical principle of beneficence comes into conflict with the principle of patient autonomy. In these situations, the nurse may believe that the patient's expressed wishes are not being respected. The following vignette illustrates this situation:

A nurse in the medical intensive care unit is caring for an older adult who has had numerous previous admissions to the unit. The patient suffers from chronic obstructive pulmonary disease. The patient is known by the physicians and nurses on the unit. Previously, this patient stated that if she were to become unable to respond and her medical prognosis were hopeless, she would not want life-sustaining interventions, such as intubation. During the patient's recent hospitalization, she suffered a cardiac arrest and was placed on life support. The patient has remained unresponsive since then. The nurse is aware that this is against the patient's previously expressed wishes. The nurse, supported by the ethical principle of patient autonomy, requests that the physician discontinue life support. The physician, supported by the ethical principle of beneficence, responds that given the apparent lack of suffering by the patient, continuation of life support constitutes "doing good."

This nurse faces a moral dilemma. Like most moral dilemmas, there is no clear solution. The best course for the nurse to follow in situations such as this is to seek to broaden the understanding of all involved by talking to the patient's family, other nurses, nurse supervisors, ethical and legal consultants, and physicians. It is often the case that these discussions lead to greater clarification of the situation and increased understanding between the parties involved. When discussions are honestly and seriously conducted, the perspectives of both nurse and physician, as well as family members, are often broadened, and understandings are reached.

It is rarely helpful to take an adversarial position, because doing so prevents one from understanding the other's perspective. However, in some instances, the nurse may find it necessary to take a firm stand against treatment of the patient. The decision by the nurse is supported by the American Nurses Association Code of Ethics, which states, "The nurse's concern for human dignity and for the provision of high quality nursing care is not limited by personal attitudes or beliefs. If ethically opposed to interventions in a particular case because of the procedures to be used, the nurse is justified in refusing to participate. Such refusal should be made known in advance and in time for other appropriate arrangements to be made for the client's nursing care" (American Nurses Association, 1985, p. 4). If no other arrangements can be made for the patient's care, then the nurse is bound by the moral principle of fidelity to provide care for the patient. Decisions to refuse to care for a patient must be carefully considered in light of the previously described ethical principle of fidelity.

The ethical principles of autonomy, beneficence, and fidelity are enacted by the nurse within a framework of care. Some nurse writers have suggested that care is the moral ideal of nursing (Watson, 1985). Watson described care as a shared experience between the nurse and the patient in which both individuals bring their unique life histories and values to the interaction. Hence, each nurse–patient interaction is unique.

From a perspective of care, the nurse does not see the patient as an object or a diseased entity, such as "the gallbladder in Room 543." The nurse instead sees each patient as a whole person. One goal of care is to understand the individual patient's different response to the illness experience. The caring nurse knows that all older adults are not alike and exhibit a wide range of responses to illness. For example, one 85-year old individual may refuse to have a foot amputated secondary to complications from diabetes, choosing to die rather than have to move from the home into a skilled care facility. Another patient of the same age with similar diagnosis and treatment recommendations may elect to have the surgery, preferring a nonambulatory, skilled care environment to death. The ethical challenge for the caring nurse is to assist each patient in making appropriate treatment choices that reflect the patient's life circumstances and values.

Advances in medicine and medical technology as well as legal and ethical issues all affect an individual's rights in health care matters, including the right to die. Older adults now have more opportunities to participate in health care decisions. Advanced directives, such as the living will, court-appointed surrogate decision makers, the Patient Self-Determination Act, and the appointment of an agent to act on one's behalf, all enable the older adult to participate in treatment decisions. To provide care for the older adult, the nurse should be aware of the nursing role and the avenues available for individuals to make their wishes known regarding end-of-life decisions. The challenge for the nurse is to balance the older patient's wishes with the legal precedents and laws regarding the right to die in the jurisdiction in which the nurse practices.

REFERENCES

American Nurses Association. (1985). *American Nurses Association code for nurses with interpretive statements.* Kansas City, MO: Author.

Annas, G. J. (1990). Nancy Cruzan and the right to die. *New England Journal of Medicine, 323*(10):670–673.

Annas, G. J., & Glantz, L. H. (1986). The right of elderly patients to refuse life-sustaining treatments. *Milbank Quarterly, 64*(Suppl. 2),96–149.

Areen, J. D. (1987). The legal status of consent obtained from families of adult patients to withhold or withdraw treatment. *Journal of American Medical Association, 258*(2), 229–235.

Beauchamp, T. L., & Childress, J. F. (1989). *Principles of biomedical ethics.* New York: Oxford University Press.

Black, H. C. (1979). *Black's Law dictionary,* 5th ed., St. Paul, MN: West Publishing.

In re Brophy v. New England Sinai Hospital, Inc., 497 N.E.2D 626, Mass. (1986).

In re Conservatorship of Morrison, 206 Cal. App3d 304, 312, 253, Cal. Rptr 530, 534 (1988).

In re Quinlan, 70 NJ 10, 355 A2d 647, (1976).

Megey, M., & Latimer, B. (1993). The patient's self determination act: An early look at implementation. *Hastings Center Report. 23*(1), 16–20.

Sabatino, C. P. (1993). "Surely the wizard will help us, Toto?" Implementing the patient self deter-
mination act. *Hastings Center Report, 23*(1), 16–20.
Schloendorf v. Society of New York Hospital, 211 NY 125, 105 NE 92 (1914).
Smith, D.H., & Veatch, R.M. (Eds.). (1987). *Guidelines on the termination of life-sustaining treat-
ment and the care of the dying.* Bloomington, IN: Hastings Center Report.
Watson, J. (1985). *Nursing: Human science and human care.* Norwalk, CT: Appleton-Century-
Crofts.

BIBLIOGRAPHY

Advance directives (editorial). (1992). *The Lancet, 340,* 1321–1322.
American Law Reports. (1986). Judicial power to order discontinuance of life-sustaining treatment.
Annotation, 48 A.L.R.67.
Florey, D. L. (1991). Advanced directives: In search of self determination. *Journal of Nursing Ad-
ministration, 21*(11), 16–21.
Yeo, M. (Ed.) (1991). *Concepts and cases in nursing ethics.* Lewiston, NY: Broadview Press.

Family Structures

Objectives

1. Identify important family-related issues to be considered in providing nursing care to older patients.
2. Delineate risk factors related to the reconfiguration of aging families.
3. Discuss the areas of family functioning to be assessed in obtaining a patient history.
4. Identify possible sources of emotional and physical support for families undergoing reconfiguration.
5. Develop a nursing care plan for a family dealing with retirement.

INTRODUCTION

THE FAMILY AS A UNIT OF STUDY IS IMPORTANT in the nursing care of older patients. With increased age come family structure changes and the patient's increased need for significant others. When illness and physical frailty are involved, even the most independent of older persons can find themselves reduced to a state of dependency. Although they might wish to be more self-reliant, they frequently find themselves needing the help of support systems, the most important of which is the family.

FAMILY AS SYSTEM

The family is an open, flexible social system that is in constant interaction with the larger physical, social, and cultural environments. The input received from the environment, which includes feedback about the family's social interactions, helps the family adapt to necessary change. When the system is in balance, homeostasis results, and the family is in a state of equilibrium.

Within the larger framework of the family there exist subsystems of family members, each with discrete but semipermeable boundaries. Examples of common subsystems include the spousal subsystem, the parent–child subsystem, and the sibling subsystem. Each of these subsystems has specific func-

Staab, AS and Hodges, LC: ESSENTIALS OF GERONTOLOGICAL NURSING,
© 1996 J. B. Lippincott Company

tions tied to specific roles that define the individual family member's purpose in the family. The effective use of semipermeable boundaries allows the discrete subsystems to engage in a healthy exchange of information with other subsystems and with the larger environment. Maintaining flexible boundaries is the key to successful family adaptation. The family, however, may resist change beyond a certain range because its members prefer to maintain comfortable patterns and roles.

Clinical Pearl

The only person who can clearly state the family makeup and how it affects him or her is the aging patient.

FAMILY PATTERNS AND PROCESSES

Nurses can gain valuable insight into the workings of an individual family system by assessing its patterns and processes when first meeting the family. By evaluating a family's communication style, the nurse can determine the relative health of the family system. For example, members in an open family system can hear and respond to each other's messages as well as accept input from the environment. Closed family systems, conversely, guard against such interchanges so as not to upset rigidly constructed boundaries.

Clinical Pearl

The communication process is the glue that keeps a family together in a healthy manner. Communication patterns provide clues to the family's ability to function.

FAMILY STRUCTURE

The foundation of structure in the family is power. Power results from a person's capacity to influence others. Traditionally, the oldest male holds the power in the American family. In other cultures, the oldest female may hold the power. For example, in Mexican American families health care decisions are made after consultation with female members in the matriarchal hierarchy. An aging grandmother with faith in the folk medicine system of care may advise her middle-age children to seek the healing powers of a *curandero* (folk healer) rather than follow the physician's advice. Therefore, the consultative process delays the physician's plan to remove a tumor while the family seeks alternate methods of care. Identifying the source of power in a family is the first step toward assessing family structure.

FAMILY ROLES

Essentially, a role is a set of behaviors expected of the occupant of a position. For example, one does not expect to see the grade school principal at the local disco demonstrating a dance. This action does not fit the role of the school principal. Similarly, the family has expectations of its members as a result of their place in the family. The eldest child is usually the most responsible. Parents have fewer expectations for the youngest child's responsibility. So the eldest child may continue to have more feelings of responsibility for the parents themselves as they grow older. In their research, Hamon and Blieszner (1990) reconfirmed the strength of filial responsibility in American society, though they did not relate the feelings of responsibility to position in the family.

Position determines formal roles within the family, and in the aging family there is some role exchange. For example, the father/provider may become more nurturing. Usually the increased nurturing results from the self-examination that often occurs with aging. After self-examination, the father/provider may decide that he was so busy working that he never got a chance to establish close relationships with his children. In young old age, he may have his last chance to do so. The father often becomes the family communicator, the one who keeps in touch with the children. This newly nurturing father often has a chance to enjoy his grandchildren more then he enjoyed his own children. His change of role may lead to more role sharing in the aging family.

The aging mother typically completes her nurturing role when the children leave home. The empty nest syndrome may be met with joyfulness instead of sadness because the change provides an opportunity for the woman to explore her potential. Of course, there are aging women who have become so embedded in the role of parent and wife that the empty nest brings unhappiness. The ability of the family to respond to change through role flexibility is of the utmost importance in successful family functioning.

FAMILY VALUES

Differing values between siblings and parents cause conflict within the family. It is particularly important that responsible children understand the aging parents' values regarding end-of-life decisions, long-term care, independence, and control. They must not only understand the values but also accept them as their parents' choices.

FAMILY FUNCTIONS

Family functions include the affective function and the socialization function. The affective function involves the family's care of the psychosocial needs of its members. The socialization function refers to the process of development or change resulting from social interaction and the learning of social roles.

As families develop, the affective function is particularly important to each person's development. Through the affective function, children learn respect, and they learn how to bond and become attached to others. Often families fulfill a therapeutic role in responding to each other's emotional needs. In aging families, the need for affective responses and feedback continues to exist, particularly as the older members age and sustain losses.

Much of the socialization function of the family is the product of a lifetime of role playing and imitation. It is in this way that the father who was a good provider inspires his son to be a good provider to his family. Aging families experience many changes in socialization. These changes often bring about a sense of loss and require new patterns of relating. Out of these family changes can come renewed growth and, in many instances, newfound happiness.

PROBLEMS WITH CHANGING ROLES ASSOCIATED WITH AGING

RECONFIGURATION

As the family ages and differentiates, the subsystems become more complex and diverse, prompting major transitions. The healthy family can weather these transitions because they are flexible enough to adapt to changing circumstances while remaining intact (Haight, 1989). A variety of family problems, from divorce to retirement, can complicate family roles during the aging process.

DIVORCE

Divorce is nearly twice as common in the 65-to-75 age group as it is in couples older than 75. Nearly 50% of people entering into marriage today will have experienced divorce by the time they begin their older adult years, and this in turn increases the likelihood that subsequent marriages will end in divorce (Kranczer, 1994). Uhlenberg, Cooney, and Boyd (1990) attributed growth in the divorce rate to several factors:

- Divorce becomes a more acceptable solution as social mores change.
- An increase in economic independence enables women to comtemplate divorce as a viable option.
- An overall increase in life expectancy makes the reality of "until death do us part" too long and intolerable a prospect for some.

In this age of divorce and remarriage, families are continually reconfigured. The problems of aging families are different for the childless, the widowed, the divorced, and the remarried (Brubaker, 1990), as described in Table 27-1.

What then are the problems faced by the older adult after a change in the family unit brought about by divorce? One potential problem is that of finances. Many older adults already live on tight budgets, with most of their assets tied up in the ownership of their house and other nonliquid possessions, such as automobiles and appliances. A divorce settlement dividing this property can result in both people experiencing a sharp decline in their financial status. With the family unit altered, older adults may be more concerned about continued love and support from their children; many even fear abandonment. This is of particular concern when one parent is estranged from one or more children.

Grieving for the loss of a divorced spouse may be as great as grieving for a deceased spouse. Uhlenberg et al. (1990) showed that divorced and separated older people experience a lower rate of satisfaction with family life, friendships, and nonworking activities. Older divorced adults also had higher death rates than their married counterparts. Separated couples tended to abandon their caretaker roles and, as a result, did not provide support for each other. This then prompted them to get their needs filled by other family members or social services.

Table 27-1

RECONFIGURED FAMILIES AND RESULTING PROBLEMS

Configuration	Problems
Married couple	Role change Task sharing Income sharing

Divorce	Decreased income
	Decreased social interaction
	  Possible relocation
	  Change in support systems
	Lost family interaction
	Need for new identity
	New daily routine

Widowhood	Grieving
	Decreased income
	Possible relocation
	Change in support systems
	Decreased social network
	  Need for new identity
	  New daily routine

Remarriage	Alienated children Need to establish new patterns and relationships Different financial systems New family configurations
Childlessness	Decreased sense of legacy Decreased primary relationships Fewer family contacts Increased institutionalization

Adapted from Haight, B.K., & Leech, K.H. (1992) Family dynamics. In M. Stanley & A. Bear (Eds.), *Health promotion in gerontological nursing practice.* Philadelphia: F.A. Davis.

DEATH OF A SPOUSE

Because women can expect to live an average of 7 years longer than their husbands, widowhood is a common problem in the aging population. In 1991, 65.7% of women age 75 and older had lost a spouse, compared with only 24.8% of men age 75 and older (Kranczer, 1994). Older adults who have lost a spouse face problems similar to those of their divorced counterparts. For example, they both experience grief.

Grief
Widows and widowers may have to do grief work that involves expressing feelings of denial, guilt, anxiety, depression, anger, and fear. These feelings may be experienced one at a time or together, and they may come and go as certain events or memories trigger them. Families who are experiencing the loss of a loved one must work together to allow each member to complete his or her own grief work.

Grief is unique for each individual. Although most grief work may be completed in 6 months to a year, some people may take twice as long before they begin to reconnect with life after their loss. Grief can become dysfunctional if it becomes a serious depression or results in thoughts of suicide. Aging families, isolated from their kin, often must have their affective needs met in other ways. For example, Siegel and Kuykendall (1990) found that men, particularly, became more depressed when sustaining a loss. However, men with church affiliations experienced less depression because church members met their affectional needs. Though the affectional needs of family members persist throughout a lifetime, the needs of aging family members may be met by others outside the family.

Because decision making is difficult during this transition, some older adults may find themselves or their families making hasty decisions. The widower may feel a strong need to leave memories behind and make a new start elsewhere. Families may fear for the safety of their bereaved and push them to relocate. These decisions and actions may not be well thought through. The older adult may not consider all the variables and their meanings. A move to a strange home and distant city to live with a child may result in more adjustment difficulties than if the widower had remained at home surrounded by familiar support systems.

Status Change

Widows and widowers go through a time of role and status change. Not only are they grieving for the lost loved one, but also they grieve for the role they once held and all the actions and meanings that went with it (Poncar, 1989). Finances may become a problem if a prolonged illness consumes most of the resources or if the individuals never performed proper estate planning. Conversely, Adlersberg and Thorne (1990) noted that widowhood may not be a time of negative transition for all older adults. Some may feel great relief to be freed from earlier responsibilities, such as the widower who nursed his spouse through a long illness or the widow of an abusive spouse. They take pleasure in finding themselves again, enjoying activities, setting new goals, and choosing a new lifestyle. Sometimes they have spent so long thinking of others that it is only with the death of the spouse that they become aware of their own needs. The surviving spouse may be hesitant, however, to acknowledge these positive aspects of widowhood for fear of family and friends' reactions.

Remarriage

Divorce and widowhood may result in another change for the family unit, remarriage. Children may be unable to accept their parent's remarriage because they believe that doing so represents a failure to grieve on the part of the remarried parent or a betrayal of filial loyalty on their part. Finances again can become an issue as troubling questions surface. "Will we retain our inheritance, or will it all be left to a stranger?" "Will we be responsible for long-term health care for this new spouse as well as for our remaining parent?" Conversely, many older adults believe they cannot remarry, often for varied reasons, some of which are loss of Social Security or health care benefits or a desire to maintain their estates. Instead, they may contemplate choosing to live with a significant other, a choice both they and their families may have difficulty accepting (see Table 27-1).

COMMUNICATION AND DECISION MAKING

Health care workers seem to forget that the aging patient is often a fully competent decision maker, who remains so until that person is declared incompetent or chooses to give up decision-making rights. Dysfunctional interactional patterns in the family's communication process, which include a failure to listen, a continuous restatement of priorities, an inability to focus on an issue, and/or the use of chitchat to avoid issues, may reinforce the nurse's misperception of the patient's incompetence.

Burden

It is also common in aging families to have conflict between children as siblings, particularly when the burden of caregiving enters the equation. Strawbridge and Wallhagen (1991) found that perceptions of unequal burdens contributed to conflict and poor mental health in families, whereas Learner, Somers, Reid, Chiriboga, and Tierney (1991) described egocentric biases when judging sibling contributions to caregiving.

It is particularly common for one child living near the parent to carry the burden of responsibility alone for many years. Finally unable to handle the burden, the child, usually a daughter, decides to place the parent in a nursing home. Suddenly, from all parts of the country, siblings appear to object to this treatment of the parent. Yet none of the objectors are willing to take over the burden of care and relieve the lone daughter of years of responsibility.

Feelings of guilt on the part of the siblings often underlie the last hue and cry for better treatment of Mom and Dad. Often these feelings of guilt translate into complaints directed at the nursing home and anger toward each other.

Roles

The literature often addresses role strain, particularly the difficulty a person feels in assuming a caregiving role. Daughters especially feel role strain when having to make relocation decisions for their mothers. It is difficult to differentiate role strain from caregiver strain caused by other stressors. For example, Scharlach, Sobel, and Roberts (1991) found that it was hard to differentiate between caregiver strain that results from changing roles and that which results from the burden of filial responsibility combined with other stressors.

Role conflict, which occurs when a particular individual perceives expectations as incompatible with his or her present role, is a more serious concern. Finley, Roberts, and Banaham (1988) found that role conflict was proportionate to the degree of filial obligation felt toward aging parents. The degree of obligation varied by parent type and the child's sex, with females feeling more role conflict if they did not fulfill the expected obligations to their parents.

Generational Values

Potential areas of conflict between generations occur when there is a clash between the old-fashioned values of the aging parents and the more modern values of the children. For example, baby boomers, who want the best even if it means buying it on credit, may lock horns with their financially more conservative parents. The clash of these different value systems creates a great potential for lack of understanding between the parties involved.

> ## Clinical Pearl
>
> *Different generations have different value systems.*

Retirement

Retirement is also a time for great change in roles and lifestyles in the family unit. Many couples enter retirement without forethought. But even with careful planning, problems can occur (Fig. 27-1). Couples may regard each other as strangers, whose habits and activities they must work to rediscover. Entering retirement, older adults may have unexpected feelings of loss. As they lose their valued role of breadwinner or successful career person, they may feel cast off and useless and react with anger and depression.

Role changes may not meet expectations. Consider, for example, the family in which the husband retires before the wife, a common occurrence when women enter the work force after years spent homemaking. Often the marital satisfaction of the working wife with a husband at home is less than that of wives when both remain employed. Lee (1988) attributed some of this decrease in satisfaction to the wife's feelings of resentment and inequity at the

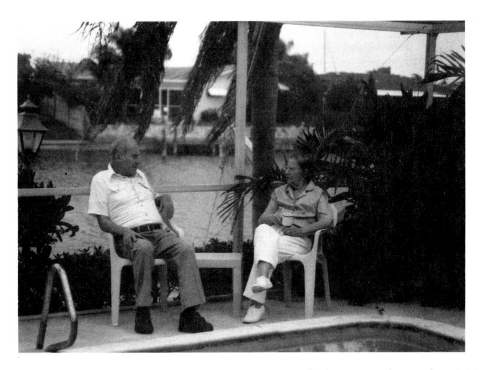

Figure 27-1. Retirement requires reassessment of identities, roles, and activities within a family unit. Even with forethought and planning, problems related to retirement can include financial strain, adjustment difficulties, and marital strain. Proper planning to include realistic expectations of family member's new roles and responsibilities before retirement helps to ease the transition.

unchanged division of household labor. Women continue to perform most of the household chores before and after retirement, while their spouses' household responsibilities tend to remain constant.

In another example of role adjustment in retirement, Silverstone and Hyman (1989) described the homemaker who goes through her adjustment period during the empty nest syndrome, resulting in a need to redefine roles and activities after her career of raising children is complete. By the time the husband retires, usually at a later time, she has resolved her confusion and uncertainty and is participating in her new lifestyle. Having a spouse feeling the same confusion and uncertainty that she has already resolved causes an upheaval in her new routine. As spouses go through these events at different periods, the marriage may feel the stress of multiple readjustments. Without empathy and understanding, significant strain can be placed on the relationship. See the nursing care plan for families dealing with retirement.

Crisis

As people grow older and their health fails, they frequently encounter health-related crises. Illness and hospitalization are both such crises. For some, the fear of illness and dependency is more frightening than the fear of death. The nurse must remember that even a routine hospital procedure can result in a permanent change of lifestyle for the older patient. Even small changes in the person's long-term routine can overwhelm what remaining coping skills the person has. More serious lifestyle changes, such as an anticipated hospitalization, can precipitate anxiety and distress depending on the person's premorbid personality.

Ethical Issues

Ethical issues abound in families as they age. Two that seem predominant for families are paternalism and decision making. Problems arise when the patient is not part of the decision-making process, either through an oversight or because others take away the right to decision making without just cause. This often happens because aging causes role change and role exchange. Previously interdependent family roles may now become dependent family roles. With this dependency, subtle changes occur in the power base of families and in the communication process. Often, children inadvertently begin to take over the decision-making process for their parents, whom they infantilize. An example of infantilization by children may occur in widowhood, where there is a major role transition. The widow may find herself assuming practical management and decision-making tasks that were performed previously by her spouse. These demands and the loss itself often put undue stress on the widow. Family members may misinterpret this stress as an inability to cope, and they may take over managing the widow's affairs without asking her if their help is needed.

▷ Clinical Pearl

The nurse can assess the power structure of the family by observing interactions, assessing culture, communication, and decision-making.

Nursing Care Plan

FOR FAMILIES DEALING WITH RETIREMENT

Nursing Diagnosis: Impaired Adjustment, related to role changes associated with retirement.

Definition: The state in which the individual is unable to modify lifestyle or behavior in a manner consistent with a change in status (Gordon, 1991).

Assessment Findings:

1. Verbalization of nonacceptance of status change
2. Nonexistent or unsuccessful ability to be involved in problem solving or goal setting
3. Extended period of shock, disbelief, or anger regarding status changes
4. Lack of future-oriented thinking

Nursing Interventions With Selected Rationales:

1. Encourage expression of feelings and concerns surrounding retirement and subsequent changes to lifestyle.
   Rationale: Verbalizing concerns enables family members to increase awareness of each other's thoughts, fears, and hopes.
2. Have patient and spouse identify positive and negative aspects of new situation.
   Rationale: Beginning the process of role change is less traumatic when both partners have a realistic and consistent view of their new circumstances.
3. Explore with the couple qualities about each other unrelated to work experience.
   Rationale: The patient is assisted in redeveloping self-confidence and value in his or her new role.
4. Explore with the patient areas of interest not yet experienced or pursued.
   Rationale: Assisting the patient in concrete goal setting and scheduling allows the patient to find meaning and structure in the new lifestyle.

Desired Patient Outcomes/Discharge Criteria:

1. Patient and spouse will identify and express feelings and concerns related to retirement.
2. Patient and spouse will develop new goals and role expectations, incorporating them into new lifestyle.
3. Patient and spouse will regain self-esteem through reassessing meaning, values, and goals and identifying those values and activities they wish to pursue in their new role.

NURSING ASSESSMENT

For nurses, there are several issues that arise in assessing and caring for the aging family. First, the nurse must assess the family unit and determine how that family is experienced by the patient. Second, the nurse must always keep in mind that the competent older adult patient is a self-reliant decision maker. Last, the nurse must consider assessment of the whole family as a system when treating the older patient. Assessment and treatment may be ineffective unless all family members are involved. The nurse must remember that changing one part of the family system will cause changes in other parts of the system. Using a systems approach, the nurse must assess the family's patterns, structure, functions, and value system using the following Patient Teaching Box as a guideline.

HISTORY AND INTERVIEW

Family Makeup

In assessing the family, the nurse must cover a wide variety of topics, from identifying the pertinent family units and the major players in that unit to retirement. When conducting an initial assessment of the family, the nurse might pose the following questions:

- Who constitutes the family?
- Who is the patient's significant other?
- Who is legally responsible for the older patient's decisions if the patient cannot make those decisions?
- Who actually helps and cares for the patient?
- Does the patient still hold the purse strings? If not, who does?

Observation of family interactions and outcomes provides key information about decision making and power within the family. The nurse might ask the following questions:

- Who decided where to retire?
- Who plans vacations?
- Who plans the menu and takes responsibility for other household chores?
- Who has primary responsibility for decision making (financial and otherwise)? How willing are you and other family members to abide by his or her decisions?

Patient Teaching Box
PARAMETERS FOR ASSESSING CHANGING FAMILY ROLES

Use the following outline to guide your systems assessment of the family and the aging patient.

Systems Assessment
- Makeup of the family
- Decision making within the family
- Processes of the family
  1. Communication
  2. Patterns of interaction
- Structure of the family
  1. Power
  2. Roles
- Functions of the family
  1. Affective
  2. Socialization

In assessing communications and interaction patterns, the nurse should ask herself:

- Do family members converse as equals?
- Do they listen to and respond to each other?
- Does their conversation convey care and concern for one another?
- Do all have an equal chance to speak?

A knowledge of family values is also important for family members to understand each other, particularly intergenerationally. Direct questions regarding differences in child rearing, job sharing, and saving patterns will provide clues to value differences. Though the nurse may observe value differences, they are not a problem unless family members are intolerant of each other's differences. Thus, intolerance of others' values is a risk factor for decreased family functioning.

Nursing assessment of the family should encompass its clearly observable affective functions as well as its more complex social functions. Nurses can gather evidence of each type of function by asking themselves the following questions:

- Do they hug and kiss freely, or do they seem isolated within themselves?
- From observing current behavior, can one determine which family members were socialized to fulfill specific roles in the family? For example, who seems most comfortable as the caregiver?

Risk Factors

Decision making, communication, and values all contribute to a systems assessment of family. However, particular problems still exist, a major one being the reconfiguration of families as they age. Whether the reconfiguration is caused by divorce, widowhood, or remarriage, assessment of risk factors created by the reconfiguration is important. To assess for reconfiguration risk factors, the nurse can assess the environment for pictures of family members and ask questions about their visiting patterns. Other pertinent questions include:

- Do you see your children as often as you did before your remarriage?
- Do your children relate well to your new spouse?
- Do you have family reunions?

Asking about the lost loved one can provide an opportunity for the grieving widow to work through many issues, thus providing the nurse with a great deal of assessment information. Divorce and other changes in marital status can place great strain on families as roles are lost and situations altered. By assisting family members in becoming aware of these changes and what they mean to them, families can pursue grief work and role restructuring in a positive way.

Retirement and one's adjustment to retirement is another area for assessment. Questions that may help evaluate retirement include:

- How do you spend the day?
- Do you and your spouse get in each other's way?

Answers provide clues for assessment of successful functioning in retirement. Those at risk in retirement may be those who cannot find substitute activities in their present lifestyle.

Finally, there is the problem of analyzing burden and determining whether burden is producing role conflict, stress, and/or strain. The nurse might ask if caring for a family member is a burden. If so, who shares the load? Is the caregiver getting any respite? Is it okay with the caregiver? Often, the questions do not even need to be asked. The caregiver, who may be isolated by the burden, may be very eager to share problems and issues with whomever they meet.

PHYSICAL EXAMINATION

The physical examination of the aging patient should focus on the assessment of present health status as well as on health-promoting regimens dedicated to preventing further illness and disability. To this end, the nurse:

1. Assesses lifestyle for healthful factors
2. Performs a review of systems to prevent exacerbated illness caused by stress
3. Creates a weekly nutrition plan and exercise program

Much of the literature links the presence of a significant other with increased emotional health for the older patient. The nurse is, therefore, encouraged to inform the patient about the health benefits of contact with a significant other.

NURSING DIAGNOSES

A thorough assessment lends itself to the making of a nursing diagnosis. With a diagnosis, a care plan can be created to direct the family's treatment. Below is a listing of selected nursing diagnoses based on changing roles in the family.

• Altered Family Processes, related to financial loss
• Spiritual distress, related to death or illness of significant others
• Anxiety, related to change in status and prestige
• Altered Role Performance, related to divorce
• Ineffective Family Coping: Disabling, related to goal conflicts
• Ineffective Family Coping: Compromised, related to retirement
• Family Coping: Potential for Growth, related to relocation

NURSING INTERVENTIONS

Nursing interventions result from a clear diagnosis and plan of care. Examples of interventions are presented for selected areas, such as patient and family education and support to families.

PATIENT AND FAMILY EDUCATION RELATED TO GRIEF

Very often, a family that is grieving is too disorganized to gather their coping abilities and resources together to resolve their problems. They may look to the nurse for guidance, and this guidance may be provided with patient education, as demonstrated in the following Patient Teaching Box.

Patient Teaching Box
INTERVENTIONS WITH SELECTED RATIONALE

The family should:
- Discuss normal changes, feelings, and problems that occur during grieving
- Discuss the grieving process and experienced stages (denial, anger, anxiety, hopelessness)
- Explore meanings and values surrounding patient's life
- Help the patient to define aspects of life that he or she wishes to maintain and those he or she would change to aid in developing a new role identity
- Explore role expectations placed on each other by family members to increase awareness of each other's perceptions, expectations, hidden agendas, and beliefs

SUPPORT

When family roles change due to reconfiguration, there is a growing need within the family for emotional and physical support from a variety of sources: community organizations or social support systems, health care professionals, and/or primary relationships. Suggested interventions under each source follows:

Community

1. Provide a list of community resources.
2. Seek out assistive programs.
3. Contact volunteer visitor programs from churches and other organizations.

Emotional

1. Provide opportunity for a life review.
2. Listen while patient talks of concerns.
3. Reinforce good themes and reframe bad themes.

REFERENCES

Adlersberg, M., & Thorne, S. (1990). Emerging from the chrysalis: older widows in transition. *Journal of Gerontological Nursing, 16*(1), 4–8.

Brubaker, T. H. (1990). Families in later life: A burgeoning research area. *Journal of Marriage and the Family*, 959.

Finley, N. J., Roberts, M. D., & Banahan, B. F., III. (1988). Motivators and inhibitors of attitudes of filial obligation toward aging parents. *Gerontologist, 28*(1), 73–78.

Gordon, M. (1991). *Manual of nursing diagnosis: 1991–1992*. St. Louis: Mosby.

Haight, B. K. (1989). Family and social support: Nursing update: The older adult. *Continuing Professional Education, 1*(16), 1–6.

Haight, B. K., & Leech K.H. (1992). Family dynamics. In M. Stanley & A. Bear (Eds.), *Health promotion in gerontological nursing practice*. Philadelphia: F.A. Davis.

Hamon, R. R., & Blieszner, R. (1990). Filial responsibility expectations among adult child–older parent pairs. *Journal of Gerontology, 45*(3), 110–112.

Kranczer, S. (1994). Changes in U.S. life expectancy. *Statistical Bulletin, 75*(3), 11–17.

Learner, M. J., Somers, D. G., Reid, D., Chiriboga, D., & Tierney, M. (1991). Adult children as caregivers: Egocentric biases in judgments of sibling contributions. *Gerontologist, 31*(6), 746–755.

Poncar, P. J. (1989). The elderly widow: Easing her role transition. *Journal of Psychosocial Nursing, 27*(2), 6–11.

Scharlach, A. E., Sobel, E. L., & Roberts, R. E. L. (1991). Employment and caregiver strain: An integrative model. *Gerontologist, 31*(6), 778–787.

Sigel, J. M., & Kuykendall, D. H. (1990). Loss, widowhood, and psychological distress among the elderly. *Journal of Consulting and Clinical Psychology, 58*(5), 519–524.

Silverstone. B., & Hyman, H. K. (1989). *You and your aging parents*. New York: Pantheon Books.

Strawbridge, W. J., & Wallhagen, M. I. (1991). Impact of family conflict on adult child caregivers. *Gerontologist, 31*(6), 770–777.

Uhlenberg, P., Cooney, T., & Boyd, R. (1990). Divorce for women after midlife. *Journal of Gerontology: Social Sciences, 45*(1), S3–11.

BIBLIOGRAPHY

Clipp, E. E., & George, L. K. (1990). Caregiver needs and patterns of social support. *Journal of Gerontology*, Social Sciences, *45*(3), S102–S111.

Lee, G. R. (1988). Marital satisfaction in later life: The effects on nonmarital roles. *Journal of Marriage and the Family, 50*, 775–783.

28

Problems With Abuse and Neglect

Objectives

1. Differentiate between abuse and neglect of the older adult.
2. Describe five categories of behavior that characterize abuse in the older adult.
3. Discuss current theories of the etiology of abuse of the older adult.
4. Identify the personality profiles of individuals and the characteristics of situations that increase the likelihood of violence.
5. Formulate a plan for nursing assessment and intervention in actual or suspected cases of abuse.

INTRODUCTION

BEGINNING IN THE 1960S, EACH DECADE has been defined by the recognition of a specific type of intrafamily violence. The 1960s saw the emergence of child abuse as a social problems; by the 1970s, spousal abuse had supplanted child abuse as the focus of attention. In the 1980s, the abuse and neglect of the older adult became the focus of much study. In the 1990s, the abuse and neglect of people of all ages continues to be of major concern.

DEFINITIONS OF ABUSE AND NEGLECT

Although research and inquiry into this complex problem continues, there is no universally agreed-on definition of abuse. Each study uses its own definition, and this hampers comparison of findings, precludes standardization of assessment tools, and may contribute to misinformation and misdiagnosis. However, most researchers agree that physical abuse, emotional abuse, and physical neglect are some of the most common manifestations of the problem. Abuse implies actions taken by the caregiver, relative, or acquaintance that

Staab, AS and Hodges, LC: ESSENTIALS OF GERONTOLOGICAL NURSING,
© 1996 J. B. Lippincott Company

cause injury or create unmet needs. Neglect implies a failure to act, which may have the same consequences.

TYPES OF ABUSE AND NEGLECT

Five categories of behavior that characterize abuse in the older adult have been identified:

- Direct physical abuse—Characterized by direct attacks that are apparently deliberate, direct physical abuse can cause physical injury. Specific examples include direct physical assaults resulting in lacerations, bruises, welts, dislocations or sprains; sexual assault; or threats with a weapon.
- Physical neglect—Comprises the failure to meet basic human needs for survival, resulting in potentially life-threatening problems, such as dehydration and malnutrition
- Financial and material abuse—Includes the theft, misappropriation, or misuse of the older adult's funds or property. Examples include withdrawal of money from the older adult's bank account without consent and sale of the elder's home or personal property without consent
- Psychological and emotional abuse—The most common type of abuse, this abuse involves the infliction of pain through verbal and emotional means. Examples of verbal abuse are yelling and screaming at or berating the elder. Emotional distancing and isolation are two other means of inflicting psychological pain on the older adult.
- Violation of rights—Denial of the basic rights of the aged, including forced institutionalization, preventing free use of the older adult's own money, and prohibiting the older adult from marrying. Also cited in this category is oversedation to make the older adult "more manageable."

STATISTICS RELATED TO ABUSE IN THE OLDER ADULT

Although the phenomenon of abuse has been described, it remains shrouded in mystery in many respects. Some researchers have labeled it the "hidden phenomenon" because it usually occurs behind closed doors and without witnesses. It is poorly understood and largely unrecorded. Estimates of the incidence of elder abuse are based on *reported* cases and range from 700,000 to 1 million per year (Pillemer & Finkelhor, 1988).

 Clinical Pearl

Assessment: In cases of abuse of the older adult, it is believed that only 1 case in 14 comes to public attention.

One of the reasons for this underreporting of abuse is the victim's failure or reluctance to report it. The older adult may not know to whom to report the abuse or may be too frightened to report it. The nurse must develop and refine needed assessment and interviewing skills to uncover this information.

Display 28-1

REASONS VICTIMS OF ABUSE DO NOT TELL

1. Perceived need to maintain family privacy and code of solidarity
2. Feelings of guilt and shame ("How could I have raised such a child?")
3. Fear of public exposure, shame, and embarrassment
4. Fear of retaliation and increased battering
5. Fear that if abuser is jailed, victim may have to testify in court against him or her
6. Knowing that abuser is the only caregiver ("Where will I be if this is taken away?")
7. May resist out of parental love
8. Thoughts that "This is God's will" or "I'll suffer now and get my reward later"
9. Feeling that he or she "deserves" such abuse
10. Learned helplessness
11. Passive personality
12. Victim unaware of abuse (particularly financial)
13. Inability to report the abuse because of mental/physical condition
14. Hoping that it will just stop someday
15. Thinking that this abuse or neglect is the norm

BARRIERS TO REPORTING

Uncovering abusive behavior is complicated by several factors. Historically, the family unit is private, and intrusions are often resented. Abuse occurs without witnesses, and the victims may not report it for fear of retaliation. Other reasons for the victim's failure to report abuse are fears of abandonment, institutionalization, or the unknown; loyalty to the family unit; and a desire to avoid the embarrassment and shame of being labeled a victim. Additionally, physical changes in the older person create obstacles to detection and reporting. Mental status changes due to disease processes and malnutrition or trauma can contribute to forgetfulness and bring into question the patient's mental competency. Contusions and fractures that result from physical abuse may be attributed to falls, which increase in frequency with age.

In the current violent "throw-away society," older adults are often viewed as unproductive. Abuse of these devalued members of society is seen as normal, expected, or harmless. Professionals in law enforcement, social work, and health care often are not properly trained to recognize this phenomenon and may even deny its existence or, if they hold unacknowledged negative feelings toward older adults, contribute to nonreporting. Perhaps nurses are among the most vulnerable to under-recognition of the problem. They may see the problem from the caregiver's perspective and overidentify with the caregiver's stress, guilt feelings, and sense of being overwhelmed by the older adult's dependency needs. The nurse may not inquire about physical signs suggestive of abuse for fear of being perceived as too intrusive. Even if the abuse is acknowledged, the nurse may not know what to do about it.

THEORIES OF ABUSE AND NEGLECT IN THE OLDER ADULT

A number of theories attempt to explain and clarify the etiology of this complex problem. Some are drawn from studies of child abuse and spousal abuse, but none of these theories has undergone empirical testing. As with other forms of domestic violence, abuse of the older adult is a manifestation of imbalance in relationships and has multiple causes.

The dependent elder impairment theory was adapted from research on child abuse and emphasizes the care-recipient's dependency and physical or mental impairments as setting the stage for abuse. Researchers have frequently noted that older adults with physical or mental impairments are at greater risk of being abused than those who lack such impairments (O'Malley, Segars, Perez, Mitchell, & Kneupful, 1984).

The stressed caregiver theory proposes that caring for an older adult is a source of stress. On the basis of a survey of 183 professionals who had reported a case of abuse of an older adult, O'Malley et al. (1984) noted that in 63% of the cases, the victim was viewed as a source of stress to the abuser. Caring for a chronically ill older person is demanding and can drain the caregiver physically, emotionally, and financially. Such unrelenting responsibility, along with preexisting stressors, may trigger abuse.

Some researchers have proposed that family violence is a set of learned behaviors with intergenerational transmission in some families. The theory of internal family dynamics states that, as a child, the abuser observed violence as an accepted reaction to stress and internalized it. The cycle of abuse then comes full circle as the caregiver who was mistreated as a child retaliates by abusing the parent.

Role reversal is at the heart of all theories of elder abuse. The ambivalence associated with taking on the responsibility of parenting a parent may trigger a crisis and precipitate abuse. The parent who was once self-sufficient is now dependent but is not a child, despite the demands for care and support. The adult child often finds no other support and must assume many responsibilities, often at great personal cost.

The pathologic personality theory focuses on the abuser. Certain personality traits, such as a low tolerance for frustration or passive–aggressive or sadistic tendencies, and the habitual use of aggression to deal with frustrations may make abusive behavior more likely (Pollick, 1987). The caregiver who is psychotic or abuses drugs or alcohol has impaired cognition and judgment, making violence more likely.

PROFILES OF THE ABUSER AND THE ABUSED

Descriptions of the abuser and the abused have emerged from exploratory and descriptive studies. The abuser is typically a relative or significant other, rather than an outsider. Because most caregiving in this country is done by women, there are implications when one attempts to profile the "typical" abuser by sex. It is unknown whether women are more likely to be abusers or if their over-representation as caregivers is responsible for their preponderance among abusers of older adults.

In an exhaustive review of the literature, Kosberg (1988) identified characteristics of individuals who may be abusive caregivers for frail and dependent older adults. Practicing nurses should carefully assess the caregiver for the presence of any of the following factors:

- Substance abuse—This abuse may distort judgment and perceptions. The substance-abusing caregiver may be unaware of the consequences of poor care or may act out negative feelings when impaired.
- Senile dementia/confusion—Many caregivers are older adults themselves and may have chronic diseases and mental status impairments. They are hardly able to care for themselves, much less a dependent older adult.
- Mental illness—Such impairments in the caregiver increase the risk of negative outcomes.
- Caregiving inexperience—Not everyone is suited to the role of caregiving. One cannot assume that a person with no experience of this nature will be able to learn how to care for a dependent older adult. Uncomfortable feelings may translate into neglectful or violent action.
- Economically troubled—Frustrations with unemployment are related to abusive behaviors. The risk of abuse is increased if the older adult is viewed as a drain on an already tight family budget.
- Abused as a child—The caregiver may act out hostile feelings as retaliation for his or her own mistreatment.
- Stress—Persons who are stressed professionally, socially, financially, or emotionally may have little energy left for the demands of caregiving.
- Unengaged outside of home—A caregiver who is isolated from family, friends, coworkers, or community resources is deprived of formal and informal sources of support.
- Dependent role—Some caregivers feel they need the role of caregiver and to have the older adult dependent upon them
- Negative personality characteristics—If the caregiver blames the older adult for problems related to the burdens of providing care, is unsympathetic to the needs of others, or is hypercritical of the older adult, the patient may be an easy target for angry or aggressive impulses and at risk for poor care. The caregiver may hold unrealistic expectations of the patient's abilities or be hypercritical of others, and this increases the likelihood of frustration and disillusionment.

The following vignettes illustrate various types of abuse the nurse may encounter in caring for the older adult:

Mr. Walters, an 82-year-old widower, lived with his stepson and daughter-in-law and their three teenage children in a mobile home in an isolated part of the country. One of the children had been in a serious automobile accident 8 months before and has been left with permanent disabilities due to brain injury. The child had recently been transferred home from a rehabilitation center after having attained his maximum rehabilitation potential. The family had moved a hospital bed for the disabled son into what had been Mr. Walters' room. They were a "proud family" and did not readily accept help from outsiders.

On the first visit, the home health nurse noted that the mobile home was infested with roaches and rodents. Screens were missing from most of the windows, and flies buzzed around remnants of several meals on the kitchen table. Unwashed dishes were piled high in the sink.

The nurse noted that the daughter-in-law was pregnant. She looked very tired and her ankles were edematous. Mr. Walters made numerous requests of the woman for such things as cigarettes and coffee. The woman dutifully complied with his requests. Mr. Walters remarked that women were here "to take care of the menfolk" and that he would "box her ears every now and then to keep her in line." During the course of the nurse's visit, Mr. Walters' stepson arrived home after working a 12-hour shift at the garment mill. The nurse noticed that the stepson immediately poured a large glass of bourbon and then shouted for Mr. Walters to get out of his favorite chair. A verbal exchange with obscenities and much fist shaking ended when Mr. Walters stormed outside. When Mr. Walters had left, his stepson confided to the nurse that Mr. Walters had physically and emotionally abused his mother. He said that he believed the injuries she suffered contributed to her death, which was officially listed as a cerebral hemorrhage. He also said he had never liked the man, that Mr. Walters had always had a bad temper and a knack for starting a fight. The reason he allowed his stepfather to stay with them was because the family was financially strapped and needed his Social Security and pension checks to help make ends meet. Besides, he asked the nurse, "Who else would have him?"

Mr. Walters' case illustrates a family with a variety of risk factors for abuse. The family culture permitted the abuse and neglect to occur because the behavior was typical of that family's interactional style. The nurse encountering this situation should carefully assess the situation and identify the factors that constitute abuse and neglect.

Mrs. Benjamin, a 78-year-old widow, lived with her daughter and son-in-law. About 3 years ago, Mrs. Benjamin suffered a stroke, which left her with mild right hemiparesis. She is able to walk with a walker but needs help with meal preparation, shopping, and handling personal finances. Recently, her daughter asked her to transfer all her resources, financial assets, and beneficiary designations to her because the family was financially strapped after two weddings. Mrs. Benjamin's assets included a substantial death benefit and trust fund from her late husband as well as stock and other investments. The daughter paid all bills and purchased all food and clothing for the household using her mother's funds. Additionally, the daughter bought a new car and several pieces of fine jewelry with these funds. When Mrs. Benjamin questioned her about the status of the funds in her account, the daughter angrily told her to "mind your own business" and then hid her walker. She confined Mrs. Benjamin to her second-floor bedroom. Unable to safely ambulate, Mrs. Benjamin was a prisoner in her own room. The only time Mrs. Benjamin saw other family members was when her meals were brought up to her cold, lonely room. Mrs. Benjamin maintained orientation to reality by listening to a small radio. Once, when she fell down the steps trying to make her way downstairs, her daughter forcefully dragged her back up without regard to the injuries Mrs. Benjamin had suffered.

Mrs. Benjamin's case illustrates emotional, physical, and financial abuse of the older adult.

Miss Read, an 82-year-old woman, was found in the closet of her apartment by a home health nurse. The woman was very frightened, but eventually the nurse was able to coax her out of the closet, and she reluctantly related her story. Miss Read said she was afraid her nephew would kill her. He had been unemployed for more than a year and had a long-standing problem with crack cocaine. About 3 months ago, he moved in with Miss Read. His mother had just died, and Miss

Read had promised her that she would look after him. He was living off Miss Read's Social Security checks, but these were mostly used to buy drugs. When he was under the influence, he would threaten to kill her, often holding a gun to her head. He always stopped short of killing her, saying, "Those checks are all you're good for." Miss Read had a bruised and swollen left eye and several bruises on her arms. She told the nurse her dentures had broken about a month before, when her nephew knocked them out of her mouth in a fit of rage. Miss Read was dressed in a threadbare house dress. She said that her jewelry and other valuables had "disappeared" shortly after her nephew had moved in. She told the nurse she was terrified of him, but she was afraid to say anything to anyone. Besides, she didn't know whom to contact. On inspection, the nurse found no food in the apartment. The water, lights, and heat had been turned off the previous month.

Miss Read's case illustrates financial and physical abuse and neglect.

Abusers may be reacting to a stressful environment that combines the demands or caregiving with other life events, such as financial difficulties, health problems, and changing job responsibilities. The caregiver's family is frequently in the "launching" stage of the family cycle, with expenditures for college tuition and weddings. It is often a time when the family income is leveling off, and the presence of an older family member with dependency needs may drain the family emotionally and financially. Many caregivers find themselves hemmed in by the pressure of simultaneously baby-sitting grandchildren and caring for a dependent older relative. In addition, the older adult's medical costs are frequently undercompensated by federal and private insurance, and these expenses compete with others incurred by the family. Feelings of resentment may grow due to the personal time restrictions and the older adult's constant presence. Mounting stress on the caregiver sets the stage for violence.

Abused older adults are typically widowed white women older than age 75, with dependency needs caused by inadequate resources or physical or mental impairments (Urquart, 1987). Certain personality characteristics, such as passivity, excessive loyalty, stoicism, and a tendency to internalize blame, may also play a role. As with spousal abuse (which can also be a form of abuse in the older adult), victims are often isolated physically, emotionally, or geographically from others. Substance abuse increases the risk of abuse, because the person may be unable to care for himself or herself and may offer little resistance to verbal and physical attacks. Conversely, some older adults may display "provocative behavior" and be overly demanding, ungrateful, ingratiating, or otherwise unpleasant. Such behavior engenders feelings of anger in the caregiver. Perhaps advanced age in itself is a risk factor, because the older adult is beset with increased vulnerability and dependency needs, especially when frail or in poor health.

 ▷ *Clinical Pearl*

Assessment: It is often difficult to differentiate between physical decline resulting from illness or the changes of aging from those changes resulting from abuse. Such differentiation can only come through repeated assessment and careful examination of each suspected case.

ASSESSMENT OF ABUSE IN OLDER ADULTS

Assessment of abuse in the older adult has been aided through the use of a number of tools, most of which incorporate a written protocol for interviewing the older adult and caregiver. The older adult's physical and mental status, the home environment, and the caregiver–patient relationship should be carefully assessed and documented.

Hamilton (1989) applied a family systems approach in the development of assessment instruments for the older adult and the caregiver. The vulnerability assessment score (VASAP) of the older adult and the stress assessment score (SASC) of the caregiver are used to evaluate the risk of abuse in the home (Fig. 28-1). An Index for Assessing the Risk of Elder Abuse in the Home (REAH) is a

A. personal data section (caregiver)				
	2 points	1 point	0 points	Score
Age	70 and over	45–69	under 45	_____
Phys. health	poor	good	excellent	_____
Ment. health	poor	good	excellent	_____
Finances	under $7000	$7–$14000	$14000 & more	_____
Dependents (not elder)	2 or more	1	none	_____
subtotal, A. personal data (sum of above, range 0 to 10)				_____
B. stress factors section (caregiver)				
1 point for a "yes," 0 points for a "no" or "don't know"				Score
Alcoholism or substance abuse?				_____
Mental retardation?				_____
History or observation of family violence?				_____
Change in lifestyle to assume care of aged person?				_____
Receives financial help from the elder?				_____
Limited time for own personal activities?				_____
Personal stresses (i.e. marital problems, empty nest)?				_____
Mostly or always at home (unable to leave aged person)?				_____
Absence of support system (family, friends, community)?				_____
Shows frustrations, resentment in care of aged person?				_____
Treats elder as a child?				_____
Has limited knowledge of the aging process?				_____
Believes any care at home is better than nursing home?				_____
Minimizes or denies dependency of aged person?				_____
Shows dependency toward the elder?				_____
Authoritative manner with the elder?				_____
subtotal, B. stress factors (sum of above, range 0 to 16)				_____
SASC (sum of subtotals A and B, range 0 to 26)				_____

Figure 28-1. SASC—Stress Assessment score of the caregiver. Used with permission: Hamilton, G. (1989). "Prevent Elder Abuse: Using a Family Systems Approach," *Journal of Gerontological Nursing, 15*(3), 23

combination of the VASAP and SASC (Fig. 28-2). By using the REAH, the nurse can gather information regarding the care requirements of the older adult and personal characteristics and environmental influences on the caregiver.

Demographic data are recorded on both the REAH and SASC, and scores are computed to ascertain the older adult's vulnerability and the caregiver's stress level (Table 28-1). In addition, the REAH and SASC each contain a list of questions that can be used to determine the patient's risk for elder abuse during the taking of the history and interview. This instrument provides an assessment of the family unit for changes over time. It is a means for identifying potential for abusive family situations, so that timely nursing diagnoses and interventions can be initiated.

The REAH is the sum of two components, the vulnerability assessment score of the aged person (VASAP) and the stress assessment score of the caregiver (SASC). Use the tables to calculate VASP and SASC (Fig. 28–1), then add them to find the REAH.

| REAH (sum of VASAP and SASC, range 0 to 41) | | | | ____ |

VASAP—vulnerability assessment score of the aged person				
A. personal data section (aged person)				
	2 points	1 point	0 points	Score
Age	85 or older	75–84	74 or younger	____
Sex		Female	Male	____
Health	Frail	Average	Robust	____
subtotal, A. personal data (sum of above, range 0 to 5)				____

B. dependency needs section (aged person)	
1 point for a "yes," 0 points for a "no" or "don't know"	Score
Intellectual or severe mental impairment?	____
Lives in home with caregiver?	____
Needs help bathing?	____
Needs help dressing?	____
Needs help toileting? (or is incontinent or has catheter)	____
Needs help eating?	____
Depends on caregiver for all social interaction?	____
Allows caregiver to assume parental role?	____
Demanding and authoritative to caregiver?	____
Is financially dependent upon caregiver?	____
subtotal, B. dependency needs (sum of above, range 0 to 10)	____
VASAP (sum of subtotals A and B, range 0 to 15)	____

Figure 28-2. REAH—An index for assessing the Risk of Elder Abuse in the Home. Used with permission: Hamilton, G. (1989). "Prevent Elder Abuse: Using a Family Systems Approach," *Journal of Gerontological Nursing, 15*(3), 23

Table 28-1

CRITERION-RELATED VALIDATION OF THE REAH COMPONENTS

(a) Vulnerability assessment, elderly person

Objective assessment		Subjective assessment		
VASAP	Rank	Low	Medium	High
12–15	Highest	0	1	1
9–11	High	0	2	7
6–8	Medium	2	10	5
3–5	Low	4	2	4
0–2	Lowest	1	1	0

Gamma correlation coefficient = 0.70, N = 40, p < 0.02

(b) Stress assessment, caretaker

Objective assessment		Subjective assessment		
SASC	Rank	Low	Medium	High
20–26	Highest	0	0	0
15–19	High	0	0	0
10–14	Medium	0	0	7
5–9	Low	3	11	9
0–4	Lowest	6	3	1

Gamma correlation coefficient = 0.86, N = 40, p < 0.01

REAH: Index for Assessing the Risk of Elder Abuse in the Home. Used with permission. Hamilton, G. (1989). "Prevent elder abuse: Using a family systems approach", Journal of Gerontological Nursing, 15(3), Slack Incorporated, p 25 March 1989.

HISTORY AND INTERVIEW

Tomita (1982) developed an assessment framework that is applicable in a medical or domestic setting. The Harborview Medical Center assessment framework addresses four areas:

- The older adult's functioning
- The physical examination
- The caregiver interview
- Collateral contacts

The purpose of the functional assessment is to determine with whom the older adult interacts frequently and on whom he or she depends for social, physical, and financial support. Mental status is evaluated to add credibility to the patient's report of abuse. During the functional assessment, the nurse asks questions concerning the nature of the patient–caregiver relationship, such as:

- Do you get along well with your caregiver?
- Are you able to discuss your needs openly with your caregiver?
- Are you both open to negotiating potentially problematic issues, such as scheduling meal times and doctor's visits?

- Do you retain control of your finances? If not, did you willingly relinquish your right to do so?

Information on high-risk situations, such as the presence of alcohol/drug abuse or mental impairments in the caregiver, may be obtained at this time. The patient's physiologic and psychological functioning are assessed by evaluating his or her ability to perform activities of daily living and instrumental activities of daily living.

RISK FACTORS

There are a number of predisposing risk factors that contribute to the incidence of elderly abuse. As was described above in the section entitled Profiles of the Abuser and the Abused, some of these risk factors manifest themselves as long-term personality traits in those involved at either end of the violent interaction. Other risk factors that play a role in the expression of violence range from those that are physiologically based to those that are specific to a given situation. Organic and psychological contributors to elder abuse that may affect victim and abuser alike include substance abuse, senile dementia (confusion or other organically based dysfunction that might impair perceptions), and mental illness.

The caregiver may succumb to abusive behavior if any of the following conditions holds:

- The caregiver is inexperienced.
- There is significant stress related to financial, professional, social, or emotional issues that may or may not directly involve the older adult.
- The caregiver was abused as a child and sees this situation as an opportunity for retaliation.
- The caregiver lives in social isolation and as a result has no access to the emotional support of family, friends, and community resources.

The assessment of abuse in the older adult is a difficult and often ambiguous procedure, because there is no definitive list of indicators. A victim of abuse is often identified based on a configuration of at-risk findings, such as:

- Injured older adult brought in to the emergency room by someone other than the caregiver
- Prolonged interval between injury or illness and presentation for medical care
- "Doctor shopping"
- Account of how injury incurred is not substantiated by physical findings
- Patient had injuries not mentioned in the history given by the caregiver
- Too many unexplained injuries
- Medication bottles indicate medications not being given/taken as prescribed
- Older adult is never allowed to speak to the nurse alone

The nurse needs to perform a complete family history and physical examination on the patient and carefully analyze the information obtained for indicators of abuse. Victims of abuse are often unrecognized, because professionals tend to discover instances of abuse only when they are actively looking for them.

PHYSICAL EXAMINATION

The physical examination is completed to elicit information as to signs and symptoms indicative of abuse and neglect. Physical signs may include dehydration and malnutrition; lacerations; or signs of beatings, such as bruises or welts, dislocations, fractures, or sprains. There may be signs of sexual assault. Mental status changes can be the result of malnutrition or withholding the person's medical care. Failure to supervise an impaired older adult can result in trauma or injury from falls or accidents. The nurse should question recurrent hospitalizations for failure to thrive or severe electrolyte disorders, such as hypokalemia or hyponatremia resulting from not eating.

▷ *Clinical Pearl*

Intervention: During the physical examination, the nurse should document verbatim all explanations given by the older adult for injuries.

CAREGIVER INTERVIEW

The interview with the caregiver is done immediately after the patient is assessed so that there is no chance for collusion. Inconsistencies in reports may be a signal that abuse is occurring. The nurse determines how the caregiver is coping with meeting the patient's needs. Information should be gathered on the caregiver's physical and mental health status as well as on the status and use of formal and informal sources of support. Questions are asked to elucidate the nature and tone of the caregiver–patient relationship and the financial status of the family. The nurse may simply reiterate some of the questions used in the functional assessment of the patient and look for caregiver corroboration of what the patient has already divulged. Collateral contacts, such as neighbors or friends, may be made before the caregiver or the patient is interviewed, or they may be made afterward. These contacts may have valuable information based on their individual appraisal of the relationship. Moreover, the nurse should remember that anyone who has contact with the patient is a potential abuser.

The assessment tool developed by Tomita (1982) is applicable in a variety of settings and provides an organized framework for documenting observations and other information. However, the tool may have limited usefulness in helping the nurse recognize potentially abusive situations and may preclude primary-level interventions.

As awareness of the problem of abuse in the older adult grows, the nurse will see refinement of existing assessment tools and development of new ones. In addition to assessing the caregiver, the patient, and collateral contacts, the nurse should carefully observe the home environment. The degree of cleanliness, the presence of vermin, the adequacy of heat/cooling, the availability of food, and any smell of urine or excreta should be noted. Unhealthy living conditions may be a form of abuse.

Clinical Pearl

Assessment: Inconsistencies in reports by caregivers and the older adult related to injuries are cause for further assessment by the nurse for potential abuse.

NURSING DIAGNOSES

A listing of potential nursing diagnoses that can be used in the care of the older adult/caregiver diad in which there is actual abuse or the potential for abuse might include the following:

- Impaired Adjustment to caregiving, related to inadequate support or knowledge
- Altered Family Processes, related to role reversal
- Altered Health Maintenance, related to inadequate support or knowledge
- Social Isolation, related to geographic location or insufficient human contact
- Self-care Deficit, related to role overload or physical/mental impairments
- Risk for Injury, related to ineffective coping or insufficient knowledge
- Powerlessness, related to physical/mental impairments or lack of knowledge
- High Risk for Injury, related to dysfunctional family interactions
- Risk for Violence, related to insufficient knowledge, inadequate coping mechanisms, or provocative behavior
- Fatigue, related to burdens of caregiving

NURSING INTERVENTIONS FOR POTENTIAL/ACTUAL ABUSE OF THE OLDER ADULT

Various intervention strategies exist for the problem of abuse in the older adult. Many interventions involve an interdisciplinary or multidisciplinary effort. The goal of primary prevention is reduction of abuse risk factors. This could be accomplished by educational programs designed to teach healthy coping patterns to caregivers and other family members involved with a dependent older adult. Such a program should include ways for the caregivers to recognize and monitor their own stress with instruction on strategies for stress reduction.

The best programs help caregivers to avoid becoming abusive by setting forth a handful of behavioral guidelines, as listed below:

- Know yourself. Don't attempt to be "Superman" or "Superwoman." Recognize mounting stress and deal with it before it gets out of hand.
- Find out as much as possible about caregiving. This can include consulting friends and confidants, clergy, or professionals who can empathize and help you problem solve.
- Check your phone book for support groups, respite care services, or in-home health care services.

- Ask for help when you need it.
- Take a course in stress management or home nursing skills if you think it will help you feel better about the way you deal with your responsibilities.
- Make time to relax. You may find deep-breathing exercises, listening to favorite music, or guided imagery tapes helpful.
- If others offer to help, don't turn them down. See if they can run errands for you, bring in a meal, help with some chores, or stay with the older adult while you get away.

Caregivers need to be made aware of available community resources that could be called on for relief from role overload. Such resources include networks of helpful relatives and friends, "guest" or respite care services offered by local hospitals, adult day-care centers, and home health care nurses and aids. Some voluntary service organizations for older adults can be excellent sources of support; the services they provide may range from supplying educational materials to offering personal counseling. Some organizations have funds available to pay for patient sitters while the caregiver attends a support group meeting. Adult protective services are available in most communities. These services promote the prevention of abuse and offer avenues for treatment in cases in which abuse has already occurred. The principles on which adult protective services are founded are listed in Display 28-2. Figure 28-3 illustrates services needed by abused and neglected older adults and their caregivers.

Other potential primary level interventions evolve from more of a grassroots level. Nurses should pay particular attention to overt and subtle ways of expressing ageism. Laughing at cruel jokes that portray older adults in stereotypical ways perpetuates myths and misinformation about this age group. Nurses should strive to empower older adults, rather than focus on their particular weaknesses and vulnerabilities. Some politically astute professionals are very interested in legislation that could mandate paid leave for those who have to care for older adult relatives at home. Such legislation could relieve some of the burdens on caregivers and ultimately focus attention on healing family problems. The general public needs education in recognizing forms of abuse in the older adult. Nurses are urged to promote development of support services for the elderly, such as congregate living units and self-help groups. Such community resources could promote communication among the various age groups in society and discourage isolation, which increases the vulnerability of older adults.

On the secondary or curative level, interventions exist in the form of nursing homes, foster homes, emergency shelters, and adult protective legislation. Forty-one states have laws that provide for case reporting in suspected abuse and criminal prosecution of guilty parties (Pollick, 1987).

The main goal of any legal intervention is to end abuse. The secondary goal is to ensure that the physical and mental well-being of the abuser and the abused are protected. Health care professionals may intervene on the secondary level through early diagnosis of abuse cases so that prompt treatment can be instituted. The safety and well-being of the older adult patient remains the primary concern, with acknowledgment of the patient's right to self-determination. Primary-level interventions are often appropriate on this level. The caregiver and others involved can be assisted to make needed role changes and to reassign duties based on a realistic appraisal of abilities and expectations.

Display 28-2
PRINCIPLES OF ADULT PROTECTIVE SERVICES

I. *Freedom over Safety.* The client has a right to choose to live at risk of harm, providing she or he is capable of making that choice, harms no one, and commits no crime.

II. *Self-Determination.* The client has a right to personal choices and decisions until such time that she or he delegates, or the court grants, the responsibility to someone else.

III. *Participation in Decision Making.* The client has a right to receive information to make informed decisions and to participate in all decision making affecting her or his circumstances to the extent that she or he is able.

IV. *Least Restrictive Alternative.* The client has a right to service alternatives that maximize choice and minimize life-style disruption.

V. *Primacy of the Adult.* The worker has a responsibility to serve the client, not the community people concerned about appearances, the landlord concerned about crime, or the family concerned about finances.

VI. *Confidentiality.* The client has a right to privacy and secrecy.

VII. *Benefit of Doubt.* If there is evidence that the client is making a reasoned choice, the worker has a responsiblity to see that the benefit of doubt is in her or his favor.

VIII. *Do No Harm.* The worker has a responsiblity to take no action that places the client at greater risk of harm.

IX. *Avoidance of Blame.* The worker has a responsiblity to understand the origins of any maltreatment and to commit no action that would antagonize the perpetrator and so reduce the chances of terminating the maltreatment.

X. *Maintenance of the Family.* The worker has a responsibility to deal with the maltreatment as a family problem, if the perpetrator is a family member, and to try to find the necessary family services to resolve the problem.

Source: G.J. Anetzberger. (1988, May). *Ethical Issues,* Paper presented at the National Conference on Elder Abuse: Linking Systems and Community Services, Milwaukee, WI, May 1988. Used with permission.

The goal of tertiary-level interventions is mitigation of the effects of abuse. Institutionalization of the older adult may provide some degree of rehabilitation in that physical and emotional trauma can be dealt with, and the healing process can begin. Group or private counseling can be an approach to promotion of attitudinal and behavioral change in the abuser. Finally, incarceration may be used as a rehabilitation alternative for the abuser. The extent of the rehabilitative effect of incarceration is questionable, particularly if it is used as the only alternative. See the nursing care plan that follows for strategies to care for the abused and neglected older adult.

Nurses provide services to older adults in a variety of settings. There are frequent opportunities to assess older adults and family systems for abuse and to plan intervention strategies on the appropriate level. The Patient Teaching Box provides information to assist the older adult avoid being a victim of abuse. Population trends intensify the need for professional awareness and recognition of the problem. Nurses are likely to encounter a higher percentage of patients older than age 65 in the coming years. Demographic trends, such as postponement of childbearing, women in the work force, and smaller family size have direct implications for future care of older adults. If alternatives to

(text continues on page 482)

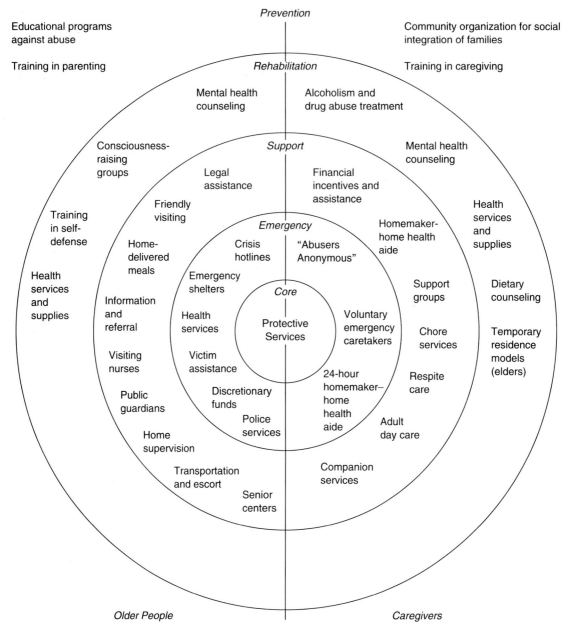

Figure 28-3. Services needed by abused older people and their caregivers. (Adapted from G. J. Anetzberger, *Report of the Elder Abuse Project: Recommendations for Addressing the Problem of Elder Abuse in Aryahoga County,* Cleveland: Federation for Community Planning, 1982.)

Nursing Care Plan

FOR PROBLEMS WITH ABUSE AND NEGLECT RELATED TO DYSFUNCTIONAL FAMILY INTERACTIONS

Nursing Diagnosis: High Risk for Injury, related to dysfunctional family interactions

Definition: Elder abuse and neglect is more likely to occur in families that are experiencing stress or that have major communication problems

Assessment Findings:
1. Signs of physical abuse
2. Signs of emotional abuse
3. Signs of family stress/violence

Nursing Interventions With Selected Rationales:
1. Maintain calm, nonjudgmental approach.
   Rationale: Both the patient and the caregiver are more likely to divulge pertinent personal information if they think it will be accepted without value judgment.
2. Encourage caregiver and care recipient to discuss what they are experiencing.
   Rationale: Putting feelings into words allows both parties to arrive at a consistent view of their situation.
3. Assist to identify alternative but assertive ways of expressing feelings and needs.
   Rationale: Both persons believe that their emotions are validated.
4. Explore ways to adjust environmental stimuli to facilitate clear communication.
   Rationale: Misunderstandings can be minimized by arranging for the clear communication of ideas.
5. Review healthy communication patterns:
   • Listen closely to others
   • Do not interrupt
   • Think before responding
   • Use "I" statements rather than "you" statements
   Rationale: Both the caregiver and the patient are more likely to engage in meaningful, nonviolent communication if they think that they are being respectfully considered in all interactions.
6. Have caregiver/care recipient role play communication techniques.
   Rationale: Rehearsing the appropriate communication skills in the presence of a third party allows the participants to get comfortable with the new rules for their interactions.
7. Discuss effect of body language on communication.
   Rationale: Making both parties aware of the ways in which feelings and meaning are conveyed nonverbally reduces the likelihood that they will inadvertently send out the wrong signals.

Desired Patient Outcomes/Discharge Criteria:
1. Patient will not show outward signs of physical abuse/neglect.
2. Patient and family will seek counseling.
3. Patient and family will discuss communication patterns.

Patient Teaching Box
HOW TO HELP THE OLDER ADULT AVOID BEING A VICTIM
OF ABUSE

Instruct the patient as follows:

Financial Abuse/Violation of Rights
1. Have your Social Security check or other regular income direct-deposited.
2. Draw up a will. If you already have one, review it annually. Be certain any revisions are carefully made.
3. Familiarize yourself with your financial status and handle your assets appropriately. You may want to consult a financial advisor or attend special classes to develop skills in this area.
4. As much as possible, plan in advance for the possibility of a disability. Seek out an attorney who specializes in estate planning and who can advise you about powers of attorney, guardianships, and conservatorship. If you need legal services and your finances are limited, contact your state legal aid society.
5. Be very careful about deeding your house or willing your assets to anyone who promises to "take care of you" or "keep you out of a nursing home."
6. If asked to sign anything, ask someone you trust to review the document before signing.

Physical and Emotional Abuse
1. Cultivate and maintain friendships with people of all ages so that you won't be totally dependent on your family for your social life or health care.
2. If an adult child with a troubled past wants to return home to live with you, think it over carefully, especially if there is a history of substance abuse, violent behavior, or mental illness. As an alternative, you may consider supporting the child in an apartment, not your residence.
3. If you have a history of volatile emotions, take a course in stress and anger management.
4. Develop a telephone network of friends who call each other daily. This can be a source of support and problem solving and can be a way to communicate problems and needs as they arise.

Adapted from: Quinn, M. & Tomita, S. (1986). *Elder abuse and neglect.* New York: Springer.

living with or being dependent on family members remain limited, more and more dependent older adults may be cared for primarily by those who are ill-equipped for such responsibility. As a result, the incidence of abuse may arise unless caregivers are educated and supported. Nurses who receive education in recognizing and intervening in abusive situations will be less afraid to take action and will know what to do.

REFERENCES

Hamilton, G. (1989). Prevent elder abuse: Using a family systems approach. *Journal of Gerontological Nursing, 15*(3), 21–26.

Kosberg, J. (1988). Preventing elder abuse: Identification of high-risk factors prior to placement decisions. *Gerontologist, 28*, 43–50.

O'Malley, H., Segars, H., Perez, R., Mitchell, V. & Kneupful, G. (1984). Elder abuse in Massachusetts: A survey of professionals and paraprofessionals. In J.J. Costa (Ed.), *Abuse of the elderly: A guide to resources and services* (pp. 57–95). Lexington, MA: D.C. Heath.

Pillemer, K., & Finkelhor, D. (1988). The prevalence of elder abuse: A random sample survey. *Gerontologist, 28,* 51–57.

Pollick, M. (1987). Abuse of the elderly: A review. *Holistic Nursing Practice, 1,* 43–53.

Quinn, M. & Tomita, S. (1986) *Elder abuse and neglect.* New York: Springer.

Tomita, S. (1982). Delectation and treatment of elderly abuse and neglect: A protocol for health care professionals. *Physical and Occupational Therapy in Geriatrics, 2,* 37–51.

Urquart, A. (1987). Elder abuse: An imperative for action. *Florida Nursing Review, 2,* 11–16.

BIBLIOGRAPHY

Sayles-Cross, S. (1993). Perceptions of familial caregivers of elder adults. *Image, 25,* 88–92.

Thompson, E., Futterman, A., Gallagher-Thompson, D., Rose, J., & Lovett, S. (1993). Social support and caregiving burden in family caregivers of frail elders. *Journal of Gerontology, 48,* S245–S254.

Weiler, K., & Buckwalter, K. (1992, September). Geriatric mental health abuse among rural mentally ill. *Journal of Psychosocial Nursing,* 32–36.

Whiteback, L., Hoyt, D., & Huck, S. (1994). Early family relationships, intergenerational solidarity, and support provided to parents by their adult children. *Journal of Gerontology, 49,* S85–S94.

Problems With
Living Arrangements
for the Older Adult

Objectives

1. Discuss the current trends related to living arrangements for the older adult.
2. Assess current and potential alternative living arrangements available to the older adult.
3. Identify factors in selecting a specific housing option.
4. Compare and contrast the various housing options available to older adults.
5. Guide others through the process of selecting housing for older adults.

INTRODUCTION

BECAUSE SHELTER IS ONE OF THE MOST basic of human needs, living arrangements are a major concern for Americans of all ages. Yet, housing involves more than the simple provision of shelter: it is at once a functional construct that fulfills basic security needs and an emotional haven that nurtures the spirit. A home is a safe, familiar place that is an ever-evolving reflection of one's self. It is the memories (in the form of pictures, furniture, and other belongings) and the people who make them that give the home a value far beyond its simple retail worth. With the advent of old age, older adults are often faced with the troubling prospect of redefining or reinventing home. Whether they choose to continue lifelong patterns or are forced by circumstances to change, it is clear that the freedom to choose where and with whom to live is crucial to older adults' ability to enjoy life.

Staab, AS and Hodges, LC: ESSENTIALS OF GERONTOLOGICAL NURSING,
© 1996 J. B. Lippincott Company

Many nurses will actively participate in these decisions as they encounter record numbers of older adults in physicians' offices, hospitals, and community health agencies. These nurses will help older adults assess their own physical abilities and limitations as well as see to it that their needs and desires are met.

ASSESSMENT OF LIVING ARRANGEMENTS FOR OLDER ADULTS

In assessing living arrangements, one must determine the extent of the older adult's functional abilities and whether or not he or she can be accommodated in the housing situation under consideration. Some important factors to consider include the person's physical and mental functioning, safety of the environment, availability of and access to transportation, presence of community support, and availability of caregivers.

PHYSICAL FUNCTIONING

The ability to ambulate, including climbing stairs, is an important qualification for residence in a large or multilevel dwelling. Patients who require the assistance of canes and walkers to get about may tire easily, so special care should be taken to ensure that the distances between commonly accessed rooms are manageable for them. Housing for the nonambulatory patient should have doorways that are large enough to allow for the passage of a wheelchair.

Housing determinations are also based on assessments of the older adult for dependency in the other activities of daily living: dressing, bathing, toileting, eating, and continence. A person who is unable to dress, bathe, or eat unaided may be encouraged to enlist the help of a part-time caregiver who visits the private home periodically. The incontinent older adult, however, usually requires care around the clock, which may make institutionalization the most viable housing option.

The older adult's inability to clean, cook, or otherwise manage a household frequently results in a referral to a home services agency or a personal caregiver. Regardless of the housing option chosen, every effort should be made to ensure that the older adult is housed in an environment that invites his or her active participation. To this end, older adults should be encouraged to perform as many of their daily activities as completely as possible.

MENTAL ABILITY

Most older Americans have intact mental abilities, but 25% of those age 65 or older have some type of cognitive impairment as a result of dementia (Spector, 1991). Dementia, no matter what the cause, is a progressive condition: its inevitable conclusion is severely impaired mental function. However, the nurse should regularly assess the older adult's mental abilities to get a more accurate depiction of remaining abilities. This information can help the nurse plan appropriate interventions to compensate for the losses.

Confusion and memory loss are also often seen in older adults. Confusion, a common sign of infection, is often seen after surgery as a result of prolonged or atypical anesthetic effects. It may also be a result of relocation to a new environment. Confusion is not a part of normal aging and should suggest to the nurse that something is wrong. The presence of confusion should be of particular concern to nurses when planning the patient's discharge from the hospital. If the confusion occurred acutely during the hospital stay and is not the result of injury to the brain, one can expect it to resolve eventually. The nurse should keep this in mind and try to avoid initiating major changes in living arrangements based solely on the presence of confusion.

Some difficulty accessing memory may be seen as a function of the normal aging process. Memory loss is a problem if it cannot be compensated for and interferes with the completion of activities of daily living or becomes a safety concern. Extensive memory loss is abnormal and suggests the presence of some pathologic condition. The nurse should be alert for changes in mental ability, including memory loss, and refer these concerns to a physician. Early referral allows for the identification and treatment of reversible cognitive impairments, thus improving the quality of life for affected persons and preventing unnecessary changes in living arrangements.

SAFETY ISSUES

Safety is a major concern when assessing living conditions. Many older adults live in unsafe housing for a variety of reasons. Relatively minor nuisances, such as excessive clutter, loose flooring or floor coverings, poor lighting, and unstable stairs, can pose safety risks for the older adult. Many of the neighborhoods or buildings in which these persons live are considered unsafe by the general public. Often these areas have declined over the years, but older adults stay because they are unwilling or unable to move. Financial constraints may prompt older adults to settle for living in these less desirable areas.

Other safety concerns are related to the older adult's physical and/or mental functioning. Persons who are unsafe ambulating or stair climbing are prime examples of those at risk as the result of impaired physical functioning. Persons who are forgetful and start fires in the kitchen or wander off and get lost pose a significant risk to themselves and others as the result of impaired mental function. Because safety is a serious concern, the nurse should determine the presence of risks and the likelihood of injury.

TRANSPORTATION

For the older adult who chooses to maintain an independent residence, reliable transportation is the link between home and a variety of social and medical services. Several factors can complicate the older adult's access to transportation.

Although many older adults retain their own automobiles, declining vision and other physical impairments may affect their ability to drive. To compensate, they may simply limit their driving to essential trips, which are made only during the day and only in good weather. As the cost of maintaining a rarely used vehicle mounts, the older adult may opt to rely on others to provide transportation. This dependence on others can severely limit the older person's lifestyle.

Creedon (1988) noted a recent housing trend of building accommodations in outlying areas, inconveniently located away from stores, hospitals, and other vital services. Older adults who no longer have the use of their automobiles may find themselves relying on public transportation to access vital services. With public transportation options decreasing nationwide, it is clear that our society is unable to meet this growing need (Creedon, 1988). Where public transportation is available, the older adult's ability to take advantage of it is severely restricted by its high cost, limited access, or inconvenient scheduling (Rosenbloom, 1993).

COMMUNITY SUPPORT

The availability of a support network is sometimes a decisive factor when making a choice from among a selection of living arrangements. Some communities have a wide variety of formal services available. Some are tightly knit with much informal caregiving, whereas others may be limited in both formal and informal support. Friends, family, and church or other organizations are all potential sources of informal support.

AVAILABILITY OF CAREGIVERS

Stone, Cafferata, and Sangl (1987) reported that 2.2 million unpaid caregivers provided aid to 1.6 million noninstitutionalized older adults during 1982. Doty (1986) stated that close to 75% of the community-living elderly who need assistance get help only from family or friends. Almost three quarters of unpaid caregivers are middle-aged women, and approximately 50% of caregivers reside with the care recipient (Stone, Cafferata, & Sangl, 1987).

SELECTING HOUSING

Selecting appropriate housing for an older adult can be a very complicated process. The nurse should guide this process, while ensuring that the desires and realistic needs of the older person are evaluated when considering the housing options available. Additionally, the nurse should attempt to focus attention on both the costs of the available options and the effect that the relocation will have on the older person.

In addition to assessing the older adult's physical and mental functioning, safety concerns, transportation issues, community support, and availability of caregivers, the nurse must also ask a host of other questions when making housing decisions. Display 29-1 provides assessment questions to help the nurse guide the decision-making process. In most cases, the older person can, and should, make the decision of where to reside (MacDonald, Remus, & Laing, 1994). This expression of self-determination should help make the older person's future more enjoyable.

LIVING ARRANGEMENT OPTIONS

Provided they can meet the expenses, older Americans have a wide variety of options when choosing where to live. A careful assessment of their needs and desires should be made, and all available options should be fully investigated. Choosing appropriate housing is particularly important for older adults, because many of them will spend the greater part of each day in that environment.

Display 29-1
ASSESSMENT OF LIVING ARRANGEMENTS OF OLDER ADULTS

A. Current situation
  1. Where is the person living?
  2. Is the current housing adequate, or are repairs necessary?
  3. Is the client living alone or with someone?
  4. How is this arrangement working?
  5. Is there a reason that the living arrangement should be altered?
      a. Inability to care for self
      b. Inability to maintain home
      c. Incompatibility or loss of housing partner
      d. Financial concerns
      e. Desire to change living arrangement
      f. Need for special services
B. Alternative situations
  1. Will the client live alone or choose to live with others?
  2. Does the client want to live in age-segregated or age-integrated housing?
  3. What services are needed or desired?
  4. What type of housing is preferred?
  5. What geographic location is desired?
  6. What is the financial situation?
  7. What are the desired characteristics of the neighborhood and dwelling itself?

LIVING IN A PRIVATE HOME

In the absence of compelling reasons to change, most older adults can remain living independently in their own homes without significantly altering their routines. However, some older adults who choose to remain in their homes find that they must make some major adjustments in their lifestyles.

Clinical Pearl

Assessment: Almost three quarters of all noninstitutionalized older adults who need assistance get this help from family and friends.

HOME SHARING

Home sharing has a variety of incarnations. An older person may choose to remain at home and have someone else move in. This arrangement may simply involve the other person sharing living expenses with the elderly homeowner; it could, however, include a formal rent agreement. Additionally, the older adult might provide a caregiver room, board, and salary as a means of maintaining a semi-independent living arrangement. These options allow older persons to remain in the familiar environment of their own homes.

Another type of home sharing involves a group of people residing in a home, providing each other with informal support and supervision. This arrangement, which is similar to the option of a more formally organized group home, allows for the sharing of living expenses.

The older adult may move into the home of another (most often with a family member) who will function as the caregiver. In this semi-independent living arrangement, the older person relocates to accommodate the caregiver. Although the people living in the home may be familiar, the home is not, often resulting in confusion and unhappiness for the displaced older adult.

Home sharing is an option with many societal benefits. When older adults can remain at home, the government is spared the often unnecessary expense of institutionalization. This, in turn, frees up beds in nursing homes, which can then be awarded to those truly in need of care. Home-sharing arrangements also allow the participants to share expenses, from the actual cost of housing to the expense of hiring a caregiver or obtaining needed services. The resultant savings for the participants makes this an economical option. Finally, home sharing has the additional benefit of flexibility and portability. Older adults may choose to share housing with any number of people (from family and friends to hired employees) in any number of locations.

HOME CARE AND OTHER HOME SERVICES

Older adults who choose to remain in the community, either in their own homes or in the homes of others, may find that they need some additional assistance to function. This assistance may be provided by services such as Meals-On-Wheels, chore workers to help with meals or cleaning, friendly visitors, telephone reassurance, transport and escort services, and visiting health professionals (nurses, aides, or therapists). These services are usually provided by a variety of agencies, which may be either publicly or privately funded from private-pay, insurance, or government sources. The local Area Agency on Aging or the Council on Aging can provide information on services available to older adults, including out-of-pocket costs and reimbursement policies.

ADULT DAY CARE AND ADULT DAY HEALTH CARE

Day-care services are useful options for functionally impaired older adults and their caregivers. Since this idea was first suggested in the mid 1970s, the number of these centers has increased from 18 in 1974 (Weissert, 1977) to 2,100 in 1989 (Burke, Hudson, & Eubanks, 1990). The option of adult care is becoming more readily available.

The area of *adult day care* can be confusing, because a variety of programs are described by similar, but not necessarily identical, terms. The National Institute on Adult Daycare (1984) defines adult day care (ADC) as a community-based group program designed to provide individualized care to functionally impaired adults. This comprehensive program provides health, social, and related support services to adults. Services are provided in a safe environment and may be available for any length of time within a 24-hour period. Conrad, Hanrahan, and Hughes' (1990) study of ADC found that this generic term is often applied to a large variety of programs ranging from social and recreational programming to those with a strong medical emphasis.

Mehlferber (1990) described three models of ADC:

- Social—Offers socialization opportunities and contact with various other support services
- Maintenance—Offers supervision, personal care, and socialization
- Restorative—Offers the services of maintenance along with monitoring and treatment of health problems

The term "adult day health care" has been applied to the provision of care in the health service–intense restorative model. Medicaid provides the main source of funding for ADC services (Burke, Hudson, & Eubanks, 1990). A program created by Congress in 1981 allows state Medicaid programs to apply for waivers to provide a range of home- and community-based services to persons who would otherwise be institutionalized. Administrators reported in an ADC survey that 51.7% of their participants would be in nursing homes or other institutions if they were not in the day program (Conrad, Hanrahan, & Hughes, 1990). The government has no statistics on the economic effect of the waiver program because this use of Medicaid funds is not reported to them (Burke, Hudson, & Eubanks, 1990).

 Clinical Pearl

Intervention: Adult day care provides structured programming in a safe environment. Its use may prevent or postpone institutionalization.

The payment for day programs may come from out-of-pocket participant fees, through Social Services block grant funding, or through grants under the auspices of the Older Americans Act. Medicare does not pay for these day programs, except in rare instances, when services are provided through a Medicare-certified outpatient facility (Burke, Hudson, & Eubanks, 1990). Additional financial support for programming is often obtained through philanthropic donations and community-based fund-raising. Most providers of these services are not-for-profit organizations, although interest is increasing in ADC as a for-profit venture.

CAREGIVING AND RESPITE

When the older adult is partially or completely dependent but remains in a private home, care must be provided. This care is most frequently provided by female family members (Montgomery & Kosloski, 1994). Caregiving imposes physical, mental, and economic stresses on caregivers, who are often struggling to balance caregiving responsibilities with employment, child rearing, housekeeping, and needs for privacy and personal time (Malett, 1993).

Although hiring a paid caregiver to share the work load is an option available to most, less than 10% of unpaid caregivers exercised this option (Stone, Cafferata, & Sangl, 1987). However, the stresses of providing care 24 hours a day, 365 days a year are often too much for any one caregiver to bear. Unless the caregiver seeks regular relief or respite from the stress of caregiving, burnout is likely to occur. One of the most devastating consequences of caregiver burn-out is institutionalization of the older person. A helpful reference for the nurse to recommend to the caregiver is *The 36-Hour Day*, which is available in most bookstores (Mace & Rabins, 1991).

Respite has several benefits (Theis, Moss, & Pearson, 1994). It allows caregivers the time to meet their own needs. Because it enables the caregivers to take a break from care provision, respite may ultimately extend the life of the caregiving arrangement, thus increasing the amount of time that an older person can remain in the community. A respite stay can also give both the older person and the caregiver a chance to preview other caregiving options before having to make a decision about their use.

Respite care can occur in a variety of settings:

- Home—When the respite provider comes to the home, the caregiver is free to leave for an agreed-on amount of time.
- Nursing home—The older adult is admitted for a temporary, predetermined amount of time, usually several days to a few weeks.
- Hospital—Space may be available on geriatric or rehabilitative units (van Werkhooven, 1992). This option is used when the older adult requires a high intensity in the level of care; however, the cost of hospitalization is often too high to make this a viable option.
- Adult day or adult day health care center—These programs provide supervision and care for older adults; services are available for varying lengths of time that total less than 24 hours per day.

The major disincentive for use of respite programs is financial, because very few designated respite services are reimbursed by private insurance or by Medicaid and Medicare, and out-of-pocket expenses can be prohibitive.

Friends and other family members may be able to arrange respite through scheduling caregiving appointments. Even a short break can be very beneficial to the primary caregiver. Additionally, use of home care services can provide much-needed caregiving breaks. The primary caregiver should be encouraged to contract for the provision of services that are difficult, uncomfortable, or distasteful to perform (eg, assistance with bathing).

SINGLE-ROOM OCCUPANCY AND OTHER HOTEL ACCOMMODATIONS

A familiar sight in the run-down areas of major cities are dilapidated hotels, which are often referred to as single-room occupancies (SROs). These hotels are usually in unsafe neighborhoods, and the residents are frequently transients who cannot afford better housing. As of 1985, the U.S. Department of Housing and Urban Development reported more than 200,00 older people living in SROs, usually below the poverty level. Many of the elderly residents have been forced by economic circumstances to live in the SROs, in which they are in constant fear for their safety. Those whom they fear are often other older adult residents with social or behavioral problems— the mentally ill, alcoholics, drug abusers, and criminals (Atchley, 1985).

Certain hotels, which call themselves retirement hotels, offer residential opportunities for older adults. These retirement hotels may be located in elegant settings and provide highly specialized services. They may be equally likely to resemble the down-scale SROs in terms of geographic location and state of disrepair. Persons may choose this type of housing due to low cost, privacy, the provision of housekeeping (and, in some instances, meal service), and location near other services (Crystal & Beck, 1992).

MOBILE HOMES AND FULL-TIMING IN RECREATIONAL VEHICLES

Mobile homes provide a fairly low-cost method of owning a home, no matter what the owner's age. Although most mobile home parks are not exclusive to older adults, it is likely that the aging of the population will also affect the demographics in mobile home parks. Mobile homes are often used in rural areas as a means of allowing an older relative to move onto another relative's property and still maintain a separate household.

Hartwigsen and Null (1989) detailed the concept of "full-timing," which is year-round residence in a recreational vehicle (RV). Full-timing may be a practical lifestyle for active older adults with friends and family in a variety of geographic locations in the United States. Full-timers can park in the yard and live with one family, until the urge to move hits. Many of the benefits of living in a mobile home are also true when full-timing. However, the fact that the full-timer often moves the RV can complicate life. The full-timer may not have a permanent address, which causes difficulty with mail delivery. In each new locale, the full-timer must become acquainted with the services available, including medical care. Full-timing can be as economical or as expensive as a person chooses, with the largest portion of expense being the cost of purchasing the RV. Other expenses include fuel, maintenance and repairs, licensure, registration, insurance, and campground/trailer park fees.

NATURALLY OCCURRING RETIREMENT COMMUNITIES

Most Americans are familiar with the phenomenon of the aging of a neighborhood or housing development. As time passes, the residences in an area fill up, those who live there age, and younger people seek residence in newly developing areas. This creates a naturally occurring retirement community (NORC). A NORC can be defined as a housing community in which more than half of the residents are at least 60 years old, even though the housing was not planned, designed, or marketed toward older residents (Hunt & Ross, 1990). Older persons may be drawn to NORCs for a variety of reasons, such as geographic location and climate, recreational opportunities, cost, or availability of services. Services often develop as needs become more evident. NORCs are usually age-integrated and often have a strong sense of community (Streib, 1990).

NORCs often develop in a single building or in areas that house fewer than 500 residents (Hunt & Gunter-Hunt, 1985). Most nonresidents would not identify NORCs as retirement communities, despite the predominance of older residents. Nevertheless, the NORC is a common environment for older Americans, with 27% of persons age 55 or older surveyed living in a community fitting the definition of a NORC (American Association of Retired Persons, 1990).

PLANNED RETIREMENT COMMUNITIES

Increasingly, older Americans reside in retirement communities that are planned and developed for and marketed to older adults. Usually they are age-segregated, with a minimum age for residence. Marketing is aimed at the young-old, that is, persons who are still very active (Hegner & Caldwell, 1991).

Planned retirement communities may be special housing developments of individual homes, multifamily dwellings (duplexes), condominiums, or apartments. Many offer several or all of the aforementioned types of housing as options within one community. Some towns are actually very large planned retirement communities that offer extensive social, recreational, health, and transportation services. Retirement villages are other examples of planned communities. These communities are usually dependent on services available through a nearby town or city (Streib, 1990).

CONTINUING CARE RETIREMENT COMMUNITIES

Continuing care retirement communities (CCRCs), also known as life-care communities, are yet another idea for housing the older adult. These communities, which were typically nonprofit and sponsored by religious or fraternal organizations, are now also being managed by hospital or nursing home corporations (Somers, 1993). CCRCs provide housing, health and long-term care, and other services.

Most CCRCs provide independent-living houses and apartments, assisted-living housing, and intermediate and skilled nursing home care. In the past, residents transferred their assets to the community on admission, in exchange for a guarantee of housing and health care until death. More recently, many CCRCs have chosen to charge a large entrance fee and a monthly fee for services. The individual's charges are based on the projected lifetime cost of care provided by the community.

Clinical Pearl

Planning: The success of continuing care retirement communities will set a precedent for a national plan to provide adequate long-term care.

Cohen, Tell, Bishop, Wallack, and Branch (1989) examined the use of nursing home services by CCRC residents. Administrators of CCRCs often express concern over the possibility that residents will use more of the high-cost, care-intensive services simply because they are available. This research suggests that despite knowing nursing home care is guaranteed, CCRC residents are no more likely to use this option than is the general public. The researchers found that CCRC residents were generally healthier than older adults in other living arrangements. Additionally, they found more short-term rehabilitative-type stays in the CCRC nursing homes.

NURSING HOMES

Nursing homes are an option for older adults who can no longer manage their own care at home or who cannot be managed in the community even with the assistance of others. Institutionalization becomes even more likely as an older adult continues to age. Institutionalization of women occurs about one and one-half times more often than for men, and persons age 85 or older are institutionalized four times more often than persons age 65 to 75 (Kemper & Murtaugh, 1991). The decision to institutionalize an older adult is rarely an easy one for older persons or for their families and caregivers. This experience may be made less burdensome once the older adult understands why a nursing home is necessary and learns how to choose the best one.

Nursing homes provide skilled nursing and intermediate levels of care. Skilled nursing care is a 24-hour-a-day service that includes social, recreational, nutritional, rehabilitative, pharmaceutical, radiologic, laboratory, respiratory, and medical services. Intermediate care is designed for persons who need assistance but who require less extensive nursing care. Often, both levels of care are provided by the same facility (Fig. 29-1).

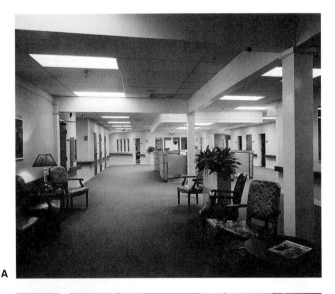

A

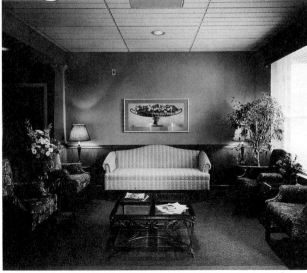

B

Figure 29-1. (A) Nursing homes can provide a pleasant and attractive environment **(B)** A tastefully furnished communal area can increase the homelike atmosphere. Riley's Oak Hill Manor South, Little Rock, AR.

OTHER HOUSING OPTIONS

Other options exist, although they are not as widely available. The following options are sometimes referred to as "sheltered care." McNicholl (1988) described the personal care home, a residence for physically, emotionally, or cognitively impaired persons who need assistance with mobility, personal care, housekeeping, and meals. Activities and supervision are provided, but medical care is not. Sheltered care is provided for persons of all ages in facilities that may be called homes for the aged, adult homes, group homes, board and care homes, or domiciliary-care facilities. Boarding houses that provide housing, housekeeping, and meals may be another venue for sheltered care. These may or may not be age-integrated. Foster care of the older adult, who moves in with a family that provides housing, housekeeping, meals, and supervision, is another aspect of sheltered care.

THE ROLE OF THE NURSE

To make an appropriate decision, the older adult (or proxy decision maker) must be provided with information on the available housing options and how these will meet the individual's personal requirements for a living environment. (Fig. 29-2). The nurse may be able to provide this information or may refer these concerns to a social worker or other appropriate resources. A list of potential sources of information on housing options and issues is provided for use by the nurse or older adult/family member (Display 29-2).

(text continues on page 499)

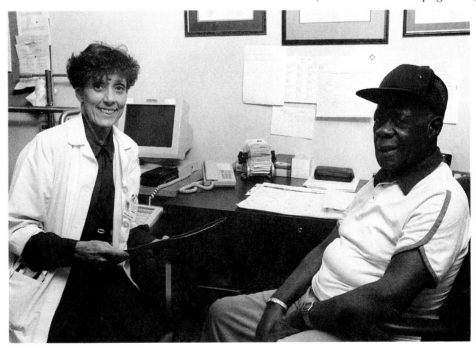

Figure 29-2. The nurse gives advice and assistance to the older adult seeking available housing options that best meet his needs.

Display 29-2
SOURCES OF INFORMATION ON HOUSING OPTIONS

American Association of Homes for the Aging (AAHA)
901 E St. NW, Ste. 500
Washington, DC 20004–2037
(202) 783–2242

AAHA is an association of not-for-profit and government nursing homes, housing programs, and programs that provide services to elders living in the community. The association's philosophy asserts that long-term care includes a continuum of services from in-home services through intensive care provided in a nursing home. The focus is on meeting individual needs and attempting to provide high quality care in any setting.

American Association of Retired Persons (AARP)
601 E St. NW
Washington, DC 20049
(202) 434–2277

AARP is an organization of persons age 50 and older whose goal is to improve the standard of life for all older Americans. A variety of programs and services are available through AARP. Information on a variety of subjects can be requested from the consumer affairs division.

American Health Care Association (AHCA)
1201 L St. NW
Washington, DC 20005
(202) 842–4444

This association includes state associations of long-term care facilities. Goals are to set standards for care provision and to encourage safe, high-quality care. Concerns involve cost, quality, affordability, reimbursement, and availability of nursing home care. Publications: *A Consumer's Guide to Long Term Care, Thinking About a Nursing Home?* and *Welcome to Our Nursing Home.*

American Mobilehome Association (AMA)
12929 West 26th Ave.
Golden, CO 80401
(303) 232–6336

AMA is an association of mobile home owners that keeps members apprised of regulations affecting them.

Beverly Foundation (BF)
70 S. Lake Ave., Ste. 750
Pasadena, CA 91101
(818) 792–2292

The foundation provides a variety of programming for use in long-term-care facilities. Publications: *Welcome to Our Nursing Home* (coloring book).

(continued)

Display 29-2

SOURCES OF INFORMATION ON HOUSING OPTIONS *(Continued)*

Children of Aging Parents (CAPS)
Woodbourne Office Campus, Ste. 302A
1609 Woodbourne Rd.
Levittown, PA 19057
(215) 945–6900

CAPS is a self-help group for adult children who are caregivers to elderly parents. Publications: *How to Start a Self Group for Caregivers, Instant Aging—Sensory Deprivation Manual, Guide to Selecting a Nursing Home.*

Cooperative Housing Foundation (CHF)
P.O. Box 91280
Washington, DC 20090–1280
(301) 587–4700

CHF works to assist in developing better cooperative housing and community services. It provides information, technical assistance, and training.

Foundation for Hospice and Homecare (FHHC)
519 C St. NE
Stanton Park
Washington, DC 20002
(202) 547–6586

The foundation accredits homemaker/home health aide services and provides consumer education programs. Publications: *All About Homecare–A Consumer's Guide.*

Intercare
P.O. Box 8561
Moscow, ID 83843
(509) 229–3259

Intercare is a group of persons interested in the long-term care of the aged, disabled, or chronically ill. It compiles statistics and is a source for information.

National Association for Home Care (NAHC)
519 C St. NE
Stanton Park
Washington, DC 20002
(202) 547–7424

This association promotes high quality of patient care, sets standards for home care, and can provide a list of home health care organizations.

National Association of Nutrition and Aging Services Programs (NANASP)
2675 44th St. SW, Ste. 305
Grand Rapids, MI 49509
(616) 530–3250

The association sets standards for meal programs and encourages communication between programs providing nutritional services for the elderly.

(continued)

Display 29-2

SOURCES OF INFORMATION ON HOUSING OPTIONS *(Continued)*

National Association of Private Geriatric Care Managers (NAPGCM)
655 N. Alvernon Way, Ste. 108
Tucson, AZ 85711
(602) 881–8008

The association provides information and referrals about geriatric care centers.

National Citizen's Coalition for Nursing Home Reform (NCCNHR)
1224 M St. NW, Ste. 301
Washington, DC 20005
(202) 393–2018

NCCNHR's purpose is to improve the quality of life of nursing home residents by improving services. NCCNHR serves as a clearinghouse for information on nursing homes and board and care issues. Publications: *Citizens' Guide to Reimbursement Issues, A Consumer Persepctive on Quality Care: The Resident's Point of View, Inappropriate Use of Physical and Chemical Restraints, The Rights of Nursing Home Residents.*

National Council on the Aging (NCOA)
409 3rd St. SW
Washington, DC 20024
(202) 479–1200

The council conducts research, serves as a national information and consultation center, and supports a variety of programs:

National Center on Rural Aging (NCRA)
c/o National Council on the Aging
(202) 479–6683

National Institute on Adult Daycare (NIAD)
c/o National Council on the Aging
(202) 479–6682

National Institute on Community-Based Long-Term Care (NICLC)
c/o National Council on the Aging
(202) 479–6680

National Institute of Senior Centers (NISC)
c/o National Council on the Aging
(202) 479–6683

National Institute of Senior Housing (NISH)
c/o National Council on the Aging
(202) 479–6680

National Voluntary Organizations for Independent Living
   for the Aging (NVOILA)
c/o National Council on the Aging
(202) 249–1200

(continued)

Display 29-2
SOURCES OF INFORMATION ON HOUSING OPTIONS *(Continued)*

National Institute on Aging (NIA)
Bldg 31., Rm 5C27
9000 Rockville Pike
Bethesda, MD 20892
(301) 496–1752

NIA conducts and supports research and training in all aspects of aging. Research reports are available. Publications: *Age Pages* and a variety of other resources. For more information write to:

NIA Information Center
P.O. Box 8057
Gaithersburg, MD 20898–8057

Nursing Home Advisory and Research Council (NHARC)
P.O. Box 18820
Cleveland Heights, OH 44118
(216) 321–4499

The council is a group of family, friends, and guardians of nursing home residents. Publications: *Patient's Bill of Rights, Selecting a Nursing Home.*

Project SHARE
336 Fulton Ave.
Hempstead, NY 11550
(516) 292–1300

Project SHARE assists with matching home sharers in Nassau County, NY. It provides advice to others wanting to establish this type of program and promotes low-cost housing for senior citizens.

National Alliance to End Homelessness (NAEH)
1518 K St. NW, Ste. 206
Washington, DC 20005
(202) 638–1526

This association seeks to end homelessness. It offers assistance to homeless individuals and conducts research and educational programs. Publications *Housing and Homelessness: A Report of the National Call to End Homelessness, SRO Handbook.*

National Shared Housing Resource Center
4314 Pine Street
Burlington, VT 05401
(802) 862–2727

This association promotes the idea of shared housing. Publications: *Consumers Guide to Home Sharing and Shared Housing News.*

Even in cases of involuntary relocation to an institution or other setting, the nurse should encourage the decision maker to accommodate as many of the older adult's desires as possible. Relocation is change, and change, even when desired, is difficult. Visiting or engaging in a trial stay at the prospective housing is suggested. By fostering a sense of control in the decision-making process and promoting a feeling of familiarity with the new environment, the nurse can make relocation a much more pleasant experience.

ROLE OF THE NURSE IN CARING FOR COMMUNITY-DWELLING ELDERLY

The nurse who works in home health/community health functions independently, usually with limited personnel or equipment resources. These nurses must be creative to meet the needs of older adults in the community. Knowledge and assessment skills of both nursing and nonnursing needs is vital to these nurses. Although the nurse practicing in the community may provide care that is often provided by other disciplines (eg, physical, occupational, or respiratory therapy), he or she must also be able to make appropriate referrals when necessary.

Often, older adults first access the community health system on discharge from the hospital or after a change in health status has led them to their physician's office. The nurse in these settings should be alert to the need for home health services and direct the older adult and his or her family to the appropriate resources as needed. Usually, a nurse screens/assesses the older adult for the services he or she will require when back in the community.

The nurse in the community serves in a variety of roles. He or she is an educator and health promoter, providing information to older adults, their families, and other interested community members. The nurse is a communicator, working to establish and maintain clear communication between the physician, the older adult and his or her family, and other professionals. Counseling and support are related roles adopted by the nurse in the community. Both older adults and their caregivers feel an emotional burden as health status changes. Identification and management of problems, promotion of self-care, and maximizing independence are important nursing roles.

Community-based nurses may also encounter the homeless older adult. Homelessness is not actually a living arrangement but, more accurately, a lack of housing. Homelessness in older adults is usually associated with low income, dementia, living alone, and having an erratic residential history (Keigher & Greenblatt, 1992). The nurse should act as an advocate for homeless older adults and refer and guide these people in an attempt to obtain a more satisfactory living arrangement.

ROLE OF THE NURSE IN THE INSTITUTIONAL SETTING

The role of the nurse in the nursing home is similar to that of the nurse within the community. Usually the decision to institutionalize an older adult is made during hospital-based discharge planning or when the caregivers decide that they are no longer able to maintain the older adult at home.

Nurses should be aware that most Americans have limited experience with nursing homes (Johnson, Morton, & Knox, 1992). As a result, they feel pressured to make a decision quickly when institutionalization becomes necessary. Many times bed availability is the decisive factor in placement, to the exclusion of investigating all other options. The nurse can help in this process by suggesting that the older adult and/or family seek recommendations from family and friends, health professionals, and clergy. Names of facilities in a selected geographic locale can be obtained from the phone book. The local Area Agency on Aging, Council on Aging, and health department as well as state agencies that address aging concerns (names vary among states) can help with specific referrals or information. The following Patient Teaching Box can help the nurse provide further guidance in this process.

Patient Teaching Box
FACTORS TO CONSIDER WHEN CHOOSING A NURSING HOME

1. Is the facility state licensed? Is it Medicaid/Medicare certified?
2. What is the thinking on care provision? Does the staff encourage independence? Are residents active in the planning of their care?
3. Is the professional nursing staff licensed? (This is a legal requirement.) Are the nursing assistants certified? Does the staff have additional knowledge, specifically about care of the elderly? What are the staffing patterns, that is, how many registered nurses, licensed practical nurses, and nurse's aides work each shift?
4. Do physicians direct each resident's care? How often do they visit? (By law, they must visit every 30 days in the first 90 days, then thereafter every 60 days.) Are physicians readily available for emergencies?
5. Does a licensed pharmacist review all patient medications periodically? Are medications handled in accordance with government regulations?
6. Are rehabilitative (eg, physical, occupational, recreational) services available?
7. What kinds of recreational opportunities are provided (current events or other groups, social programs, trips, volunteer opportunities, exercise classes, arts and crafts or hobbies, movies)?
8. What other services are available (respiratory therapy, podiatry, dentistry, optometry, personal care services)?
9. How is the food? How does it look? Do the residents like it? Is food available for snacks or at other times when a resident is hungry? Are special dietary needs and preferences addressed? Is there a registered dietitian on staff or available as a consultant? Is the kitchen clean and well run?
10. Are there clear disaster/emergency policies and plans?
11. Does an arrangement exist for transfer to an acute care facility if this type of care is needed?
12. Is infection control monitored? Is hand washing encouraged? Are gloves available? Do staff wash hands and use gloves?
13. What is the physical facility like? Is the layout convenient? Is the environment appropriate for older adults (appropriate lighting, grab bars in halls and bathrooms, adequate room for wheelchair access)? Is the facility clean, are the grounds well kept, and is equipment in good repair? Does the facility have an odor problem?
14. How are problem behaviors (wandering, yelling, and incontinence) handled? Are diapers used?
15. Is the facility religiously affiliated? How are spiritual needs met?
16. Are visitors welcome? When can they visit? Are children allowed? May family or friends participate in facility-sponsored activities? Is there a resident and/or family council? Are families encouraged to be involved with the resident and his or her care?
17. What are the qualifications of the facility administrators? Are they accessible? Do people seem to be able to talk to them?
18. How do the residents appear? Are they clean, well groomed, and dressed in street clothes? Do they interact with other residents, staff, and visitors? Do they appear happy?
19. How do the staff appear? Are they clean and appropriately dressed? Do they interact with residents and other staff? Are they polite to others on the phone and in person? Do they smile and laugh?
20. How have they fared on recent state health department surveys? Do they acknowledge their problems and are they trying to improve their facility? (These public records are available at the health department for review.)

The nurse can suggest that the telephone be used to initiate contact with a potential home. Level of care, cost, accepted reimbursement, and bed availability can be determined over the phone. In-person visits can then be scheduled at promising facilities. Drop-in observation at mealtimes or during other daily activities may be helpful as well. If possible, the older adult should visit potential facilities as part of the decision-making process. When this is not feasible, it is suggested that the older person be allowed to visit before making a permanent move. Another possibility to investigate is that of "trial," or short-term admission, which allows the person to try out the home before making a permanent move.

If problems are experienced in the nursing home, the nursing staff, director of nursing, administrator, or social worker should be able to help. Additional assistance is available from a nursing home ombudsman, who can be reached through the local Area Agency on Aging or state office on aging. The ombudsman is able to investigate complaints and initiate corrective action as a resident advocate. Many states employ additional nursing home investigators who do complaint investigation.

The nurse can help older adults and family members deal with the emotional reactions that result from the decision for nursing home placement. When the older adult is admitted to the nursing home, he or she may feel depersonalized as a result of losing family and work roles and being forced to follow the facility's rules and schedules. The older adult may become frustrated, angry, or depressed about the situation and may feel humiliated by the dependency on others and the lack of privacy.

Families also have to contend with an array of emotions. They often feel guilty about placing a relative in a nursing home, even when this clearly is the best option. Depression and feelings of inadequacy are often experienced. Family members may also feel embarrassment when their loved one behaves in socially inappropriate ways (which is especially seen in older adults with dementia). Anger and resentment over the cost of care or the need to rearrange life responsibilities around nursing home activities may also surface.

No matter what the emotion, nursing home residents and their families should be encouraged to share their feelings. Nurses are often the first people to note signs of emotional stress. Referral to support groups, which create an open environment wherein the person feels free to express emotions, can prove extremely useful. Nurses must help guide family members and nursing home residents in establishing new relationships with each other and with other nursing home residents and their families.

Nurses can help smooth the transition to the nursing home by attempting to take into account the older adult's personal preferences and attempting to accede to these as often as the facility schedule permits. Additionally, nursing home staff find it helpful to know something about the older adult as a person. The nurse should encourage the older adult and the family to bring in pictures and important items from the older adult's past. Bringing a favorite piece of furniture, pictures, or other items can personalize the room and make it seem more comfortable and familiar. Having comfortable clothing like the older adult wore at home can help with the adjustment. The nurse should reinforce that the nursing home is just that—a home. Through these and similar efforts, the nurse can help make the atmosphere comfortable and homelike.

REFERENCES

American Association of Retired Persons. (1990). *Understanding senior housing for the 1990s*. Washington, DC: Author.

Atchley, R. C. (1985). *Social forces and aging* (4th ed.). Belmont, CA: Wadsworth.

Burke, M., Hudson, T., & Eubanks, P. (1990). Number of adult day care centers increasing, but payment is slow. *Hospitals, 64*(21), 34, 36, 38, 40, 42.

Cohen, M. A., Tell, T. J., Bishop, C. E., Wallack, S. S., & Branch, L. G. (1989). Patterns of nursing home use in a prepaid managed care system: The continuing care retirement community. *Gerontologist, 29*(1), 74–80.

Conrad, K. J., Hanrahan, P., & Hughes, S. L. (1990). Survey of adult day care in the United States. *Research on Aging, 12*(1), 36–56.

Creedon, M. A. (1988). Housing for elderly persons: Its implications for nursing. In *Strategies for long-term care* (Pub. No. 20-2231) (pp. 263–271). New York: National League for Nursing.

Crystal, S., & Beck, P. (1992). A room of one's own: The SRO and the single elderly. *Gerontologist, 32*(5), 684–692.

Doty, P. (1986). Family care of the elderly: The role of public policy. *Milbank Quarterly, 64*(1), 34–75.

Hartwigsen, G., & Null, R. (1989). Full-timing: A housing alternative for older people. *International Journal of Aging and Human Development, 29*(4), 317–328.

Hegner, B. R., & Caldwell, E. (1991). *Geriatrics: A study of maturity* (5th ed.). Albany, NY: Delmar.

Hunt, M. E., & Gunter-Hunt, G. (1985). Naturally occurring retirement communities. *Journal of Housing for the Elderly, 3,* 3–21.

Hunt, M. E., & Ross, L. E. (1990). Naturally occurring retirement communities: A multiattribute examination of desirability factors. *Gerontologist, 30,* 667–674.

Johnson, M. A., Morton, M. K., & Knox, S. M. (1992). The transition to a nursing home: Meeting the family's needs. *Geriatric Nursing, 13*(6), 299–302.

Keigher, S. M., & Greenblatt, S. (1992). Housing emergencies and the etiology of homelessness among the urban elderly. *Gerontologist, 32*(4), 457–465.

Kemper, P., & Murtaugh, C. M. (1991). Lifetime use of nursing home care. *New England Journal of Medicine, 324*(9), 595–600.

MacDonald, M., Remus, G., & Laing, G. (1994). Research considerations: The link between housing and health in the elderly. *Journal of Gerontological Nursing, 20*(7), 5–10.

Mace, N. L., & Rabins, P. V. (1991). *The 36-hour day* (2nd ed.). New York: Warner.

Malett, J. (1993). Caring for the caretakers: The patient's family. *Journal of ET Nursing, 20*(2), 78–81.

McNicholl, A. M. (1988). Congregate living and the institutional campus. In *Strategies for long-term care* (Pub. No. 20-2231) (pp. 239–244). New York: National League for Nursing.

Mehlferber, K. (1990). The role of the nurse in adult day care. In C. Eliopoulos (Ed.). *Caring for the elderly in diverse care settings* (pp. 284–289). Philadelphia: J. B. Lippincott.

Montgomery, R. J., & Kosloski, K. (1994). A longitudinal analysis of nursing home placement for dependent elders cared for by spouses vs. adult children. *Journal of Gerontology, 49,* 562–574.

National Institute on Adult Daycare. (1984). *Standards for adult daycare*. Washington, DC: National Council on Aging.

Rosenbloom, S. (1993). Transportation needs of the elderly population. *Clinics in Geriatric Medicine, 9*(2), 297–310.

Somers, A. R. (1993). "Lifecare": A viable option for long-term care for the elderly. *Journal of the American Geriatrics Society, 41,* 188–191.

Spector, W. D. (1991). Cognitive impairment and disruptive behaviors among community-based elderly persons: Implications for targeting long-term care. *Gerontologist, 31*(1), 51–59.

Stone, R., Cafferata, G. L., & Sangl, J. (1987). Caregivers of the frail elderly: A national profile. *Gerontologist, 27*(5), 616–626.

Streib, G. F. (1990). Retirement communities: Linkages to the locality, state, and nation. *Journal of Applied Gerontology, 9*(4), 405–419.

Theis, S. L., Moss, J. H., & Pearson, M. A. (1994). Respite for caregivers: An evaluation study. *Journal of Community Health Nursing, 11,* 31–44.

United States Department of Housing and Urban Development. (1985). *American Housing Survey for the U.S.: 1985*. Current Housing Report Series No. H-150-85. Washington, DC: U.S. Government Printing Office.

van Werkhooven, M. (1992). The frail elderly population. In M. M. Burke & M. B. Walsh (Eds.). *Gerontological nursing: Care of the frail elderly* (pp. 1–48). St. Louis: Mosby.

Weissert, W. G. (1977). ADC programs in the United States: Current research projects and a survey of 10 centers. *Public Health Reports, 92,* 49–56.

BIBLIOGRAPHY

Forschner, B. E. (1994). Long-term benefits: A retirement community grows by reaching out to area residents. *Health Progress, 75*(1), 70–71, 74.
Paul, M. (1993). A little help, a lot of independence: Retirement community advances the cause of aging with dignity. *Health Progress, 74*(4), 43–45.

30

Problems With Community Resources

Objectives

1. Identify a framework for assessing community resources available to the older adult.
2. Identify the components of financial programs that support older adults in the community when meeting their health care needs.
3. Discuss several health care policy and reimbursement issues that directly affect the older adult living in the community.

INTRODUCTION

THE AVAILABILITY OF COMMUNITY RESOURCES is critical for the older adult, who may need the assistance of a variety of social service agencies and health insurance programs. These programs may provide 1) health insurance that reimburses for health maintenance, illness prevention, and long-term care or 2) financial assistance to pay for home health care, provide support for the caregiver, and meet basic needs of daily living, such as housing, food, and pharmaceuticals.

The role of the professional nurse requires knowledge of the services and function of various social agencies whose responsibility is to assist in the financial support of the older adult. Because the way in which each functions is tailored to meet the specific needs of the community, nurses must be knowledgeable of the range and scope of services provided.

When examining the community resources for the older adult, it is imperative that a general view of all financing policies of the health care delivery system be described. These policies are founded on the four critical variables of equity, access, quality, and cost containment. These four concepts serve useful

Staab, AS and Hodges, LC: ESSENTIALS OF GERONTOLOGICAL NURSING,
© 1996 J. B. Lippincott Company

criteria for reviewing the community resources available for the delivery of health care. These concepts are specifically defined as follows:

- *Equity*—Fairness in the distribution of health care regardless of age, race, disability, or economic status
- *Access*—Ability of any individual to enter the health care system regardless of geographic proximity to health care services
- *Quality*—Attainment of predetermined standards of care measured during or after the delivery of health care
- *Cost containment*—Efforts by third-party payers, such as private insurance companies, the state, or the federal government, to decrease the expenditures for health care delivered to individuals, groups, or the population as a whole

The establishment of Medicare occurred at a time in this country when equity and access were two issues at the forefront of social policy. In the 1980s emphasis shifted to cost containment, forcing policy choices and directives in the budgeting, allocation, and distribution of health care resources to older adults. Along with the recent emphasis on cost containment, renewed concerns have arisen about the quality of health care for the older adult, especially in terms of cost/benefit analysis. Special interest groups, such as the American Association of Retired Persons (AARP), have made notable efforts to ensure quality health care for their constituent members. In describing and lobbying for community resources, AARP addressed health policy development, political action of health care recipients, and the amount and availability of money to finance the delivery of health care in the United States.

CARE OF THE OLDER ADULT IN THE COMMUNITY

The older adult receives health care in a variety of community settings, each requiring a different form of reimbursement and level of care. The provision of this myriad of services is fraught with potential imbalances in equity and access across states and at various levels of government. As an example, some of the living arrangements are designed based on an available reimbursement program rather than on specific patient needs. The prevailing strategy was to provide equal access to quality health care for the older adult, and the emphasis was on patient needs rather than on the availability of money to support the service. However, in today's cost-containment environment, the older adult's selection of living arrangements is limited to the following options:

- Independent living with periodic hospitalizations for acute illnesses
- Independent living with occasional to daily assistance from a public health or home health nurse, with periodic hospitalizations for acute episodes when necessary
- Dependent living with a relative or in a residence for older adults that provides 24-hour surveillance or delivery of nursing care
- Dependent living in a long-term–care center with skilled nursing care delivered 24 hours daily

No matter which of these living situations is selected, it is clear that the older adult will need financial support for the expenses of daily living, such as meals, housing and transportation, and health care delivery. The cost of health care increases as the level of dependency increases and varies depending on the residential choice of the older adult.

Because older adults consume more health care and their numbers are ever increasing, federal and state governments are continually searching for ways to decrease costs. These efforts generate several problems with community resources.

The degree of patient disability, which affects the amount and kind of health care delivered, must be considered within each category of community living. Three groupings of disability are used as a guide for measuring health care use or to plan for discharge into the community from an acute care facility. Note that each of the three groupings could apply to the older adult within any of the four community placement categories. These groupings are:

- Independent—Cares for all activities of daily living (ADLs) even when suffering from a short-term acute illness.
- Frail—Has one of the following medical diagnoses: cerebrovascular accident, chronic disabling disease, confusion, falls, dependence in ADLs, impaired mobility, incontinence, malnutrition, polypharmacy, pressure sores, prolonged bed rest, restraints, sensory impairment, or socioeconomic/family problems
- Severely impaired—Has severe dementia and ADL dependence or terminal illness (Winograd et al., 1991)

Given the number of variables that can influence the level of care needed and the amount of financing that may or may not be available to pay for it, it is evident that the nurse must be versed in health policy issues for the older adult. Generally, the greater the impairment, the higher the cost of care and the more difficult it will be to find community placement and financing for that care.

Clinical Pearl

Planning: When planning discharge for an older adult from an acute care setting, the nurse must assess the degree of disability present so that referral and community placement will be consistent with health care needs.

HEALTH POLICY DEVELOPMENT OF COMMUNITY RESOURCES FOR THE OLDER ADULT

Generally, the United States lacks a cogent and clear statement defining a specific health care policy for the older adult. Instead, policymakers at both the state and federal levels of government have passed laws, written regulations for health care delivery, repealed existing programs, or decreased funding to certain programs in a nonsystematic fashion. Historically, legislation supporting health care delivery that becomes law at the federal or state level represents the values and beliefs of legislators and their constituents rather than reflects a distinct health policy. As a result, health policy for older Americans exists as a jigsawed set of laws rather than as a written official policy describing the mission and objectives of the health care delivery system. This approach results in a system of fragmented care, problems with access, and a reliance on high-tech interventions rather than on health maintenance and long-term care. This approach to health policy development constitutes a major difference between the United States and other industrialized nations, many of which have clear policy guidelines.

As the number of older adults continues to grow, there will be an ever-increasing need for public policy discussion and definitive policy decisions. Without such a focus, the health care needs of the older adult will be in a constant state of flux and driven more by cost-containment concerns than by any interest in delivering quality care to older Americans. This approach to policy development has already had a monumental effect on all health care delivered either in inpatient settings or through community resources.

CONTEMPORARY PROBLEMS AND CONCERNS IN THE PROVISION OF HEALTH CARE TO THE OLDER ADULT

In the 1990s, containing costs for health care will be a primary concern. This issue is of the utmost importance for the older adult who must plan health care financing and make intelligent choices when selecting a supplemental health insurance plan. The cost-containment dilemma demands that the professional nurse understand these issues in order to facilitate discharge planning, impart information regarding reimbursement, and make correct referrals to appropriate community agencies. After an acute care hospitalization, cost containment is a factor in long-term care admissions and other community placement. Specifically, referrals to home health agencies or long-term care is frequently made based on reimbursement available to older adults and their families.

Professional nurses are becoming increasingly more responsible for referring the older adult to community resources on discharge. It is critical for the nurse to contact the family soon after an admission to an inpatient facility to determine if a social service agency has been assigned to the family and what services, if any, the patient will require on discharge. This information should be a part of the complete nursing assessment of the newly admitted patient. If this information is not part of the medical record, it is imperative that it be gathered during discharge planning. If there is anticipatory need for special referrals for home health care or expansion of previous care, planning should commence soon after admission and well before actual discharge.

The nurse should inform families of the older adult about health insurance purchases and the extent of coverage of suggested policies. For example, questions are often asked about the amount of out-of-pocket financing for medication and other pharmaceutical services. Information pertaining to various expenditures is of critical importance to older adults and their families.

The financing of health care is accomplished through various methods of third-party reimbursement (insurance). Third-party reimbursement is carried out either by private insurers or government programs of insurance, such as Medicare and Medicaid. For persons younger than age 65, health insurance is usually obtained through an employer as an employee benefit. Older adults (older than age 65) have the distinct advantage of being a beneficiary of a universal, publicly financed health insurance system referred to as Medicare. Essentially, this program pays a part of their medical bills, regardless of income, and ensures access to all available medical care (Feder, 1990).

Medicare

Medicare, the nation's largest insurance program, is administered at the level of the federal government. Because it is a federal agency, it offers uniform benefits for all those 65 years and older. As part of Lyndon Johnson's Great Society, this program was enacted into law in 1965 as Titles XVIII and XIX amendments to the Social Security Act of 1965.

Medicare was based on the belief that those older than 65 years had the greatest need for health care services, the least private coverage, and the least income to pay for health care. In 1972, Medicare was expanded to include coverage of the disabled under Social Security and individuals with end-stage renal disease. The total growth of Medicare continues to be phenomenal. The number of participants grew from 28 million in 1980 to 35 million in 1992 ("Statistical Abstracts," 1994). In 1990, Medicare expenditure reached $108.9 billion and accounted for two thirds of all federal health expenditures (Advisory Council on Social Security, 1991). This figure grew to more than $129 billion by 1992, indicating the exponential growth of this insurance program ("Statistical Abstracts," 1994). Because Medicare is financed through general revenues, the tremendous growth in costs has been attributed to the federal budget deficit and represents a drain on tax revenues. Spending for health care greatly exceeded inflation in the last decade. Thus Medicare, like other aspects of financing health care, reflects this inflation and the ever-spiraling costs on which recent cost-containment initiatives are based.

Payment for Medicare insurance premiums occurs in many ways. The hospital insurance portion (referred to as Part A) is funded through a payroll tax on employers and employees. The supplementary medical insurance for outpatient care and physician services (referred to as Part B) is financed through a combination of general revenues and premiums paid for out of pocket by the beneficiaries of the program. The older adult is still responsible for paying premiums on the portion of insurance that covers outpatient care and physician services.

Feder (1990) pointed out that Medicare was established to ensure that the older adult had affordable health insurance protection. This objective has been successful due to improvements in access to care, support of increased technology, and longer life expectancy for the older adult. However, the beneficiaries' ability to pay premiums and to share costs for physician and hospital care has become ever more tenuous as health care costs have risen.

During the 1980s, new federal directives and rising health care costs contributed to a marked increase in cost sharing for the beneficiaries of Medicare. As a result, beneficiaries' out-of-pocket expenses almost doubled during this time (Feder, 1990).

Older adults spend as large a portion of their income on health care as they did before the passage of Medicare. More than one fifth of older adults spend more than 15% of their incomes on the out-of-pocket costs of medical care. This does not include long-term care. More than one tenth spend more than 20% of their total income on out-of-pocket expenses. About half of these expenses involved services that Medicare covers. The remainder pays for acute care services that Medicare excludes, most notably, prescription drugs. Although the older adult may have better access to care with Medicare, the out-of-pocket payments for the program remain proportional to the amount spent before Medicare was passed (Feder, 1990).

> ### ▷ *Clinical Pearl*
>
> *Assessment: One of the problems of financing care for the older adult is the out-of-pocket fees for supplemental insurance and prescription drugs. If the nurse assesses that the older patient is unable to pay for medications, then he or she must refer the patient to the appropriate social agency for assistance to pay for necessary treatment.*

Medicaid

There are several major differences between Medicare and Medicaid. Medicare is both funded and administered by the federal government to provide health care benefits to Americans 65 years of age and older; Medicaid, however, is designed to provide assistance to the medically indigent of all ages. Both laws were passed simultaneously. Unlike Medicare, Medicaid was delegated to the states for funding and administration. This resulted in considerable inconsistencies in equity and coverage among the programs of various states. Each state was thus left with the responsibility for establishing eligibility and coverage standards in order to receive federal matching funds to compensate for initial discrepancies.

Older adults become beneficiaries of Medicaid when they are unable to pay their share of supplementary insurance under Medicare. Most often, Medicaid payments cover the elderly poor receiving care in a long-term–care facility. The growth in the Medicaid expenditures has surpassed that for Medicare, resulting in considerable budget deficits at both the state and federal government levels. In 1980, there were 20 million recipients of Medicaid. This number grew to 22 million by 1988.

Medicaid frequently provides financing of long-term care of the older adult. Because of the availability of financial assistance for this care, increased Medicaid funding and nursing home use are linked. Total nursing home costs from all payers amounted to $32 billion in the 1980s, with percentage increases surpassing the Consumer Price Index. Therefore, the costs to Medicaid of providing nursing home payments have increased at a rate far greater than the rate of inflation or the price of consumer goods. Medicare's share of reimbursement for persons older than 65 demonstrates this sharp increase in payment for nursing home care. In 1990, Medicare paid almost $16 billion. Considering this decade's enrollment and demands, it has been projected that Medicare will pay $27 billion in the year 2005 and $45 billion in 2020 (Schick & Schick, 1994).

Medicaid was primarily developed to pay for acute care services, not long-term care. However, since its inception in 1965, states gradually expanded the eligibility requirements for and benefits covered by Medicaid. This increased coverage suggests one reason for the increased demand for nursing home care. Some states have decreased Medicaid expenditures as a means of controlling the overuse of long-term-care facilities. This trend was accentuated in 1981 with the passage of the Omnibus Budget Reconciliation Act, which provides more flexibility in setting Medicaid policies and decreases the federal government's Medicaid assistance to state programs. With other cost-containment pressures being instituted to decrease or shorten hospitalizations, there is even more pressure to provide long-term care at a time when the federal government is attempting to decrease its share of financing.

In addition to shifting more of nursing home costs to the states, other approaches to controlling Medicaid costs have been attempted. For example, some states have instituted stricter eligibility requirements for admission to a nursing home. Other states are attempting to regulate the number of nursing home beds by placing a limit on the expenditures for this care. The Medicaid program has been especially useful to those older adults living in the community who cannot afford out-of-pocket supplemental insurance for Medicare. Therefore, access and equity have been maintained by those older adults who are in poverty.

 Clinical Pearl

Intervention: When planning for discharge into the community of an older adult who requires nursing home care, the nurse may encounter difficulty in placement because of a shortage of beds and lack of funding. Discharge planning should be made early in the hospitalization to allow time for processing of the application for Medicaid funding and/or securing a nursing home bed.

Catastrophic Health Insurance

Catastrophic health insurance (CHI) was originally passed by the House and Senate and signed into law in 1988. The bill represents the greatest expansion of Medicare since 1965, provides new benefits for recipients, and eradicates limits on covered hospital days. In particular, the CHI program offers:

- Unrestricted number of hospital days
- Financing for hospitalization with a dual premium structure that includes a flat premium and an additional mandatory income-related premium
- Self-financing by the actual recipients of care, thereby requiring no new taxes for the program
- A state-supported Medicaid program to pay (buy-in provision) the premium, deductibles, and co-insurance payments of those Medicare beneficiaries with incomes below the poverty line
- Coverage of outpatient prescription drugs (Phillip & Biordi, 1990)

The payment mechanism for this legislation required that beneficiaries pay all program costs through an increase in Part B (physician reimbursement) and a new income-related sliding scale applied to supplemental premiums. This law initiated not only a means test for payment, but also payment by the beneficiaries themselves for expanded benefits.

Early in the development of CHI, there were indications that the bill lacked popular support. One controversial item was the conspicuous omission of reimbursement of potentially expensive high-cost and out-of-pocket payment items. These included long-term care, prevention/wellness care, dental care, and eyeglasses (Holstein & Minkler, 1991).

Lobbying groups of older adults were very active during the debate of this law. There was a lack of unanimous support from all political groups representing Medicare recipients. The bill was originally supported by AARP. However, the Gray Panthers, traditionally concerned about the health needs of low-income older adults, actively opposed the bill. Two organizations, the National Council of Senior Citizens and the National Association of Retired Federal Employees, originally supported the bill and then switched their positions. The most organized and public opposition came from the National Committee to Preserve Social Security and Medicare, often referred to as the "Roosevelt Group." Members of Congress were overwhelmed by the protests of Medicare recipients who regarded the CHI as poorly conceived and grossly unfair to seniors. Much of their outrage centered on the cost, which although more expensive than before the bill was passed, provided fewer benefits. The groundswell of opposition was overwhelming (Holstein & Minkler, 1991).

During efforts to repeal this legislation, the beneficiaries and constituents of members of Congress were persistent in their communication. Rice, Desmond, and Gabel (1990) used a telephone survey to ask recipients of Medicare their feelings about CHI. These findings revealed that older adults 1) lacked knowledge of the legislation, 2) did not support the legislation, and 3) greatly feared a program riddled with deductibles, co-insurance, and self-pay policies.

With the groundswell and lack of support, the legislation was finally repealed in November 1989. The repeal may have been costly to the older adult in several ways. In CHI, provisions for co-payment of prescriptive medications were repealed. Holstein and Minkler (1991) believe the repeal will bring about a renewed financial burden to elderly women, who tend to use several prescriptive medications and have less money to pay for them. Repeal has led to a significant increase in the cost of Medigap policies designed to cover supplemental insurance. In 1990, older adults paid more than $10 billion per year in premiums. If this amount continues to escalate, it is likely to be an economic burden.

Medigap Policies

Policies purchased by the older adult to cover those medical interventions not covered by Medicare are becoming increasingly expensive. As a result, many poor older adults have their supplemental insurance paid for by Medicaid. Individual states vary in their willingness to provide financial assistance to the poor under these circumstances. The Congressional Budget Office found that 12% of those older than age 65 have incomes below the federally established poverty line and that 20% have incomes below 125% of the poverty level. Only about 9% of all Medicare enrollees are eligible for state-administered Medicaid coverage to pay the deductibles and cost-sharing provisions of Medicare. Unfortunately, depending on the state provisions, only one third of enrollees below the poverty line are eligible for Medicaid (Phillip & Biordi, 1990).

Approximately 72% of Medicare enrollees supplement their policy with Medigap insurance. In public hearings, these policies have been criticized by members of Congress as being expensive with limited benefits and high administration costs. Additionally, several television news programs have featured Medigap insurance salesmen who have preyed on older adults, selling them multiple, expensive, and unnecessary policies. Unfortunately, the purchase of these policies often results in duplication of coverage for some services and lack of coverage for others (Phillip & Biordi, 1990).

In addition, the Committee on Finance in the U.S. Senate also found that older adults with low incomes were more likely than those with high incomes to be without Medigap insurance. For example, nearly 30% of older adults with incomes below $9000 lacked either supplemental or Medicaid coverage as compared with the elderly whose incomes were above $25,000. The likelihood of being without Medigap insurance increases with age, along with higher morbidity rates, use of pharmaceuticals, and the need for medical care. In summary, of all Medicare enrollees, 80% are dually eligible for Medicaid coverage, and the remaining 20% have no other coverage other than Medicare (Phillip & Biordi, 1990).

The older adult in the community acute care setting and long-term care has a variety of health care financing problems. The financing alternatives for the four possible categories of community placement are listed in Table 30-1. As

---

Table 30-1

FINANCING HEALTH CARE FOR THE OLDER ADULT BASED ON FOUR CATEGORIES OF CARE IN THE COMMUNITY

Category 1	Category 2	Category 3	Category 4
Status			
Independent living with periodic hospitalizations during acute episodes of illness	Independent living with home health assistance and hospitalizations for acute care episodes	Dependent living with relatives or in a residence with 24-hour surveillance and assessment, but not skilled care	Depdendent living in a long-term-care center offering skilled nursing care
Financing			
Inpatient: Out-of-pocket deductible for each hospital stay, may be covered by Medigap insurance, Medicaid, or out of pocket. Most costs covered by Medicare for predetermined length of stay.	*Inpatient:* Hospitalization similar to first category. *Home health care:* Medicaid recipient fully covered depending on individual state's policy of reimbursement; Medigap insurance may cover, depending on individual policy. Medicare reimburses home helath care visits.	*Inpatient:* As in Category 1. *Home health Assistance of Relative:* No compensation for relative caring for older adult; if home health visits are made, financing done according to Category 2. *Residential Setting:* Medicaid or out of pocket.	*Inpatient:* As in Category 1. *Long-term Care:* Medicare covers a certain number of days of skilled nursing care. Medicaid covers costs at a predetermined rate dependent on individual state's policies. *Out of pocket:* For those not qualifying for Medicaid, costs are financed out of assets and home equity.
Outpatient: Co-payment, Medicaid, or Medigap insurance.			

noted in this table, acute care in a hospital has better coverage than long-term care, unless the recipient is covered by Medicaid. Use of out-of-pocket financing continues to be an important consideration for the older adult, as demonstrated by the negative response to CHI when payment for the program by the beneficiaries was soundly and quickly defeated. Out-of-pocket expenditures rose from $996 per year per older adult (average) in 1980 to $2,322 in 1991 (Schick & Schick, 1994). That average is expected to reach $2,583 by early in the next century (Thomas & Kelman, 1990). Even though the general economic status of the older adult has improved due to increased Social Security benefits and Medicare and Medicaid, the percentage of those older than age 65 living in poverty has not changed. Those older adults living alone are five times more likely to live in poverty than are couples. Those living alone tend to be women and minorities. The U.S. government continues to finance persons older than age 65 at a rate higher than that for any other age group. Public spending for persons older than age 65 is 3.5 times greater than for those younger than age 65. It is estimated that 40% of the costs of Medicare/Medicaid are incurred during the last 3 months of life because of the health care costs associated with dying and terminal illness (American Medical Association Council on Scientific Affairs, 1990).

ALTERNATIVE METHODS OF DELIVERING HEALTH CARE TO THE OLDER ADULT

Newly developed health care delivery systems are available to the older adult. These systems use different financing mechanisms and offer a variety of services not offered by the more traditional fee-for-service institutions and practitioners.

HEALTH MAINTENANCE ORGANIZATIONS

Congress passed a law in 1973 that laid the foundation for instituting health maintenance organizations (HMOs). This law was instrumental in developing an alternative form of health care delivery that differed from the traditional fee-for-service arrangements. The fee-for-service providers are those practitioners in the community and health care institutions who charge for every service of care delivered. For example, if an older adult visits a physician for care and monitoring of diabetes, the fee for the outpatient visit would be charged to either the patient or the insurance company. If the same patient visited an ophthalmologist, the fee would be separately billed to the patient or insurance carrier (Medigap or Medicaid). With the passage of the Health Maintenance Act of 1973, financial assistance was given to develop HMOs or to provide services on a capitation basis rather than for an individual fee. Capitation reimbursement means that the enrollee pays a monthly fee for a previously established service. The recipient is not charged extra for frequency of services used, as long as the service is provided by the HMO. This legislation grew out of the federal government's desire to decrease the cost of health care while encouraging competition between health insurance plans and providers.

Originally, the HMO legislation supported the development of these plans and required that certain services such as those listed below be provided:

- Physician services
- Inpatient and outpatient services
- Medically necessary emergency health services
- Short-term outpatient evaluative and crisis intervention mental health services
- Medical treatment and referral services for alcohol and drug abuse
- Laboratory and x-ray services
- Home health services
- Preventive services

Between 1976 and 1985, the Medicare program was expanded to permit beneficiaries a choice of health care services through an HMO or a fee-for-service plan. In addition, legislation supported supplemental health services, including intermediate and long-term care, vision and dental care, mental health services not included under basic services, and provision of prescriptive drugs. To encourage more enrollees older than 65 years to use the HMO as Medigap, an amendment to the Health Maintenance Act of 1973 was passed in 1976. This amendment added a provision requiring that those HMOs receiving reimbursement from Medicare and Medicaid be federally qualified.

The phenomenal growth of HMOs since 1973 has mirrored the concern for increased health care costs. By 1984, more than 15 million persons of all ages had enrolled in HMOs. By 1990, that number had grown to 40 million enrollees. This growth is attributed to the substantial increase in charges by fee-for-service insurance carriers. HMO fees have not been as inflationary. HMOs have maintained lower costs primarily by decreasing hospital days and using salaried physicians who link cost-saving methods of health care delivery. Physician fees are further decreased by HMOs by using physician specialists only by referral (Stein, Linn, Edelstein, & Stein, 1989).

Clinical Pearl

Assessment: When making referrals and planning for discharge from an acute care setting, nurses working with older adults must know the patient's economic status. Patients at poverty level or those unable to pay out-of-pocket expenses will need a referral to an appropriate social agency to begin the process of application for available Medicaid and other social benefits.

PREFERRED PROVIDER ORGANIZATIONS

An alternative kind of health care system that delivers care to the older adult is the preferred provider organization (PPO). The PPO is a corporation somewhat similar to the individual practice associations contracted to an HMO. The PPO receives health insurance premiums from enrolled members and has individual contracts with physicians and hospitals to provide care. The PPO functions as a gatekeeper to health care delivery. Most importantly, the PPO contracts with hospitals for care at an agreed-on price that tends to be lower than prevailing charges for the traditional fee-for-service insurance. Physicians are paid a fee for service generally at a discounted rate but are not paid by capitation, as frequently occurs in an HMO. Capitation payment to physicians is a monthly salary earned for their provision of service. If the patient uses a non-PPO physician or enters a hospital without a suitable referral, there is a substantial penalty to be paid by the subscriber, usually in the form of a high deductible. In contrast to the HMO, there is no payment of care outside of the PPO, and the entire cost is paid out of pocket if care is selected from a non-PPO source. The PPO is an example of a plan that provides cost savings to the health care system while delivering care at a discounted rate.

SOCIAL/HMOS

Since 1985, Medicare has been experimenting with a new alternative health plan referred to as a social/HMO (S/HMO). The plan covers the usual hospital and physician services covered by Medicare, with chronic benefits including nursing home, personal care, homemaker services, prescription drugs, eyeglasses, and dental care. Several of these services are not mandated to be offered in a basic HMO plan; their provision under S/HMOs signifies a major expansion of benefits to the older adult. These services are financed by Medicare through a single monthly capitation payment and premiums from subscribers to the plan. The plan has been discussed and debated for years as health care planners have considered the most cost-effective way to deliver comprehensive care to the Medicare population. This comprehensive plan would include ways to coordinate multiservices, control utilization, and integrate financing for long-term care (Newcomer, Harrington, & Friedlob, 1990).

Marketing of the social/HMO and the HMO has been used to inform older adults of the plans, foster their desire to enroll in these plans, and terminate the fee-for-service insurance plans. Several studies have examined the effectiveness of marketing and have measured consumer satisfaction with alternate forms of health care reimbursement systems. Newcomer et al. (1990) polled enrollees of four social/HMOs to find out their reasons for enrolling and their degree of awareness of the choices they had for selecting an alternative plan. They found that enrollees who felt vulnerable to anticipated health care problems tended to join the social/HMO. Those perceived vulnerabilities could either be fear of not being able to afford the costs of comprehensive health care or an actual health problem. Enrollees in the social/HMO were found to be very knowledgeable of competing plans. In addition, they found if the enrollee did not pay out of pocket for any health plan such as Medicaid, they lacked the incentive to join the social/HMO. They also found that advertising was the most effective way to tell Medicare recipients about the plan; it was more useful than family and friends as a source of information. Finally, those selecting social/HMOs did so because of the extensive benefits provided for fewer out-of-pocket payments (Newcomer et al., 1990).

Researchers will continue to monitor and measure the popularity and effectiveness of alternative plans as long as they are available for consumers. As an example, Stein et al. (1989) found that the only difference in levels of satisfaction in the recipients of Medicare between fee-for-service and HMO plans was in the physician–patient relationship. For those who paid a private fee for service, the physician–patient relationship was more positively rated. At the same time, the recipients of fee for service realized this type of care was more costly.

Similarly, studies have examined the use of health care services by the older adult as a function of the type of health care plan. In comparing PPO, HMO, and fee for service for Medicare patients, Thomas and Kelman (1990) found that the PPO enrollees had a shorter mean length of stay in acute care facilities than did HMO and fee-for-service patients. Specifically, they found that patients subscribing to fee-for-service plans had similar lengths of stay to the HMO enrollees. This finding is contrary to previous findings.

Due to the pressure of cost constraint and the ever-spiraling health care expenditures in the United States, it appears that offering alternative health care insurance plans will be a continual factor facing the recipients of Medicare as well as health care providers. A nurse is often asked about the choices that an older patient may have to make regarding these plans of care. It is imperative that the professional nurse be knowledgeable about the plans and be prepared to assist the patient in making informed choices from among them. The Patient Teaching Box presents a plan that should assist the nurse with this intervention.

CASE MANAGEMENT

Although case management is considered an alternative form of health care delivery, the recipients of this type of health care may be covered by any of the previously identified alternative health care plans. Most frequently, case management is linked to a managed care concept, which is an inherent part of the HMO concept. Case management had been defined in many ways. Case managers may function in:

- Assisting with patient intakes
- Service planning
- Referral and system linkage
- Monitoring of services and noting changes in patient status
- Advocacy on behalf of patients (Fleishman, Mor, & Piette, 1991)

Patient Teaching Box
CHOICES OF MEDIGAP HEALTH INSURANCE

The following information should be given to an older adult who is in the process of selecting health insurance to supplement Medicare:

1. All recipients of Medicare will need supplemental insurance if they do not qualify for Medicaid.
2. Supplemental insurance must be purchased to cover the costs of traditional care, such as reimbursement, community physician, and hospital fees. This plan is commonly referred to as a Medigap plan to cover fee-for-service health care.
3. Supplemental insurance plans referred to as preferred provider organizations (PPOs) can also be purchased. These plans require that the subscriber pay premiums and patronize physicians and hospitals that are part of the plan. Depending on the plan, referrals to specialists may be closely monitored.
4. Health maintenance organizations (HMOs) are additional supplemental plans that may also be purchased. Each HMO offers a variety of services and provides certain benefits. It is critical that the older adult examine what is being purchased, because no two plans are alike. The new social/HMOs, which offer long-term–care coverage, usually charge higher premiums.

These caregivers provide assistance to persons in the community who may need a variety of health care services; however, the major focus is on need assessment and access to certain types of health care. Case management is defined as a professional service, the central function of which is the arrangement and coordination of health or social services (Eggert, 1991). A case manager does not necessarily have to deliver care, but he or she is responsible for recommending, arranging, and planning the financing of the care in the community. The case management approach is an ideal one because it is designed to assist the older adult in the community who may need help in providing self-care. The intended purpose of case management is to provide services that allow the patient to be cared for at home as opposed to in a long-term-care facility. The outcome is a decrease in cost to the older adult.

COST-CONTAINMENT MEASURES

Cost of health care for the older adult residing in the community continues to be a primary problem due to limited or controlled health care resources. Recent changes in the provision of care to the older adult that involve using nurses to interface with the health care system are designed to decrease the cost of care and/or limit its use.

CASE MIX REIMBURSEMENT

Case mix is a recent cost-containment approach some states use to manage the health care expenses of older adult Medicaid recipients entering nursing homes. The purpose of this system is to adjust payments to the nursing home depending on the level of care required. This approach allows the patient to pay the facility rates that are commensurate with the actual services rendered rather than a uniform flat fee for semiskilled of skilled nursing home care. The particular level of case mix determination for individual patients is made after basic assessments. Patient assessments are established related to patient needs or functional disabilities and/or services that are necessary to deliver required care. In several states, the case mix determination is made by public health nurses and social welfare agencies.

A clear advantage to the reimbursement agency is that payment is based on actual care delivered and focuses on patient needs. High-needs patients generally gain better access to nursing home care. Institutions can more effectively plan for the delivery of appropriate care. One disadvantage of case mix is the complexity of assessment. Community groups interested in the welfare of the older adult complain that the classifications of case mix frequently do not account for the psychosocial needs of the patient and only weigh biologic factors of care. Use of standard forms may inflate the level of disability in order to increase the level of reimbursement to the institution (Schlenkler, 1991).

Two other methods are used by states to monitor the reimbursement to nursing homes for recipients of Medicaid. The first is called facility-specific ratings, defined as rates based on the facility's past average cost per day. These rates are subject to ceilings. Generally, the rates for average cost per day are the lowest, rather than the highest, rates. The second method is class rate, which assesses level of patient care needs but does not consider facility costs.

DIAGNOSIS-RELATED GROUPS

Diagnosis-related groups (DRGs) were initiated to control Medicare costs incurred by older adults during acute care hospital stays. Before the institution of DRGs, few limitations were placed on the length of a Medicare patient's hospital stay. As a result, hospital stays were extended, sometimes unnecessarily, and Medicare was billed for the care that was delivered. Using this model of reimbursement, Medicare billing was similar to other traditional forms of health insurance. In 1982, Congress enacted a prospective payment system as part of the Tax Equity and Fiscal Responsibility Act. This legislation set limits on Medicare reimbursements for hospital costs at a per-case level and placed a limit on the annual rate of increase for Medicare's reasonable costs per charge. In 1983, Congress enacted the prospective payment system for most hospital services covered by Medicare, and in 1994 Medicaid began paying on a DRG system. This change in policy has essentially transformed Medicare and Medicaid from disinterested financiers of health care into wise purchasers of efficient quality health care.

The DRG payments are made based on the type of illness treated during the hospital stay. Originally, 467 DRGs were identified based on retrospective studies of discharge diagnoses and hospital charges. Each DRG is given a relative cost weight by which the dollar amount to be paid is based on national cost averages. Payment for these groupings is fixed before admission to a hospital and does not take into account actual costs of care. If a patient's length of stay exceeds an upper limit, referred to as an outlier threshold, the hospital receives an additional amount that may fall below actual costs. If the patient is discharged before the allotted number of days, the hospital receives full funding for the DRG. This encourages health care institutions to be more efficient in the delivery of their care.

Since the beginning of the implementation of DRGs, the results have been dramatic. During the first year, the average length of stay was greatly decreased and admission rates fell. The introduction of DRGs created concern in the professional nursing groups that the increase in acuity of patients' conditions would result in greater stress for nurses. Several years of implementation have demonstrated the nurses' ability to give care within the limits of DRGs. Many traditional third-party payers have also adopted a prospective method of reimbursement. This indicates that this approach to cost containment will be a vital part of health care policy.

Several methods of payment for delivery of health care have been described. It is anticipated that professional nurses will continue to play a critical role in informing the older adult of the possible choices in selecting health care plans to supplement their Medicare coverage. The nurse will be a key referral agent in helping the older adult gain access to assistance from social agencies in the community where the older adult resides. The nurse must be aware of these resources and the ever-increasing types and varieties of health insurance plans that are constantly developed to cover services and reimbursement not allowed in Medicare.

As nurses deliver care in the last part of the 1990s and into the next century, containment of health care costs will be even more important. Innovations in cost-effective health care will continue to be devised, thus creating new opportunities for all nurses to practice in different settings. As cost containment becomes increasingly central to the nation's stance on health policy, renewed debate will erupt over how the policy of cost containment affects and will continue to affect the older adult's access to quality care.

REFERENCES

Advisory Council on Social Security. (1991). *Report on Medicare Projections by the Health Technical Fund to the 1991 Advisory Council on Social Security*. Washington, DC: U.S. Government Printing Office.

American Medical Association Council on Scientific Affairs. (1990). Societal effects and other factors affecting health care for the elderly. *Archives of Internal Medicine, 150*, 1184–1189.

Eggert, G. M. (1991). Case management: A randomized controlled study comparing a neighborhood team and a centralized individual model. *Health Services Research, 26*, 471–501.

Feder, J. (1990). Health care of the disadvantaged: The elderly. *Journal of Health, Politics, Policy and Law, 15*, 259–269.

Fleishman, J. A., Mor V., & Piette, J. (1991). AIDS case management: The client's perspective. *Health Services Research, 26*, 447–470.

Holstein, M., & Minkler, M. (1991). The short life and painful death of the Medicare Catastrophic Coverage Act. *Journal of Health Science, 221*, 1–6.

Mechanic, D. (1987). Challenges in long term care policy. *Health Affairs, 6*, 22–34.

Newcomer, R., Harrington, C., & Friedlob, A. (1990). Awareness and enrollment in the social/HMO. *Gerontologist, 30*, 86–93.

Phillip, T. A., & Biordi, D. L. (1990). Financial ruin or financing catastrophic health coverage: Who pays? *Journal of Professional Nursing, 6*, 94–102.

Rice, T., Desmond, K., & Gabel, J. (1990, Fall). The Medicare Coverage Catastrophic Act: A post mortem. *Health Affairs*, 75–78.

Schick, F. L., & Schick, R. (1994). *Statistical handbook on aging Americans, 1994 edition*. Phoenix: Oryx Press.

Schlenkler, R. E. (1991). Nursing home costs, Medicaid rates, and profits under alternative Medicaid payment systems. *Health Services Research, 26*, 623–649.

Statistical Abstract of the United States 1994. (1994). Washington, DC: The National Data Bank. U.S. Department of Commerce, U.S. Government Printing Office.

Stein, S. R., Linn, M. W., Edelstein, J., & Stein, E. M. (1989). Elderly patients' satisfaction with care under HMO versus private systems. *Southern Medical Journal, 82*, 3–8.

Thomas, C., & Kelman, H. R. (1990). Health services use among the elderly under alternative health services delivery systems. *Journal of Community Health, 15*, 77–92.

Winograd, C. H., Gerety, M. B., Chung, M., Goldstein, M. K., Dominquez, F., & Vallone, R. (1991). Screening for frailty: Criteria and predictors of outcome. *Journal of American Geriatric Society, 39*, 778–784.

BIBLIOGRAPHY

Cherner, S. L. (1991). *The universal health care almanac*. Phoenix: Silver & Cherner, Ltd., R. C. Publications.

Harrington, C., & Swan, J. C. (1987). The impact of state Medicaid nursing home policies on utilization and expenditures. *Inquiry, 24*, 157–172.

Kahn, K. L., Keller, E. B., Sherwood, M. J., Rogers, W. H., Draper, D., Bentow, S. S., Reinish, E. J., Rubenstein, L. V., Kosecoff, J., & Brook, R. H. (1990). Comparing outcomes of care before and after implementation on DRG-based prospective payment system. *Journal of the American Medical Association, 264*, 1984–1988.

Source Book of Health Insurance Data. (1992). Health Insurance Association of America.

Future Trends in the Care of the Older Adult

Objectives

1. Describe six factors that will directly influence the health care delivery system for older Americans in the future.
2. Discuss the importance of measuring patient health outcomes as they relate to the development of nursing interventions for the older patient.
3. Outline the national health policies that directly influence the health care of older Americans.
4. Contrast and compare the following components of a community-based long-term–care system: case management, in-home services, continuous-care centers, and adult day-care centers.
5. Discuss the importance of nurses being advocates for older Americans in the political process.

INTRODUCTION

THE FUTURE OF HEALTH CARE DELIVERY for the aging American population lies in the continued development of both hospital-based and community-based health and human service resources. The primary purpose of this health care delivery must be to provide support systems that facilitate and prolong independent living for older Americans, who may have multiple and increasingly complex health and human service needs.

FACTORS INFLUENCING HEALTH CARE FOR THE OLDER ADULT

In looking to the future, we must be aware of the current status of the health care system serving older adults and the various factors that will directly influence the development of new and more comprehensive services. Professional nurses will be expected to address the following six factors in the future:

- Meeting the increasing demand for health care
- Providing access to needed services
- Ensuring the quality of care
- Measuring health outcomes
- Preserving the quality of life
- Containing the costs associated with providing comprehensive care

MEETING THE INCREASING DEMAND FOR CARE

The number of persons 65 or older in the United States has grown steadily since the early 1900s and will grow at an accelerated rate in the future. As the population ages, the demand for health care and social services will continue to escalate. With the predicted substantial increase in the number of these citizens, access to needed services will become a major issue. A continued emphasis will be placed on the development of comprehensive community-based services for the older American population.

PROVIDING ACCESS TO NEEDED CARE

Older people are more likely to develop chronic health problems, necessitating frequent use of health care and social services. For many older adults, gaining access to these services presents a complex problem and often plays a key role in determining whether they can remain in the community or require institutionalization (Kemper, Applebaum, & Harrigan, 1987). Historically, older adults have had difficulty obtaining access to needed care for a variety of reasons, including living on a fixed income or other financial restraints, the lack of needed services, and the lack of adequate transportation (Kane & Kane, 1987).

As the cost of providing health care escalates, many elderly find that Medicare entitlements are helpful but fall short of meeting the expense of carefully following a prescribed medical regimen. The problems surrounding access to care are further exacerbated when the senior citizen has no knowledge of existing resources. These resources, if they exist at all, may be maldistributed by geography or specialty.

ENSURING QUALITY OF CARE

Because enhancing the quality of care for patients and their caregivers is the ultimate goal of professional nursing, the nurse must constantly monitor the quality of services delivered and the resulting health outcomes. Of particular importance is the question of whether nurses can consistently render quality service according to professional standards of practice.

MEASURING HEALTH OUTCOMES

The trend in measuring the effectiveness of nursing interventions for the older adult is directly influenced by the systematic measurement of health outcomes. The art of determining the quality of nursing care by measuring health outcomes is highly valued by consumers and health professionals alike. Several critical elements must be considered when examining the quality of care being provided, including record-keeping methods and research studies designed to test interventions. It is important for professional nurses to collect and analyze information related to the effectiveness of all nursing interventions. This information can then be used to improve nursing care.

In addition to being the direct care providers of the future, nurses will take on a leadership role in health care by comprehensively assessing their older adult patients to design an individualized care system. The nurse of the future will practice in and often manage the multidisciplinary care system needed for older adults. This system will address the patient's needs from sociologic, biologic, and psychological perspectives.

PRESERVING THE QUALITY OF LIFE

An aging population brings with it major concerns about the prevalence of chronic conditions that may diminish the quality of life of the older adult. Quality of life is based on an individual's values, beliefs, expectations, and personal assessment of the situation (Zawadski, 1984). Older adults who are able to care for themselves and remain in their own home environments view the quality of their lives positively, even though they may experience chronic problems, such as debilitating arthritis (Kane & Kane, 1987).

Providing the resources to sustain older adults in their quest for independent living arrangements can challenge not only the individuals themselves but also their families and communities. The trend seems to indicate that as individuals age, some choose to move from their private homes to congregate living or senior citizens' residential communities. They do this for at least two reasons: first, to maintain their independence and individual identities, and second, to have easy access to varying degrees of supportive care within these residential communities. However, few of these settings offer the comprehensive health care and social services needed to maximize independence at truly affordable rates. For many senior citizens, congregate living arrangements eventually dissolve, primarily because personal financial resources for health care, if available, are insufficient to cover increasing costs. This frequently results in the more cost-effective alternative of placing the older adult in a nursing home.

In the future, nurses will be required to use innovative strategies to maintain the patient in a community-based setting. They will use the resources of support services, home health care, and adult day-care services to create a network of support necessary for community and home-based maintenance.

CONTAINING THE COSTS OF HEALTH CARE

Health care costs for all Americans continue to escalate. The trend toward higher health care costs is particularly burdensome for the elderly, who often endure multiple health problems and live on fixed or limited incomes. Most of the money spent by the federal government on health care pays for services provided to those with known medical problems or to the institutionalized older adult. Health care costs frequently go essentially unconstrained. For example, medications are frequently ordered without regard to the effect that paying for them will have on the elderly patient's budget. Patients who are unable to meet the expenses incurred may discontinue needed prescriptions, to the detriment of their long-term health. The result is that their conditions worsen, which ultimately leads to greater expenditures of precious health care resources by the older adult as their health status worsens.

 Clinical Pearl

Cost Containment: Nurses need to carefully assess the medications of their patients to ensure that their prescribed medical regiment is being carefully followed and that medications are obtained as cheaply as possible.

Previous attempts to control the costs associated with long-term care have focused on identifying core services to satisfy needs and on developing providers for these services (Kemper, 1988; Weissert, 1988). Most of these services, such as home health, resource identification, and referral, and nutrition services are intended to lower the costs associated with premature institutionalization by helping the frail individual to remain at home. Unfortunately, the costs associated with many community-based long-term–care service projects are frequently no lower than nursing home costs (Kemper, 1988).

NATIONAL HEALTH POLICIES THAT DIRECTLY INFLUENCE CARE

Throughout the late 1950s and early 1960s, legislators struggled to develop comprehensive entitlement programs to alleviate the health problems that were faced by many of their older constituents. However, the true extent of the problems confronting the older adult was not clearly understood. The Older Americans Act, adopted by the federal government in 1965, established a network of local, state, and federal agencies whose primary responsibilities are to 1) identify the needs of the older population and 2) develop community resources to meet those needs.

A 1973 amendment to the Older Americans Act provides for the establishment of Area Agencies on Aging at state and regional levels. The Area Agencies on Aging conduct assessments of the needs of their older citizens and develop services to meet their needs. Advisory committees on aging at the local level cooperate with the appropriate Area Agency on Aging in planning and implementing programs. The work of the local advisory groups and their Area Agencies on Aging is coordinated by state human service departments. Ultimately, these organizations are responsible to the federal Department of Health and Human Services for the development of comprehensive services.

Funds are allocated to each state under the Older Americans Act for the planning, implementation, and evaluation of services. Each state is then free to allocate the funds it receives through the regional Area Agencies on Aging. The Area Agency on Aging is then responsible for either providing needed services or for arranging contracts with local providers for the needed services. Examples of services commonly offered at the state and local levels are home-delivered meals, congregate nutrition services, case management, chore services, home health care, homemaker services, senior centers, transportation, friendly visiting services, and telephone assurance. Telephone assurance programs stay in contact with the frail elderly through daily friendly telephone calls. Many telephone assurance programs use specially trained volunteers to elicit information about the older citizen's well-being and to initiate referrals when unmet needs are identified. There is no charge for the services offered through the Area Agency on Aging for those who cannot afford to pay, although contributions are accepted from willing participants. The network established through the Older Americans Act has proved to be an effective system for the identification of the needs of the older adult. It has also provided a framework for the continued development of resources at the local level to meet those needs.

A growing awareness that financial barriers often block older Americans' access to health care expressed itself in many health policy proposals in the early 1960s. After several years of debate at the local, state, and national levels, the Social Security Act was amended by Congress in 1965 to create Medicare and Medicaid. These two programs have profoundly affected the health care of the older adult in several ways.

Medicare, commonly referred to as amendment Title XVIII, was designed as a federal health insurance program. It is available to those citizens age 65 and older and to those who are eligible to receive Social Security benefits. This federally subsidized insurance program was originally designed primarily to provide hospital and physician services. There are two major components to Medicare, with complementary packages of services to be found in both Medicare Part A and Medicare Part B (see Chapter 30).

Medicare Part A provides basic hospital insurance coverage and is available to eligible citizens age 65 and older. Basic services covered by Part A include hospital care, posthospital extended care, and home health benefits. Medicare Part B requires the participant to pay a modest monthly premium and covers physician services, hospital outpatient services, physical therapy, diagnostic tests, and ambulance services.

Even with Medicare, older citizens may still find themselves encumbered by health care costs for preventive care, deductibles, and copayments on hospital expenses, fees that are in excess of the Medicare payments, and premiums and other co-insurance fees. For many seniors, the fear of spending their life savings and resources during an extended illness often becomes a harsh reality.

Medicaid offers a blend of federal and state resources to help the financially indigent of all ages meet the costs of health care. Each state defines its own criteria for eligibility and benefits within limits set by the federal government. Eligibility for Medicaid is generally tied to having expended all other insurance benefits and the vast majority of one's personal financial resources. Once eligibility has been established, Medicaid benefits can include:

• Skilled nursing home care
• Home health care
• Physician care

- Inpatient and outpatient hospital services
- Laboratory services
- Radiologic services
- Limited coverage for the cost of physician-prescribed medications (this Medicaid benefit is unavailable in some states)

EVOLVING HEALTH CARE DELIVERY SYSTEMS

COMMUNITY-BASED LONG-TERM CARE

Community-based long-term care programs have developed over the past 30 years to: 1) address the preference that older citizens have for receiving care in their own homes and communities rather than in more restrictive institutional settings and 2) decrease public expenditures on long-term care. As inpatient costs continue to escalate, new models for managing older adults' health care problems in the community are being developed. These will continue to evolve as third-party payers, policymakers, and health care agencies struggle to find cost-effective alternatives to institutional care. Community-based long-term care projects attempt to coordinate primary, secondary, and tertiary health care services with additional human services. These services are designed to meet the unique needs of seniors living in their own homes.

Many models for community-based service-delivery systems for older adults have been developed since 1960 (Weissert, Cready, & Pawelak, 1988). The designers of these models have attempted to address the traditional barriers to care faced by senior citizens, such as lack of access to care, insufficiency of affordable and high quality services, and the cost of providing the care each senior citizen needs to maintain a quality life. These systems were developed in concert with the Older Americans Act to improve access to community-based health care and social services. The services they provide consist of information regarding community services, referral for needed care, and limited direct care.

This traditionally problem-oriented focus has resulted in a lack of attention to the value of health promotion and preventive care models. These models usually target service delivery to the frail elderly, who are at risk for nursing home placement. They also aim to improve the quality of life of older adults by helping them remain in their own homes, thus obviating the need for nursing home care (Brown, Blackman, Learner, Witherspoon, & Saber, 1985; Kemper, 1988; Weissert, Cready, & Pawelak, 1988).

The cost of these community-based models was expected to produce savings that would ultimately offset the high cost of nursing home care; however, studies have not conclusively revealed short- or long-term significant cost savings. What has been shown is that the quality of life for the senior citizen can be significantly enhanced by promoting independence and avoiding premature institutionalization.

CASE MANAGEMENT

Nursing case management is a process by which resources and services are organized and coordinated to respond to individual health care needs (Flynn-Hollander, Zimmerman, & Valentine, 1990). There is a developing body of research demonstrating that effective nursing case management can enhance the

> ### Clinical Pearl
>
> *Nursing Case Managers: Preliminary studies examining the efficacy of nursing case managers reveal that they are highly successful at assessing older patients' needs and attaining both successful patient-oriented clinical outcomes and fiscal efficiency (Flynn-Hollander, Zimmerman, & Valentine, 1990).*

achievement of expected health outcomes, which translates into earlier discharge dates of older patients from hospital settings. Whether the care to be coordinated is in an institutional setting or a community-based setting, the nurse case manager is a proven asset to the health care team.

IN-HOME HEALTH SERVICES

Services provided in the older adult's home by a skilled nurse can range from conducting a physical assessment to administering chemotherapy. In-house health agencies provide services for four general groups of individuals: 1) recovering older patients who need help returning to optimal functioning; 2) chronically ill older patients who need assistance in adapting to changes in status and preventing deterioration; 3) the frail elderly; and 4) the terminally ill. Often a nurse provides direct care and coordinates the services of a wide array of additional providers. Some home health agencies are designed to be run as for-profit organizations, and others are operated as public services on a not-for-profit basis. Many hospitals have developed home health agencies to serve their communities. In the future, most nurses will find their employment in home health care or community-based programs rather than in acute care. A large majority of their services will be directed toward home- and community-based older adults and their caretakers.

CONTINUOUS-CARE CENTERS

An innovation in the concept of extended care facilities is the development of retirement communities, which can meet a wide variety of needs for their residents. These communities provide three basic levels of services, each of which

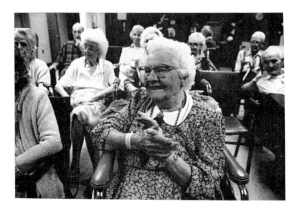

corresponds to circumstances of each resident. The strength of these communities lies in their ability to integrate a variety of resources and personnel to meet the needs of older adults. Senior citizens taking advantage of these types of facilities are those who range from completely independent persons to those requiring intensive custodial care.

Older adults who choose these types of communities as a means of transition from their traditional living arrangements may initially purchase, rent, or lease their basic living unit at the appropriate care level for their needs. For example, a senior citizen might move into a furnished apartment and function independently for a number of years. Eventually, the individual will utilize intermediate levels of care, which might include moving to a smaller living unit and taking advantage of the services of an increasing number of health and human service providers. The final step may entail gaining access to an infirmary/hospital-like setting, where more institutional inpatient services can be arranged. These residential facilities provide a framework for thoughtful, economical, and rational utilization of health care resources in the context of everyday living arrangements. In the future, the nurse will play a key role in assessing and making arrangements for older adults as they make the transition from one setting to another.

ADULT DAY-CARE CENTERS

Another service available in a number of communities is adult day care. These facilities are designed to provide a therapeutic environment for the elderly during the routine working day. They enable caregivers to be employed and achieve some respite from the daily demands of giving care; additionally, they often provide caregiver support and counseling.

Some adult day-care facilities serve the basically well and ambulatory older adult. These provide structured crafts programs and other social activities. Other adult day-care facilities are designed for the medically and/or mentally impaired older adult. These therapeutic adult day care facilities may specialize in caring for victims of stroke and Alzheimer's disease. Unlike the facilities that provide for the basically well older adult, therapeutic day care facilities are usually staffed with persons experienced in caring for senior citizens and nurses who have extensive training in providing gerontological nursing. Individualized plans of care, which foster independence and self-care, are collaboratively developed by the nurse and other service providers. In the future, nurses will be the designers and directors of adult day-care centers.

A MULTIDISCIPLINARY MODEL FOR COMMUNITY-BASED LONG-TERM CARE

A model health care system should be based on current trends in the development of community-based services for the well older adult, those requiring intermediate care, and frail senor citizens. The health care system model of the future may use a multidisciplinary team of health and human service providers. Team services will also focus on health promotion and disease prevention, monitoring chronic problems, and monitoring the need for coordinating services.

(text continues on page 531)

Table 31-1	EXAMPLES OF PRIMARY, SECONDARY, AND TERTIARY COMMUNITY-BASED SERVICES TO BE PROVIDED BY HEALTH PROFESSIONS TEAM MEMBERS	

Team Member	Primary Care Community-Based Services
Nursing	Coordinate team care planning
	Perform individual health assessments
	Conduct individual and/or group, individual, and caregiver health education
	Administer immunizations (flu, Pneumovax, and tetanus)
	Direct special services, such as group exercise programs for arthritic patients and group diabetes education classes
	Conduct individual patient health counseling
	Provide training and counseling for caregivers
	Recommend changes in care plans
Pharmacy Education	Provide individualized and group medication
	Conduct pharmacy tours
	Periodically send out a medication newsletter
	Organize and direct a community-based medication brown-bag program addressing health issues
	Assist in caregiver education and training
	Assemble and maintain a variety of patient medication information
	Recommend changes in care plans
Nutrition	Provide behavior modification education
	Provide individualized meal planning
	Give cooking demonstrations
	Teach community nutrition education
	Teach patient group education classes
	Provide home visits for in-home cooking demonstrations and food storage and safety education
	Conduct grocery store tours
	Assist in caregiver education and training
	Provide nutrition label reading education
	Individualized dietary counseling
	Recommend changes in care plans
Social Work	Provide group therapy/support group
	Provide individual assessment/counseling
	Provide family counseling

(continued)

Table 31-1	EXAMPLES OF PRIMARY, SECONDARY, AND TERTIARY COMMUNITY-BASED SERVICES TO BE PROVIDED BY HEALTH PROFESSIONS TEAM MEMBERS *(Continued)*	
Team Member	**Primary Care Community-Based Services**	
	Provide financial counseling/budget planning	
	Act as a patient advocate	
	Teach stress management	
	Recommend changes in care plans	
Team Member	**Secondary Care Community-Based Services**	
Nursing	Conduct history and physical examinations	
	Provide crisis interventions	
	Assess mental status as related to physical condition	
	Conduct health maintenance screenings	
	Initiate assessment for acute problems	
	Initiate and follow up on physician referrals	
	Recommend changes in care plans	
Pharmacy	Conduct assessment to include:	
	Medication history (prescription and nonprescription medications)	
	Compliance assessment	
	Medication cost/month	
	Medication management systems	
	Review current pharmacy services	
	Identify polypharmacy problem	
	Provide pharmacokinetic information	
	Conduct home visits	
	Assess for allergies/drug intolerance	
	Recommend changes in care plans	
Nutrition	Services to be provided will include:	
	Diet history and food frequency recalls	
	Diet history evaluation for nutrient content	
	Dietary compliance assessment	
	Assessment of current weight	
	Assessment of possible problems hindering eating	
	Recommendation of modified diets	
	Recommend actions for changes in care plans	

(continued)

Table 31-1	EXAMPLES OF PRIMARY, SECONDARY, AND TERTIARY COMMUNITY-BASED SERVICES TO BE PROVIDED BY HEALTH PROFESSIONS TEAM MEMBERS *(Continued)*

Team Member	Secondary Care Community-Based Services
Social Work	Perform a financial screening
	Do a family profile
	Do an activities of daily living screening
	Administer the mini-mental examination
	Provide a short psychiatric evaluation schedule
	Do a home environmental safety assessment
	Recommend changes in care plans

Team Member	Tertiary Care Community-Based Services
Nursing	Monitor chronic diseases (under protocol)
	Prescribe medications under protocol for commonly seen health problems (advanced nurse practitioner)
	Make minor adjustment to stabilize medications and treatments under protocols
	Draw and evaluate lab data
	Conduct home visits for follow-up purposes
	Recommend changes in care plans
Pharmacy	Monitor drug efficacy
	Recommend changes in care plans
Nutrition	Monitor weight and nutritional status
	Make nutrition referral and counsel regarding daily caloric count and food diary
	Recommend changes in care plans
Social Work	Monitor family situation/individual's psychosocial status
	Ensure that all available human service resources are utilized
	Recommend changes in care plans

(continued from page 528)

The proposed service delivery model addresses the problem of access in a number of ways:

- It uses a readily accessible team of health and social service providers. This enables each individual patient to have multiple problems evaluated and needs met during each visit.
- Team members assess each patient's knowledge/use of existing resources to determine which resources are being accessed.

• Model service is made available in areas in which the target population resides.

A major goal of the model multidisciplinary team is to promote wellness by increasing the older patient's knowledge of existing health care and human service resources and by assisting with adaptation to the aging process. The service-delivery component of the model would be designed to incorporate a nursing case management approach to care planning, implementation, and evaluation.

THE NURSE ADVOCATE'S ROLE IN FUTURE HEALTH CARE SYSTEMS

Many senior citizens are capable of productively finding their own way through the health care and human service systems. These individuals often act as their own advocates. However, for many senior citizens, the complexities of today's health care system prove to be overwhelming. Additionally, within the health care system there is a propensity toward dehumanization of older Americans, a condition that further prevents them from receiving the care they need. Nurses can serve as patient advocates in ensuring that effective communication exists between the older patient who has health care needs and the various providers who are attempting to meet those needs.

Nurses are fortunate to be educationally prepared to provide guidance and counseling to older patients and their families regarding a multitude of problems. Nurses must be sensitive to the fact that, as older Americans are forced into a state of dependency, they become more dependent, thereby creating a vicious cycle (Weiner, Brok, & Shadowsky, 1987). When planning for the future, nurses need to be advocates for senior citizens and include them when developing proposed services from the earliest stages of development through the evaluation phase. Older adults eager to participate in their own destiny will readily provide guidance for the design, implementation, and evaluation of services. If necessary, they will participate in the redesign of services rather than allow service to be thrust on them by others. As advocates for seniors, nurses need to educate the general public about the myths of aging. The fact is that, given the opportunity to make contributions to their society, older citizens will freely share their wisdom and lend their support in the development of services tailored to meet their unique needs. The nurse advocate of the future will plan and implement health care services that enhance the older adult's independence and promote the availability of accessible, affordable, and high-quality nurse-directed health services.

The concept of advocacy can be naturally extended into the realm of health policy planning and implementation. In the area of health policy development for senior citizens, nurses must represent themselves as advocates for older health care consumers.

Clinical Pearl

Political Awareness: Legislation is pending that will create many opportunities for nurses with advanced education and clinical experience to receive direct reimbursement for planning and providing care to senior citizens.

An example of legislation that directly influences nursing is the amending of Medicare and Medicaid programs to enable direct payment to nurses for the provision of care to the older adult. By remaining informed regarding complex health issues, nurses can anticipate the direction of a developing health care program. Through the process of working with their elected officials, nurses can help shape the program/policy for older Americans.

Political action by senior citizens is manifested in the Gray Panthers and the American Association for Retired Persons (AARP). The Gray Panthers are an active and politically astute group of senior citizens who have traditionally championed equal rights for the elderly. AARP is an association with millions of dues-paying members across the nation. The AARP offers many services to its members, such as group insurance, specially designed travel packages, and financial counseling. In addition to these benefits, AARP members are kept well informed regarding health policy developments that could influence the care they receive. As a political action group, AARP is a large and well-organized, well-funded, articulate advocate for older Americans.

REFERENCES

Brown, T. E. Jr., Blackman, D. K., Learner, R. M., Witherspoon, M. B., & Saber, L. (1985). *South Carolina long-term care project: Report of findings*. Spartanburg, SC: South Carolina State Health and Human Services Finance Commission.

Flynn-Hollander, S., Zimmerman, J., & Valentine, B. (1990, Summer). Health care in transition: Nursing case management. *Stanford Nurse*, 8–12.

Kane, R. A., & Kane, R. L. (1987). Long-term care: Principles, programs, and policies, New York: Springer.

Kemper, P. (1988). The evaluation of the national long term care demonstration. *Health Services Research, 23*(1), 161–174.

Kemper, P., Applebaum, R., & Harrigan, M. (1987). Community care demonstrations: What have we learned? *Health Care Financing Review, 8*(4), 87–100.

Weiner, M. B., Brok, A. J., & Shadowsky, A. M. (1987). *Working with the aged*. Norwalk, CT: Appleton-Century-Crofts.

Weissert, W. G. (1988). The national channeling demonstration: What we knew, know now, and still need to know. *Health Services Research, 23*(1), 175–198.

Weissert, W. G., Cready, C. M., & Pawelak, J. E. (1988). The past and future of home- and community-based long-term care. *Millbank Quarterly, 66*(2), 309–385.

Zawadski, R. T. (1984). Research in the demonstrations: Findings and issues. Community-Based Systems of Long Term Care, *Home Health Care Services Quarterly, 4*(3–4), Kinghampton, NY: Hayworth Press, 209–227.

BIBLIOGRAPHY

American Association of Retired Persons. (1989). *A profile of older Americans*. Prepared by the Program Resources Department, American Association of Retired Persons, and the Administration on Aging, U.S. Department of Health and Human Services. Washington, DC:

Donabedian, A. (1973). *Aspects of medical care administration*. Cambridge, MA: Harvard University Press.

Eggert, G. M, Friedman, B., & Zimmer, J. G. (1990). *Models of intensive case management*. Haworth Press.

The health care cost squeeze on older Americans. (1992). Families U.S.A., Washington, DC.

APPENDIX
Interpreting Laboratory Values for Older Adults

Interpreting laboratory results is one of the most difficult aspects of providing health care to older adults. Aging produces many changes in organ systems, even in the absence of disease. Therefore, it is reasonable to expect that at least some laboratory values for healthy older adults will be different from those of healthy young adults.

Many different mechanisms can effect the changes we see in laboratory test reference ranges in older adults. These mechanisms include the following:

1. *Limited excretory capacity* is clearly relevant. For example, the decrease in renal function that accompanies age affects the glomerular filtration rate, serum creatinine, and blood urea nitrogen. Another example is biliary excretion, which may affect bilirubin values.
2. *Hormonal effects* can affect other laboratory parameters as well as alter reference ranges for the hormones themselves. These alterations are most obvious when there is an abrupt change in reference ranges at the time of menopause. For example, serum phosphate rises sharply in women after menopause, whereas a steady age-related decline is seen in men.
3. *Serum protein changes* have many important effects. The steady decline with age of albumin alters the reference ranges of substances substantially bound to albumin. There are similar age-related changes in other carrier proteins. However, these age-related falls in carrier proteins are overshadowed by the magnitude of falls that result nonspecifically from illness. It is necessary to correct for these protein changes to accurately interpret other laboratory values in older patients (Hodkinson, 1990).
4. *Homeostasis* may deteriorate with advancing age and give rise to wider reference ranges for metabolites that are less well controlled. Although there are many reference ranges that remain constant with age and although there is no general deterioration of metabolic homeostasis with aging, the older adult does seem to be more liable to homeostatic disturbances when he or she becomes ill (Hodkinson, 1990).
5. *Selective effects of mortality* may have relevance to lipid reference ranges in old age. For example, because high cholesterol is a risk factor for coronary heart disease, it is postulated that the reference ranges for cholesterol are lower in older adults due in part to the early death of individuals with high values of cholesterol and coronary heart disease in middle age. Familial longevity may also be directly associated with lower cholesterol levels (Hodkinson, 1990).
6. *Intake of nutrients* is the main determinant of some blood constituents, vitamins, and iron in particular. Be aware that lower reference ranges due to decreased dietary intake cannot be interpreted as evidence of deficiency. Deficiency is substantiated when the lower values are shown to be associated with impaired health status, and dietary supplement results in elevated values. In the same vein, the lower ranges should not be regarded as changes of aging but simply indicators of lower dietary intake.
7. *Occult disease* may cause alterations in reference ranges rather than a true age-related change. Some of these alterations can be due to definite disease, such as Paget's disease or multiple myeloma or benign or clinically insignificant diseases.
8. The *influence of medication* on reference ranges can be significant. There are a large number of known drug effects on laboratory tests and probably many more that are undetermined. Medications may have a direct influence on laboratory analysis or cause physiologic effects that can alter the test value. Effects include underestimation of lab values due to inhibitory effects, overestimation due to cross-reactivity, competitive binding, organ toxicities leading to decreased excretion, or other alterations in production, regulation, excretion, or cellular sensitivity to the substance being tested. Medications may also interfere with the evaluation method being used. Drugs include alcohol and illegal substances.

Because interpreting laboratory values in older adults is so complex, it is now the standard in health care to refer to **reference ranges** of laboratory values instead of normal ranges. Reference range refers to 95% distribution of the test results in the reference population. The **reference population** is a population of comparable subjects who are of appropriate race, sex, and age and who have a defined health status (Duthie and Abussi, 1990).

There are several cautions to consider. It will be virtually impossible to find a reference range that mirrors a particular patient with a particular set of health conditions for comparison with every patient you will have, even though this would be an ideal situation. You will have to use established reference ranges from well populations. These reference ranges differ from those for young adults and should be recognized as indicators for potential disruptions in homeostasis that older adults encounter. These ranges for older adults may indicate that the patient is closer to a condition of risk or serious impairment. Alternatively, a range for older adults may indicate a state of increased tolerance or benign change (Jeppesen, 1986).

Your challenge will be to recognize and understand the effects of illness, other diseases, and various therapies on the laboratory values you will be interpreting. The question, "What test result is significant and raises suspicion of disease?" is part of that all-important integration and correlation of information available to the health care team for the diagnosis and treatment of the older adult (Kelso, 1990).

For this index, Henry's text, *Clinical Diagnosis and Management by Laboratory Methods*, 18th edition, was used as a source for standard values. Other standards are referenced and can be found in the bibliography that follows the Appendix.

The reference ranges for older adults are those ranges within which 95% of values for persons over age 70 fall. The major source is Anderson's (1989) article and other sources, as referenced.

Further nursing implications and etiology can be found in the chapter that deals with the specific body system and health problem and in the Age-Related Changes section of each chapter.

Interpretation of Laboratory Values

Lab Test	Relative Risk		Etiology	Nursing Implications
	Young Adults	Older Adults		

URINALYSIS

Lab Test	Young Adults	Older Adults	Etiology	Nursing Implications
1. Protein	Negative	0–1+ A 1+ with negative sediment may be of no clinical significance (Faubert et al., 1989).	May be changes in kidney basement membrane, renal pathology, or subclinical urinary tract infection (Durakovic & Milorad, 1983). Also may increase with fever, strenuous exercise.	Always collect a fresh, concentrated, un-contaminated specimen. Rule out renal pathology, subclinical urinary tract infection, DM.
2. Glucose (Glu)	Negative	Negative (1+ common)	Not known	Upper limits of normal may be low. Glycosuria may not occur until plasma glucose exceeds 300 mg/100 mL. Urine glucose checks in the elderly are highly unreliable (Garner, 1989).
3. Specific gravity (SG)	1.016–1.022	Maximum lower value 1.024 by age 80 (Goldman, 1986).	33%–50% decline in number of nephrons impairs kidney's ability to concentrate urine.	Always evaluate these low values in terms of dietary restrictions of sodium or protein or use of diuretics (Jeppesen, 1986).
4. Creatinine clearance (CrCl)	M 104–140 mL/min F 87–107 mL/min	M 100–150 mL/min Must be calculated to take into account age-related decrease in glomerular filtration rate (GFR); $$CrCl = \frac{(140 - age) \times body\ wt\ (Kg)}{serum\ Cr \times 72\ Kg}$$ Women are 85% of this (Hering & Carlson, 1982).	Decline in muscle mass with age results in less creatinine production and, as a result, serum levels do not rise in proportion to the fall in renal function (GFR), ie, a normal serum creatinine can translate into a 50%–60% of normal CrCl (Rowe et al., 1976).	CrCl, not serum creatinine alone, should be the criterion for renal function to prevent drug toxicity when giving drugs excreted via the urinary system (Gambert & Duthie, 1983).
5. Acetone (ketones)	Negative	Negative	N/A	Positive values seen in uncontrolled DM, malnutrition, starvation.

BLOOD CHEMISTRY

6. Albumin	3.2–4.5 g/dL	M 2.3–4.7 g/100 mL F 2.6–5 g/100 mL (Kain et al. 1990). Decreases with advancing age. Before 65, levels in men higher than women. After 65, values equalize and decline at the same rate.	Makes up more than 1/2 of total serum protein. Albumin increases oncotic pressure and carries hormones, fatty acids, and other insoluble substances. Elevated levels may accompany dehydration and multiple myeloma. A decrease in serum albumin means that the reference ranges of substances that are substantially bound to albumin may be altered even though the unbound fraction remains unchanged (Hodkinson, 1990). Decreased serum albumin produces edema and is present in diarrhea, immune disorders, and metastatic cancer. May also be a sign of chronic infection, malnutrition, or nephrotic syndrome.
		Decline thought to be associated with age-related changes in liver function—liver size, blood flow, enzyme production (Goldman, 1986). Change is statistical but of no or minimal clinical significance.	
7. Bilirubin (Bili)	0.1–1.2 mg/dL	0.1–1.2 mg/dL	Serum bilirubin is affected by hemoglobin metabolism, liver function, and biliary tract dynamics. Bili and its degradation products are pigments and produce the normal color of sputum, bile, stool, and urine. An elevated Bili will produce jaundice. Obstruction of biliary excretion may produce light-colored stool and dark urine. It is also important to know direct and indirect Bili values to establish differential diagnoses. Elevation of one or all three Bili levels may indicate known or suspected hemolytic disorders, confirm observed jaundice, or determine cause of jaundice—liver dysfunction, hepatitis, biliary obstruction, carcinoma (Cella & Watson, 1989).
		No significant change with age in the absence of associated disease (Gambert & Duthie, 1983).	
8. Blood urea nitrogen (BUN)	8–23 mg/dL	Increases; higher in men—sometimes as high as 69 mg/100 mL M 10–38 mg/100 mL F 10–30 mg/100 mL	BUN is influenced by hydration satus, tumors, infection, dietary intake of protein, GI bleeding, liver function, and renal function. An increased or decreased BUN must be correlated with other relevant clinical and laboratory information.
		Declines in cardiac output and renal blood flow lead to decreased GFR, and this in turn leads to an increase in BUN. This retention counters and exceeds a decrease in blood urea production due to body composition changes.	

(continued)

Lab Test	Young Adults	Older Adults	Etiology	Nursing Implications
9. Calcium (Ca)	9.2–11 mg/dL	M 8.9–10.9 mg/100 mL F 9.1–10.7 mg/100 mL	Decline in estrogen in postmenopausal women leads to elevations. Intestinal absorption of Ca has been shown to decrease with age.	In postmenopausal women, an upper level of 10.7 or even 11 may be normal in the absence of symptoms, evidence of hyperparathyroidism, or other causes (Caird, 1973). Evaluate if cardiac arrhythmias present, or in renal disease. Diuretic therapy may elevate.
10. Carbon dioxide (CO$_2$)	22–26 mEq/L	No change	N/A	—
11. Chloride(Cl)	95–103 mEq/L	No change	N/A	—
12. Creatinine (Cr)	0.6–1.2 mg/100 mL	0.4–1.9 mg/100 mL must be related to age and creatinine clearance. Consistently higher in men than in women due to differences in muscle mass.	Total daily endogenous production of creatinine decreases due to decline of body muscle mass. However, due to decrease in renal function, creatinine values can remain at normal to high levels. Therefore, a creatinine clearance is essential to calculating drug doses.	Creatinine clearance essential to prevent drug toxicity. Increased level may indicate severe renal dysfunction and is present in trauma. Decreased levels associated with muscular dystrophy.
13. Potassium (K)	3.8–5.0 mEq/L	Slight increase. M 3.7–5.3 mEq/L F 3.5–5.6 mEq/L	N/A	Avoid salt substitutes, largely composed of potassium. Monitor serum K levels if patient taking diuretics—K-sparing or K-wasting or anticoagulants. Increased levels due to decreased secretion, increased intake, medications. Decreased levels due to increased secretion, decreased intake, and medications. Always evaluate if cardiac arrhythmias present.
14. Sodium (Na)	136–142 mEq/L	Basically no change. Interval widens slightly to 137–148 mEq/L.	N/A	If increased, rule out cardiac disease, Cushing's disease, renal disease. If decreased, rule out Addison's disease, congestive heart failure (CHF), diarrhea, dehydration, IV over-hydration. Also possible with diuretic therapy.
15. Uric acid	M 4.0–8.5 mg/100 mL F 2.7–7.3 mg/100 mL	2.6–9.2 mg 2.0–8.2 mg (although reports are not consistent).	No clinical significance.	Thiazide diuretics are the most common cause for increased levels. Also elevated in infection. Levels greater than 7.7 may indicate gout (Jeppesen, 1986).

PROTEINS

16. β globulin	2.3–3.5 g/100 mL	Increase slightly	None
17. Total serum protein	6.0–7.8 g/100 mL	M 5.4–7.8 g/100 mL F 5.3–7.8 g/100 mL	Slight decline is normal with aging. Increased β globulin may balance decreased albumin, resulting in no change.	Evaluate in terms of its components in order to make diagnostic implications (Dybkaer et al., 1981). Decreased total protein may indicate malnutrition, liver disease, chronic infection, or renal disease

CARBOHYDRATES

18. Glucose (fasting)	70–110 mg/dL	M 52–135 mg/100 mL F 58–135 mg/100 mL	Pancreatic insulin supply declines and release is slower with age. With decline in lean body mass, less tissue is available for glucose uptake. Some cellular resistance to insulin develops with age (Williams, 1983).	Drugs such as alcohol, monoamine oxidase inhibitors, and beta blockers can lead to a rapid fall in glucose. A rise in glucose can quickly precipitate nonketotic hyperosmolar acidosis. A drop triggers confusion as brain cells are deprived of glucose. Consider patients' nutrition, weight, activity, infection, stress, healing lesions, and presence of acute chronic disease before initiating treatment. Presenting symptoms of DM may be none to life-threatening. Patient usually presents with visual disturbances or neuropathic complications. Patient education very important (Riesenberg, 1990).
19. Glucose tolerance test	Fasting 70–110 30′ 30–60 60′ 20–50 120′ 5–15 180′ fasting level or below	Higher peak at 2° with slower decline. Rise at 1° equals 9 mg/100 mL ± 5 mg/100 mL for each decade of life (Gambert & Duthie, 1983).		

LIPIDS

20. Cholesterol (total)	150–250 mg/100 mL	M below 260 mg/d F below 280 mg/dL. M: increases to age 50, then decreases. F: Lower than men till 50, then increases till 70, and decreases after 70 (Miller, 1990).	Drop in estrogen that accompanies menopause triggers cholesterol rise.	After menopause, women's risk of cardiovascular problems increases to the level of men's.
21. Triglycerides	<250 mg/dL; 500 g/dL abnormally high	M 198–327 mg/100 mL F 191–316 mg/100 mL M: Increase to age 50, then a decline. F: Continues to rise with age (Coodley, 1989).	Not known	Family history, weight, presence of other risk factors, activity level, medications, and diet should be considered when evaluating cholesterol, triglycerides, and high density lipoprotein (HDL) levels. A low HDL is seen as a risk factor in heart attacks, especially in postmenopausal women. A low HDL is associated with other risk factors—obesity, low activity, alcohol consumption, and smoking (Cauley et al., 1982). Consider interventions to lower cholesterol and raise HDL.

(continued)

Lab Test	Relative Risk		Etiology	Nursing Implications
	Young Adults	Older Adults		

THYROID FUNCTION TESTS

Lab Test	Young Adults	Older Adults	Etiology	Nursing Implications
22. Thyroxine (T_4)	5.5–12.5 μg/dL	Decreases slightly (Rock, 1985).	Secretion and degradation rates decrease with age, but little change in concentration in circulation.	Abnormal values in thyroid tests are usually related to altered states of binding proteins, concurrent use of medications, or the presence of non-thyroid disease.
23. Triiodothyronine (T_3)	80–200 ng/dL	Decreases 25% (Rock, 1985).	Partially due to decreased peripheral conversion of T_4 to T_3.	Hyperthyroidism may be masked in the elderly, with the absence of ocular findings or generalized hyperactivity. Signs and symptoms may appear in only one major organ system. Weight loss is a significant sign. Recognizing hypothyroidism presents unique problems—distinguishing nonspecific signs and symptoms of thyroid disease from changes found in normal elderly without thyroid disease.
24. Thyroid-stimulating hormone (TSH)	<5–7 mU/L	Increases slightly (Rock, 1985).	May represent subclinical hypothyroidism in which concentrations of circulating T_4 are not yet decreased (Rock, 1985).	

LIVER FUNCTION TESTS: ENZYMES

Lab Test	Young Adults	Older Adults	Etiology	Nursing Implications
25. Acid phosphatase (ACP)	0.13–0.63 U	0.0–1.6 U—slight change	N/A	Because information about enzymes is used to assess the status of the heart, liver, and muscles, it is important to know whether changes occur due to age.
26. Alkaline phosphatase (ALP)	20.130 U	M 21.3–80.8 U (Anderson, 1989) or 118–138 U (Kelso, 1990). F 19.9–83.4 U or 129–160 U One study suggests normal range be 107–142 U. Wide range of acceptable values reported. Upper limits of normal gradually but significantly increase with age, with a more pronounced rise in females.	Etiology as varied as the ranges. May be due to liver disease; renal changes which cause decreased vitamin D, in turn causing demineralization and elevated AP (Jeppesen, 1986); bone disease (Paget's) or minor bone trauma (Kelso, 1990); or malabsorption (Gambert & Duthie, 1983). May be normal changes of aging, such as hormonal, loss of recognition mechanisms, development of enzyme inhibitors, decreased enzyme production due to organ failure or metastatic disease, and decreased catabolism of the enzymes leading to prolonged activity (Jeppesen, 1986).	The wide range in normal values affords much latitude in interpretation. Laboratory values at either extreme of a reference range do not necessarily indicate problems. Remember that all laboratory values must be evaluated within the context of the patient's health history and profile. Obvious acute incidents such as a myocardial infarction (MI) will cause abnormally high levels during and immediately after the event.
27. Aspartate aminotransferase (SGOT, AST)	8–33 U	5–40 U. None or slight increases with advancing age. Levels for women remain lower than for men (Jeppesen, 1986).	Not known	Elevations occur when there is cellular damage to the tissues in which the enzyme is found—liver, myocardial, skeletal muscles, kidneys, pancreas, brain (Cella & Watson, 1989).

Test	Normal Values	Age-Related Changes	Comments
28. Alanine aminotransferase (SGPT, ALT)	4–36 U	Not known	Elevated serum ALT levels are considered a sensitive index of liver damage. Also seen in disorders such as muscular dystrophy (MD), MI, CHF, and renal failure (Cella & Watson, 1989).
29. Lactate dehydrogenase (LDH)	80–120 U/L	Not known	Numerous drugs may produce elevated levels. Elevations used to confirm MI, differentiation of MI from pulmonary infarction, confirmation of chronic liver, lung, renal disease (Cella & Watson, 1989).
30. Creatinine phosphokinase (CK, CPK)	M 55–170 IU/L F 30–135 IU/L	Age-related loss of muscle mass or decline in liver function.	May see pronounced elevations in acute MI, severe angina, after cardiac surgery, early MD, and with certain medications (Cella & Watson, 1989).
31. Amylase	30–220 U/L	Not known	Elevations seen in pancreatic inflammation, morphine sulfate administration. Decreased levels seen in disorders involving loss of functional pancreatic tissue.
HEMATOLOGY			
32. Hemoglobin (Hgb)	M 13.5–18 g/100 mL F 12–16 g/100 mL 10–17 g/100 mL 9–17 g/100 mL Declines gradually with age. Values for women are lower than for men in all age groups. If stringent criteria are applied to reference population, some say there should be no change and that 12 g/100 mL should be the recommended lower level for older men and women (Lipschitz, 1990a).	No change or some decline in active bone marrow, thus there is a possible decline in hematopoiesis. If no decline in hematopoiesis, there is at least a reduction in reserve capacity. Therefore, the ability to respond to increased demands can be compromised (Lipschitz, 1990a). Commonly, coexisting chronic disease, with or without inflammation, is thought to account for low Hgb levels. Active destruction, changes in enzymatic function within red blood cells, or decreased survival time of red blood cells has been suggested as a possible cause (Kelso, 1990).	Always compare with previous values. A wider range of values is appropriate and prevents 10% of women and nearly 50% of men from being classified as anemic by narrower ranges of normal (Kelso, 1990). However, just because Hgb declines with age, do not automatically assume that a low value is normal. Compare against previous values and look for other signs of anemia: decreased hematocrit count, pale skin, pale conjuctiva, clinical evidence of blood loss, cognitive changes.
33. Hematocrit (HCT)	M 40–54% F 38–47% 38–54% 35–49% Decline parallels changes in Hgb.	As above.	As above.

(continued)

Relative Risk

Lab Test	Young Adults	Older Adults	Etiology	Nursing Implications
34. Red blood cells (RBCs)	M 4,600,000/mm^3–6,200,000/mm^3 F 4,200,000/mm^3–5,400,000/mm^3	M & F: 3,000,000/mm^3–5,000,000/mm^3	As above.	Changes in RBC indices are important in diagnosing different anemias. Mean corpuscular volume (MCV) measures individual cell size. Increased with folic acid deficiency, vitamin B$_{12}$ deficiency, cirrhosis, aplastic anemia; decreased with chronic iron-deficiency thalassemias, anemia of chronic disease. Differentiates anemias as normocytic, microcytic, or macrocytic. Mean corpuscular hemoglobin concentration (MCHC) measures average concentration of Hgb in RBCs. Increased indicates spherocytosis, decreased indicates hypochromia, chronic iron deficiency anemia. Mean corpuscular hemoglobin (MCH) measures average weight of Hgb. Increased indicates macrocytosis, decreased indicates microcytosis or hypochromia.
35. White blood cells (WBCs)	4,500/mm^3–11,000/mm^3	M 3,600/mm^3–12,700/mm^3 F 3,100/mm^3–12,000/mm^3	No real change in range due to age. Therefore, any discrepancy is consistent with a disease process. The most common WBC disorders in older adults are neoplastic diseases. Other causes include lack of production, increased destruction, increased splenic sequestration, metastasis to bone marrow, normal count with impaired function (DM, chronic renal failure) (Capizzi et al., 1990).	Changes may be reflections of or contributions toward alterations in immune status and antimicrobial activity. Protect elders from infection; encourage pneumococcal, tetanus, and influenza vaccines. Rule out malignancies, immune disorders, drug toxicity, malnutrition, sepsis (Cavalieri, et al., 1992).
36. Lymphocytes	1.0–4.8 × 10^9/L	T-lymphocytes and B-lymphocytes fall (Jeppesen, 1986).	Defective cell-mediated (T-cell) and antibody-mediated (B-cell) responses, increased antibody function, and increases in products of dysregulation. Involution of the thymus gland (decrease in size, impaired competence) believed to be principle cause for immunologic deficiency (Jeppesen, 1986).	Net effect of changes is increased susceptibility. Increased incidence of infections, malignancies, lymphoproliferative, and autoimmune diseases (Jeppeson, 1986).

37. Erythrocyte sedimentation rate (ESR)	M <15 mm/hr F <20 mm/hr	M <30 mm/hr F <42 mm/hr Increases may equal 0.22 mm/hr per year of aging (Jeppesen, 1986).	Appears to be nonspecific, although age-related increases in globulin and fibrinogen may contribute to elevated levels (Jeppesen, 1986).	ESR rate is used to evaluate the activity and progression of inflammation in disease. It refers to the rate at which erythrocytes settle out of coagulated blood in 1 hour. However, it is a test viewed with limited diagnostic value. An isolated high value may be of no clinical significance unless correlated with other abnormal clinical signs. If still elevated after 2 weeks, further investigation is warranted. Helpful in diagnosing polymyalgia rheumatica, multiple myeloma, or temporal arteritis. Normal ESR does not preclude an underlying disease.
38. Iron (Fe) (and transferrin)	M & F 60–150 µg/dL	Both decrease with age for men and women: 93 µg/dL ± 5.0 (Lipschitz, 1990a).	It is suggested that decrease is due to decreased intake, decreased absorption from the GI tract, ineffective erythropoiesis (impaired iron incorporation) or decline in bone marrow cellularity (Gambert & Duthie, 1983). Transferrin is a transport protein. It regulates iron absorption and transport in the body. Its decrease with age decreases iron's ability to bind.	The majority of anemias in the elderly will be those most commonly associated with inadequate iron supply for erythropoiesis. However, iron stores increase in both men and women as age increases. Therefore, *nutritional* iron-deficiency is rare in older adults. GI blood loss, the anemia of inflammation and chronic disease, (due to infection, immune reaction, tissue necrosis, neoplasm), anemia due to protein-energy malnutrition, and marrow failure are the most prevalent causes in older adults (Lipschitz, 1990b). Increase dietary intake; iron supplements may help, but elderly may not respond to iron therapy. Increased Fe levels seen in aplastic anemia, hemolytic anemia, hemochromatosis, pernicious anemia, and acute hepatitis; decreased levels seen in iron-deficiency anemia. Abnormal protein levels may result in decreased transferrin levels.
39. Total iron binding capacity (TIBC)	250–400 µg/dL	May decrease with age. 307 µg/dL ± 13.0 (Lipschitz, 1990a).	Reflects transferrin content in serum. Estimates amount of transferrin available to bind.	Increased levels with iron-deficiency anemia, alcoholism, acute hepatitis. Decreased levels with hypoproteinemia and iron-overload conditions.

(continued)

Lab Test	Young Adults	Older Adults	Etiology	Nursing Implications
40. Ferritin	M 15–200 µg/L F 12–150 µg/L	M greater than 100 µg/l after age 50. F greater than 80 µg/L after age 60 (Cella & Watson, 1989). Ferritin levels continuously rise in men starting at 30 years old. In women, levels remain low until middle age, then rise continuously after menopause (Jeppesen, 1986).	As listed above for Fe.	The primary iron storage compound. A good indicator of available iron stores and the most sensitive test for detecting iron-deficiency anemia. Level directly related to amount of stored iron. Decreased levels seen in chronic iron-deficiency anemias. Increased levels seen in megaloblastic and hemolytic anemias.

COAGULATION TESTS

Lab Test	Young Adults	Older Adults	Etiology	Nursing Implications
41. Platelets	150,000–450,000 × 10^9/L	No appreciable change in numbers, but characteristics change—decreased granular constituents, increased platelet release factors.	Potential for decreased amount of active bone marrow resulting in decreased production.	Also a reduced capability to regenerate platelets after severe loss. Thus regeneration after drug or radiation therapy may be slowed. Care of elderly patients after such interventions should be planned accordingly, in terms of potential for or actual bleeding (Jeppesen, 1986).
42. Fibrinogen	200–400 mg/dL	Believed to increase with age. In fact, they seem to parallel ESR increases (Jeppesen, 1986).	May be related to dietary intake of fat or fiber (Jeppesen, 1986).	
43. Prothrombin time (PT)	10–13 seconds	No change in healthy elders.	N/A	Shortened bleeding times are corrected with aspirin (Jeppesen, 1986).
44. Partial thromboplastin time (PTT)	60–70 seconds	No change in healthy elders.	N/A	Bleeding precautions for patients with extended bleeding times. Check coagulation levels if signs of bleeding occur—pallor, positive occult blood test, increased bruising, GI bleed, cognitive changes, hematuria, bleeding gums, etc. Also check vitamin K level.

ARTERIAL BLOOD GASES

Lab Test	Young Adults	Older Adults	Etiology	Nursing Implications
45. PO$_2$	95–100 mg/Hg	11–15% decrease	Steady decline of lung function with age—structure of chest wall, exchange capabilities, alveolar ventilation, pulmonary rigidity, and vascular bed resistance (Cavalieri et al., 1992).	Due to listed changes in lung function, older adults are typically more fragile and therefore more susceptible to respiratory problems. Will develop respiratory ailments quicker, stay sick longer, and may not recover fully. Be vigilant for changes in respiratory status, signs of infection, cardiac problems, cognitive changes, especially in COPD patients. Remember that you have less time to intervene than with a younger patient before a catastrophic event occurs.
46. PCO$_2$	35–40 mmHg	2–3% increase (Jeppesen, 1986)	As above.	
47. pH	7.38–7.44	No change	N/A	

APPENDIX REFERENCE LIST

Anderson, G. D. (1989). A fresh look at assessing the elderly. *RN, 52*(6), 28–39.

Caird, F. J. (1973). Problems of interpretation of laboratory findings in the old. *British Medical Journal, 4,* 348–351.

Capizzi, R. L., Powell, B. L., & Cruz, J. D. (1990). White cell disorders. In W. R. Hazzard, R. Andres, E. L. Bierman, & J. P. Blass (Eds.), *Principles of geriatric medicine and gerontology.*

Cauley, J. A., Laporte, R. E., Kuller, L. H., & Black-Sandler, R. (1982). The epidemiology of high density lipoprotein cholesterol levels in post-menopausal women. *Journal of Gerontology, 37*(1), 10–151.

Cavalieri, T. A., Chopra, A., & Bryman, P. N. (1992). When outside the norm is normal: Interpreting lab data in the aged. *Geriatrics, 47*(5), 66–70.

Cella, J. H., & Watson, J. (1989). *Nurses manual of laboratory values.* Philadelphia: F. A. Davis.

Coodley, E. L. (1989). Laboratory tests in the elderly: What is abnormal. *Postgraduate Medicine, 85,* 333–338.

Durakovic, Z., & Milorad, M. (1983). Proteinuria in the elderly. *Gerontology, 29,* 121–124.

Duthie, E. H. & Abbusi, A. A. (1991). Laboratory testing: current recommendations for older adults. *Geriatrics, 16* (10), 41–50.

Dybkaer, R., Lauritzen, M., & Krakauer, R. (1981). Relative reference values for clinical chemical and haematological quantities in "healthy" elderly people. *Acta Medicus Scandanavia, 209,* 1–9.

Eliopoulos, C. (1990). Appendix B: Reference for laboratory values. In *Health assessment of the older adult* (pp. 302–309). Redwood City: Addison-Wesley Nursing.

Faubert, P. R., Shapiro, W. B., Porush, J., & Kahn, A. (1989). Medical renal diseases in the aged. In W. Reichel (Ed.), *Clinical aspects of aging* (3rd ed) pp. 228–247. Baltimore: Williams & Wilkins.

Gambert, S. R. & Duthie, E. H. (1983). Laboratory testing in the elderly. *Wisconisn Medical Journal, 82,* (8), 19–20.

Garner, B. C. (1989). Guide to changing lab values in elders. *Geriatric Nursing, 10,* 144–145.

Goldman, R. (1986). Aging changes in structure and function. In D. Carnevali & M. Patrick (Eds.), *Nursing management for the elderly* (2nd ed). pp. 73–101. Philadelphia: J. B. Lippincott.

Henry, J. B. (1991). *Clinical diagnoses and management by laboratory methods* (18th ed). Philadelphia: W. B. Saunders.

Hering, P. J. & Carlson, R. E. (1982, July 2). Serum creatinine and renal function in the elderly (letter to the editor). *Journal of American Medical Association,* p. 31.

Hodkinson, H. M. (1990). Alterations of laboratory findings. In W. R. Hazzard, R. Andres, E. L. Bierman, & J. P. Blass (Eds.), *Principles of geriatric medicine and gerontology* (2nd ed). pp. 241–246, New York: McGraw-Hill.

Jeppesen, M. E. (1986). Laboratory values for the elderly. In D. Carnevali & M. Patrick (Eds.), *Nursing management for the elderly* (2nd ed.), pp. 102–142. Philadelphia: J. B. Lippincott.

Kain, C. D., Reilly, N., & Schultz, E. D. (1990). The older adult: A comparative assessment. *Nursing Clinics of North America, 25* (4), 833–851.

Kelso, T. (1990). Laboratory values in the elderly—are they different?, *Emergency Medical Clinics of North America, 8,* 241–254.

Leukenottee, A. G. (1994). Older adult laboratory values. *Pocket Guide To Gerontological Assessment* (pp 286–288). St Louis: Mosby–Yearbook, Inc.

Lipschitz, D. A. (1990a). Aging of the hematopoietic system. In W. R. Hazzard, R. Andres, E. L. Bierman, & J. P. Blass (Eds.), *Principles of geriatric medicine and gerontology* (2nd ed.), pp. 655–661. New York: McGraw-Hill.

Lipschitz, D. A. (1990b). Anemia in the elderly. In W. R. Hazzard, R. Andres, E. L. Bierman, & J. P. Blass (Eds.), *Principles of geriatric medicine and gerontology* (2nd ed.), pp. 662–668. New York: McGraw-Hill.

Melillo, K. D. (1993). Interpretation of laboratory values in older adults. *Nurse Practitioner, 18*(7), 59–67.

Miller, N. E. (1990). Aging and plasma lipoproteins. In W. R. Hazzard, R. Andres, E. L. Bierman, & J. P. Blass (Eds.), *Principles of geriatric medicine and gerontology,* (2nd ed.), pp. 767–776. New York: McGraw-Hill.

Riesenberg, D. (1990). Diabetes mellitus. In C. K. Cassel, D. E. Riesenberg, L. B. Sorenson, & J. R. Walsh (Eds.), *Geriatric Medicine* (2nd ed.). New York: Springer-Verlag.

Rock, R. C. (1985). Interpreting thyroid tests in the elderly: Updated guidelines. *Geriatrics, 40* (12), 61–68.

Rowe, J. W., Andres, R., Tobin, J. D. et al. (1976). The effect of age on creatinine clearance in men: A cross-sectional and longitudinal study. *Journal of Gerontology, 31,* 155–163.

Scott, R. B. (1993). Common blood disorders: A primary care approach. *Geriatrics, 48*(4), 72–80.

Williams, T. F. (1983). Diabetes mellitus in older people. In W. Reichel (Ed.), *Clinical aspects of aging* (2nd ed), pp. 411–415. Baltimore: Williams & Wilkins.

BIBLIOGRAPHY

Eliopoulos, C. (1990). Appendix B: Reference for laboratory values. In *Health assessment of the older adult.* pp. 302–309. Redwood City: Addison-Wesley Nursing.

Leukenottee, A. G. (1994). Older adult laboratory values. *Pocket guide to gerontological assessment.* pp. 286–288. St Louis: Mosby–Yearbook, Inc.

Melillo, K. D. (1993). Interpretation of laboratory values in older adults. *Nurse Practitioner, 18*(7), 59–67.

Scott, R. B. (1993). Common blood disorders: A primary care approach. *Geriatrics, 48*(4), 72–80.

Index

NOTE: A *t* following a page number indicates tabular material, an *f* following a page number indicates a figure, a *b* following a page number indicates a patient teaching box, and a *d* after a page number indicates a display.